INTRODUCTION TO BASIC NEUROLOGY

HARRY D. PATTON, M.D., Ph.D.

Professor and Chairman, Department of Physiology and Biophysics,
University of Washington School of Medicine

JOHN W. SUNDSTEN, Ph.D.

Associate Professor of Biological Structure,
University of Washington School of Medicine

WAYNE E. CRILL, M.D.

Associate Professor of Physiology and Biophysics and of
Medicine (Neurology), University of Washington School of Medicine;
Chief of Neurology, Seattle Veterans Administration Hospital

PHILLIP D. SWANSON, M.D., Ph.D.

Professor of Medicine and Head of Neurology,
University of Washington School of Medicine

W. B. SAUNDERS COMPANY

Philadelphia, London, Toronto

W. B. Saunders Company: West Washington Square
Philadelphia, PA 19105

1 St. Anne's Road
Eastbourne, East Sussex BN21 3UN, England

1 Goldthorne Avenue
Toronto, Ontario M8Z 5T9, Canada

Introduction to Basic Neurology   ISBN   0-7216-7113-6

Last digit is the print number: 9   8   7   6   5   4

PREFACE

This volume is a belated response to the epidemic of curricular revision that spread through medical education in the late sixties. Triggered by a multitude of factors, including student demands for "relevance" and public pressure for accelerated output of physicians, the curricular revolution struck deeply at the basic science–oriented Flexner model, which had dominated medical education for half a century. Often motivated more by revolutionary zeal than by incisive logic, medical institutions throughout the nation were soon competing frantically to achieve the most radical departure from the Flexner system. This feverish lemming race to the sea seems now to be abated, but the fallout of these convulsive years is still very much with those of us who teach beginning medical students. In many institutions (including ours) the two major consequences of the revolution were, first, drastic reduction (up to 50 per cent or more) of time allotted to basic science instruction and, second, increased emphasis on interdisciplinary treatment of introductory medical science, an organ or organ-system rather than a disciplinary approach usually being the organizing principle.

Taken together these two basic changes made the conventional basic science textbooks inadequate or at best inappropriate for use by first-year medical students. Firstly, they are too long and too deep for the drastically pared "core curricula." Secondly, they are intended for students whose classwork is supplemented and enriched by laboratory experience, a luxury severely curtailed by the new time restraints. Finally, most classical textbooks follow an organization suitable to Flexnerian across-the-board courses in a single discipline, not to the multidisciplinary "scrambled eggs" format of the organ-system core curricula. The present volume is an attempt to cope with the altered requirements of the Neocurricularian Epoch.

We have attempted to present the salient features of basic neurological science with sufficient parsimony that the beginning student can learn by (rather than be overcome by) reading. Emphasis is placed on encouraging the student to acquire a working comprehension and intuitive grasp of basic material without the distraction of rigorous documentation of all the data covered. At the same time we have avoided the stark and sterile syllabus format because we firmly believe that students can best master, retain, and use basic material when it is fitted into a logical intellectual framework. Indeed, the need for such stimulation is intensified by the paucity of laboratory experience in modern medical curricula.

Secondly, we have attempted where feasible to meld together information derived from different disciplinary approaches, and each of us has dared to venture outside his special sphere of training. However, we have not made a fetish of the multidisciplinary approach, the virtues of which we believe have been overrated by curricular revisionists. We have made the most of those situations in which data from the various disciplines complement and reinforce one another. But we have steadfastly avoided unnatural blending of data for the mere sake of disciplinary egalitarianism, especially when such forced intrusions would break the chain of thought and thus distract, rather than help, the reader. Despite the interdisciplinary sallies, we suspect that students will have little difficulty in identifying the disciplinary affiliations of the authors without reference to the title page.

Finally, we have tried to compensate for some of the educational elements that have fallen victim to the compression of the time scale of basic science instruction. The numerous drawings and the anatomical atlas in the appendix represent efforts to compensate partly for shortened time in the laboratory. Even so, we find that some laboratory work is essential, especially for neuroanatomy and neuropathology; ours occupies approximately 35 hours. The glossary of word roots is intended to help the student cope with the immense vocabulary of neurological science, a Herculean chore even in the Archecurricularian Era, when more time and exposure permitted a less hasty introduction to medical argot.

The title requires a word of explanation if not of apology. This is an introductory textbook of *basic neurology,* not of neurology. We have made no attempt to deal systematically with disease of the nervous system but rather to cover most of the material that we believe a student should understand before he undertakes a serious study of neurological disease. One omission is neuropathology, a subject that we find is best presented in the laboratory along with normal neuroanatomy.

The authors are indebted to Janet Palmquist, Vicki Neff, and Doris Ringer for cheerfully and magically converting handwritten manuscripts into legible prose and to Mrs. Remedios Moore, whose editorial assistance has given our prose a measure of precision and quality that would otherwise have been lacking. Finally, we acknowledge our debt to Helen Halsey, Phyllis Wood, and Joy Godfrey for their carefully executed illustrations and to Roy Hayashi for his excellent photographs of the gross brain specimens.

H.D.P.
J.W.S.
W.E.C.
P.D.S.

CONTENTS

v

Chapter 8

Chapter 9

Chapter 10

Chapter 11

CHAPTER 1

DEVELOPMENT AND GROSS TOPOGRAPHY OF THE CENTRAL NERVOUS SYSTEM

JOHN W. SUNDSTEN

FORMATION OF THE NEURAL TUBE

INTERNAL DEVELOPMENT:
Gray and White Columns

EXTERNAL GROSS MORPHOLOGY

VENTRICULAR SYSTEM

The central nervous system (CNS) consists of the brain and spinal cord. These structures are housed in bony cavities provided by the cranium and vertebral column and are well protected by both a covering complex of membranes and a cushioning and supporting series of cavities and spaces filled with cerebrospinal fluid (Fig. 1–1). The membranes are, from within outward, the *pia mater, arachnoid,* and *dura mater* (Figs. 1–1 and 1–2). The collective term for them is *meninges*. The pia and arachnoid are sometimes together referred to as the *leptomeninges,* and the dura is sometimes termed the *pachymeninges*.

The *pia mater* is closely applied to the brain, spinal cord, and roots of cranial and spinal nerves; it has a basement membrane but no intervening space. It is analogous to the layer of connective tissue that binds

soft tissues and organs (viscera) found in the thoracic, abdominal, and pelvic cavities (*e.g.,* visceral peritoneum and visceral pleura). The *arachnoid* membrane is attached to the pia by many "weblike" connective tissues, the trabeculae, and is separated from it by cerebrospinal fluid in the subarachnoid space.

The tough, protective *dura mater* is closely applied to the arachnoid; the serous surfaces of the two membranes slide smoothly over one another, so that the subdural space is only a potential space. During hemorrhage, it may be opened and filled with blood (subdural hematoma). The *cranial* dura is normally fused with the inner layer of periosteum lining the bones of the cranial cavity, whereas the *spinal* dura is separated from the periosteum of the vertebral canal by epidural fat and

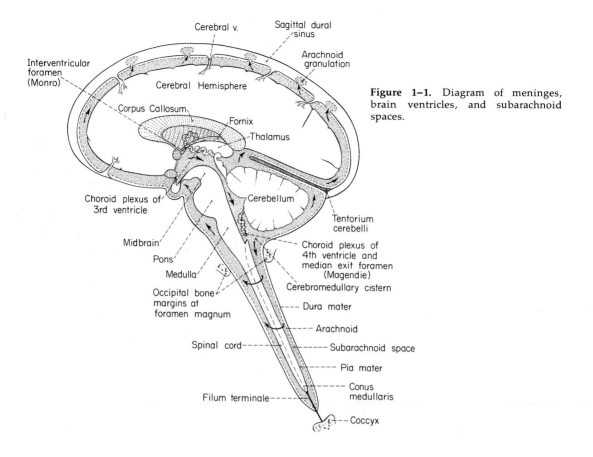

Figure 1–1. Diagram of meninges, brain ventricles, and subarachnoid spaces.

blood vessels. Because of the areolar nature of the epidural space in the vertebral canal, it provides a common site for metastatic processes or infections that can result in compression of the spinal cord. In contrast, since the epidural space in the cranium is only a potential space, metastases are not common; but skull fractures can readily tear meningeal vessels there and cause epidural hematomas. Subdural hematomas can result from tearing of bridging veins.

A ventricular system of cavities and channels filled with cerebrospinal fluid (CSF) also protects the brain and spinal cord and is readily seen in a sagittal section of the adult brain (Figs. 1–1 and 1–3). The cavities, their openings into the subarachnoid space, and their relationships with the major gross morphological divisions of the brain are most easily understood if one first gains an appreciation of the embryonic development of the CNS.

FORMATION OF THE NEURAL TUBE

By the 19th day of embryonic life a *neural plate* has formed as a specialized thickening of ectoderm (Fig. 1–4). As the neural plate continues to thicken, it folds, and a tubular structure "pinches off" from the overlying ectoderm and becomes the *neural tube.* At the posterolateral margins of the neural tube, *neural crest* cells migrate away from the tube and become posterior root ganglia, cranial nerve ganglia, and autonomic nervous system ganglia. Neural processes grow proximally and distally from the posterior root ganglion cells to form the posterior roots. They conjoin with the anterior roots emerging from the anterior aspect of the spinal cord and brainstem to form the spinal and cranial nerves (Fig. 1–5). The nerves develop in concert with tissue masses that they will

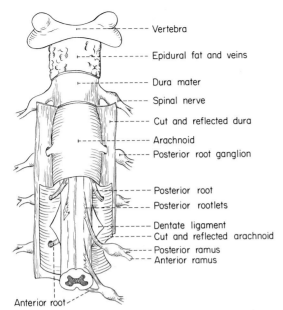

Figure 1–2. Posterior view of spinal cord and meninges. (Adapted from Wolf-Heidegger, *Atlas of systematic human anatomy*, New York, Hafner Publishing Co., 1962.)

eventually innervate: dermatomes (skin) and myotomes (muscles). The manner by which this occurs and the arrangement of peripheral fibers forming nerves will be described later.

Sometimes the neural groove fails to

close over completely into a tube, most frequently at either its rostral or caudal limits, and congenital defects result. When the failure occurs rostrally, *anencephaly* may ensue, in which the brain develops very poorly and becomes necrotic as it is exposed to amniotic fluid. The resultant infant has a "froglike" head and usually dies shortly after birth. When the spinal portion of the groove fails to close, usually in the lumbosacral region, the anomaly is called a *spina bifida*. This term actually covers several possible defects, in all of which the vertebral arch fails to fuse properly. There may be a defect of the bony spinal canal without protrusion of the spinal cord or meninges (*spina bifida occulta*), or a sac containing either the meninges (*meningocele*) or the meninges and spinal cord (*meningomyelocele*) may protrude posteriorly. In the latter deficiency the overlying membrane is very thin and

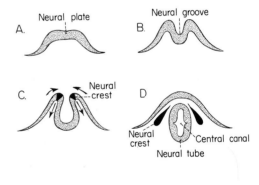

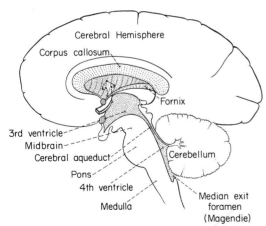

Figure 1–3. Ventricular system, as seen in sagittal view of the brain (see also Figure 1–15). The arrow indicates the continuity of the lateral ventricles (one in each hemisphere) and the single third ventricle via the interventricular foramen. The lateral ventricles are not actually seen in the midline view unless the septum pellucidum (membrane between the corpus callosum and fornix) is removed.

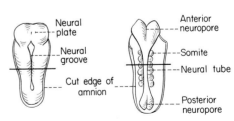

Figure 1–4. *Above,* Formation of neural tube. *A,* Neural plate develops. *B,* Neural groove forms. *C,* Neural groove deepens and neural crests appear at the lip margin. *D,* Neural groove becomes neural tube with the neural crests at its sides.

Below, Two dorsal views of this development are shown. At the *left,* the stage represented shows both the neural plate and groove being formed. At the *right* the neural groove has not finished closing over into a tube and shows anterior (rostral) and posterior (caudal) neuropores. The horizontal lines represent the approximate levels of sections *C* and *D.*

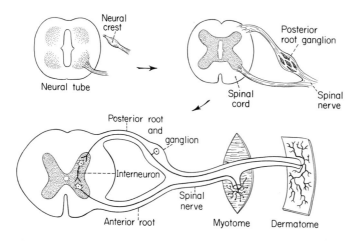

Figure 1–5. Migration of neural crest associated with a segment of spinal cord to form a dorsal root ganglion, and subsequent formation of a spinal nerve innervating a myotome and a dermatome.

nonepithelialized; thus infection, and not infrequently death, may occur. Other abnormalities of the central nervous system often occur along with the above, but the most notable is *hydrocephalus,* in which there is a dilatation of the ventricle.

INTERNAL DEVELOPMENT: Gray and White Columns

A general pattern is revealed in the interior of the neural tube as the differentiation of the CNS parenchyma takes place (Fig. 1–6). Neuroepithelial matrix cells in the *ependymal layer* (immediately next to the cavity of the neural tube) multiply by mitosis and at a certain moment become committed as either *neuroblasts* or *glioblasts (spongioblasts)* and migrate away from the ependymal layer to form the central nervous system. The neuroblasts migrate

first and form clusters of cell bodies (*nuclei*) and bundles of axons (*tracts*). The glioblasts form the glial supportive elements of the CNS, the oligodendrocyte and the astrocyte.

An important landmark in the developing neural tube is the *sulcus limitans,* a shallow depression in the wall of the neural canal that courses longitudinally and divides the developing tube into approximately equal anterior and posterior halves (Fig. 1–7). Anterior to the sulcus the developing neurons are clumped together as *basal plate elements;* they eventually form the adult *anterior gray matter.* The largest groups of these nerve cells are motoneurons, and they project their axons out of the neural tube via anterior roots, to innervate effector end organs, *i.e.,* striated muscles (innervated directly) and smooth muscles and glands (innervated via au-

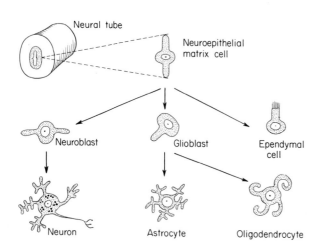

Figure 1–6. Lineage of cells of the central nervous system, showing the origin of neurons, glial cells, and ependymal cells from the primitive neuroepithelial cells in the developing neural tube.

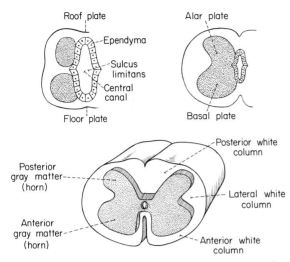

Figure 1–7. Development of spinal cord gray and white columns and narrowing of primitive neural tube cavity.

for spinal reflex behavior, for more complex neural interconnections from the spinal cord with the brainstem and cerebellum, or for the relaying of afferent input to sensory pathways ascending to the forebrain (Fig. 1–8).

The *gray matter* formed by the primitive alar and basal plate elements is often referred to as the posterior and anterior *horns* because of its H-like morphological appearance in cross section. The *white matter* (or white columns) of the spinal cord is located superficial to the gray. It is composed of axons of neurons originating either in the spinal cord gray matter, particularly the posterior gray, or in the dorsal root ganglia, and of axons descending from more rostral areas of the CNS. In later chapters, both the fiber systems in the white columns and the nuclear subdivisions of the spinal gray will be covered in more detail. At this time it is sufficient to appreciate the general origin and morphological plan of the developing neural tube.

tonomic ganglia). Many interneurons in the anterior gray matter also make complex connections with the motoneurons.

Posterior to the sulcus limitans, *alar plate elements* develop into neurons forming the *posterior gray matter*. These receive input from primary afferent fibers entering the spinal cord via the posterior roots. Recall that all the primary afferent neurons originate from neural crest elements that migrated out to form the posterior root and cranial nerve ganglia. These ganglia project axonal processes distally (peripherally) to somatic (*e.g.*, skin) and visceral (*e.g.*, hollow organ) structures. Here at the periphery, afferent information is initiated at the fiber endings by transduction of mechanical and chemical events in the physical environment to electric potentials. The information is then conducted to the CNS, eventually over the posterior roots, as mentioned above, and into the posterior gray matter. This gray matter also receives input from, and gives input to, other neurons at the same spinal cord level (intrasegmental connections), neurons at other spinal cord levels (intersegmental connections), and neurons in more rostral parts of the CNS (suprasegmental connections). It is through these alar plate neurons and their connections, then, that the first information processing takes place in the CNS, whether it is

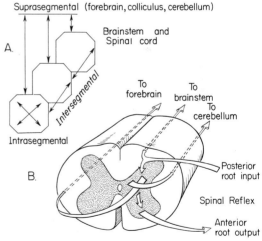

Figure 1–8. General summary of connectivity. *A*, Diagram of intrasegmental, intersegmental, and suprasegmental interconnections. *B*, Major channeling of afferent information to the interneuron pool for spinal reflexes and to the brainstem, forebrain, and cerebellum. The crossed pathway to the forebrain represents the spinothalamic tract; the ipsilateral path in the lateral funiculus represents the spinocerebellar tract; and the ipsilateral path to the brainstem represents the posterior column path to the medullary gracile and cuneate nuclei.

EXTERNAL GROSS MORPHOLOGY

The neural tube undergoes marked gross anatomical changes as it develops into the CNS, its rostral end becoming the *brain*, and its caudal end the *spinal cord*. The adult CNS remains as a tube, but a far more complex one because of the internal development of nuclear groups and fiber systems and changes in its external morphology from the differential growth of certain areas along the neuraxis. The pertinent changes begin at the rostral end of the neural tube; a primitive brain vesicle develops and undergoes a series of expansions and foldings, leading to the definitive *cerebral hemispheres, diencephalon, midbrain, pons, medulla,* and *cerebellum* (Figs. 1–9 to 1–11). At first, the tube expands and becomes partially constricted into three parts, the *forebrain (prosencephalon), midbrain (mesencephalon),* and *hindbrain (rhombencephalon).* The *forebrain* grows most rapidly, resulting in a cephalic flexure, so that the definitive forebrain forms an angle to the midbrain. Ultimately, outpocketings occur from the forebrain on both sides and develop into left and right cerebral hemispheres *(telencephalon).* These expand rostrally and caudally, covering over much of the cranial portion of the tube, and comprise the *cerebral cortex* and *basal ganglia.* The major basal ganglia (Fig. 1–12) are the *caudate, putamen,* and *globus pallidus.* Another nuclear mass, the *amygdala,* is developmentally one of the forebrain's basal ganglia, but it is functionally related to the limbic system (Chap. 27). Two other nuclear groups functionally related to the basal ganglia are the *subthalamic nucleus* and the *substantia nigra* (the latter is located in the midbrain).

That part of the forebrain from which the outpocketings occur is the *diencephalon.* The diencephalon becomes the adult *thalamus* and *hypothalamus.* The *mesencephalon* becomes the definitive *midbrain,* and the *hindbrain* divides by a series of changes into the *pons* and *cerebellum* (together, the

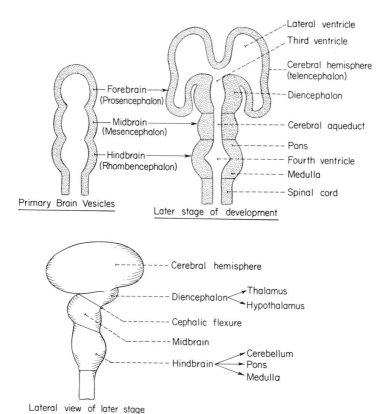

Figure 1–9. Development of the forebrain, midbrain, and hindbrain. The two sketches at the top also show the ventricles. A side view of the developing central nervous system is shown below.

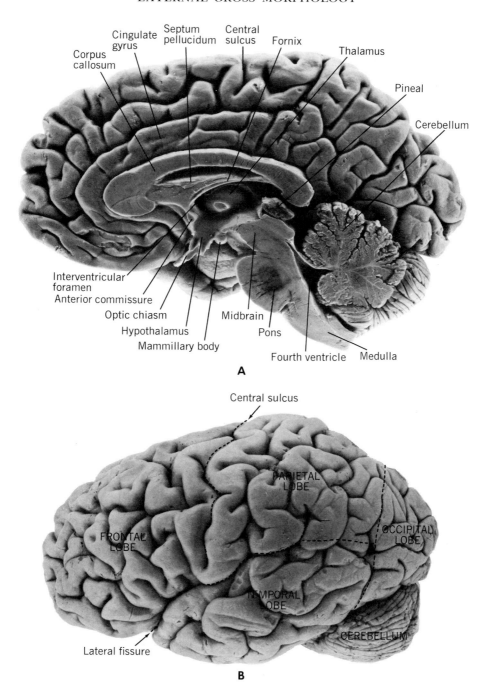

Corpus callosum Cingulate gyrus Septum pellucidum Central sulcus Fornix Thalamus Pineal Cerebellum

Interventricular foramen Anterior commissure Optic chiasm Hypothalamus Mammillary body Midbrain Pons Fourth ventricle Medulla

A

Central sulcus

PARIETAL LOBE OCCIPITAL LOBE FRONTAL LOBE TEMPORAL LOBE CEREBELLUM

Lateral fissure

B

Figure 1–10. *A,* Sagittal view of an adult brain specimen. *B,* Lateral view of an adult brain specimen.

metencephalon) and the *medulla* (*myelenceph-alon*). The *brainstem* is a term usually used for the combined midbrain, pons, and medulla. Caudally, the brainstem is continuous with the spinal cord.

Whereas individual structures of the forebrain will be discussed in more detail in later chapters, their development as shown by frontal sections is illustrated in Figure 1–12 in order that their relative positions can be clearly visualized in at least a summary fashion. The appearance of the forebrain in cross section is made complex not only by the extensive growth of these different parts of the cerebral hemispheres but also by the appearance of the *corpus callosum,* a massive bundle of fibers interconnecting homotypical cerebral cortical points, and the *internal capsule,* a large fiber bundle interconnecting the thalamus with the cortex and providing a route for cortical cells to project their axons to the basal ganglia, brainstem, and spinal cord. These major subdivisions of the adult brain are indicated in the sagittal view of a gross specimen shown in Figure 1–10. Note also the position of two prominent landmarks: the *tentorium cerebelli,* a dense layer of dura separating the forebrain from the cerebellum at the level of the midbrain, and the *foramen magnum,* marking the approximate division between brainstem and spinal cord. These landmarks are of clinical importance, since one can use them conceptually to approximate major regions of the CNS—the forebrain (supratentorial), brainstem and cerebellum (infratentorial), and spinal cord—at which lesions can occur. Throughout the following chapters it will become apparent that the signs and symptoms of neurological disease may vary according to which one of the three regions is involved.

VENTRICULAR SYSTEM

It is important to remember that the neural tube is hollow throughout its development, a situation that is also true in the adult brain and spinal cord, although in the latter the central canal is frequently obliterated. The cavity is filled with cere-

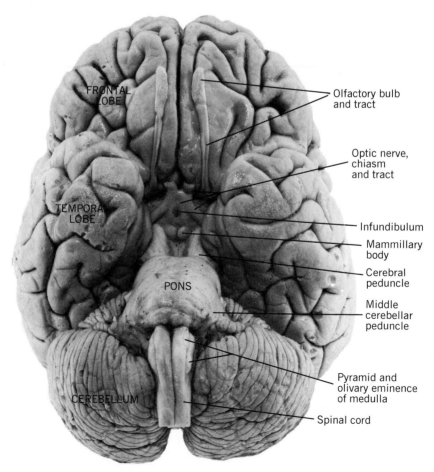

Figure 1–11. Ventral view of an adult brain specimen.

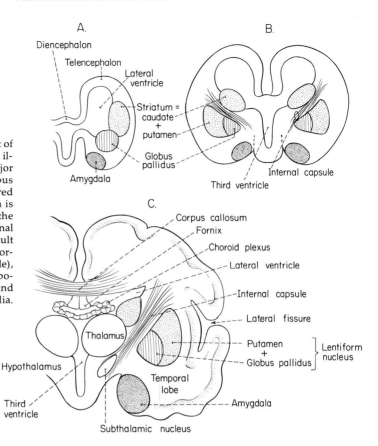

Figure 1–12. *A* and *B,* Development of the forebrain in frontal sections, illustrating the position of the major basal ganglia. *A,* The striatum, globus pallidus, and amygdala have appeared in the telencephalon. *B,* The striatum is divided into its component nuclei, the caudate and putamen, by the internal capsule. *C,* Frontal section of the adult forebrain, showing fiber systems (fornix, corpus callosum, internal capsule), diencephalon (thalamus and hypothalamus), choroid plexus of lateral and third ventricles, and the basal ganglia.

brospinal fluid (CSF) and is continuous with the subarachnoid space through three exit foramina of the fourth ventricle (Figs. 1–1 and 1–5). The CSF cushions and protects the brain and spinal cord from mechanical shock and may also have nutritive functions (see Chapter 2).

In a typical transverse section through the developing neural tube, the central canal is seen to be relatively large compared

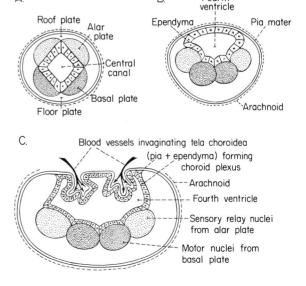

Figure 1–13. *A* to *C,* Stages in the development of the fourth ventricle and the choroid plexus. Note that the roof plate is stretched out as the ventricle expands, and it thus allows the formation of the choroid plexus.

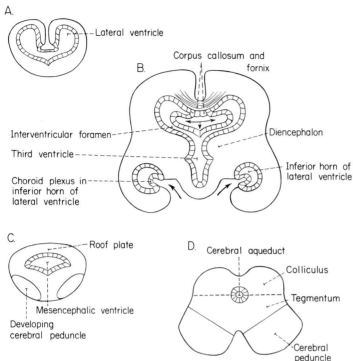

A.

Lateral ventricle

B.

Corpus callosum and fornix

Interventricular foramen

Third ventricle

Choroid plexus in inferior horn of lateral ventricle

Diencephalon

Inferior horn of lateral ventricle

C.

Roof plate

Mesencephalic ventricle

Developing cerebral peduncle

D.

Cerebral aqueduct

Colliculus

Tegmentum

Cerebral peduncle

Figure 1–14. *A* and *B,* Frontal sections through the developing forebrain, showing portions of lateral and third ventricles and choroid plexus. The arrows in *B* are in the subarachnoid space, marking sites at which blood vessels will invaginate to form the choroid plexus of the lateral and third ventricles. The continuity of the ventricular system is illustrated in Figure 1–15. *C* and *D,* The developing midbrain, showing the formation of the cerebral aqueduct, colliculi, tegmentum, and cerebral peduncles.

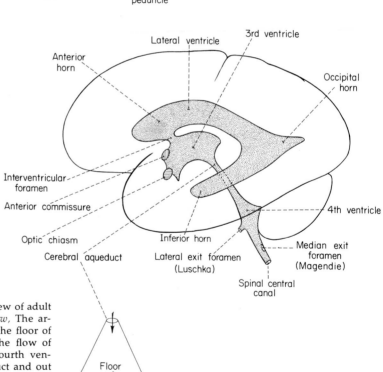

Lateral ventricle

3rd ventricle

Anterior horn

Occipital horn

Interventricular foramen

Anterior commissure

Optic chiasm

Cerebral aqueduct

4th ventricle

Inferior horn

Lateral exit foramen (Luschka)

Median exit foramen (Magendie)

Spinal central canal

Floor of 4th ventricle

Lateral exit foramen

Median exit foramen

Figure 1–15. *Above,* Lateral view of adult ventricular system *in situ. Below,* The arrows in the posterior view of the floor of the fourth ventricle indicate the flow of cerebrospinal fluid: into the fourth ventricle from the cerebral aqueduct and out through the two lateral and one median exit foramina.

to that of the adult and is lined with *ependyma*. The change from a large hollow tube to the small central canal in the adult spinal cord takes place as neurons develop and the entire tube is almost filled with neuron cell bodies, axons, and glia (Fig. 1–7). The remaining small central canal is, however, patent throughout infancy, and CSF can flow into it from the fourth ventricle. In the caudal part of the medulla and in the midbrain the central canal is also small, but in the rest of the brainstem — *i.e.*, the pons and rostral part of the medulla — the posterior part of the neural tube bulges out laterally to form a thin roof consisting of apposed layers of ependyma and pia mater (Fig. 1–13). The *fourth ventricle* is thus formed, and into its caudal portion blood vessels invaginate, forming the *choroid plexus.* A similar choroid plexus occurs in the developing cerebral hemispheres where the *lateral ventricles* are formed and in the roof of the diencephalon overlying the midline *third ventricle* (Fig. 1–14). The third ventricle remains somewhat as it appears in the developing neural tube and communicates with the lateral ventricles through the *interventricular foramina* (of Monro). Connection is maintained with the fourth ventricle by way of the narrow *cerebral aqueduct* passing through the midbrain. A schematic drawing of the adult ventricular system is shown in Figure 1–15.

The cerebrospinal fluid (Chap. 2) is formed by the choroid plexus. It circulates out into the subarachnoid space through three openings in the fourth ventricle, two lateral and one caudal, to bathe the entire central nervous system (Figs. 1–1 and 1–15). The fluid is absorbed into the venous system through numerous *arachnoid villi* on the dorsal surface of the brain that thicken into granulations in the adult and protrude into the *superior sagittal sinus* (see Figure 1–1).

ADDITIONAL READING

Langman, J. *Medical embryology:* human development, normal and abnormal. 2nd edition, Baltimore, The Williams & Wilkins Co., 1969, Chap. 15.

Moore, K. L. *The developing human: clinically oriented embryology.* Philadelphia, W. B. Saunders Co., 1973, Chap. 18.

CHAPTER 2

THE CEREBROSPINAL FLUID AND THE BLOOD–BRAIN–CEREBROSPINAL FLUID BARRIER SYSTEM

PHILLIP D. SWANSON

The cerebrospinal fluid (CSF) is the fluid surrounding the brain and spinal cord in the subarachnoid space and filling the cerebral ventricles (Fig. 2–1). It can easily be obtained from humans by the technique of lumbar puncture. With the patient lying on one side, with his legs and back flexed, a 20- or 22-gauge needle is inserted between the L3 and L4 spinous processes. After the needle has entered the subarach-noid space, and after the stylet has been removed, clear, colorless fluid flows from the needle at rates that depend upon the pressure within the subarachnoid space.

Perhaps the most important function of the cerebrospinal fluid is to support the brain and spinal cord within the skull and vertebral canal. It can be calculated that the buoying effect of the CSF will reduce the effective net weight *in situ* of a 1500-g

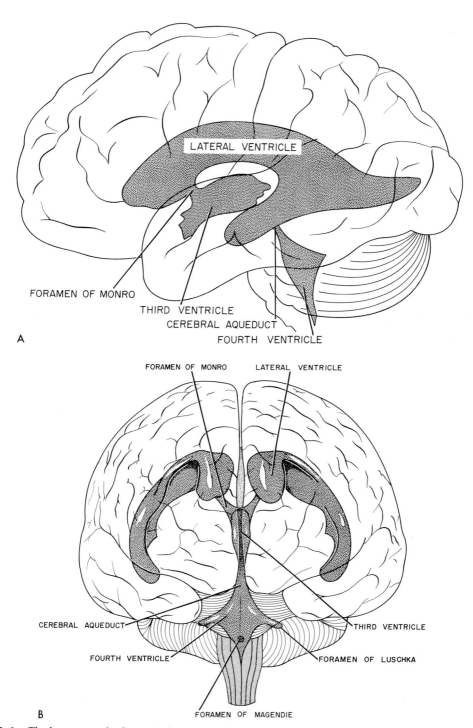

Figure 2–1.   The human cerebral ventricular system shown in lateral (*A*) and anteroposterior (*B*) views. (From Curtis *et al., An introduction to the neurosciences,* Philadelphia, W. B. Saunders Co., 1972.)

brain and spinal cord to less than 50 g. This buoyancy prevents the nerve roots and vessels that enter and leave the nervous system from being stretched in response to acceleration of the head. The cerebrospinal fluid may also play an important role in the regulation of the fluid environment surrounding neuronal and glial cells and may provide a route for some materials to enter or leave the brain. These latter functions are still being defined for individual substances.

COMPOSITION OF THE CEREBROSPINAL FLUID

The cerebrospinal fluid differs most strikingly from serum in being almost free of protein (see Table 2–1). The protein content is even lower in ventricular fluid than it is in fluid obtained at lumbar puncture. Most of the protein is albumin, whereas less than 16 per cent is globulin. The globulin fraction is important, however, since an elevation of gamma globulin can occur in certain disorders, including multiple sclerosis. Of the major immunoglobulins that make up the gamma globulin fraction, IgG is most likely to be elevated. General increases in CSF proteins can occur in other conditions, including spinal block, either intrinsic or extrinsic tumors, and a variety of other neurological conditions.

The glucose level in the CSF is lower than in serum and is reduced further in bacterial, fungal, or tumor meningitis.

TABLE 2–1.   Representative Chemical Values in Adult Human Lumbar Cerebrospinal Fluid (CSF) Compared with Values in Serum

	CSF	Serum
Proteins (mg/100 ml)	10–45	5500–8000
Glucose (mg/100 ml)	60	75–105
Osmolality (mOsm/l)	289	280–300
Na^+ (mEq/l)	147	136–145
K^+ (mEq/l)	2.9	3.5–5.0
Ca^{++} (mEq/l)	2.3	4.5–5.5
Mg^{++} (mEq/l)	2.4	1.5–2.5
Cl^- (mEq/l)	113	98–106
Inorganic phosphorus (mEq/l)	0.5	1–1.5
pH	7.31	7.38–7.44 (blood)

CSF concentrations of various ions also differ from their serum concentrations and from the concentrations expected in a plasma ultrafiltrate. Sodium ion (Na^+) is present at a slightly higher concentration than in serum, whereas levels of potassium (K^+) and calcium (Ca^{++}) ions are reduced (Table 2–1).

The pH in CSF is lower than in blood and is usually held at about 7.31. Alterations in consciousness occur when the CSF pH drops. Carbon dioxide (CO_2) diffuses freely between blood and CSF, so that CSF acidosis is most likely to occur with hypercapnia due to chronic pulmonary disease.

The CSF normally contains no more than five mononuclear leucocytes per cubic millimeter. Elevation in CSF white cell counts (i.e., pleocytosis) accompanies meningitis due to viruses, bacteria, fungi, and occasionally neoplasms that have seeded into the meningeal spaces. Mononuclear cells predominate in viral meningitides, except at the outset, when there may be more polymorphonuclear cells. Bacterial meningitis is usually associated with a predominantly polymorphonuclear response, though meningitis due to tuberculosis is an exception. Malignant tumors that spread within the subarachnoid space may be detected by finding neoplastic cells on stained specimens of CSF.

FORMATION OF THE CEREBROSPINAL FLUID

Cerebrospinal fluid is constantly being formed and removed. The principal site of formation is generally considered to be the choroid plexuses in the lateral, third, and fourth ventricles. Clinical support for the view that CSF is formed within the ventricles comes from the occurrence of enlarged ventricles (hydrocephalus) when there is obstruction to CSF flow due to tumor or other causes.

Rates of formation of CSF can be directly determined by the technique of ventriculocisternal perfusion. Through a cannula placed in a lateral ventricle, artificial CSF containing a high-molecular-weight substance, such as inulin, is pumped at a constant rate. Outflow is collected from the cisterna magna, and the rate at which fluid is produced is determined from the dilution of the concentration of the substance. Rates of production vary with the size of the animal and range from 2.2 μl per minute in rats to 20 μl per minute in cats and 300 to 400 μl per minute in man. These rates are independent of intracranial pressure, though recent experiments with choroid plexus isolated in an intraventricular chamber showed that rates of formation can be reduced by elevation of perfusion pressure.

The choroid plexuses consist of villi with cuboidal, or low columnar, epithelium surrounding a large central capillary (Fig. 2–2). By electron microscopy, tight junctions at the apical end of the cells can be demonstrated to restrict the movement of large molecules from the blood into the cerebrospinal fluid. In human embryos it is estimated that the choroid plexus accounts for 63 per cent of the ventricular surface area. The plexuses receive their blood supply from the anterior and posterior choroidal arteries.

The theory of a secretory role for the choroid plexus has been favored for many years. The most convincing early experimental evidence in support of the choroid plexus as the principal site of formation of CSF was obtained early in the 20th century by the neurosurgeon Walter Dandy when he was able to prevent the development of hydrocephalus in experimental animals by removing the choroid plexuses from the cerebral ventricles. The precise proportion of CSF formed by the choroid plexuses is difficult to estimate and may be as high as 80 to 85 per cent; the remainder enters the ventricles from the ependymal lining or diffuses from the brain into the subarachnoid space. A few investigators maintain that the choroid plexuses play only a minor role in the formation of the CSF.

Harvey Cushing noted that *in vivo*, drops of serous material formed on the surface of human choroid plexus and formation stopped after a choroidal artery was clipped. It is now possible to sample fluid from the choroid plexus in a chamber that can be perfused. The fluid can be analyzed and its rate of formation can be studied under different experimental conditions. The composition of the choroid plexus fluid is indistinguishable from that of CSF

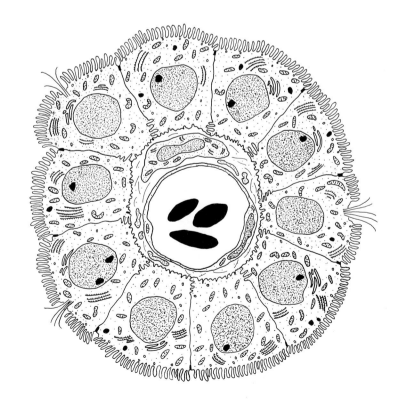

Figure 2–2. Diagram of a mammalian choroidal villus in cross section. The cuboidal cells have numerous microvilli as well as tufts of cilia on their apical surfaces. Lateral and basal cell membranes are infolded. A basement membrane (not drawn) lies beneath the epithelium. The space between the central capillary and the epithelial basement membrane contains a pial cell, pial cell processes, and collagen fibrils. Approximate magnification, ×3200. (From Dohrmann, *Brain Res.*, 1970, *18*, 197–218.)

obtained from within the ventricles. These fluids differ somewhat from fluid obtained by lumbar puncture in that their protein content is lower.

Formation of CSF is an energy-dependent process, and the rate of production is therefore reduced by dinitrophenol, which is an uncoupler of mitochondrial oxidative phosphorylation. Cardiac glycosides inhibit active transport of Na^+ and K^+ in many tissues, presumably by reducing the activity of the (Na^+, K^+)-ATPase enzyme system. These agents also are potent blockers of CSF formation. The volume of CSF is reduced 50 per cent or more when the choroid plexus is perfused with ouabain at a concentration between 10^{-3} and 10^{-4} M. These findings support the view that active transport processes are important for CSF formation.

Another potent inhibitor of CSF production is the carbonic anhydrase inhibitor acetazolamide. This enzyme catalyzes the reaction

$$CO_2 + H_2O \overset{\text{carbonic}}{\underset{\text{anhydrase}}{\rightleftharpoons}} H_2CO_3 \rightleftharpoons H^+ + HCO_3$$

Inhibition of carbonic anhydrase may reduce CSF production by its vasoconstrictor effect on choroidal arteries, though this is not the only mechanism that has been suggested.

The evidence that production of CSF is an active secretory process can be summarized as follows:

(1) Fluid is transported against osmotic and hydrostatic pressure gradients.
(2) Newly formed CSF contains more Na^+ and less K^+ than a dialysate of plasma does.
(3) Formation of CSF is blocked by metabolic inhibitors and by inhibitors of active transport of Na^+ and K^+.

There are no neurological disorders that are known to be due to interference of CSF formation.

SUBSTANCES TRANSPORTED BY THE CHOROID PLEXUS

The choroid plexus is now being regarded as an organ that not only elaborates cerebrospinal fluid but also transports some substances into and others out of the CSF. It is thus an important regulator of the CSF composition and has even been regarded as a miniature kidney (Pollay, 1974). Na^+ ion is probably the main ion that is actively transported from the blood into the CSF through the action of the (Na^+, K^+)-activated ATPase system. K^+ ions are transported in the opposite direction. Glucose can move in either direction across the choroid plexus, probably by a process of *facilitated diffusion*. The process is saturable and probably involves a specific carrier system. It has been suggested that interference with this system in bacterial meningitis may be partly responsible for reduction of CSF glucose levels. There is some evidence that the choroid plexus may clear amino acids and certain anions from the CSF. Thiocyanate ion (SCN^-) and iodine are accumulated by choroid plexus preparations and thus are removed from CSF by saturable processes. Clearance of other substances, such as the neurotransmitter metabolites homovanillic acid and 5-hydroxyindolacetic acid, as well as amines, such as 5-hydroxytryptamine, is also by saturable processes.

CIRCULATION OF THE CEREBROSPINAL FLUID

The cerebrospinal fluid circulates from its site of origin in the ventricles. From the lateral ventricles, fluid passes into the third ventricle through the foramina of Monro, then through the narrow aqueduct of Sylvius, into the fourth ventricle, and finally out into the subarachnoid cisterns through the two lateral foramina (foramina of Luschka) and the caudal foramen (foramen of Magendie) into the subarachnoid cisterns. The fluid then flows over the surface of the hemispheres and passes into the superior sagittal sinus through the *arachnoid granulations* or *villi* (Fig. 2–3). It has been suggested that one-way pores exist in the arachnoid villi that permit passage not only of fluid but also of particles as large as red blood cells. Electron microscope studies have failed to confirm the existence of morphologically identifiable pores. It now appears that the red

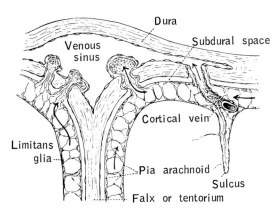

Dura
Subdural space
Venous sinus
Cortical vein
Limitans glia
Pia arachnoid
Sulcus
Falx or tentorium

Figure 2–3. Drawing of leptomeninges, illustrating the subarachnoid space through which cerebrospinal fluid percolates. Fluid may escape by way of arachnoid villi, thin sacculations that invaginate the dural venous sinuses, or by way of venules that drain into the sinuses. Arachnoid and pia mater are joined by filaments, the pia being closely applied to the brain, the arachnoid following the dura, separated from it by a potential subdural space. In its course out of the brain, the vein is separated from the pia by the Virchow-Robin space. (Modified from Weed, *J. med. Res.*, 1914, 31, 56–92.)

cells become sequestered in the villi, where they are broken down within 2 to 6 days of entry by the action of enzymes located in lining membranes. The enzyme heme oxygenase is present in arachnoid and in the choroid plexus and catalyzes the formation of bilirubin from heme. Levels of this enzyme increase within a few hours after blood has been introduced into the subarachnoid space.

HYDROCEPHALUS

Obstruction of the pathways of circulation of the cerebrospinal fluid can result in enlargement of the ventricular system (hydrocephalus) because of continued secretion of cerebrospinal fluid. Hydro-

cephalus can be produced by an ependymoma or other tumors within a ventricle or by congenital stenosis of the aqueduct of Sylvius. Obstruction at the exit foramina can also occur, as well as inflammation in the cisterns following either subarachnoid hemorrhage or bacterial meningitis. Such arachnoiditis can prevent the fluid from flowing over the surface of the brain to the venous sinuses. Operationally, hydrocephalus has been categorized as (1) either obstructive or nonobstructive and (2) either communicating or noncommunicating. Obstructive hydrocephalus results from lesions interfering with the flow of CSF and located either within the ventricles or in the subarachnoid space. Nonobstructive hydrocephalus occurs in only one situation: in the presence of a papilloma of the choroid plexus that secretes cerebrospinal fluid faster than it can be absorbed. Hydrocephalus is *communicating* when it can be shown that communication exists between the lateral ventricles and the lumbar subarachnoid space. One usually demonstrates this by introducing air into the lumbar subarachnoid space and showing by x-ray its appearance in the lateral ventricles. Whereas either aqueductal stenosis or third or fourth ventricle tumors would produce obstructive, noncommunicating hydrocephalus, basilar arachnoiditis would produce obstructive, communicating hydrocephalus (Table 2–2).

INTRACRANIAL PRESSURE

Intracranial pressure is normally measured by placement of a manometer on the lumbar puncture needle while the patient is fully relaxed. Up to 150 to 180 mm of CSF is usually considered normal. Since the brain, cerebrospinal fluid, and intra-

TABLE 2–2. Classification of Types of Hydrocephalus

	Obstructive	Nonobstructive
Communicating	Basilar arachnoiditis secondary to subarachnoid hemorrhage or bacterial meningitis.	Secreting papilloma of choroid plexus.
Noncommunicating	Aqueductal stenosis. Obstruction to third or fourth ventricles by tumor. Closure of exit foramina.	None.

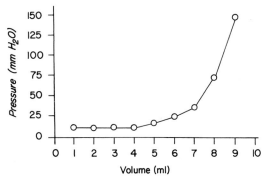

Figure 2–4. Intracranial pressure-volume relationship in monkey. One ml of fluid was added each hour to a supratentorial extradural balloon.

cranial vessels are contained within a space that is essentially surrounded by nondistensible bone, expanding lesions, such as brain tumors, brain abscesses, or subdural hematomas, can raise the intracranial pressure by adding volume to this space. It may take a considerable period of time for a slowly growing tumor to cause increased intracranial pressure. Presumably this compensation is achieved by reduction of the volumes of cerebrospinal fluid and venous vessels. Experiments in which the intracranial volume has been artificially increased show that, after the volume has increased beyond the "limits of compensation," even a small additional increase in the intracranial contents will cause a large increase in pressure (Fig. 2–4).

When an expanding lesion is located in the cerebral hemispheres, not only does the cerebrospinal fluid pressure increase, but also neurological symptoms are produced by encroachment on the brainstem and adjacent structures at the level of the tentorium. Depression of consciousness and dilatation of the pupil (due to compression of the midbrain and stretching of the third cranial nerve) are important clinical signs of "tentorial herniation."

BLOOD-BRAIN AND BLOOD–CEREBROSPINAL FLUID BARRIER SYSTEMS

The existence of these barrier systems is presumed from the observations that (1) many substances appear to take longer to penetrate from the blood stream into the brain substance or into the cerebrospinal fluid than they do into other organs; and that (2) after the concentrations of substances in the brain or CSF have reached their maximums, they are still lower than the concentrations in other organs. It should be immediately pointed out that if the "barrier" concept is accepted, it should not be equated with a simple anatomical barrier. The rates of movements of different substances into the brain and CSF may be very different, and the mechanisms underlying these different rates of penetration are also diverse. For some substances, such as those of high molecular weight, there may be a morphological barrier; for others, the slower rate of penetration may depend on rates of diffusion or transport by specific control systems.

The mechanisms for movement of materials into the brain (blood-brain barrier) are not necessarily identical to those for movement into the CSF (blood-CSF barrier). Morphologically, in the vicinity of the cerebral capillaries there is no equivalent of the epithelial cell of the choroid plexus. At the junction of the blood and brain there is presumably no need for net production of a volume of fluid equivalent to the CSF. However, there is probably a greater need for an efficient glucose-transport mechanism. At both sites there may be a need for restrictions on movements of proteins, ions, and other substances from the blood stream and for control of the pH in the environment of the central nervous system. At both sites, morphological barriers and mechanisms of diffusion, facilitated diffusion, and active transport exist for such control.

Diffusion

A number of substances, including ethanol, volatile and nonvolatile anesthetics, and urea, penetrate rapidly into the brain and into the CSF. These substances probably diffuse across the membrane and cell barriers. Rates of diffusion depend on molecular size and charge, and especially on lipid solubility.

If a molecule can exist in both ionized and un-ionized forms, the un-ionized form usually moves more effectively into the brain or CSF. Water moves rapidly into or out of the brain by diffusion. In conditions of hyposmolarity or hyperosmolarity brought about by electrolyte or water imbalance, cerebral swelling or shrinkage can result from shifts in water content.

Penetration of High-Molecular-Weight Substances into the Brain and Cerebrospinal Fluid

The polysaccharide inulin (mol wt 500) and the proteins horseradish peroxidase (mol wt 40,000), ferritin (mol wt 460,000), microperoxidase (mol wt 2000), and al-

bumin (mol wt 69,000) do not easily enter the brain from the vascular system. Electron microscopy of the distribution of electron-dense particles has shown that these large materials do not pass beyond the tight junctions between cerebral capillary endothelial cells (Fig. 2–5). Similar tight junctions between apical portions of choroid plexus epithelial cells may serve as a similar barrier to passage into the CSF.

Significance of the Blood-Brain Barrier

The control of which substances move into the brain from the blood stream must

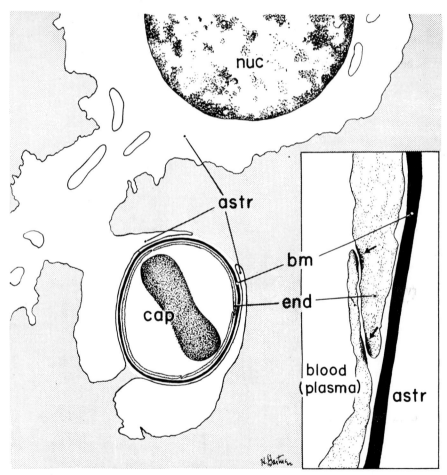

Figure 2–5. Diagram of the relationship between glial cells and the vascular system in brain. The clear space represents an astrocyte (*astr*) containing a nucleus (*nuc*); its perivascular feet almost surround a capillary (*cap*), which contains an erythrocyte. The capillary membrane is surrounded by a basement membrane (*bm*). The inset shows the junction between two endothelial cells (*end*), which is sealed by terminal bar condensations indicated by arrows. The basement membrane is continuous and is shared by endothelium and the adjacent glial cell. Magnification, × 6500 for left drawing; × 90,000 for inset. (Drawing adapted from photomicrographs in Maynard *et al., Amer. J. Anat.,* 1957, *100,* 409–433.)

be important for normal brain function. Glucose passes into the brain rapidly from the blood, and it is most certainly true that the brain derives its glucose, oxygen, and other necessary substances from the blood through capillaries and not from the cerebrospinal fluid. Practically all neurons in the brain are much closer to the capillaries than to cerebrospinal fluid. Occlusion of an artery to the brain for a short period of time results in destruction of most of the tissue. It is only the outer subpial region (molecular layer of the cerebral or cerebellar cortex or white matter of the brainstem and spinal cord) and the inner subependymal (periventricular) region that may be spared and that may, therefore, be able to depend on the cerebrospinal fluid for some of its substrates. Other substances, however, such as proteins and certain ions, take much longer to equilibrate with brain tissue than glucose does.

Although a great deal has been written about movement of dyestuffs into the brain, a more contemporary example of the blood-brain barrier is the commonly used clinical procedure known as the *brain scan*. This procedure is used to localize certain pathological processes that affect the nervous system, especially brain tumors. A radioactive material is injected into the patient intravenously. The material most widely used at present is [^{99}Tc] technetium pertechnetate. This substance has a half-life of 6 hr and is obtained as the sodium salt ($NaTcO_4$). Other substances have also been used, including radioiodinated human serum albumin and mercury-chlormerodrin compounds. With a rectilinear scanner, which picks up gamma rays that are given off by the radioactive agent, the counts can be recorded on x-ray film. Normally, very little radioactivity is picked up over the cerebral hemispheres, but a great deal of radioactivity is seen in areas in which muscle and other tissues absorb the radioactive compound. When there is a breakdown in the blood-brain barrier, as in neoplasms or necrosis of the brain, radioactivity may be picked up in that area and will show up as a darkened region on the brain scan. Presumably, the radioactive ion is able to cross the capillary into either the extracellular or intracellular spaces of the tumor or of the infarcted area.

RELATIONSHIP BETWEEN THE CEREBROSPINAL FLUID AND THE BRAIN'S EXTRACELLULAR FLUID

Not long ago, in the days when electron microscopic pictures were accepted as realistically representing living tissue, it was widely believed that the brain was unique in having practically no extracellular space. To accommodate the uncomfortable fact that there were far too many sodium ions in the brain than could be reasonably believed to be within nerve cells, scientists suggested that glial cells served as a functional extracellular space and that, in order to pass from the blood stream into a neuron, a nutrient such as glucose would have to pass first through a glial cell.

This seemed a rather unwieldy system, and physiologists were relieved when electron micrographs showed that some extracellular space could be discerned after tissue was fixed by a freeze-substitution method. More direct studies have been possible with organisms that have glial cells that are large enough to be impaled by microelectrodes without damage. These systems include the ganglion of the leech and the optic nerve of the mud puppy. These cells contain a high internal K$^+$ concentration and their membrane potentials are at the equilibrium potential for K$^+$ ions. This makes it possible to estimate changes in intracellular K$^+$ concentration when the outer concentration is known. It has been shown that altering the composition of the bathing medium by, for example, substituting sucrose for Na$^+$ ions, produces a conduction block in the mud puppy's optic nerve without altering the internal K$^+$ concentration in the glial cell. Restoring Na$^+$ to the medium rapidly reverses this block. This, and other evidence, suggests that molecules, including inulin, choline, dextran, and sucrose, and ions, such as Na$^+$ and K$^+$, can diffuse rapidly in intercellular clefts. Moreover, removal of glial cells from the leech ganglion does not prevent the neurons from conducting

THE CEREBROSPINAL FLUID AND THE BRAIN'S EXTRACELLULAR FLUID   21

normal impulses; thus the glial cell is not critical for controlling the environment around the neuron.

Several lines of evidence support the contention that the fluid around neurons resembles in composition the cerebrospinal fluid. It is known that chemical substances injected into the subarachnoid space diffuse much more rapidly into brain tissue than when they are administered through the blood stream. This is true of radioactive cations and of other substances, including high-molecular-weight substances such as inulin and horseradish peroxidase. In composition the fluid around neurons resembles the cerebrospinal fluid more than plasma. Pappenheimer and his associates measured the alveolar ventilation in a goat whose ventricle was perfused with artificial CSF—a sensitive bioassay method—and found that the respiratory neurons behaved in a much more physiological fashion when the composition of the artificial fluid was made to resemble cerebrospinal fluid than when it was made to resemble plasma. A clinical example is a patient who is comatose because of acidosis. The plasma pH may be restored to normal, but the patient remains comatose since the pH of the cerebrospinal fluid is still low and has not yet equilibrated with the pH of the plasma.

Many factors influence the penetration of materials into the brain, including transport processes (which may be specific for certain substances, such as glucose), lipid solubility, size of the compound, pumping of the compound out of the cerebrospinal fluid, and binding to plasma proteins.

Movement of Substances between the Cerebrospinal Fluid and the Brain's Extracellular Fluid

There is little doubt that most substances, when placed into the subarachnoid space or into ventricular fluid, have little difficulty in diffusing into the interstitial fluid of the brain. This is true even of the high-molecular-weight substances, whose entry into the brain or CSF from the blood stream is restricted. This exchange probably occurs between adjacent pial or ventricular ependymal cells and the extracellular channels between cellular elements. One question that is being asked by investigators is whether ions and molecules normally move in only one direction, e.g., from the brain to the cerebrospinal fluid (CSF as a "sink"), or whether some may move in the reverse direction, from the cerebrospinal fluid to the brain (CSF as a "source"). One approach has been that of Cserr (1974), who has carried out an experiment (described in the following paragraphs) with the spiny dogfish, whose medulla oblongata is exposed to cerebrospinal fluid on the fourth ventricular surface only.

The plasma concentration of the (usually radioactively labeled) substance being examined is maintained at a constant level for the duration of the experiment. The medulla oblongata is sliced parallel to the floor of the fourth ventricle, and the content of the substance is determined in each section. If the substance diffuses from the blood stream into the brain and then moves into the CSF, the concentration should be lowest near the ventricular surface. Conversely, if the CSF functions as a source of the material, its concentration should be highest near the ventricular surface.

In this preparation, inulin, mannitol, sucrose, and sulfanilic acid have been demonstrated to be cleared from the brain by the sink action of CSF. In contrast, urea appears to move more rapidly into the CSF than into the brain, and during the period before equilibrium is reached, the tissue concentration profiles indicate movement from the CSF into the brain.

ADDITIONAL READING

Brightman, M. W.   The distribution within the brain of ferritin injected into cerebrospinal fluid compartments. II. Parenchymal distribution. *Amer. J. Anat.*, 1965, *117*, 193–220.

Cserr, H. F.   Relationship between cerebrospinal fluid and interstitial fluid of brain. *Fed. Proc.*, 1974, *33*, 2075–2078.

Cserr, H. F.   Physiology of the choroid plexus. *Physiol. Rev.*, 1971, *51*, 273–311.

Davson, H.   *Physiology of the cerebrospinal fluid.* Boston, Little, Brown & Co., 1967.

Kuffler, S. W.   Neuroglial cells: Physiological properties and a potassium-mediated effect of neuronal activity on the glial membrane potential. *Proc. roy. Soc. (Lond.)*, Ser. B, 1967, *168*, 1–21.

Kuffler, S. W., and Nicholls, J. G.   How do materials exchange between blood and nerve cells in the brain? *Perspect. Biol. Med.*, 1965, *9*, 69–76.

Pollay, M. Transport mechanisms in the choroid plexus. *Fed. Proc.*, 1974, *33*, 2064–2069.

THE NEURON, GLIA, AND MYELIN

JOHN W. SUNDSTEN

The neuron is the structural and functional unit of the nervous system, a cell highly specialized for the generation and conduction of electrical impulses. It contains all the usual cytoplasmic components necessary for the maintenance of cellular life and in addition has special membrane properties that account for its electrical characteristics. As a starting point, we can assume that there are at least four major functions carried out by the central nervous system neuron through its different parts: (1) It receives input from other neurons, chiefly by way of its dendrites and soma. (2) It can make computations, particularly summation of inhibitory and excitatory postsynaptic potentials, eventually leading to the generation of an action potential through depolarization of the membrane in the region of the initial segment of the axon. (3) It conducts the action potential along the axon to the axon terminals. (4) It transfers information by synaptic transmission at the terminals to other neurons, muscle cells, or gland cells. In other words, the neuron is highly specialized to handle information, whether initiated in the external or the internal environment, or

within the CNS. The structure this cell has evolved to carry out such functions is unique, and its salient features are covered in the sections that follow.

MORPHOLOGY OF THE NEURON

The cell body (soma) of the central nervous system (CNS) neuron consists of a nucleus and cytoplasm. Extending from its surface are several cylindrical processes whose contents are continuous with the cytoplasm. These processes are the (often numerous) *dendrites* and the single *axon*, which usually gives off several collateral branches (Fig. 3–1). Neuron cell bodies and their processes vary greatly in dimension. The diameters of the somas can be several microns in small neurons, such as the stellate cells in the cerebral cortex, or may be as much as 100 μm, as in the motoneurons. Most of the several billions of neurons in the CNS are small. Generally, dendritic processes reach no more than a few millimeters from the cell body, though some in the brainstem may extend farther. Axons show the greatest differences in

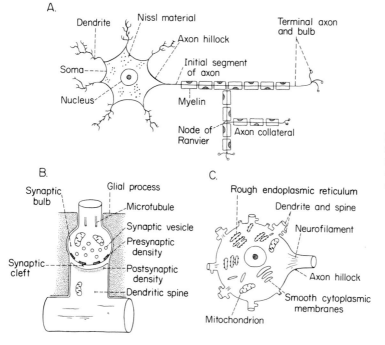

Figure 3-1. *A,* A multipolar neuron, as seen under the light microscope. *B,* A synapse, and *C,* the neuron soma, as shown by electron microscopy.

length, ranging from several micrometers to several feet. An example of the latter is a corticospinal neuron associated with the movement of the big toe; its soma resides in the cerebral cortex of the brain and its axon ends in the caudal part of the spinal cord. Also, as will be seen later, some of the longest fibers are the large sensory fibers from the hands and feet that extend all the way to the brainstem.

The neuron's cell body is the metabolic center of the cell and contains all the requisite cytoplasmic systems that would be expected in any dynamic cell. Numerous *mitochondria* meet the high energy requirements of the cell. They are particularly concentrated in synaptic regions, where they supply the energy needed for the transmission process. The neuron is also an active protein synthesizer and thus has a liberal complement of intracytoplasmic membranes along with *ribosomes* (particles of ribonucleoprotein). Aggregates of ribosomes form the characteristic *Nissl* material seen with the light microscope. The Nissl material extends into dendrites, though it is not as dense there as in the soma; it does not go out into the axon.

Through electron microscopy it has been shown that the intracytoplasmic

membranes form networks of channels and cysternae, called the *endoplasmic reticulum (ER)*. When the membranes are folded into stacks and associated with ribosomes they form *rough,* or *granular ER,* which form the Nissl substance just mentioned. When the membranes have a curved lamellar appearance, expanded at their ends but without ribosomes attached, they form the *Golgi networks.* These structures probably concentrate and package cell products, such as synaptic vesicles. *Microtubules* are believed to form a rapid centrifugal transport system to distant parts of the cell. That is quite a task for neurons such as those in the long tract systems mentioned earlier. A smooth *ER* is also present in the cytoplasm and sometimes can be seen to interconnect areas of rough *ER* or *Golgi networks.* Thus, it may be that the intracytoplasmic membranes form a single organelle that takes on different appearances and functions in different parts of the cell. *Neurofilaments* consisting of protein threads are found throughout the cell, and in the dendrites and axons are arrayed parallel to the long axis. They may give some structural support to the neuron, though their role is by no means clearly understood.

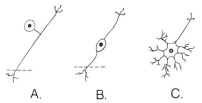

Figure 3–2. Morphological types of neurons. *A,* The unipolar (pseudounipolar) neuron is typical of all dorsal root ganglia and general sensory ganglia associated with cranial nerves. *B,* The bipolar neuron occurs in the cranial nerves for special senses. *C,* The multipolar neurons differ widely in shape; the motoneuron type is shown here. Other types are illustrated in Figure 3–3.

The receiving portion of the neuron consists of its dendrites and cell body, and can be either simple or complex, depending on the diversity of cell processes and synaptic sites. There are three basic morphological types of neurons that are named after the "polarity" their processes give to the cell body: *unipolar* (or *monopolar*), *bipolar,* and *multipolar* (Fig. 3–2).

The unipolar and bipolar neurons are afferent neurons conveying electrical impulses toward the central nervous system and are thus found in the spinal and cranial nerves of the peripheral nervous system. The unipolar neuron does not have typical dendritic processes but instead has a single process attached to the cell body that divides into two parts. The unipolar neuron is often called *pseudounipolar* (a somewhat cumbersome term) because in development there were originally two processes that later fused together in a T-shaped fashion at their junctions with the cell body. This cell type is illustrated by the sensory receptor neuron. One branch of the process is distributed to the spinal cord (or to the brainstem if it is in a cranial nerve), and the other to the periphery (skin or deep tissue), where only its distalmost patch of membrane behaves functionally as a dendrite. The bipolar neuron is also of a simple design. It is a phylogenetically older type of cell that evolved into the unipolar type. Two processes exit from the cell body, a dendritic process and an axonic process. This cell is also a sensory receptor neuron and is found only in cranial nerves associated with the special sensory modalities

of olfaction, vision, audition, and equilibrium. Both the unipolar and bipolar cells conduct action potentials from receptor endings to the central nervous system and are referred to as *primary afferents* (see Chapter 4).

The third type of neuron, the multipolar neuron, has a single axon but, in contrast to the other two types, has many dendrites. Neurons of this type are the most numerous of neurons found and form most of the gray matter of the central nervous system. They are divided into subtypes according to the pattern of dendritic branching and the size and shape of cell body. The motoneuron is the typical example (Fig. 3–1), though many others can be considered to have multiple poles, such as the pyramidal and stellate cells in the cerebral cortex, granule and Purkinje cells in the cerebellar cortex, interneurons in general, and dense groupings of neuron somas throughout the central nervous system, called *nuclei* (Fig. 3–3). All the multipolar neurons integrate (add and subtract) many inputs from different fiber terminals, so that an appropriate output in the form of action potentials is conducted down the axon. Clearly, structurally and functionally the multipolar neuron is far more complex than the bipolar and unipolar neurons. Essentially each one is a very sophisticated computer. An even more humbling fact is that our CNS has several billions of them at any one moment either silently "waiting" for input, or idling, or discharging rapidly.

Even though the first-order afferent neurons are of simpler design than the others, their task is of major importance: they are the first link in the chain of

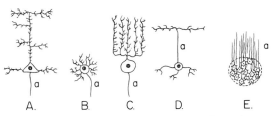

Figure 3–3. Various representative configurations of multipolar neurons: *A,* pyramidal cell; *B,* stellate cell; *C,* Purkinje cell; *D,* granule cell; *E,* a nucleus of multipolar cells. *a* indicates axon. Dendrites have been omitted from *E* for clarity.

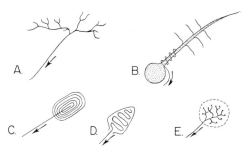

Figure 3–4. Major types of afferent nerve endings found in skin. Nonencapsulated endings: *A,* free nerve endings; *B,* endings encircling a hair follicle. Encapsulated endings: *C,* Pacinian corpuscle; *D,* Meissner's corpuscle; *E,* nondescript encapsulated bulb.

events that translates the physical properties of the environment into something we can sense. A dramatic example of this is shown by clinical cases in which the primary afferents associated with pain are either damaged or absent, so that bruising, breaking, and burning has disastrous effects on the part affected. Normally we are endowed with a full complement of sensory receptor neurons that can transduce the physical environment into neural impulses (see Chapter 7).

Such receptor neurons have specialized membrane properties at their distal endings. In some instances they have definite, identifiable structural receptor elements, as in the retina. More often, naked nerve endings (*i.e.,* endings bare of myelin coverings) themselves transduce the mechanical and chemical environmental energies into electrical energy that can be actively conducted by nerve fibers. The naked nerve endings may either end freely in an innervated structure, such as the skin or adventitia, or terminate in a capsular investment of epithelial cells (Fig. 3–4). Examples of *nonencapsulated* naked nerve endings are those for pain (which are widely distributed) and those associated with hair follicles. The latter endings are

categorized as tactile, since they are sensitive to slight displacement of hairs.

Some of the *encapsulated* receptors have an ordered appearance. For example, the *Pacinian corpuscle* has a concentric, "onion-skin" arrangement of connective tissue around the naked endings. Pacinian corpuscles are numerous in deep structures and skin and are particularly sensitive to vibratory stimuli, since they adapt rapidly. In *Meissner's corpuscle* the nerve fiber winds its way in a tortuous fashion through a connective tissue investment. Meissner's corpuscles are numerous on the hairless (glabrous) skin of the hands and feet and are a variety of tactile receptors. In other types of sensory endings the naked terminals are covered by connective tissue capsules shaped like *bulbs* or *discs*. Bulbs and discs have a rather wide distribution (*e.g.,* subcutaneous tissue, serous and mucous membranes, penis, joint capsules, etc.), but no evidence has yet been found for their constancy or specificity. Specific endings exist in muscles, however, associated with the intrafusal muscle fibers forming neuromuscular spindles (Fig. 3–5). The endings are of two types: a primary, or *annulospiral*, ending wrapped around the middle of the intrafusal fiber, and a secondary, smaller, or *flower-spray*, ending associated with the intrafusal fiber at a distance from the central region. Both are stretch receptors and, along with the gamma efferents to the intrafusal muscle fibers of the neuromuscular spindle, serve to regulate muscle tone. In the tendons, specific endings of another type, the *Golgi tendon organs*, act to prevent excessive stretch on the muscle (see Chapter 6).

In summary, receptors widely ranging in type, from naked endings to encapsulated naked endings to highly specialized endings, exist as an interface between the organism and its environment and set up in response to mechanical and chemical

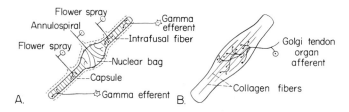

Figure 3–5. Encapsulated afferent endings associated with (*A*) muscle spindle and (*B*) Golgi tendon organ. Two types are shown in the intrafusal muscle fiber: the annulospiral endings in the equatorial nuclear-bag region and flower-spray endings on either side. The gamma efferent fibers are also shown.

stimuli the chains of events that bring about the appropriate reflex responses and neural coding that are interpreted as sensation.

THE SYNAPSE

One of the most distinctive features of neurons is the morphology of the axon terminals (*bulbs, end-feet,* or *boutons*) forming the *synapse*, the functional junction between nerve cells (Figs. 3–1, 3–6, and 3–7). The axon terminal contains synaptic vesicles that release a chemical transmitter substance (*e.g.,* acetylcholine [ACh], and in some fibers a catecholamine, such as noradrenalin or dopamine). The transmitter passes through a presynaptic membrane into a synaptic cleft of 200-Å width, crosses to the postsynaptic cell, and polarizes its membrane on contact (see Chapter 8). Transmission of information is unidirectional across the synapse.

The ultrastructural details of the synapse have received considerable attention in the past few years, although the functional significance of some of the morphological findings has not been clarified. Most synapses fall into two major morphological types (Fig. 3–6). In one (Type I) the synaptic vesicles are rounded and range from 300 Å to 600 Å. Postsynaptic membrane density is more pronounced than presynaptic membrane density, so that the synapse has an asymmetrical appearance. In the other (Type II) the vesicles are flattened or ellipsoid and smaller, ranging from 100 Å to 300 Å. Membrane densities at both presynaptic and postsynaptic sites are of comparable thickness, so that the synapse appears symmetrical. Type II synapses have a less prominent postsynaptic density and a narrower syn-

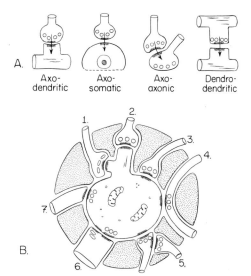

Figure 3–7. Types of synapses, as seen with the electron microscope. *A,* Simple synaptic connections. *B,* Complex glomerular synaptic arrangement around a central dendritic shaft. The glomerular capsule is formed by neuroglial cells (*stippled*). *1,* Inhibitory contact with the base of the spine; *2* and *3,* contacts on the spine and shaft of the dendrite; *4,* an *en passage* synapse; *5,* serial synapse, axoaxodendritic; *6,* reciprocal synapse (inhibitory and excitatory) between two dendritic processes; *7,* a dendrodendritic synapse.

aptic cleft than do Type I synapses. The general assumption is that the flattened vesicles of the Type II synapses contain inhibitory transmitters, whereas the rounded vesicles of the Type I synapses contain excitatory transmitters. Type I synapses are more prominent on the distal part of dendrites and on dendritic spines, whereas Type II synapses are more likely to be found on the proximal dendritic trunks and somas.

This characterization of synapses is useful, but it should be recognized that it is not final. Vesicle size and densities seen with the electron microscope can depend on technical factors. Furthermore, although there is good evidence that the Type I synapse is excitatory, for example, at parallel fiber input to the Purkinje cell's dendritic spines (see Chapter 21), there is also a *Type II excitatory* synapse between climbing fibers and the Purkinje cell's dendrites. The basket cell input to the Purkinje cell body is Type II inhibitory, as would be expected from the general rule. The eventual understanding of the

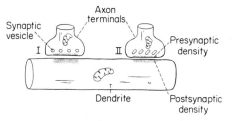

Figure 3–6. Type I and Type II axodendritic synapses, as visualized with the electron microscope.

synaptic apparatus—that is, the structure and function of presynaptic, cleft, and postsynaptic components—is of more than passing interest, as it is the site at which information is chemically transmitted to the next neuron, or effector cell.

The *neuropil* is a general term used to describe areas of the central nervous system with many fibers, presynaptic and postsynaptic; it is a region with many synapses. To clarify the connections found in a neuropil area, we have categorized a given synapse according to which parts of the two neurons' membranes make contact (Fig. 3–7A). Thus synaptic inputs, from axons to dendrites, are called *axodendritic*. Synapses of this type are most numerous. *Axosomatic* synapses are between axons and cell bodies and are far fewer in number, and *dendrodendritic* synapses have been identified between dendrites in some parts of the CNS. *Axoaxonic* synapses also occur in some neurons at the initial segment of the axon and at axon terminals, though they are rarer than the types just mentioned. It has been proposed that axoaxonic synapses may be one means of accomplishing presynaptic inhibition. Certainly the anatomical locations of the synaptic sites at the initial segment and at the terminal of the axon are suitable ones to bring about inhibition, *i.e.*, either by preventing development of the action potential or by preventing the triggering of transmitter release.

Synaptic networks in any given neuropil are, however, far more complex than the simple one-to-one, input-output relation between two cells in a linear series that is usually represented graphically for didactic reasons. Dendritic expansion through branching and spine formation greatly increases membrane surface area to provide thousands of input sites. The synaptic packing can become very geometrical, as in glomeruli (Fig. 3–7B) and other composite contact formations. Within such complexes many types of synaptic arrangements may be found, from a simple axodendritic or dendrodendritic contact to *serial* contacts (*e.g.*, axoaxodendritic) or *reciprocal* contacts, where two synapses are made in opposite directions between the same two processes. Further, a mixture of inhibitory and excitatory synapses may be present in neighboring regions of membrane. The great complexity of the neuropil then can be seen even in the reflection of a single isolated region of inputs. The unravelling and clarifying of the networks and patterns of the neuropil still remain a formidable barrier to our understanding of the function of the central nervous system.

NEUROGLIA

A great number of the differentiating neuroepithelial cells develop, not into neurons, but into two types of *neuroglial* cells, *oligodendrocytes* and *astrocytes* (see Figure 1–6). These cells were originally

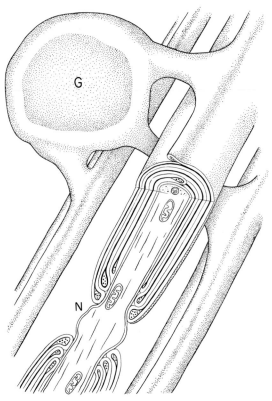

Figure 3–8. Myelinated coverings of fibers in the central nervous system. Oligodendrocyte (*G*) has three footlike processes going to different axons. The oligodendrocyte's cytoplasmic membrane is indicated in three dimensions in the center of the figure to show the concentric wrappings that form myelin (*dark lines*). Note that the loops of glial cytoplasm end at the node of Ranvier (*N*), leaving it unmyelinated. (Modified from Bunge *et al.*, *J. biophys. biochem. Cytol.*, 1961, *10*, 67–94.)

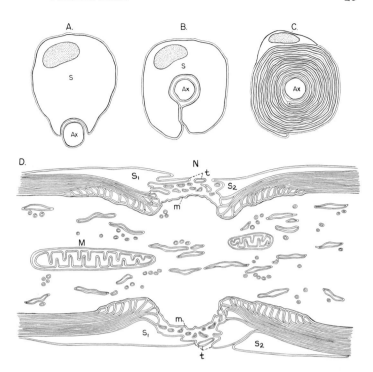

Figure 3–9. Myelinated covering of axon in the peripheral nervous system. *A, B,* and *C,* Sequential stages in myelin formation around an axon (*Ax*) by the cytoplasmic membrane of a Schwann cell (*S*). *D,* Longitudinal view of a myelinated axon. The outer layers of cytoplasm of the two Schwann cells that are myelinating the axon are indicated (*S₁* and *S₂*). The plasma membrane (*m*) of the axon is labeled at the node of Ranvier (*N*). Mitochondria (*M*) are also shown. Note the tongues of Schwann cell cytoplasm (*t*) overlapping at the node; this does not occur in the central nervous system (see Figure 3–8). (After Robertson, *Progr. Biophys.,* 1962, *10,* 343–418.)

conceptualized as simple "neural glue" holding the nervous system together but are now known to have farther-reaching functions. They appear to be scattered throughout nerve tissue without any clear pattern, though the *oligodendrocytes* are closely associated with large neurons, in a kind of satellite position around the cell body, and also are in high concentration in white matter. These cells are responsible for the myelination of CNS fibers (Fig. 3–8). *Myelin* is a lipoprotein formed by concentric wrappings of the oligodendrocytes' cell membrane with most of the cytoplasm "squeezed" out (Figs. 3–8 and 3–9). One oligodendrocyte will myelinate several axons but only for the distance of an internode (*i.e.,* up to a millimeter). A gap of bare axon, called the *node of Ranvier* (see Figures 3–8 and 3–11), appears between the myelinations produced by two adjacent oligodendrocyte wrappings. It is here that axon collaterals arise, usually at right angles (see Figure 3–1). In peripheral nerves the *Schwann cell* (a neuroepithelial cell derivative) myelinates fibers in a similar manner (Fig. 3–9), but it myelinates an internode of only one fiber instead of several. *Unmyelinated* fibers are also associated with either oligodendrocytes or

Schwann cells, but the typical concentric cell membrane wrappings are not formed. The bare axons simply "rest" in an indentation in the cell membrane (Fig. 3–10). It is the rule that several unmyelinated axons are associated with one oligodendrocyte or Schwann cell.

Fiber size is directly proportional to conduction speed of the nerve impulse, and for a given diameter a myelinated fiber conducts faster than does an unmyelinated one. This is because the myelin sheaths are discontinuous at the nodes of Ranvier and thus conduction of the impulse is saltatory (by "jumps") rather than continuous. Because of the insulating effect of myelin, current flow (via ions) across the axon membrane sufficient to cause an action potential can take place only at the nodes. In unmyelinated fibers the current flows across the membrane all along the axon continuously; therefore, conduction is slower. Note also that myelin is absent at the initial segments and at the terminals of all axons. The membrane properties at these sites are specialized for the development of action potentials and the initiation of the transmission process, respectively. Both phenomena require that ions move with relative im-

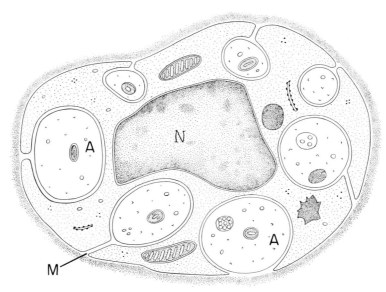

Figure 3–10. Unmyelinated axons indenting the cytoplasm of a Schwann (or glial) cell. *A,* axon; *N,* nucleus; *M,* mesaxon. (After Elfvin, *J. Ultrastruct. Res.,* 1958, *1,* 428–454.)

punity across membranes, and this situation would not obtain if myelin were present.

This close relationship between the oligodendrocyte, myelin, and nerve conduction is of particular importance since the proper functioning of the CNS depends on the intactness of the relationship. A case in point would be a demyelinating disease such as multiple sclerosis. The primary event can be envisioned as affect-

ing the integrity of the oligodendrocytic cell itself; subsequently demyelination takes place. The impairment in neural conduction then is presumably through altered properties of the now demyelinated axons.

The *astrocytes* are more randomly dispersed and not necessarily associated only with neurons. Some are closely related to the pia mater on the external surface of the brain, and some have end-feet that

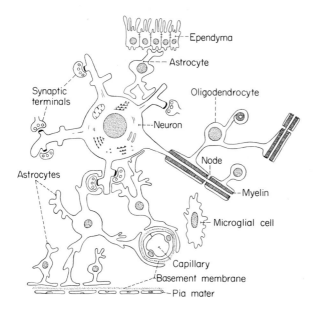

Figure 3–11. Nonneuronal cells in the central nervous system. The ependymal cells have cilia protruding on their ventricular side; an astrocyte is interposed between the ependyma and a neuron. Other astrocytes are shown with end-feet on a capillary, or on the pial surface as well as on the neuron. The two oligodendrocytes are associated with myelinated axons. Near the capillary is a microglial cell (probably phagocytic). A few axodendritic synapses are also shown. (Modified from Warwick and Williams, *Gray's anatomy,* Philadelphia, W. B. Saunders Co., 1973).

form cuffs around capillaries within the brain (Fig. 3–11). In both instances a basement membrane separates the meso-dermal (pial and vascular) from the neuroectodermal (glial) components. Col-lectively the pial-glial membranes form a supporting structure, and the vascular-glial junctions form a barrier to the ready entrance of some materials into neurons (see Chapter 2). Cajal noted long ago that the astrocytes are especially prominent in areas of neuropil where synapses are fre-quent, and now it is generally assumed that they also insulate or isolate synaptic zones from one another (Figs. 3–1, 3–7, and 3–11). Glia never intervene between pre-synaptic and postsynaptic components of the synapse, but clearly are in contact with the neuronal membranes surrounding the synaptic region.

The astrocytes also have a role to play in disease and injury. When neurons are destroyed, astrocytic proliferation occurs along with the invasion by phagocytic cells (*microglia*—though these are actually derived from mesoderm and *not* there-fore a type of glial cell). The origin of phagocytic cells in the CNS is not entirely settled. For example, astrocytes, or per-haps undifferentiated glioblasts, can also become phagocytic. The significant point is that the debris is cleared out by phago-cytic action and the remaining region, now absent of functional neurons, is scarred over with a fibrillary astrocytic "skeleton" (*gliosis*).

DEGENERATION AND REGENERATION OF NERVE

Two basic pathological changes take place in a nerve cell when it is damaged, and these can readily be described in the instance in which the axon is severed: *anterograde* and *retrograde* degenerative processes in parts of the cell *distal* and *proximal* to the cut, respectively (Fig. 3–12). The *anterograde* (or Wallerian, or *ortho-grade*) changes occur in all of the axon, from the damaged site through the termi-nal endings, since this portion of the cell is now removed from the metabolic center in the cell body. The axon begins to degen-

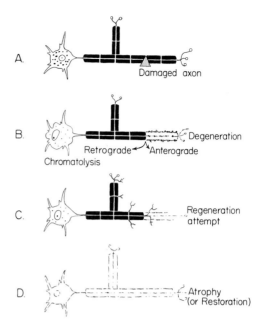

Figure 3–12. Neuronal degeneration. *A,* Normal neuron is damaged by a lesion. *B,* Anterograde de-generation is characterized by clumping of myelin and beading of axon. Retrograde change is exempli-fied by chromatolysis and swelling of cell body. *C,* Neuron attempts to regenerate by sending out axon sprouts. *D,* Neuron atrophies; under appropriate conditions it could regenerate.

erate within a few hours after the injury and breaks up into beaded segments after several days. During this process changes go on within the axoplasm, such as swelling and hypertrophy of neurofilaments at the terminals. Subsequent to the breakdown of the axon, the myelin sheath (in myelinated fibers) also disintegrates into clumps of debris. Initially, the oligodendrocyte (the Schwann cell in the peripheral nervous system) digests its own myelin wrappings within its own cytoplasm. Eventually, the degenerating products are phagocytozed by undifferentiated glial cells and/or micro-glial cells invading the area from blood vessels, and the area is replaced by an as-trocytic scar. This may take months, de-pending on the size of lesion. If very large, as from occlusion of a large vessel, such as the middle cerebral artery, then an astro-cytic scar may wall off the infarcted area rather than replace it.

Researchers have used many of the de-generative changes, such as the beading of axons, clumping of myelin, changes in size and changes at the terminals, to trace pathways in the CNS. For example, the Nauta technique, a method of silver staining that can be applied to the degenerating smaller unmyelinated fibers and terminals, has enabled investigators to provide a far better wiring diagram of the CNS than was previously possible. This and other staining methods are summarized at the end of this chapter.

Retrograde changes in the nerve cell proximal to the damaged area are present but are less dramatic and are more variable than the anterograde ones just described. The length of axon proximal to the cut may degenerate if the damage is severe. The response in the cell body is more prominent. Several changes occur in the cellular organelles, directed initially at repair and restoration of functions in the cell. The nucleus swells and moves to an eccentric position next to the cell membrane. The Nissl material (RNA) is dispersed and therefore is stained more lightly; thus the term *chromatolysis* is used in a generic sense to describe the over-all changes in the cell body during retrograde degeneration. The mitochondria swell, and the Golgi apparatus proliferates. If such responses of the cellular organelles to injury are successful, they can restore the cell to its pretraumatic state, provided that the original damage is far distal on the axon and that a sufficient number of intact axon collaterals remain proximally. In other words, the greater the amount of cell membrane left intact, the greater the chances are that the neuron can maintain its integrity. In the CNS, the length of axon distal to the transection will never be replaced (see later), and if the damage is severe enough and close enough to the cell body, then the whole neuron will atrophy. How much is "enough" depends on age, size of neuron, and unknown factors that make some networks or chains of relays in the nervous system more or less susceptible to injury.

In both the central and peripheral nervous systems injured fibers will attempt to grow back to their original destinations by sprouting many branches from their cut ends. Unfortunately, in the CNS the formation of glial scars prevents the sprouts from extending a sufficient distance to establish a functional connection with a postsynaptic cell. Even when the astrocytic scar is prevented from forming or is removed, there is no orderly channel for the growing axon to grow into as there is in the peripheral nervous system. In the latter, the Schwann cell itself does not die when its axon is injured, as is true of the oligodendrocyte in the CNS. In the peripheral nervous system the inner myelin wraps of the Schwann cell disintegrate, but the outermost cell membrane (the *neurilemma*) remains intact, forming a functional tube, or at least a column of debris, along which the sprouting axons can grow. Thus if the distance is not too great, and especially if the ends of a cut peripheral nerve can be approximated, there is a good chance of recovery of some functions.

Such random growth of new axons down neurilemmal sleeves would appear as a fairly ineffectual means of reestablishing motor and sensory functional contacts. However, there are many more fibers growing from the cut nerve end than there were originally. That is, each axon sends out many new sprouts, and adjacent healthy nerves apparently also send out new branches, particularly in the actual denervated area. Thus the problem is perhaps more one of "overkill." By mechanism(s) not yet understood, the denervated area will chemically recognize the appropriate fiber if it arrives there. The fibers that do not find innervation sites ultimately atrophy. Complete restoration of motor and sensory function of course does not always happen. With major damage there will be less specific return of muscle function, more in the direction of a mass action for a given movement, and sensation though present is likely to be less discretely localized and of somewhat greater threshold.

GENERAL CLASSIFICATION AND USEFULNESS OF STAINS

At about the beginning of the century, several staining methods for nerve tissues were developed; modifications of them are still used today. They can be roughly divided into four major groups according to the part of the neuron stained (myelin, axon, whole neuron, soma). The *Weigert* method selectively stains the lipids in normal myelin sheaths. It was used with great success by the early comparative neuroanatomists in their attempts to map the various pathways in normal preparations; of course the smaller unmyelinated fibers were undetected. Many variations of it are still very useful for descriptive purposes and are referred to as *myelin sheath* stains. The *Marchi* method demonstrates degenerating myelin sheaths. It has been used in studies of the course of myelinated fibers that have been interrupted either by experimental lesions or by pathological diseases. This method has the disadvantages of being difficult to use and subject to artifact. Also, only degenerating myelinated fibers are stained, and this is a severe limitation, since most of the CNS is built up of either very thinly myelinated fibers or unmyelinated fibers. It is mentioned here because it has historical interest and because much of our understanding of CNS pathways stems from its usage. This knowledge is subject to revision and addition as more precise methods are evolved.

A contemporary method, the *Nauta* method, has been evolved out of various silver impregnation methods. It has allowed researchers to trace not only the smaller unmyelinated axons but also their degenerating terminals. In the past decade this experimental degeneration technique has provided a great deal of information on the interconnections of structures within the CNS by small fibers. It is probably fair to say that with this method and its variations the knowledge of the connectivity of the CNS is being rewritten. Another old method, the *Golgi* technique, has been revised by some workers and put to good use. It is worth noting here that the famous Spanish histologist Ramón y Cajal used this method almost exclusively to describe the entire nervous system, and with Golgi received the first Nobel prize in 1904. For some as yet unknown reason, the Golgi silver impregnation technique selects only a few whole nerve cells at random; thus under appropriate conditions, the neuron soma, dendrites, and axons can be seen in their entirety. It is particularly good in evaluations of dendritic fields, and some investigators have attempted to trace pathways with it.

One of the most common methods for looking at normal material is the *Nissl* method. A basic aniline dye (*e.g.,* cresyl violet, thionin) is used in this technique to stain the Nissl material (RNA) in the cell body and to a lesser extent in the basal part of the dendrites. It is commonly used in combination with Luxol fast blue, which shows myelin sheaths, as a routine method for studying sections of both normal and pathological material. Another stain commonly used by the neuropathologist is the *Holzer* stain, which is a selective method for showing astroglia.

The electron microscope as a research tool has been put to good advantage by the morphologist interested in the fine structural detail of nerve cells, particularly their synaptic contacts. It is used both in the study of normal material and in experimental degeneration studies. Neuroanatomical research also utilizes fluorescence microscopy, autoradiography, and other contemporary methods, including electrophysiological ones, but all are too detailed to repeat here.

ADDITIONAL READING

Bourne, G. H., ed. *The structure and function of nervous tissue,* Vol. 1, Structure I. New York, Academic Press, 1968.

Nauta, W. J., and Ebbesson, S. O. E., eds. *Contemporary research methods in neuroanatomy.* New York, Springer-Verlag, 1970.

CHAPTER 4

THE PERIPHERAL NERVES, SPINAL CORD, AND BRAINSTEM

JOHN W. SUNDSTEN

The peripheral nervous system, as its name implies, is outside, or external to, the central nervous system (CNS). Thus it can be thought of as comprising all nerve tissue in the body except the brain and spinal cord. Its structure and organization are properly covered in texts dealing with the histology and gross morphological aspects of the nervous system. Here, its major components are summarized, particularly those that provide an understanding of how neurons are collected together and arranged into peripheral—and to a lesser extent visceral—nerves. This objective necessitates at least an overview of the morphology of the spinal cord and its continuation rostrally into the brainstem, since these are the structures to which the peripheral nerves are attached and to which they ultimately send information or

from which they receive it. The peripheral nervous system then basically consists of: the posterior (afferent) and anterior (efferent) nerve roots of the spinal cord, the posterior root ganglia and cranial nerve ganglia containing cell bodies of afferent neurons, autonomic ganglia containing cell bodies of sympathetic or parasympathetic elements, plexuses, and spinal and cranial nerves containing afferent and efferent fibers with their respective endings.

Events in the external and internal environments are first detected by receptors that are categorized according to where the input is initiated: *exteroreceptors* in the skin, *proprioceptors* in deep tissue (muscles, tendons, and joints), and *interoceptors* in the viscera. Subsequent to the activation of these receptors by appropriate stimuli, information is conducted via *afferent* fibers

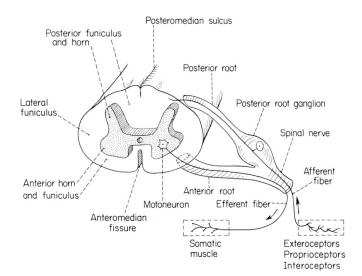

Figure 4–1. Segment of spinal cord showing formation of spinal nerve and destination of afferent and efferent fibers. White matter (funiculi) and gray matter (horns) of spinal cord are indicated.

into the CNS (Fig. 4–1). Note that the use of *afferent* and *sensory* synonymously is only partially correct. All fibers conveying impulses to the CNS are afferent, but only those afferent fibers that enter into pathways in the CNS related to conscious sensation are properly called *sensory.* Many afferents enter into interneuron pools in the spinal cord and brainstem that are involved in reflex connections or that project information to the cerebellum. Such information is not "sensed." Literally, *afferent* simply means going *toward* something, in this case, the CNS. *Efferent* (motor) fibers, that is, fibers distributed to muscles and glands, arise from columns of motoneuron nuclei in the spinal cord and brainstem and exit through their respective foramina leading *away* from the CNS. Both the efferent and the afferent fibers combine to form peripheral nerves, as is discussed below.

Peripheral nerves are distributed to regions derived from either the body wall or the body cavities; the former include the skin and muscles, and the latter, the viscera. Thus, peripheral nerves innervate either somatic or visceral structures. It is important to note that both afferent and efferent fibers are found within most peripheral nerves, whether they are somatic or visceral nerves. Damage to a nerve, then, would likely cause impairment of both sensory and motor functions. The distribution of peripheral nerves is more

readily understood by a grouping together of the individual fibers into different *functional categories,* according to their origin and the normal direction of the impulses they conduct, that is, *visceral afferent, visceral efferent, somatic afferent,* and *somatic efferent fibers* (Fig. 4–2). Such functional categorization becomes more complex in cranial nerves with the addition of special sensory receptors (for taste, olfaction, vision, and audition) and muscle groups derived from branchial arches (muscles of facial expression and mastication and muscles of the pharynx and larynx). However, the basic pattern is the same. A summary of the functional categories appears in Figures 4–13 to 4–15 and can be referred to in later chapters when specific examples are discussed.

THE SPINAL NERVE

The manner in which a *spinal nerve* is formed from posterior (dorsal) and anterior (ventral) roots is shown in Figures 4–1 and 4–2. Note that the anterior roots are composed only of efferent fibers, whereas the posterior roots are composed only of afferent fibers. The cell bodies for the afferent fibers, whether somatic or visceral, are located in the posterior root ganglia. These ganglion cells are of the *pseudounipolar* type (see Figure 3–2), with a central (proximal) process going to the

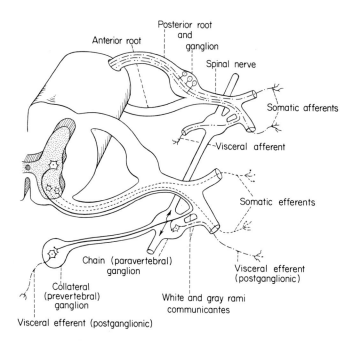

Figure 4–2. Diagram of spinal cord, spinal nerves, and sympathetic components, emphasizing the route taken by *somatic efferent* and *afferent* fibers, and *visceral efferent* and *afferent* fibers. For clarity, afferent paths are shown in the upper and efferent paths in the lower spinal nerve.

CNS and a peripheral (distal) process going into a peripheral nerve, whereby it is distributed to skin, to deep structures, or to the viscera. Since afferent information is conducted from the receptor all the way to the spinal cord by action potentials, we can consider the centrally and peripherally distributed process of the dorsal root ganglion cell as an axon; thus, functionally, only the receptor ending is considered as a "dendrite." The cell bodies of the motoneurons that form the anterior root are located in the anterior gray columns of the spinal cord and certain brainstem nuclei and will be discussed in more detail in later sections.

Recall that the region of the spinal cord giving rise to a single pair (*i.e.*, one on each side) of anterior and posterior roots is called a *spinal cord segment. Segmental levels* are referred to in the cord and brainstem for describing either the position of anatomical pathways or the location of lesions along the rostrocaudal dimension of the neuraxis. Developmentally, the segmental basis is accurate throughout, but, because of the complexity of the internal aspects of the brainstem, the level there is more approximate. Since different nuclei and fiber systems appear at different medullary, pontine, or midbrain levels, a lesion might be spoken of as occurring at the level of a prominent internal structure, such as the inferior olivary nucleus, or might be described as occurring at the level of a given cranial nerve nucleus. In contrast, spinal cord segmental levels are clearly numbered in the same manner as their corresponding posterior and anterior roots and spinal nerves, there being 8 cervical levels, 12 thoracic, 5 lumbar, and 5 sacral (Fig. 4–3).

DISTRIBUTION OF THE SPINAL NERVE

A typical cross section of a spinal cord in the vertebral canal, with attached spinal nerve, is shown in Figure 4–4. Recall that the spinal nerve contains both afferent and efferent fibers and that it divides into a *posterior ramus,* supplying the posterior, or back, musculature and skin, and an *anterior ramus,* supplying the anterior body wall and appendages. Note also that a portion of the autonomic nervous system, the sympathetic chain, is attached close to the origin of the anterior ramus of the spinal nerve.

The autonomic nervous system and its patterns of innervation of visceral structures, that is, smooth muscles, cardiac muscle, and glands, will be discussed more fully in Chapter 11. At this time certain of

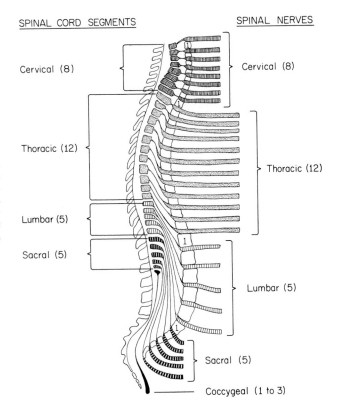

SPINAL CORD SEGMENTS   SPINAL NERVES

Cervical (8)

Thoracic (12)

Lumbar (5)

Sacral (5)

Cervical (8)

Thoracic (12)

Lumbar (5)

Sacral (5)

Coccygeal (1 to 3)

Figure 4–3. Relationships between spinal cord segments, vertebral bodies and spines, and spinal nerves exiting in the intervertebral foramen. The first cervical, thoracic, lumbar, and sacral vertebral bodies are indicated. (Adapted from *Bing's local diagnosis in neurological diseases,* Haymaker, ed., St. Louis, The C. V. Mosby Co., 1969.)

its features are mentioned, since they are a part of the general topic of the formation of nerves. The sympathetic ganglia are attached to the anterior ramus of the spinal nerve by *white* and *gray rami communicantes.* Information from the central nervous system is conveyed to the ganglion cells by *preganglionic fibers* that collectively form the *white* (myelinated) *ramus communicans.* The *preganglionic fibers* may (1) synapse at

the ganglion entered, or (2) ascend or descend to other chain ganglia by way of the interconnecting *sympathetic trunk,* or (3) leave without synapsing and form *splanchnic* nerves that are distributed to *collateral ganglia* in the abdominal cavity (Fig. 4–2). The cell bodies of the sympathetic neurons in the chain ganglia give rise to *postganglionic* fibers that return to the spinal nerve via the *gray* (unmyelinated) *ramus communi-*

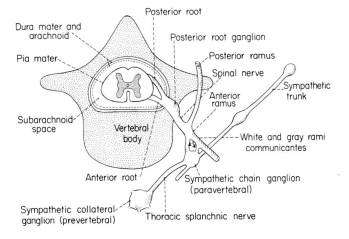

Figure 4–4. Spinal cord in the vertebral canal, with attached roots, spinal nerve, rami, and sympathetic chain.

Posterior root

Dura mater and arachnoid

Pia mater

Subarachnoid space

Vertebral body

Anterior root

Sympathetic collateral ganglion (prevertebral)

Thoracic splanchnic nerve

Posterior root ganglion

Posterior ramus

Spinal nerve

Anterior ramus

Sympathetic trunk

White and gray rami communicantes

Sympathetic chain ganglion (paravertebral)

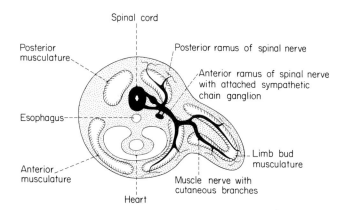

Figure 4–5. Segment of developing embryo, showing the formation and distribution of a spinal nerve. Limb bud and nerves are shown on one side only.

cans. Postganglionic fibers from the collateral ganglia do not form named nerves but instead reach visceral structures by many short fiber bundles, often coursing along blood vessels.

The plan of spinal nerve distribution is fairly simple when seen in a cross section through one of the developing embryonic somites where the posterior and anterior roots have already combined to form the spinal nerve (Fig. 4–5). The posterior ramus of the spinal nerve extends through the posteriorly placed muscle mass of the back, whereas the anterior ramus supplies both the anterior musculature and that in the limb buds. Note that the spinal nerves are "mixed" (composed of efferent and afferent fibers) and that the cutaneous nerves penetrate muscle to reach the overlying skin. In the adult, afferent fibers may separate from a plexus or a peripheral nerve and form a "pure" cutaneous nerve.

Each of the body somites gives rise to a cutaneous unit, or *dermatome*, and a muscle unit, or *myotome*. In the early developmental stages a spinal cord segment innervates its respective muscle mass and dermatome by way of its own spinal nerve (see Figure 1–5). By definition a *dermatome* is the area of skin innervated by the fibers in a single posterior root. As will be shown later, however, each dorsal root centrally distributes information to more than one spinal cord segment by way of its ascending and descending collateral branches. Also, in the adult the formation is more complex, because each dermatome overlaps its adjacent ones (see Figure 4–8) and in the extremities is stretched out as shown in Figure 4–6A (compare with Figure 13–2, which shows a dermatome map in more detail). A simplified general plan of dermatomal landmarks in the hypothetical adult (Fig. 4–6B) serves as an adequate guide to

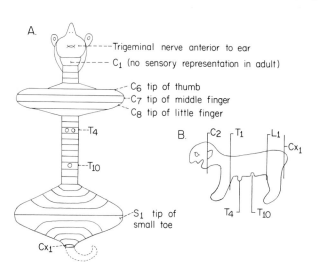

Figure 4–6. *A*, Primitive dermatomes before limb rotation, formation of outlets, and loss of tail. *B*, Definitive dermatomal landmarks in the hypothetical adult. (See also Figure 13–2 for a map of dermatomes in the adult.)

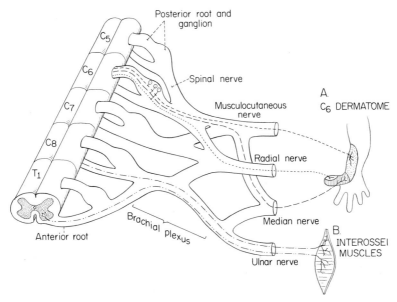

Figure 4–7. The manner in which root fibers are collected in a plexus to be distributed with peripheral nerves. At *A* is shown the C6 dermatome on the anterior aspect of the right forearm and thumb. It is innervated by its posterior root fibers, which reach it via three peripheral nerves, the musculocutaneous, radial, and median. In the example at *B,* the interossei muscles are innervated by a single nerve, the ulnar, which has fibers from cord segments C8 and T1.

some key points that can easily be remembered.

Motor innervation also becomes more complex as individual muscles develop and migrate from the primitive muscle mass, taking their nerve supply with them, but in the thoracic region the arrangement of muscles (*e.g.,* intercostal muscles) and their innervation remain close to the developmental pattern. In the appendages the segmental pattern of motor innervation is less apparent but is present regionally. For example, shoulder muscles are innervated by spinal cord segments C4 to C6, forearm muscles by segments C6 to C8, and hand muscles by segments C8 to T1.

In the extremities several peripheral nerves or their branches may innervate a single dermatome or muscle, and any one nerve may innervate more than one dermatome or muscle. This comes about by the intervention of a *plexus* between the spinal nerve trunk (fibers associated with a single spinal cord segment) and the peripheral nerve (fibers from several spinal cord segments). In other words, a plexus provides a reasonably economical means of sorting out posterior and anterior roots,

exchanging them, and directing them into the formation of the peripheral nerve itself. In the example shown in Figure 4–7, note that the C6 dermatome, on the anterior aspect of the forearm and thumb, is innervated by three peripheral nerves, the *musculocutaneous, radial,* and *median* nerves, but that all those afferent fibers enter the C6 spinal cord segment. Note that any one of those nerves, each of which has afferents in it associated with several cord segments, would be distributed to several dermatomes, and that adjacent dermatomes overlap (Fig. 4–8). In Figure 4–7, an

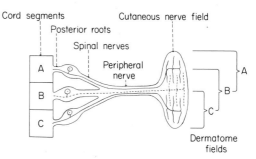

Figure 4–8. Sensory innervation of a cutaneous nerve field, showing dermatomal overlap.

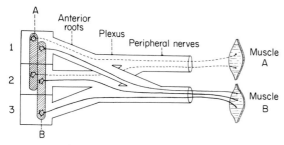

Figure 4–9. Motor innervation of skeletal muscle. Motoneuron pools (*A* and *B*) overlap (*1, 2, 3* spinal cord segments) and innervate muscles *A* and *B*.

example of the innervation of a muscle group, the *interossei*, is also illustrated. A single peripheral nerve, the *ulnar*, carries efferent fibers arising from both spinal cord segments C8 and T1. In general, muscles receive fibers from more than one spinal cord segment because the motor neuron cell bodies extend as nuclear masses in the anterior gray of the spinal cord over rostrocaudal distances that cross the segmental boundaries (Fig. 4–9). Although not shown in the figure, any one of the nerves indicated would also carry efferent fibers to more than one muscle.

It is important not to confuse *dermatome fields* with *cutaneous nerve fields* of innervation. The area map of the former is much different from that of the latter (see Figure 13–2) because peripheral nerves, particularly those in the extremities, carry fibers from several spinal cord segments that are distributed to several dermatome regions. The sensory impairment in a *peripheral nerve lesion* would then cross dermatomal lines. Further, note that since there is considerable overlap of a dermatomal field by adjacent ones, damage to a single posterior root would probably not result in a detectable loss of sensation. Such loss could come about through damage to several consecutive roots or spinal cord segments. However, *irritation* of a single posterior root, such as by the herpes zoster virus invading a single posterior root ganglion, can result in clinically observable signs and symptoms referred to a specific dermatome field. Thoracic roots are commonly involved. If, for example, the T4 ganglion is affected, then the initial burning pain and later vesicular eruption would have a segmental

distribution confined to the T4 dermatome in the area of the chest wall on a level with the nipple. In summary, this distinction between dermatomal field and cutaneous nerve field comes about because of the redistribution of fibers that takes place in the plexus between spinal nerves and the peripheral nerves, notably the brachial plexus, associated with the upper extremity, and the lumbosacral plexus, associated with the lower extremity.

A patient with a peripheral lesion and one with a tumor impinging on various roots would present quite different kinds of symptoms. A specific case will illustrate: A 45-year-old man was admitted to the hospital because of weakness in his hands. Over the previous few months he had noted some loss of muscle mass in each of his hands. He noted on direct questioning some numbness in the little finger of each hand as well as on the ulnar aspect of the ring finger on each hand. On examination the patient was found to have marked wasting of the first dorsal interosseous muscle and weakness of abduction of the fingers of both hands. He had good bulk of the muscles of the thenar eminence and could appose and abduct his thumbs without difficulty. There was loss of sensation to pinprick over the distribution noted above. In this patient, the differential diagnosis lay between involvement of the cervical roots (C8) and involvement of the ulnar nerves. Weakness and wasting of interosseous muscles might occur in either situation. The thenar muscles are supplied by the same roots, and would probably be involved in a root lesion, but, since they are innervated by the median nerve, would not be affected by damage to the ulnar nerve. Sensory signs on the ulnar half of the ring finger also indicate damage to the ulnar nerve as opposed to the C8 root. Laboratory investigations would include measurement of conduction velocity in the ulnar nerve and might demonstrate a conduction block across an area of nerve compression.

GROSS MORPHOLOGY OF THE SPINAL CORD

The spinal cord is continuous with the medulla of the brainstem and exits from

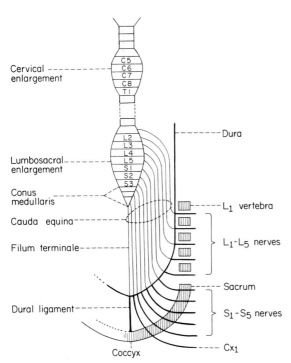

Cervical enlargement

C5
C6
C7
C8
T I

---- Dura

L2
L3
L4
L5
S I
S2
S3

Lumbosacral enlargement

Conus medullaris

Cauda equina

Filum terminale

Dural ligament

---- L₁ vertebra

L₁-L₅ nerves

---- Sacrum

S₁-S₅ nerves

---- Cx₁

Coccyx

Figure 4–10. Spinal cord enlargements and the cauda equina.

the cranium through the *foramen magnum.* The same meningeal sleeve that surrounds the brain also covers the spinal cord and firmly attaches to the coccyx caudally by a ligament composed of a condensation of dura (Fig. 4–10). A threadlike remnant of embryonic neural tube (*filum terminale*) passes through this ligament, fusing with it. The dura mater is fused laterally with the periosteum of the *intervertebral foramina,* the site at which the posterior and anterior roots join to form spinal nerves, and passes uninterrupted into the connective tissue (epineurium) surrounding the spinal nerves. The spinal cord itself is located in the meningeal sleeve of membranes and is, in turn, secured firmly to the dura laterally by means of *dentate ligaments,* which are condensations of pial membrane found at regular intervals along the entire length of the cord. This description should make it clear that the spinal cord does not whip around within the vertebral canal but is firmly secured to its dural covering and is well protected by the cerebrospinal fluid in the subarachnoid space. However, note that since the cord is firmly encased in a

bony cavity and is surrounded by sturdy dura mater, it is susceptible to damage (hemorrhage, neoplasm, and so forth), as it is a relatively soft structure and has no place in which it can give way.

The diameter of the spinal cord is not uniform throughout its length. Most apparent are two enlarged regions that occur in the lower cervical and in the lumbosacral cord (see Figures 4–3 and 4–10). These *spinal cord enlargements* are due to the additional neurons in both the posterior and anterior gray columns at these levels associated with the innervation of the upper and lower extremities. In other words, because of the extremities' requirement for greater sensory input and motor output, the lower cervical and lumbosacral levels of the spinal cord are larger than the upper cervical and thoracic segmental levels. Another gross anatomical factor that should be emphasized is that the spinal cord ends at approximately vertebral level L2. This happens because in the course of development the vertebral column grows to a greater extent than the spinal cord does, and the coccygeal segments of the neural tube atrophy. Therefore, the posterior and anterior roots from most of the lumbar and all the sacral cord segments extend farther caudally, as the *cauda equina,* than the spinal cord itself does (see Figures 4–3 and 4–10). This anatomical point is of clinical significance, for it enables one to withdraw cerebrospinal fluid from the subarachnoid space without damaging the spinal cord. The removal of CSF (spinal tap, lumbar puncture) is commonly done at the intervertebral level L4 to L5.

ENTRY ZONE OF THE POSTERIOR ROOTS

The posterior root fibers (*first-order neurons* or *primary afferent neurons*) enter the spinal cord as a series of slender bundles, or *rootlets.* All remain on the *ipsilateral* (same) side. At the entry zone, which is in the posterolateral sulcus of the spinal cord, the thinly myelinated and unmyelinated fibers are collected together and enter the spinal cord a little bit lateral to the larger, heavily myelinated fibers (Fig. 4–11). This anatomical distinction has its functional

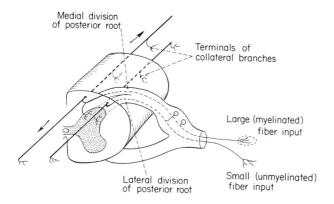

Figure 4–11. Medial and lateral divisions of the posterior root, containing large and small fiber afferents, respectively. Ascending and descending collateral branches of the primary afferents and their terminals are also indicated. Note that they all terminate on the *ipsilateral* side.

counterpart in a separation of sensory modalities, which is discussed fully in later chapters. At this time it is sufficient to point out that the smaller fibers are part of the afferent pain pathway, and it is here at the entry zone of the root that the pain pathway is for the first time taking a unique course. The larger myelinated fibers that are part of the touch and position sense pathways enter the spinal cord more medially. The fibers conveying information relevant to different qualities of the somatic sensory input, up to this anatomic locus, have been intermixed throughout the course of the afferent fibers in the peripheral nerves, plexuses, spinal nerves, and posterior roots.

When the smaller fibers enter the cord, they send out primary ascending and descending collateral branches extending only over one or two spinal cord segments in the *posterolateral fasciculus* capping the posterior gray matter. Many synapses onto neurons in the posterior gray matter are made along the way via secondary collateral branches. The larger fibers enter more medially and also have primary ascending and descending branches but, in contrast, extend over many segments. Indeed, some of them are very long and can be traced all the way into the caudal part of the medulla in the brainstem before terminating. To reach the medulla, these fibers travel in the *posterior white columns*, giving off their secondary collaterals mainly in the first few segments after entering the cord. Other fibers in this group ascend and descend only a short distance, give off many collaterals, and terminate in the posterior gray matter. These fibers in the posterior

white matter establish synaptic contact with interneurons or, in some instances, with motoneurons directly, thus providing the anatomical substrate for a variety of spinal cord reflexes.

Similarly, the collaterals from the smaller, unmyelinated fibers entering the posterior gray matter form reflex connections via interneurons. Such reflex connections are not confined to the segmental levels receiving direct input because some of the neurons in the gray matter give rise to fibers that make intersegmental connections. The overall effect of the ascending, descending, and intersegmental connections is such that afferent input at one level can, if appropriate, be transmitted to gray matter at many cord levels. An obvious functional example of this is the quick reflex movements of legs, arms, and trunk that one makes without really thinking about it when stepping hard on a very sharp object.

In addition to providing synaptic interconnections for spinal reflexes, the posterior gray columns contain nuclear groups that project their axons out into the *lateral white columns*, forming major tracts ascending to higher levels, such as the thalamus and cerebellum (*e.g.*, spinothalamic tracts and spinocerebellar tracts). These so-called *tract cells*, or *relay nuclei*, in the posterior gray and the ascending pathways will be described in more detail later (Chap. 13). The collateral branching and terminals of the two major inputs—the myelinated fibers in the medial division of the posterior root and the unmyelinated fibers in the lateral division of the posterior root—are summarized in Figure 4–11.

SOMATOTOPIC ARRANGEMENT OF FIBERS

The fibers ascending through the white columns of the spinal cord are *somatotopically (topographically)* organized. That is, the fibers are arranged such that portions of the body about which they convey information are represented in an orderly fashion. As fibers enter the spinal cord at successively higher levels, they come to lie in relation to the fibers that are already there rather than just to be mixed in with them at random (Fig. 4–12). In the *posterior white columns*, these fibers are still primary (first-order) afferent neurons whose cell bodies are in the dorsal root ganglia. They are somatotopically organized as follows: The fibers coming into the spinal cord sacral segments are located most medially; the more rostrally entering fibers are simply added on to those already present, so that, progressing laterally, the lumbar, thoracic, and, finally, the cervical inputs are represented. In other words, the lower extremity is represented medially and the upper extremity laterally.

In the *lateral white columns*, a somatotopic arrangement of ascending (and descending) fibers is also found, but for the *spinothalamic tract* the order is reversed as compared to that in the posterior columns. The reason for this is simple: The first-order afferent neuron ends in the posterior gray matter and a second-order (or third-order) neuron gives rise to the ascending fibers found in the lateral white columns. Starting then caudally, we find that neurons in the sacral segments cross the midline and

are joined on their medial surface by similar neurons coming from more rostral segments, the cervical representation coming in last, *i.e.*, most medially. It is as if the axons emerging from the posterior gray matter at successively higher segments are "pushing" out more laterally the spinothalamic fibers already present from lower levels. In the *spinocerebellar* tracts, the somatotopic arrangement has been "pushed" into a somewhat posterior-to-anterior arrangement, with the sacral input represented in fibers located most posteriorly. Finally, the descending *corticospinal* fibers have a medial-to-lateral pattern; the cervical fibers are conveniently positioned medially, and the lumbar fibers, which must descend farther before entering the gray matter, are positioned laterally.

In summary, fibers entering the cord and ascending directly to the medulla in the posterior columns, those leaving the posterior gray horns, *e.g.*, in the spinothalamic and spinocerebellar tracts, and those descending to the cord from higher centers, *e.g.*, in the corticospinal tracts, enter and leave their respective cord segments in a "logical" laminated fashion without becoming intermixed. An analogous situation obtains in the wiring of an amplifier or in the annual rings of a tree. Such somatotopic patterns and location of tracts within the white matter will be more apparent after each one is studied in more detail. Even at this point it should be clear that, because of the different arrangements and positions of fibers, the encroachment of lesions into different levels or portions of CNS structures would cause a patient to present different somatotopic distributions of motor and/or sensory defects.

THE INTERNAL BRAINSTEM

The cranial nerves attach to the brainstem, their afferent fibers for the most part entering more posteriorly than their efferent fibers, in much the same way that the spinal nerve root attaches to the spinal cord. Although in its development the brainstem is initially similar to the spinal cord, insofar as its alar and basal plate neurons receive afferents and send out

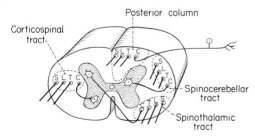

Figure 4–12. Topographic arrangement of fibers in major ascending and descending tracts. Segmental levels of input: *C*, cervical; *T*, thoracic; *L*, lumbar; and *S*, sacral.

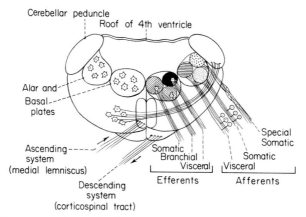

Figure 4–13. Schematic cross section of the brainstem, showing approximate location of motor nuclei and sensory receiving nuclei of cranial nerves and their respective efferent and afferent fibers. On the left side the primitive alar and basal plates have not yet divided into subgroups of nuclei as they have on the right. Contralateral input to the cerebellum is also indicated, as well as fibers ascending in the medial lemniscus and corticospinal fibers descending in the pyramids. The cranial nerves can be grouped according to the functional categories of their efferent and afferent fibers and associated brainstem nuclei (see also Figures 4–14 and 4–15 and Appendix II):

Somatic Efferent
Oculomotor (III) ⎫
Trochlear (IV) ⎬ extrinsic muscles of the eye
Abducens (VI) ⎭
Hypoglossal (XII) — tongue muscles
Branchial Efferent
Mandibular division of trigeminal (V₃) — muscles of mastication
Facial (VII) — muscles of facial expression
Glossopharyngeal (IX) ⎫ muscles of pharynx and
Vagus (X) ⎬ larynx
Visceral Efferent (parasympathetic)
Oculomotor (III) — intrinsic muscles of eye
Facial (VII) ⎫
Glossopharyngeal (IX) ⎬ salivation

Vagus (X) — secretion, smooth muscle contraction, and cardiac deceleration
Visceral Afferent
Facial (VII) ⎫ general visceral afferents
Glossopharyngeal (IX) ⎬ and taste afferents; the
Vagus (X) ⎭ olfactory nerve (I) is sometimes included in this category also

Somatic Afferent
Trigeminal (V) — somatic sensation from the head (VII, IX, and X also have a few components innervating the ear)
Special Somatic Afferent
Optic (II) — vision
Vestibulocochlear (VIII) — equilibrium and audition

efferents, respectively (see Figures 1–7 and 1–8), other changes make its definitive appearance (see Appendix II) quite different. For example, in the caudal pons and rostral medulla the roof plate expands to form, along with blood vessels, a choroid plexus; the cerebellum arises with its attendant nuclear masses and fiber systems; and other nuclear groups and fiber systems appear in relation to development of special senses, reflex centers, and forebrain structures. As a result (Fig. 4–13), well-outlined nuclear groups receiving the primary afferents of the cranial nerves are dispersed somewhat, though they remain basically in the posterolateral part of the tegmental field. Similarly, the motoneuron groups are less continuous intersegmentally than are those seen in the spinal cord; clearly marked nuclei are formed at differ-

ent levels in the medulla, pons, and midbrain. These motoneuron nuclei remain for the most part in a position anteromedial to the above-mentioned nuclei receiving the primary afferent fibers. Collectively, the cranial nerve nuclei are shown schematically in the posterior and lateral views illustrated in Figures 4–14 and 4–15 and in the cross sections in Appendix II. This overview will be referred to again later in more detail when specific ascending pathways, sensations, and movements are discussed.

CRANIAL NERVES

Although there are differences among the individual *cranial* nerves, these twelve pairs of nerves are basically composed of

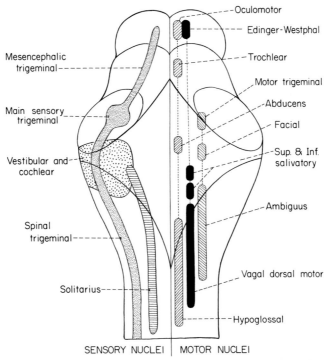

Figure 4–14. Cranial nerve nuclei in surface projection on a schematic posterior view of the brainstem. The cerebellum has been removed by a cut through the cerebellar peduncles, so that the floor of the fourth ventricle is revealed. Caudally, the medulla is severed at about the transition to the spinal cord. Rostrally, the superior and inferior colliculi of the midbrain are indicated. The cranial nerve sensory nuclei are shown on the left side and the motor nuclei on the right. These motor and sensory nuclei are grouped according to the functional categories indicated in Figure 4–13.

Somatic Efferent
    Oculomotor nucleus (III)
    Trochlear nucleus (IV)
    Abducens nucleus (VI)
    Hypoglossal nucleus (XII)
Branchial Efferent
    Trigeminal motor nucleus (V)
    Facial motor nucleus (VII)
    Nucleus ambiguus (IX, X)
Visceral Efferent
    Edinger-Westphal nucleus (III)

    Superior salivatory nucleus (VII)
    Inferior salivatory nucleus (IX)
    Dorsal motor nucleus of vagus (X)
Visceral Afferent
    Nucleus solitarius (VII, IX, and X)
Somatic Afferent
    Spinal, main, and mesencephalic nuclei of the trigeminal (V)
Special Somatic Afferents
    Vestibular and cochlear nuclei (VIII)
    Note: None of the visual (II) system is shown.

fibers of the same types as are found in *spinal* nerves. The major difference is that some are entirely motor or sensory in function, resembling spinal anterior and posterior roots, respectively, rather than spinal nerves where afferents and efferents are intermixed. Note also that the second cranial (optic) "nerve" is actually a *tract* that has been drawn out from the CNS during development. The cranial nerves will be taken up in more detail later in the

context of different sensations and movements. Following is a general statement of their attachment sites and a few of their major functions (see Figure 4–16).

Olfactory Bulb and Tract (I). The olfactory bulb lies on the olfactory sulcus between orbital gyri of the frontal lobe, and its tract extends posteriorly in this sulcus. The primary olfactory (first cranial) nerves are usually torn away during removal of the brain because they are small

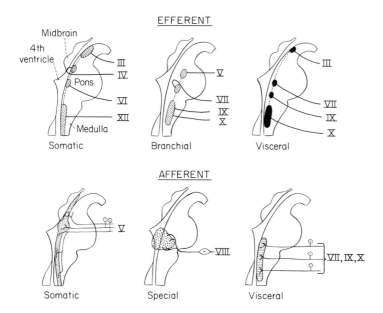

Figure 4–15. Cranial nerve nuclei in surface projection on a side view of the brainstem. The nuclei are categorized as in Figures 4–13 and 4–14. (See also listing beneath Figure 4–14.)

bundles entering the olfactory bulb from the olfactory epithelium in the nose by passing through the cribriform plate.

Optic "Nerve" (II). Both optic nerves are partly united in the *optic chiasm*, which straddles the diencephalon immediately in front of the stalk (infundibulum) of the *pituitary gland*. The fibers constituting the optic pathway observed grossly are continuations of the axons of ganglion cells lo-

cated in the retina. Posterior to the optic chiasm, they are arbitrarily referred to as *optic tracts* and anterior to it as *optic nerves*.

Oculomotor Nerve (III). The third cranial nerve emerges at the medial side of the cerebral peduncle in the *interpeduncular fossa* and then lies between the posterior cerebral and superior cerebellar arteries. The third nerves supply most of the extrinsic, striated muscles (responsible for

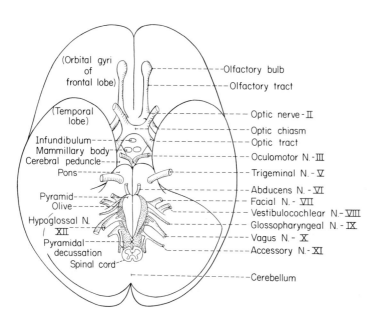

Figure 4–16. Cranial nerves as seen in a ventral view of the brain. (The hypoglossal nerve is shown only once.)

eye movement) and all of the intrinsic, smooth muscles (controlling accommodation and pupillary size) of the eyes.

Trochlear Nerve (IV). This is the only nerve to emerge on the dorsal aspect of the brainstem and to cross completely as it exits. It appears in the groove between the inferior colliculi, then curves around the sides of the midbrain. It functions in eye movements (pulling the eye downward when it is turned inward and rotating it medially when it is turned outward) along with the third and sixth nerves.

Trigeminal Nerve (V). The fifth cranial nerve is attached to the side of the brainstem at the junction of the pons and the middle cerebellar peduncle, through the middle of which it passes. It has a small motor root on its medial aspect. It supplies sensory fibers to the face and motor fibers to the muscles of mastication.

Abducens Nerve (VI). The sixth cranial nerve emerges anteriorly at the caudal border of the pons near the midline. It functions in eye movements (abducts the eye) along with the third and fourth nerves.

Facial Nerve (VII) and Vestibulocochlear Nerve (VIII). Both the seventh and eighth cranial nerves are attached at the same level as the abducens nerve but farther laterally, between the lower border of the pons and the lateral margin of the medulla. The seventh nerve supplies the muscles of facial expression. The eighth cranial nerve functions in audition and equilibrium.

Glossopharyngeal Nerve (IX), Vagus Nerve (X), and Accessory Nerve (XI). The ninth, tenth, and eleventh cranial nerves are attached by a series of rootlets arranged in a craniocaudal line just posterolateral to the inferior olive. The glossopharyngeal and vagus nerves are closely related. They supply the muscles of the pharynx and larynx, respectively, and convey visceral afferent information from the same general regions. The vagus nerve is also a major parasympathetic nerve, supplying the heart, lungs, and gastrointestinal tract in the thoracic and abdominal cavities. The accessory nerve has only a temporary gross attachment to the vagus and is essentially a cervical spinal nerve that ascends from the spinal cord through the foramen magnum and joins the tenth nerve. It supplies the sternocleidomastoid and trapezius muscles in the neck region.

Hypoglossal Nerve (XII). The twelfth cranial nerve emerges by a series of rootlets in the groove between the pyramid and the inferior olive. It supplies the muscles of the tongue.

The origins of cranial nerves can be seen in the atlas of cross sections (Appendix II).

EXAMPLES OF CRANIAL NERVE DAMAGE

Some examples of cranial nerve damage are described here as illustrations rather than complete surveys. Not all nerves are included, and some will be dealt with in more detail later.

Oculomotor, Trochlear, and Abducens Nerves. Since these all innervate the extrinsic eye muscles, they will be considered together. Damage to the nerves may occur within the brainstem (intramedullary) and/or after the nerves have exited from the brainstem (extramedullary). Location within the brainstem is suggested by the presence of additional signs caused by interruption of ascending or descending pathways. Because of the relatively long course taken by the nerves within the cranium before they enter the orbit, it is more common for cranial nerve palsies to be due to lesions extrinsic to the brainstem. An important example is a paralysis of the third nerve by compression or stretching against the *tentorium cerebelli* by an expanding supratentorial lesion (*i.e.*, in either the anterior or middle cranial fossa), such as a brain tumor. The cardinal sign of dysfunction of any of the nerves supplying the extraocular muscles is deviation of the eye, causing double vision (diplopia). It should also be mentioned that damage to the parasympathetic fibers associated with the third nerve (oculomotor) results in increased pupillary size and loss of pupillary reflex to light.

Trigeminal Nerve. Headache and facial pain are extremely common and usually result from irritation of the trigeminal nerves. A specific type of facial pain is *trigeminal neuralgia (tic douloureux)*, a major affliction related to the fifth nerve. This consists of paroxysms of pain localized to one of the divisions (usually the first or second) of the trigeminal nerve. The pain usually starts at certain trigger zones (commonly near the eye, nose, and alveolar margins) at the slightest stimulus and lasts only a few seconds, as a rule, but is severe ("excruciating," "stabbing," "cutting," "grinding," or "tearing"). The cause of this disease is not clear but has recently been suggested to be compression of the nerve by an adjacent tortuous artery. It can be dealt with medically or, if necessary, neurosurgically.

Facial Nerve. Unilateral facial weakness is the most obvious concomitant of seventh nerve damage. "Bell's palsy" is a common affliction in which individuals of any age rapidly develop weakness of one side of the face because of dysfunction of the facial nerve. The cause may be viral or allergic. When the paralysis is severe, the patient cannot contract facial muscles to exhibit facial expression on the afflicted side, and even at rest the face is asymmetrical. Since complete eye closure is impossible, a serious related problem may be corneal drying, leading to ulceration. Bell's palsy usually improves spontaneously.

In the central nervous system, damage to corticobulbar fibers descending to the facial nucleus will also cause paralysis of the facial muscles, but more so in the lower part of the face because the muscles in the upper part (responsible for eye closure and wrinkling of the forehead) are controlled by a part of the facial nucleus in the pons that receives fibers from both cerebral cortices. Hemiparesis due to the descending corticospinal motor fibers anywhere above the midpons (Chap. 19) is commonly accompanied by such partial facial paralysis because of involvement of corticobulbar fibers.

Hypoglossal Nerve. Damage to the twelfth nerve results in atrophy and loss of function of the tongue muscles on the same side. When the tongue is protruded, it will deviate to the same side as the damaged nerve, because normally the tongue muscles on one side act in a manner that "pushes" the tongue to the opposite side.

ADDITIONAL READING

Warwick, R., and Williams, P. L. *Gray's anatomy.* Philadelphia, W. B. Saunders Co., 1973, Chap. 7.

CHAPTER 5

RESTING AND ACTION POTENTIALS OF NEURONS

HARRY D. PATTON

THE NERVE IMPULSE

The function of neurons is to transmit messages. These messages, known as *nerve impulses*, are transient changes in the physicochemical state of the cell membrane. One can initiate nerve impulses artificially by passing an electrical current through the cell membrane, or, in an afferent fiber, naturally by subjecting its peripheral terminal (or *receptor*) to the appropriate natural stimulus, *e.g.*, mechanical distortion, a change in temperature, or light. The ability of a cell to undergo such transient physicochemical changes in response to a stimulus is called *excitability*. Muscle and gland cells, as well as neurons, are excitable cells.

An impulse, once initiated in an elongated excitable cell, propagates automatically, without further dependence on the initiating stimulus, over the entire cell membrane. At any one site on the cell the change persists for only a millisecond ($^1/_{1000}$ sec) or less but rapidly spreads, wavelike, from point to point along the membrane. The property of self-propagation of a locally initiated impulse is called *conductivity*. Excitability and conductivity are properties unique to nerve, muscle, and gland cells.

Accompanying the transient alterations underlying the impulse is a readily detectable electrical change, called the *action potential*. The action potential is best operationally defined by describing how it is measured. This is illustrated in Figure 5–1. The horizontal cylinder diagrammatically

49

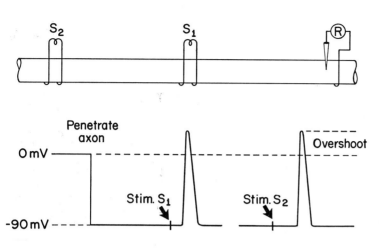

Figure 5–1. Intracellular recording of resting and action potentials of an axon. *R* is a voltage recorder connected to a micropipette, which is shown penetrating the membrane and establishing electrical contact with the interior of the axon. S_1 and S_2 are stimulating electrodes connected to current-generating devices. The graph below shows the voltage recorded at *R*; the sign indicates the polarity of the micropipette relative to the external medium. At the beginning the pipette tip is in the external medium and no voltage is recorded. When the axon is impaled, action potentials produced by threshold stimulations through S_1 and S_2 are registered. (From Ruch and Patton, eds., *Physiology and biophysics,* Philadelphia, W. B. Saunders Co., 1965.)

represents an axon; its borders represent the axon membrane, shown for simplicity without the myelin sheath.

The axoplasm, the nerve's intracellular substance, is electrically conductive because salts are among its constituents. The extracellular fluid is also a good electrical conductor. The membrane is not a perfect insulator, but it has a much higher resistance than does either the intracellular or extracellular medium. On the right, the wedge-shaped structure represents a glass capillary tube tapered to a tip diameter of about 0.5 μm. The capillary is filled with a conducting solution, usually saturated aqueous KCl solution. The fluid in the large end of the capillary is connected by a silver wire to one pole of a voltage-recording instrument (*R*), usually a cathode-ray oscilloscope. The extracellular fluid is connected with the other input. Since this fluid is everywhere isopotential, the recording instrument shows no deflection when the capillary is lowered into it (see left portion of voltage graph in the lower portion of Figure 5–1). Because the capillary tip is minuscule, it can be inserted through the axon membrane without causing serious damage; around the tip the membrane appears to seal and thus to prevent significant ionic interchange between the axoplasm and the extracellular fluid.

When an axon is thus impaled so that the fluid in the pipette makes electrical contact with the axoplasm, the recording

instrument immediately registers a voltage, usually of 50 to 90 mV, the value varying in different excitable tissues (see lower graph in Figure 5–1). Irrespective of the absolute value of the recorded potential, the polarity is always the same: the intracellular pipette is *negative* to the electrode connected to the extracellular fluid. This means that the resting axon membrane has a voltage across it, the inside being negative to the outside. This voltage is called the *resting potential,* in contradistinction to the *action potential,* to be described presently. The resting potential of an axon, or muscle fiber, is stable and invariant; in the absence of any stimulus to the cell, it remains unchanged for hours. Unlike the action potential, the resting potential is not unique to excitable cells. All cells have a resting potential; and, although its absolute value varies greatly among cells (the red blood cell, for example, has a resting potential of only 10 mV), its polarity is always "inside negative."

An action potential is elicited when a stimulus is applied to the axon membrane. In Figure 5–1 the stimulus is a brief (perhaps 0.5-msec) electrical shock applied to the axon through two electrodes (S_1) in contact with its external surface; the curlicue connecting the two electrodes is symbolic of a current-delivering device, such as a battery. Most of the current generated by the device passes through the extra-

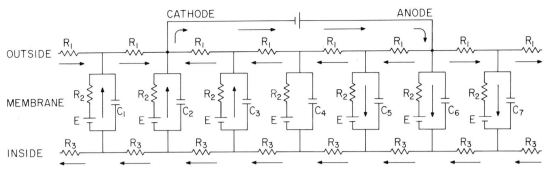

Figure 5–2. Electrical analog of cell membrane. At R_2 are resistors representing the frictional resistance to ionic movement through pores in the membrane. C_1 to C_7 are capacitors representing the nonporous parts of the membrane. At E are batteries with negative poles directed inward, representing the resting membrane potential. R_1 and R_3 are resistors representing the resistances of extracellular and intracellular fluids; R_3 resistors are of higher value than those at R_1. The battery at the top represents an external stimulator connected to the outside of the membrane. Arrows show direction of current flow through extracellular fluid, membrane elements, and intracellular fluid. Transmembrane inward current at anode A increases voltage across condensers C_5, C_6, and C_7. Outward current at cathode C lowers voltage across C_1, C_2, and C_3. Maximal voltage changes occur at C_6 and C_2. (From Fulton, ed., *Textbook of physiology*, Philadelphia, W. B. Saunders Co., 1955.)

cellular medium between the electrodes because of its low resistance; but when the pulse is sufficiently intense, some of the current passes through the membrane at the anode (remember that by convention current passes from anode to cathode), horizontally through the axoplasm, and outward through the membrane at the cathode (see Figure 5–2).

The effect of outward current flow is to diminish the resting membrane potential at that site; *i.e.*, the axoplasm, normally about 90 mV negative to the exterior, moves to a value less negative—to 70 or 80 mV. Such a reduction of membrane resting potential is called *depolarization*. Conversely, the effect of inward current flow at the anode is to increase the transmembrane potential, and the increase is called *hyperpolarization*. Both of these passive changes of membrane potential caused by transmembrane current flow are local—they are maximal at the sites of the stimulating electrodes and diminish exponentially with distance. For this reason they are not detected by the recording micropipette piercing the axon several centimeters from the stimulus site.

To understand why outward currents depolarize and inward currents hyperpolarize the membrane, recall that at rest the axoplasm is some 90 mV negative to the exterior. Thus the membrane has the equivalent of a small battery across it with the negative pole located inside.

Current generated by this battery flows from positive to negative—from outside to inside—across the membrane. Current generated by the electrical stimulus flows also from outside to inside at the anode; it reinforces the "membrane battery" and increases the voltage. At the cathode the stimulus current passes from inside to outside, *i.e.*, it opposes the "membrane battery" and lowers the voltage. A satisfactory electrical analog model of a small patch of membrane consists of a resistance and a capacitor in parallel with a battery (the resting potential) in series with the two. A larger patch of membrane is represented by a number of such elements connected by resistors representing the resistances of the intracellular and extracellular fluids, as in Figure 5–2. Such a circuit behaves in response to current flow just as the axon membrane behaves. The voltage decreases at sites where current flow reinforces the battery. Also, the influence of current flow on voltage is local and diminishes exponentially with distance from the source of current flow. Because the response of nerve membranes to transmembrane current flow is similar to that first studied in underwater cables, it is referred to as the *cable-property of membranes*. A more detailed description of cable properties is found in Ruch, T. C., and Patton, H. D., eds., *Physiology and biophysics*, Philadelphia, W. B. Saunders Co., 1965.

When the stimulus pulse is sufficiently strong, the recorder (R), after a few milliseconds, registers a rapid transient change in voltage, shown in the bottom record of Figure 5–1. The transmembrane potential moves rapidly toward zero (*i.e.*, the membrane depolarizes). Not only is the resting potential completely dissipated, but the change of voltage "overshoots" zero by some 20 to 30 mV, so that for a brief instant the inside of the membrane reverses polarity, becoming positive, rather than negative, to the extracellular fluid. The membrane then promptly repolarizes, and the resting potential resumes its initial stable value, inside negative, and remains so until the next stimulus is applied. This transient voltage change, amounting to 110 to 120 mV and occupying 0.5 to 1.0 msec, is the *action potential*. The capacity to respond thus to an applied transmembrane current is unique to excitable tissues. Other cells, such as the red blood cells and neuroglial cells, respond only passively to transmembrane currents; the magnitude of voltage change never exceeds the applied voltage.

Further experiments, not indicated in the diagram, indicate that the action potential is initiated at the cathode, where outward current flow depolarizes the membrane, and that it ensues only when the magnitude of depolarization reaches a definite *threshold* value, which varies from 10 to 40 mV in different excitable tissues. The threshold of a mammalian axon is about 10 mV depolarization; an action potential is triggered by any event that causes the transmembrane potential to move from its resting value of 90 mV inside negative to 80 mV inside negative. Moreover, depolarizations of more than the threshold (10 mV) trigger an action potential identical in magnitude and time course to that produced by threshold depolarization.

Thus the action potential is an "all-or-nothing" event. Threshold and all-or-nothing behavior are unique properties of excitable cell membranes and are lacking in those of glial cells, red blood cells, and squamous epithelial cells. Such behavior suggests that the resting nerve fiber stores the energy for the action potential and requires only the triggering influence of a threshold depolarization to release it. The axon may be likened to a gunpowder fuse: It requires a threshold elevation of temperature to release the energy of the pre-stored gunpowder; the threshold may be attained by the application of either a paper match or an acetylene torch, but the response of the fuse is the same. The axon differs from a fuse, however, in that it rapidly restores its energy by repolarization and is only then ready for the next triggering. A mammalian axon fully restores its charge in only about 1 msec (*refractory period*) and can thus generate trains of action potentials up to frequencies of 1000 per second.

Another important property of the axon is illustrated in Figure 5–1. A stimulus applied at S_2, located farther from R than is S_1, elicits an action potential identical to that generated by stimulation at S_1 except that the latency, i.e., the time between the application of the stimulus and the beginning of the action potential, is longer. The difference in latency suggests that an action potential, once initiated by depolarization, propagates itself at uniform speed from the site of initiation along the membrane, again like the action in a gunpowder fuse. Systematic investigation reveals that this is so; the latency is a direct function of conduction distance.

The speed of impulse conduction (i.e., latency : conduction distance) varies directly with the size of the fiber; it is faster for large axons than for small axons. Among myelinated mammalian axons speeds vary from about 6 m/sec for small axons (1 μm in diameter) up to 120 m/sec for the largest axons (20 μm in diameter). Because speed is directly related to diameter, one value can be readily calculated from the other. For myelinated mammalian axons the relation is $S = 6D$, where S is the speed in meters per second and D is the fiber diameter in micrometers (including the myelin sheath). Unmyelinated fibers less than 1 μm in diameter conduct much more slowly, down to 0.5 m/sec or less. Three distinct, although interrelated, questions are implied in the experiments illustrated in Figure 5–1: (1) How is the "inside negative" resting transmembrane potential generated? (2) How does threshold depolarization generate the "all-or-nothing" action potential in excitable cells? (3) How does the action potential propagate itself? These three questions will now be dealt with in order.

ORIGIN OF THE RESTING POTENTIAL

Solute Composition of Extracellular and Intracellular Fluids

Animal tissues have no significant supply of free electrons; bioelectrical charges are carried by ions of dissolved electrolytes. It is therefore reasonable to infer that the "inside negative" resting potential found across all membranes results from an unequal distribution of ions in the intracellular and extracellular compartments. The first step then is to examine the solute compositions of the intracellular and extracellular fluids. Although the small, 90-mV resting transmembrane potential could be (and, in fact, is) produced by ionic imbalances far too small to be directly detected by chemical analysis, nevertheless an examination of the compositions of the two fluids is rewarding, for it provides clues toward the establishment of a testable hypothesis concerning the origin of the resting potential.

The major inorganic cations of body fluids are Na^+ and K^+, and the major inorganic anions are Cl^- and HCO_3^-. Listed in the first two vertical columns of Table 5–1 are the concentrations of these ions (in millimoles per liter) in the extracellular and intracellular fluids of mammalian muscle; consideration of the other two columns may be postponed.

TABLE 5–1. Compositions of Extracellular and Intracellular Fluids of Mammalian Muscle

	Extra-cellular (mmol/l)	Intra-cellular (mmol/l)	Ion_o / Ion_i	Equilibrium Potential (mV)
Cations				
Na^+	145	12	12.1	66
K^+	4	155	1/39	−97
Others	5	−	−	−
Anions				
Cl^-	120	4	30	−90
HCO_3^-	27	8	3.4	−32
Others	7	155*	−	−
Potential	0 mV	−90 mV	−	−

*Value for organic anions (see text).

An examination of the first two columns reveals at once that, despite its exquisite thinness, the muscle cell membrane is nevertheless an effective selective barrier to ionic movement and that it sustains on its two sides solutions of markedly different ionic compositions. The extracellular fluid contains mainly Na^+, Cl^-, and HCO_3^-, with only a trace of K^+. On the other hand, the intracellular compartment contains mainly K^+ and little Na^+. Also, the intracellular fluid contains very little inorganic anion (Cl^- and HCO_3^-); apparent electrical balance is achieved by a considerable concentration of organic anions (mainly glutamate and aspartate), asterisked in the table. Note that in both the extracellular and intracellular compartments anions and cations balance. The balance reflects the inadequacy of chemical determination to reveal directly the source of the resting potential, for since the intracellular fluid is 90 mV negative to the extracellular fluid, either it must contain a small excess of anions, or the extracellular fluid must contain a slight excess of cations, or both. However, the data permit the elaboration of an hypothesis concerning the origin of the resting potential. To develop this hypothesis requires a brief review of the behavior of ions in solution. The discussion that follows is for simplicity largely qualitative and designed to provide an intuitive, rather than a quantitatively exact, description. Students desiring a more rigorous treatment should consult the references listed at the end of this chapter.

Concentration Gradients

The fact that ions of the same species are unevenly distributed across the cell membrane is noteworthy. This uneven distribution is emphasized in the third column of Table 5–1, which lists for each species (except the intracellular organic anions) the ratio of concentration outside the membrane (extracellular) to that inside the membrane (intracellular). Figure 5–3 illustrates a simple case in which a membrane, freely permeable to water and to a solute, S, separates two compartments, x and y. A convenient, and perhaps cor-

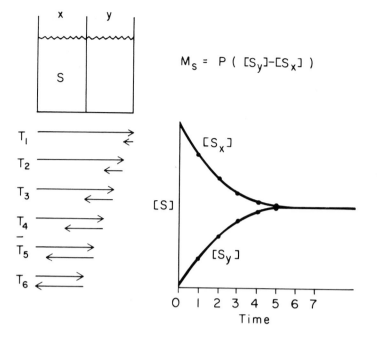

$$M_S = P ([S_y]-[S_x])$$

Figure 5–3. Diffusion and the influence of concentration gradient on the distribution of a solute across a permeable membrane. See explanation in text.

rect, way to visualize the membrane is as a sheet containing numerous microscopic perforations, or pores, large enough to admit H_2O and S molecules. S is dissolved in compartment x and at repeated equal, but infinitely small, intervals its concentration is measured in both x and y compartments.

The arrows below the compartmentalized container illustrate diagrammatically the movement, or flux, of S in the two directions across the membrane at successive intervals. (The movement of solvent H_2O molecules might also be diagrammed, but for the present discussion this would not alter the conclusions and, for simplicity, is ignored.) During the first interval between the dissolving of S in compartment x and T_1, S moves mainly from left to right (x to y); only a small countermovement from y to x occurs (see T_1). This is because the flux in either direction is determined by the probability of S molecules, in their random movement, striking a pore in the membrane; since all the S molecules are in x at the outset, the main movement is from x to y. Nevertheless, after some S molecules have penetrated to y, a small but finite probability exists that some will encounter a pore on the y side and return to x. The net movement in the interval T_1 is

represented by the difference in the lengths of the two arrows.

Plotted in the graph in the lower-right part of the figure are the concentrations of S, indicated as $[S]$*, in x and y at successive intervals. At T_1 $[S_x]$ has decreased and $[S_y]$ has increased by an equal amount. During the next interval (see T_2) the movement from x to y is less than that during the first interval because the reduced concentration in y diminishes the probability of S particles striking a pore on the x side. But the traffic from y to x has increased relative to T_1 because $[S_y]$ has increased. The net exchange is still from x to y, but the change is less than during T_1; at T_2 the slopes of the concentration curves (in the two compartments) are less than at T_1 (see graph). At each subsequent interval, the net movement becomes smaller as the concentrations in the two compartments approach equality, which occurs at T_6; then the movement of S is forever the same in both directions, the net flux is zero, and the concentrations are invariant. The system is said to be in a *steady state*, and the process that leads to it

_____

*Throughout this text square brackets are used to represent concentration of the substance named.

is called *diffusion*. The underlying determinant of diffusion is a difference in concentration—a *concentration gradient*. This is expressed quantitatively by the statement $M_S = P ([S_y] - [S_x])$, where M_S = the net flux in millimoles per square centimeter per second, $[S_y] - [S_x]$ = the concentration gradient,* and P = the permeability, a constant characteristic of the membrane and its thickness.

To prevent the establishment of a steady state in a system with a fully permeable membrane requires the expenditure of energy. Hence, a concentration gradient may be viewed as the equivalent of a force moving solute particles from regions of high concentration into regions of lower concentration until equal concentrations are attained. Obviously in cells some other force must be active, for Table 5–1 clearly indicates that the concentrations of solutes are not equal on the two sides of the cell membrane.

Voltage Gradient

In Figure 5–4 is diagrammed a system that differs from that in Figure 5–3 in two respects: (1) The solute in x is an electrolyte ionizing into cations (C^+) and anions (A^-), and (2) the membrane is permeable to H_2O and to C^+ but is impermeable to A^-. Such a *semipermeable membrane* may be

---

*Actually it is a negative concentration gradient, for the gradient has a direction from low concentration to high (uphill), whereas the flux is from high concentration to low (downhill).

visualized as a sheet containing microscopic perforations that permit the passage of H_2O and C^+ but prevent the penetration of A^-, possibly because of their shape or size. As in the simple diffusion model, C^+ particles tend to move from x to y along their concentration gradient and some, by random movement, follow this path. However, A^- particles are constrained to x by the anion-impermeable membrane. Consequently, each time a C^+ moves into y an unbalanced A^- is left in y. The excess of A^- in x creates a voltage across the membrane, negative on the x side, that tends to attract C^+ back into x.

The arrows below symbolize the movements of C^+ particles at successive intervals. At T_1 many have moved into y along the concentration gradient, but more have returned to y than in the diffusion model of Figure 5–3 because many are attracted back to x by the voltage gradient. The net flux of C^+ is thus less than in the diffusion model, and the change in concentration smaller (see graph). The voltage (V) at T_1 is created by the widowed and unrequited anions (A^-) in x. The remaining arrows indicate that this exchange continues until T_3, resulting in decreasing net fluxes as the voltage attracting C^+ back into x increases and as the concentration gradient moving C^+ into y decreases. At T_3 the movements in the two directions become equal because the concentration gradient force tending to move more C^+ into y is exactly balanced by that of the opposing voltage gradient attracting C^+ into x. After T_3 the concentrations in x and y are stable because the net flux is zero. The

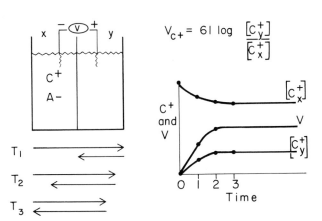

Figure 5–4. Influence of voltage gradient on distribution of charged ions across a semipermeable membrane that permits penetration of solvent and cations (C^+) but prevents transfer of anions (A^-). Compartment x might be likened to the intracellular fluid containing K^+, which can permeate the cell membrane, and organic anions, which are too large to traverse membrane pores.

voltage is also stable because no further separation of charges occurs since the flux is zero. Such a system is said to be in *electrochemical equilibrium,* a special kind of steady state. Note that in contradistinction to the steady state in the diffusion model, the concentrations are not equal; the tendency to equalize is exactly balanced by the voltage gradient.

Such a system in equilibrium is described quantitatively by the *Nernst equation:*

$$V_{C+} = \frac{K}{Z} \log_{10} \frac{[C^+_y]}{[C^+_x]}$$

where V_{C+} = the voltage at equilibrium, or the *equilibrium potential,* of C^+; Z = the valence of C^+; $[C^+_y]$ and $[C^+_x]$ are concentrations of C^+ in y and x at equilibrium; and K is a constant, with a value of 61 at mammalian body temperature.* The equation simply states that the equilibrium potential of an ion is directly proportional to the logarithm of the ratio of the ion concentrations on the two sides of the membrane. Knowing the concentrations, one can calculate the equilibrium potential. This has been done in the fourth column of Table 5–1 for each of the inorganic ions; the calculated values indicate the membrane potential expected if each ion were in simple electrochemical equilibrium.

K+ and the Resting Potential

The calculated equilibrium potentials permit us to make some educated guesses concerning the origin of the resting potential. Ignoring, for the moment, the glaring difference between the measured resting potential and the equilibrium potential for Na+, we infer from the identity of the predicted and actual values for Cl− that Cl− is passively distributed in accordance with the Nernst equation and that we need assume no other forces than concentration gradient and voltage gradient to

explain its distribution. The equilibrium potential for K+ is also close to the resting potential, being only 7 mV greater. Indeed, so close are the two potentials that, early in this century, before methods of measuring membrane potentials with resolution and accuracy were available, Bernstein postulated that the resting potential is the equilibrium potential for K+ and that the intracellular organic anions constitute the particles to which the membrane is impermeable. According to Bernstein's hypothesis V_m (resting membrane potential) $= V_{K+} = 61 \log \frac{[K^+_o]}{[K^+_i]}$, where $[K^+_o]$ and $[K^+_i]$ are the concentrations of K+ outside the membrane (extracellular) and inside the membrane (intracellular).

Another reason for suspecting K+ is that the resting potential is quite sensitive to variations in extracellular concentration of K+ (Fig. 5–5). If an axon or muscle cell is bathed in solutions of consecutively increasing concentrations of K+, the membrane potential progressively decreases. This behavior is predicted by the Nernst equation, for as $[K^+_o]$ is increased, $[K^+_o]/[K^+_i]$ approaches 1 and the log of the ratio approaches 0; therefore V_{K+} approaches 0. Moreover, through a considerable range of concentrations the resting potential varies linearly with log $[K^+_o]$, just as the Nernst equation predicts. However, at low values of $[K^+_o]$, near the normal extracellular K+ concentration, the relation departs from linearity and each increment in $[K^+_o]$ produces less decrease in resting potential than would be predicted by the Nernst equation. This behavior, coupled with the disquieting 7-mV discrepancy between the measured and predicted membrane potentials in normal extracellular fluid, suggests that Bernstein's hypothesis approximates, but does not completely tally with, fact.

Distribution of Na+

An even more shattering blow to the hope that ion distributions in the extracellular and intracellular fluids can be explained wholly in terms of electrochemical

---

*The Nernst equation can also be applied to anions, but then K is negative since Z is negative; if one wants to keep K positive, one must reverse the ratio to read log $[A^-_x]/[A^-_y]$.

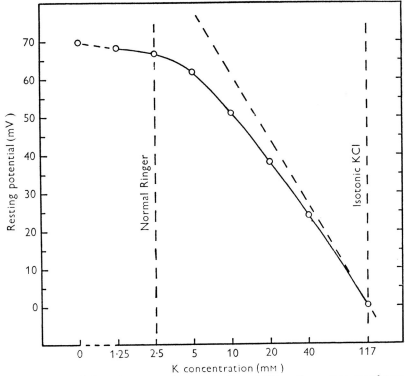

Figure 5–5. The influence of changing external concentration of K$^+$ on the resting membrane potential of a frog nerve fiber. The ordinate is the resting potential (in absolute units without designation of polarity). The abscissa is external concentration of K$^+$; the scale is logarithmic. (From Eccles, *The neurophysiological basis of mind*, Oxford, Clarendon Press, 1953.)

equilibrium is the alarmingly anomalous distribution of Na$^+$. At the prevailing concentrations Na$^+$ has a calculated equilibrium potential of $+66$ mV, *i.e.*, 66 mV "inside positive," or 156 mV removed from the resting potential. The discrepancy is too large to be dismissed as an experimental error. Stated another way, at a resting potential of 90 mV "inside negative" and with the [Na^+_o] at 145 mmol/l (a value easily determined accurately), the Nernst equation requires an intracellular concentration of Na$^+$ of 483 mmol/l. This is about 40 times the measured intracellular concentration of Na$^+$! Bernstein dealt with this dilemma in a bold, if somewhat cavalier, fashion by asserting that the cell membrane is impermeable to Na$^+$, in which case the Nernst equation would not apply. We now know from experiments with radioactive Na$^+$ that Na$^+$ does penetrate resting cell membranes, but

to do Bernstein justice, we must admit that he was almost right, for resting cells are only very sparingly permeable to Na$^+$. Nevertheless, the anomalous distribution of Na$^+$, coupled with clear evidence that it can be exchanged across the cell membrane, compels us to conclude that some mechanism other than concentration and voltage forces governs the distribution of Na$^+$. Further, this mechanism must perform active metabolic work to maintain [Na^+_i] at a low level since both voltage and concentration gradients tend to force Na$^+$ into the cell.

Low [Na^+_i] is maintained by a *Na$^+$ pump*, a term chosen to imply that that work is done. The Na$^+$ pump utilizes metabolic energy derived from the breakdown of adenosine triphosphate (ATP) and creatine phosphate to extrude, against the voltage and concentration gradients, Na$^+$ ions which leak into the cell. The pump thus

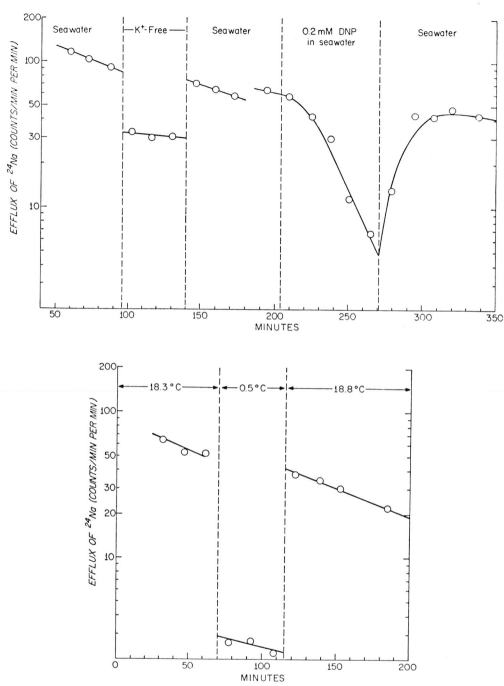

Figure 5–6. Sodium efflux in a squid axon. The axon is first soaked in a radioactive-Na$^+$ solution for a long time until the axoplasm contains a significant content of radiosodium. The axon is then washed and transferred to a bath of flowing seawater, which is sampled at intervals for measurement of the quantity of radiosodium extruded. The graph shows this "washout" as a function of time. The downward slope (linear on the log scale of the ordinate) occurs because internal concentration of radiosodium drops as it leaks out and is washed away. The effects of replacing seawater with a K$^+$-free bathing medium and of adding dinitrophenol, a metabolic poison, to the bathing medium are inscribed on this linear decline. The lower graph shows the effect of lowering bath temperature. (After Hodgkin and Keynes, *J. Physiol.*, 1955, *128*, 28–60.)

maintains a far lower [Na^+_i] than that predicted by the Nernst equation. Indeed, nearly all of the efflux of Na$^+$ from resting cells is accomplished by the action of the pump.

Evidence for Na$^+$ pumping derives from experiments in which the efflux of Na$^+$ is measured from cells preloaded with radioactive Na$^+$. First, the rate of efflux is highly dependent on temperature, a finding consistent with a metabolic origin of pump energy (Fig. 5–6). Secondly, when cells are treated with a metabolic poison that prevents the formation of ATP (*e.g.*, dinitrophenol, cyanide, or fluoride), the efflux of Na$^+$ is reduced to low levels (Fig. 5–6). [Na^+_i] increases and (since Na$^+$ replaces intracellular K$^+$) the resting membrane potential declines. Finally, the rates of efflux of Na$^+$ are temporarily restored in the poisoned axons by intracellular injection of ATP (Fig. 5–7).

Once the existence of ion pumping is admitted, one is prompted to reconsider the relatively small, but nevertheless significant, 7-mV deviation of the K$^+$ equilibrium potential from the resting potential. Recall that the equilibrium potential is greater than the measured resting potential; this means that [K^+_i] is higher by about 35 mmol/l than the Nernst equation would predict for a potential of -90 mV (*i.e.*, [K^+_o]/[K^+_i] is smaller than expected. This condition can be explained if K$^+$ is actively pumped into the cell. There is reason to believe that the same mechanism that pumps Na$^+$ out of the cell against concentration and voltage gradients also pumps K$^+$ into the cell against its concentration gradient, maintaining [K^+_i] at a higher level than that predicted by the Nernst equation (which describes the simple electrochemical equilibrium system uncomplicated by energy-expending pumps). Coupled "inward K$^+$"–"outward Na$^+$" pumping is supported not only by the high equilibrium potential of K$^+$ but also by the observation that Na$^+$ extrusion drops by about two-thirds when the normal extracellular medium is replaced by a K$^+$-free solution (Fig. 5–6). Apparently the efficiency of the Na$^+$ pump requires extracellular K$^+$ for its return trip. Some ingenious models of the Na$^+$-K$^+$ pump have been proposed (Fig. 5–8), but the actual mechanism is obscure.

In summary, Bernstein's prescient hypothesis was nearly correct; he asserted that the resting potential is a K$^+$ equilibrium potential and that the anomalous distribution of Na$^+$ is due to impermeability of the membrane to Na$^+$. Now, six decades later, we state that the resting potential is *close* to the K$^+$ equilibrium potential and that the membrane is *sparingly* permeable to Na$^+$. In addition, the existence of active ion pumping, an important concept not included in Bern

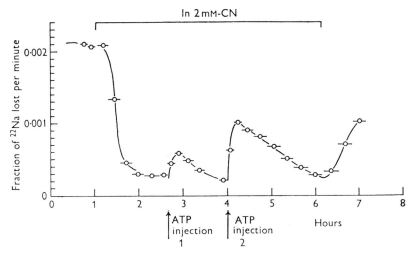

Figure 5–7.   The effect of intracellular injection of ATP on the efflux of Na$^+$ in a squid axon poisoned with cyanide. The experimental method is the same as that employed in Figure 5–6. (From Hodgkin, *The conduction of the nervous impulse*, Springfield, Ill., Charles C Thomas, 1964.)

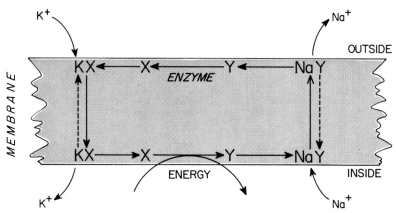

Figure 5–8. A hypothetical "carrier" mechanism for the Na$^+$-K$^+$ pump of cell membranes. Na$^+$ is assumed to combine with a molecule, Y, at the internal surface of the axon. NaY then diffuses through the membrane along its concentration gradient. At the outer surface an enzyme splits Na$^+$ from Y and converts Y to X, which has affinity for K$^+$ in the extracellular fluid. KX diffuses to the interior surface, where X is reconverted to Y through energy supplied by intracellular oxidative mechanisms. X and Y are supposed to be confined to the membrane and to diffuse only when combined with an ion. (From Ruch and Patton, eds., *Physiology and biophysics,* Philadelphia, W. B. Saunders Co., 1965.)

stein's simple mechanistic hypothesis, is accepted in modern theory. We will now examine in more detail some of the consequences of adding a pump to the Bernstein model diagrammed in Figure 5–4.

Membrane Permeability and Steady-State Voltage

On the left in Figure 5–9 is reproduced the simple electrochemical-equilibrium model of Figure 5–4; the graph below shows the development of the voltage across the membrane in the heavy line V_{C^+}. On the right is the same model with a C^+ pump added; the pump returns some of the C^+ to the x compartment after it has diffused into y. The arrows below have the same connotation as before, except that the movement from y to x is now fractionated into a passive component (*solid arrow*) and a pumped component (*dotted arrow*). For simplicity the pumping rate is assumed to be constant (although this is not quite correct), and hence the dotted arrow is always the same length.

Because the pump assists transport from y to x, the net flux and the voltage increment (*dotted line* in graph) are less at T_1 than in the equilibrium model. At T_2

the discrepancy is even greater, and at T_3 steady state is reached at a value less than the equilibrium potential. The effect of the pump, therefore, is to produce a steady-state potential less than that predicted by the Nernst equation. It is easy to see that if the dotted arrow were drawn longer, connoting a greater pumping rate, the steady state would be achieved earlier and at an even lower voltage. In this circumstance at the steady state a greater proportion of the movement from y to x will be accounted for by pumping; *i.e.*, the ratio between the lengths of solid arrow and dotted arrow is decreased. Indeed the discrepancy between equilibrium and steady-state values is a function of the ratio of passive flux to pump flux. *The more active the pump, relative to passive movement, the lower the steady-state voltage and the greater its deviation from true equilibrium voltage.*

It is because of the K$^+$ pump that the resting potential is lower (90 mV inside negative) than the equilibrium potential for K$^+$ (97 mV inside negative). The discrepancy is not large because the membrane is freely permeable to K$^+$, and passive factors allow a significant influx of K$^+$. This emphasizes the important point that one factor affecting the value of the steady-state potential is the ease with which the pumped ions can move passively across the membrane, *i.e.*, the *permeability*

Membrane Permeability

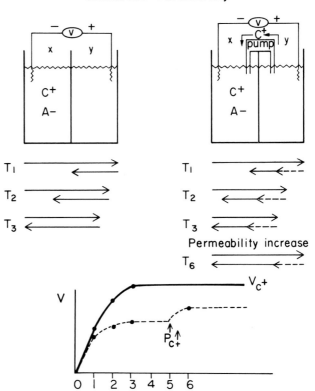

Figure 5–9. Comparison of voltage generation in electrochemical equilibrium model and in the same model containing an active cation pump. For description see text.

of the membrane to the ions. Membrane permeability can be visualized as a kind of frictional resistance to the movement of ions through membrane pores; it is thus a limiting factor in the rate of passive transfer and thereby a *determinant of the magnitude of the steady-state potential*. This relation is extremely important, for, as will be demonstrated presently, change in membrane permeability (presumably by change in the number of selective pores through which ions can move) accounts for most naturally occurring membrane potential changes, including the action potential of excitable cells.

The influence of permeability on steady-state potential is illustrated diagrammatically in Figure 5–9. In the graph the arrow labeled $P_{C+} \uparrow$ signifies that the permeability to C^+ has suddenly increased. The directional arrows labeled *Permeability increase* indicate the new steady state achieved at T_6. Because it is now easier for C^+ to penetrate the membrane and move from x to y, the arrow to the right is longer

than that at T_3. But it is also easier for C^+ to move in the opposite direction, so the steady state is achieved by an increase in the solid arrow pointing to the left. Since the action of the pump (*dotted arrow*) is not significantly influenced by the change in permeability, the ratio of passive exchange to that due to the pump is increased. Accordingly the new steady-state voltage is closer to the equilibrium value (see T_6 on dotted line of graph). The rule is that, when membrane permeability to a pumped ion increases, the membrane potential moves closer to the equilibrium potential of that ion. Conversely, when either pumping activity increases or permeability decreases, membrane potential deviates even farther from the equilibrium value.

The influence of ionic permeability on membrane potential explains why the resting membrane potential is far removed from the equilibrium potential for Na^+ but is only slightly (7 mV) less than the equilibrium potential for K^+, even though both ions are pumped by the same mechanism.

The resting membrane is about 50 times more permeable to K^+ than to Na^+; indeed, about 99.9 per cent of Na^+ efflux is due to pumping, whereas a significant portion of K^+ influx is by diffusion.

In all the foregoing discussion an implicit assumption is that the Na^+-K^+ pump is electrically neutral with the active Na^+ extension to the active K^+ influx (see Figure 5–8). Such a *neutral pump* does not contribute directly to the membrane potential, which results only from the relative membrane permeabilities to the two ions. In fact in most tissues such balanced pumping does not appear to hold, the ratio of Na^+ pumped out:K^+ pumped in being about 3:2. In this case, the pump, by extruding more positive charges than it moves into the cell actively, generates a potential over and above that determined by membrane permeabilities. Such an imbalanced mechanism is called an *electrogenic Na^+-K^+ pump*. The magnitude of the contribution of electrogenic pumping varies in different tissues. In squid axon only about 3 mV of the 65 mV resting potential is ascribable to imbalanced electrogenic pumping. In other tissues the contribution is larger. In any case the more important concept to grasp is that of the role of membrane permeability because most of the important electrical events of excitable cells result from changes in membrane permeability rather than from variations in pump activity.

GENERATION OF THE ACTION POTENTIAL

The foregoing discussion immediately suggests an attractive hypothesis for the generation of the action potential, *viz.*, that ionic permeability of excitable membranes is voltage-dependent and is so changed by threshold depolarization that a new voltage level results. Since the polarity of the membrane potential is reversed during the peak of the action potential, *i.e.*, the inside is positive to the outside, an increase in permeability to Na^+ is a likely explanation, for Na^+ is the major ion present in the extracellular and intracellular fluids with a positive equilibrium potential. Supporting this hypothesis is the observation that the overshoot of the action potential is highly dependent on $[Na^+_o]$: As $[Na^+_o]$ is decreased in logarithmic steps, the overshoot decreases linearly (Fig. 5–10); and in Na^+-free media nerve and muscle cells become inexcitable. Note that, whereas the resting potential is dependent on concentration of K^+, it is little influenced by changes in concentration of Na^+. As early as 1902, Overton postulated that Na^+ plays a critical role in the generation

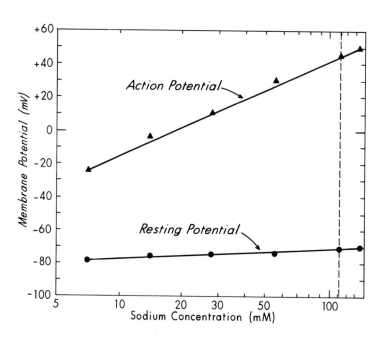

Figure 5–10. Effect of varying extracellular concentration of Na^+ on resting and action potentials of a frog axon. The ordinate gives the potential of the intracellular fluid relative to extracellular fluid; the scale is linear. The abscissa gives extracellular concentration of Na^+; the scale is logarithmic. The vertical dotted line at right indicates normal $[Na^+_o]$ for the frog. The line labeled *Action Potential* plots the peak of the action potential; the amplitude of the action potential is thus the difference between the lines delineating the action potential and the resting potential. (After Huxley and Stämfli, *J. Physiol.*, 1951, *112*, 496–508.)

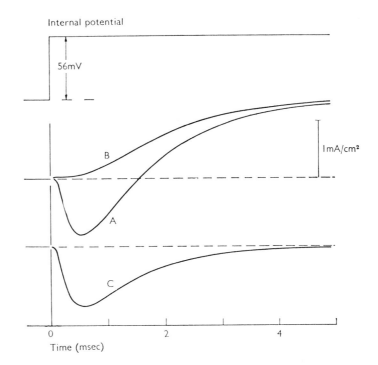

Figure 5–11. Records of transmembrane currents in a squid axon subjected to a voltage-clamp depolarization of 56 mV. The upper trace marks the application of the depolarizing voltage step. Trace *A* shows the currents resulting from this voltage step: inward currents are downward; outward currents are upward. In *B* the seawater surrounding the axon was replaced by a Na⁺-free solution; the remaining outward current is carried by K⁺. Trace *C*, obtained by subtraction of curve *B* from curve *A*, plots the time course of the isolated inward current carried by Na⁺. Note that the Na⁺ current is transient and disappears in 5 msec, even though the voltage is still held at the depolarized level. The K⁺ current shows no such inactivation at this time. (From Hodgkin and Huxley, *J. Physiol.*, 1952, *116*, 449–472.)

of the action potential, but the full mechanism was discovered by Hodgkin and Huxley during the period 1950 to 1960, an achievement for which they were awarded the Nobel Prize in 1963.

A full description of Hodgkin and Huxley's sophisticated quantitative techniques is beyond the scope of this book, but their line of attack and conclusions can be summarized. They employed a device known as a voltage clamp, which permitted them to measure differentially the transmembrane currents carried by Na⁺ and by K⁺ ions at different values of membrane potential held constant by the voltage clamp. A sudden depolarization of the axon membrane initiates an inward current that then reverses to a prolonged outward current (Fig. 5–11*A*). Hodgkin and Huxley found that the early inward current is carried by an influx of Na⁺ ions, for in Na⁺-free media it disappeared, leaving only the more slowly developing outward current. They readily identified the outward current with an efflux of K⁺ ions (Fig. 5–11*B*). The Na⁺ current can be determined by subtraction of curve *B* from curve *A*, as shown in Figure 5–11*C*.

Having identified the carriers of the two currents, Hodgkin and Huxley were able to calculate the membrane permeabilities (or more properly conductances) to these ions at various membrane potentials and to establish that a threshold depolarization produces a transient increase in Na⁺ permeability of about 500-fold (Fig. 5–12). During this phase Na⁺ enters the cell readily along its voltage and concentration gradients. By carrying positive charges into the cell the influx of Na⁺ causes further depolarization, and this, in turn, causes more depolarization and a further increase in permeability to Na⁺. This event, known as the *Hodgkin cycle*, can be diagrammed as follows:

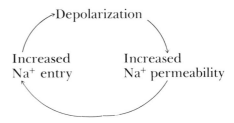

The Hodgkin cycle accounts for the abrupt rising phase and overshoot of the action potential in unclamped axons; during the period of immensely augmented Na⁺ permeability, the membrane potential

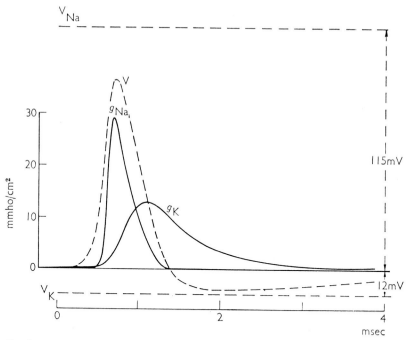

Figure 5–12. Conductances and voltage changes in a squid axon during an action potential. *V*, voltage change in absolute units, *i.e.,* the resting potential corresponds to zero on the voltage scale; the dotted line at the top represents the equilibrium potential of Na$^+$ and that at the bottom, the K$^+$ equilibrium potential. The curves labeled g_{Na} and g_K plot the time courses of changes in Na$^+$ and K$^+$ conductances, which are proportional to membrane permeabilities to these ions. (From Hodgkin, *The conduction of the nervous impulse,* Springfield, Ill., Charles C Thomas, 1964.)

veers precipitously toward the equilibrium potential for Na$^+$ (65 mV inside positive).

The peak of the action potential is limited, for two reasons. First, the voltage-sensitive Na$^+$ permeability change is transient; *i.e.,* the membrane pores opened by depolarization to admit Na$^+$ ions close rapidly even though the depolarization is maintained (Fig. 5–11C). This decay is called *inactivation of Na$^+$ permeability.* Even after the source of artificial depolarization is removed, the pores admitting Na$^+$ remain closed and insensitive to voltage change for a short time (about 1 msec), and this delay in recovery is the refractory period. The waning of Na$^+$ permeability also prevents the action potential from reaching the Na$^+$ equilibrium potential and limits the overshoot to 20 or 30 mV.

The second reason for the limited peak of the action potential is related to the late, outward current in voltage-clamped axons (Fig. 5–11A), which is due to a voltage-sensitive increase in K$^+$ permeability. In clamped preparations in Na$^+$-

free media, the K$^+$ current can be seen in isolation (Fig. 5–11B); it begins at about the same time as the Na$^+$ current but develops more slowly and only reaches its peak when Na$^+$ permeability is waning. The voltage-sensitive K$^+$ permeability mechanism is also much less sensitive to inactivation than is that for Na$^+$ and may even persist for a time after removal of the clamping voltage. The effect of increased permeability to K$^+$ is to hasten repolarization after the peak action potential, for during this time K$^+$ flows out of the cell, and the membrane potential shifts toward the equilibrium potential for K$^+$. In some preparations the action potential is followed by an afterhyperpolarization, *i.e.,* by a tail of slightly greater than resting potential (Fig. 5–12V). This is due to the pores' persistence in admitting K$^+$, an action causing the membrane to "seek for" the K$^+$ equilibrium potential, which is about 7 mV greater than the resting potential.

The voltage sensitivity of ionic permeability is unique to excitable cells. All cells have Na^+-K^+ pumps and resting potentials, but only nerve, muscle, and gland cells are capable of undergoing dramatic changes of permeability upon depolarization. The critical role of permeability mechanisms in excitability makes excitable cells vulnerable to certain drugs and toxins that block voltage sensitivity. Such agents are useful as local anesthetics, for, although they do not alter resting potentials, they render axons as insensitive to voltage change as red blood cells already are.

Procaine blocks both the voltage-sensitive Na^+ and K^+ pores. Tetrodotoxin, a poison found in the puffer-fish, blocks only the voltage-sensitive Na^+ channels, and leaves the voltage-sensitive K^+ mechanism intact. The same poison is found in some species of newts (tarichatoxin). Structurally different from tetrodotoxin but with a similar blocking action on Na^+ channels is saxitoxin, a poison produced by some species of dinoflagellates. Dinoflagellates are responsible for "red tides," during which shellfish contaminated by them become lethally poisonous because of their content of saxitoxin. The selective action of these toxins proves that the Na^+ and K^+ channels are separate and independent voltage-sensitive pores. Conversely, tetraethylammonium (TEA) ions block the voltage-sensitive K^+ channels but do not affect the Hodgkin cycle. TEA poisoning does not block excitability, but prolongs the time course of action potentials, reflecting the absence of the repolarizing influence of the K^+ conductance change.

The critical events underlying the action potential are diagrammed in Figure 5–12, which shows the time courses of the Na^+ (g_{Na}) and K^+ (g_K) permeabilities along with the voltage changes (V) during an action potential. The net effect of an action potential is the influx of a small quantity of Na^+ and the loss of a small quantity of intracellular K^+. So small are the quantities exchanged that axons can conduct many thousands of impulses even at high frequencies before being crippled by accumulation of intracellular Na^+ and loss of intracellular K^+. With the lower frequencies characteristic of normal function, the Na^+-K^+ pump reliably removes Na^+ and replaces K^+, thus maintaining the membrane battery at its normal resting level. It should be emphasized that the pump operates at a rate infinitely slow relative to the time course of the action potential and plays no direct role in the action potential. The action potential is directly ascribable to the voltage-sensitive permeability mechanisms. The role of the pump is to maintain the ion concentrations and membrane potential at levels compatible with excitability. It is the work of the pump that accounts for the all-or-nothing property of excitable cells, for it stores the charges that determine the amplitude of the action potential. The depolarizing stimulus merely triggers the Hodgkin cycle.

CONDUCTION OF THE ACTION POTENTIAL

An action potential is generated by depolarization of the membrane to the threshold value. After this the Hodgkin cycle and the K^+ permeability changes assume control of events, and the action potential proceeds automatically without further dependence on the stimulus. Moreover, once initiated in a patch of axon membrane, the action potential propagates relentlessly and inevitably along the axon until it has moved along the entire cell. Since depolarization to the threshold level is the *sine qua non* for generation of an action potential in a resting membrane, the question of self-propagation, or conduction, reduces to one of how the generated action potential can depolarize to threshold value the resting membrane not affected by the initial artificial depolarization. Because of the cable properties of nerve, the latter depolarization is confined to only a few millimeters at best.

For an unmyelinated axon such as the giant axon of the squid, the mechanism of propagation occurs as diagrammed in Figure 5–13B. During the peak of the action potential in a segment of nerve, the membrane potential reverses polarity, the inside being positive to the outside. This is indicated in the middle of the axon in Figure 5–13B by the minus signs outside the axon and the plus signs inside. The reversal of polarity leads to local current

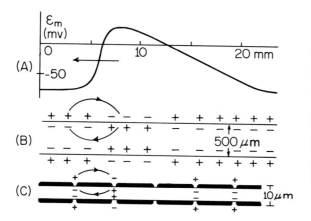

Figure 5–13. Mechanisms of conduction in unmyelinated squid axon (*B*) and myelinated mammalian axon (*C*). Trace *A* shows the action potential propagating from right to left. Arrows indicate the direction of current flow through membrane in front of the action potential. Similar current flow (not shown) occurs in the wake of the action potential, but it does not reexcite the repolarized membrane because permeability to Na⁺ is still inactivated and the membrane is refractory. (From Ruch and Patton, eds., *Physiology and biophysics*, Philadelphia, W. B. Saunders Co., 1965.)

flow from positive to negative, as indicated by the arrows. The outward current flow through the resting membrane in front of the action potential (which is depicted as moving from right to left) depolarizes the membrane and triggers its Hodgkin cycle. The newly activated membrane in turn explodes into an action potential, generates local currents, and depolarizes the next segment; and so on, until the action potential has moved along the full length of the axon.

The speed of propagation is a function of diameter. This is because the membrane behaves like a resistive-capacitative (*RC*) circuit, as diagrammed in Figure 5–2. When current flows through such a circuit, the change in voltage does not occur immediately but follows a time course that varies directly as the product of $R \times C$. Thus a low-resistance circuit changes voltage more rapidly than does a high-resistance circuit. Since a large axon has a lower longitudinal resistance than does a smaller axon, it depolarizes more rapidly and its conduction speed is faster.

But depending solely on diameter is a prodigal way to achieve speed. The squid, in order to attain a less-than-breakneck conduction speed of about 25 m/sec, pays the exorbitant price of growing axons half a millimeter or more in diameter. Bundles of large numbers of rapidly conducting axons such as are found in mammalian nervous systems would, were speed accomplished solely by increasing axon size, be inordinately bulky and metabolically taxing. The mammal has economically

solved this problem by manipulating the capacitance as well as the resistance of axons. Mammalian axons are wrapped with myelin, which is an excellent insulator. The membrane is exposed only at the nodes of Ranvier, spaced at intervals proportional to diameter up to about 2 mm in large axons.

Capacitance denotes the number of charges on a condenser required to maintain a given voltage; it decreases as the thickness of the insulator increases. At the nodal gap (about 1 μm long) the naked membrane thickness is about 100 Å and the capacity is relatively high, but in the much more extensive (2-mm) internodal region the myelin may be 2 μm thick and decrease the capacity about 200-fold. As a consequence the relatively long internode stores at resting potential only as many charges as the minuscule node. Thus there is far less charge to be neutralized during conduction and considerably greater conduction speed than there would be if the axon were naked throughout. In mammalian myelinated axons, transmembrane current flow occurs only through the nodes of Ranvier, and conduction is thus from node to node, as shown in Figure 5–13*C*. This is called *saltatory conduction*, from the Latin verb *saltare*, meaning *to hop*. The conduction speed is immensely increased by nature's prudent use of simple electrical laws. The squid must spawn an axon 0.5 mm in diameter to achieve a speed of 25 m/sec. This is about the conduction speed of a mammalian myelinated axon only 4 μm in diameter.

SUMMARY

All living cells exhibit a resting potential across their 100-Å-thick lipoprotein membranes. The magnitude of the resting potential varies, but the polarity is always "inside negative." Muscle cells have a resting potential of about 90 mV.

All cells also have a transmembrane difference in ion concentrations; the extracellular fluid contains high concentrations of Na^+ and Cl^- ions and low concentrations of K^+ ions, whereas the intracellular fluid contains high concentrations of K^+ ions and low concentrations of Na^+ and Cl^- ions. The major anions of intracellular fluid are organic ions (*e.g.*, aspartate and glutamate), to which the membrane is impermeable.

The resting potential is mainly dependent on the distribution of K^+ ions and thus is only a few millivolts less than the equilibrium potential for K^+. Cl^- is passively distributed across the membrane and is at equilibrium. Both K^+ and Na^+ ions are pumped across the membrane; Na^+, outward, and K^+, inward. The resting potential is far removed from the Na^+ equilibrium potential because the resting membrane is only slightly permeable to Na^+; nearly all of the Na^+ efflux is due to the pump. The membrane is far more permeable to K^+ than to Na^+; hence the resting potential is only slightly lower than the K^+ equilibrium potential (97 mV inside negative).

Excitable cells (nerve, muscle, and gland) have the specialized and unique capability of changing ionic permeability as a function of transmembrane voltage; this unique property underlies the action potential. Depolarization transiently increases Na^+ permeability. When depolarization reaches the threshold value (about 10 mV for nerve cells), Na^+ enters the cell, depolarizing the membrane more and further increasing the Na^+ permeability—the Hodgkin cycle. The membrane potential shifts precipitously toward the equilibrium potential for Na^+ (65 mV inside positive)—the rising limb of the action potential. At the peak of the action potential, the membrane is "turned momentarily inside out," the inside being positive to outside. The voltage-sensitive Na^+ permeability mechanism is transient and rapidly becomes inactivated. Inactivation curtails the peak of the action potential and contributes to repolarization of the membrane to the resting level, inside negative. The second factor leading to repolarization is a voltage-sensitive increase in K^+ permeability that begins apace with Na^+ permeability increase but develops more slowly, reaching a peak after Na^+ permeability has dropped almost to resting level. Elevated K^+ permeability moves the membrane potential toward the K^+ equilibrium potential (97 mV inside negative). Inactivation of Na^+ permeability causes the refractory period, which limits the frequency of impulses a cell can generate to about 1000 per second. During the action potential the cell gains a minute amount of Na^+ and loses a minute amount of K^+. During rest periods the Na^+-K^+ pump extrudes the added Na^+ and restores the lost K^+.

The action potential, once initiated, is self-propagating and spreads like a wave over the membrane. In unmyelinated axons the stimulus to the polarized membrane is current flow generated by the action potential itself—the so-called *local circuit*. Conduction speed is determined by diameter; large fibers conduct more rapidly than small fibers because they have a lower internal resistance. In myelinated fibers the myelin sheath acts as an insulator and prevents transmembrane current flow in the internodes; the movement of charges occurs only at the nodes of Ranvier, spaced at intervals of about 2 mm in large fibers. Conduction of the impulse is saltatory, *i.e.*, the impulse hops from node to node. For a given fiber diameter saltatory conduction is more rapid than simple local-circuit conduction because the myelin sheath of internodes reduces capacitance, and the reduced capacitance in turn diminishes the number of charges held across the membrane at a given resting potential. For myelinated fibers the relation of speed to diameter is $S + 6D$, where S is speed in meters per second and D is external diameter (including myelin) of the axon in micrometers. The squid axon, operating on local-circuit flow, has a size of 500 μm but a conduction speed of only 25 m/sec. This speed is reached by mammalian myelinated fibers with diameters of only 4 μm.

ADDITIONAL READING

Hodgkin, A. L. Ionic movements and electrical activity in giant nerve fibers. *Proc. roy. Soc. (Lond.)*, 1957, Ser. B, *148*, 1–37.

Hodgkin, A. L. *The conduction of the nervous impulse.* Springfield, Ill., Charles C Thomas, 1964.

Katz, B. *Nerve, muscle, and synapse.* New York, McGraw-Hill Book Co., 1966.

Woodbury, J. W. The cell membrane: ionic and potential gradients and active transport. Chap. 1 in *Physiology and biophysics*, Ruch, T. C., and Patton, H. D., eds., Philadelphia, W. B. Saunders Co., 1965.

Woodbury, J. W. Action potential: properties of excitable membranes. Chap. 2 in *Physiology and biophysics*, Ruch, T. C., and Patton, H. D., eds., Philadelphia, W. B. Saunders Co., 1965.

CHAPTER 6

MUSCLE AND NEUROMUSCULAR TRANSMISSION

HARRY D. PATTON

FUNCTION OF MUSCLES

Mammals react to environmental changes adaptively by three mechanisms: glandular secretion, movement, and postural adjustment. For the latter two mechanisms the ultimate executant organ is muscle. Skeletal muscles are attached by tendons to bones and may, by shortening, change the spatial relation of these bones, producing movement. A contraction in which muscle shortens against a constant load is called an *isotonic contraction*. On the other hand, a muscle may contract without shortening and offset an external force imposed on the muscle. For example, when the body is standing quietly erect, the quadriceps femoris, the large extensor

of the knee, contracts to prevent buckling of the knee joint in response to gravity. A contraction in which the muscle does not shorten but develops tension is called an *isometric contraction*. Contraction of cardiac muscle and smooth muscles of hollow visceral structures compresses the contents of the heart and viscera. If the organ is closed, the contraction is isometric and internal pressure rises. If there is a means of egress for the contents, *e.g.*, an open cardiac valve, the muscle fibers shorten and the contents are moved to a region of lower pressure.

A skeletal muscle is wholly regulated by the nervous system; it responds slavishly when, and only when, it is "instructed" to do so by the nervous system. Unlike skeletal muscles, cardiac muscle and many smooth muscles are not paralyzed by denervation; they are intrinsically rhythmic and continue to contract in the absence of their nerve supplies. Although they are not dominated by their nerve supplies, both cardiac and smooth muscles are neurally regulated; after denervation, they lose their capacity to vary their contractions adaptively in response to changing conditions. For example, the acceleration of heart rate in exercise, an adaptive response that increases the flow of oxygenated blood to the working muscles, is impaired by cardiac denervation.

CONTRACTION OF SKELETAL MUSCLE

Structure of Skeletal Muscle

A skeletal muscle (Fig. 6–1) consists of many thousands of cylindrical *muscle fibers*, each about 60 μm in diameter and varying in length from a few millimeters to many centimeters, depending upon the muscle. The membrane surrounding the muscle fiber is structurally similar to that of an axon and possesses the same exceptional functional properties of excitability and conductivity. Each muscle fiber contains bundles of smaller cylindrical *myofibrils* (Fig. 6–1) about 1 μm in diameter and extending the length of the fiber. A fiber may contain more than a thousand fibrils. Each fibril, in turn, comprises many fine parallel *filaments* coursing longitudinally. The filaments are of two types, *thick* (100 to 120 Å) and *thin* (60 to 70 Å), and their relative arrangements in the fibril are responsible for the characteristic transverse striations seen in electron and polarized-light micrographs of muscle.

Each fibril is divided into many sarcomeres, about 2.5 μm long in resting muscle, by transverse dark lines called *Z lines* (Fig. 6–2D). Securely anchored to the Z lines and extending less than half the length of the sarcomere in orderly parallel array are the thin filaments. In the middle part of the sarcomere the thick filaments are interdigitated between the free ends of the thin filaments, one or two thin filaments lying between each pair of thick

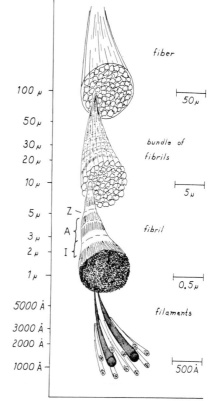

Figure 6–1. Constituent parts of skeletal muscle. (After Buchthal and Kaiser, *Biol. Meddr.*, 1951, *21*, 1–318.)

filaments, depending upon the plane of section (Fig. 6–3). The region occupied by thick filaments is called the *A band* (for *anisotropic*). In electron micrographs the A band appears dark because of the close packing of thick and thin filaments, except in its center, where the ends of thin filaments do not meet and only the thick filaments bridge the gap. The light, central region lacking thin filaments is called the *H band* (for *hell*, the German word for *bright*). At either end of the sarcomere between the Z line and the A band only thin filaments occur; the light, terminal areas are called *I bands* (for *isotropic*).

The Sliding-Filament Hypothesis

As shown by electron micrographs the A band remains nearly constant in width, no matter whether the fiber is contracted,

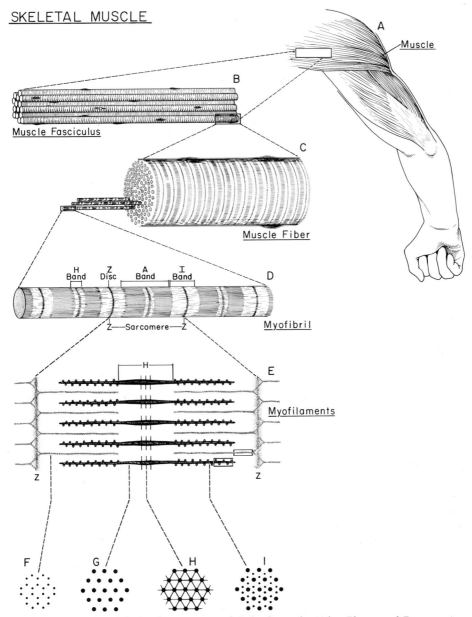

SKELETAL MUSCLE

A — Muscle

B — Muscle Fasciculus

C — Muscle Fiber

D — Myofibril

Z — Sarcomere — Z

H Band / Z Disc / A Band / I Band

E — Myofilaments

H

Z Z

F G H I

Figure 6–2. Histological and molecular structure of skeletal muscle. (After Bloom and Fawcett, *A textbook of histology*, Philadelphia, W. B. Saunders Co., 1968.)

relaxed, or stretched. In contracted muscle, the I and H bands decrease in thickness. These observations force the conclusion that the shortening of contracting muscle is not due to either shortening or folding of the filaments, as had previously been postulated; in fact, the filaments appear not to change length appreciably during either contraction or stretching of the muscle. Muscle shortening must then result from a sliding of thin filaments between the thick filaments, thus shortening the sarcomere at the expense of the I and H bands.

Highly magnified electron micrographs show fine bridges projecting laterally from the thick filaments, linking them with the interdigitated thin filaments. It is postu-

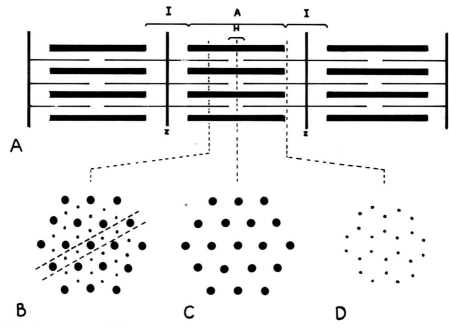

Figure 6–3. Arrangement of filaments in a myofibril. *A,* Longitudinal section shows bands as related to overlapping filaments. *B* to *D,* Cross sections taken at indicated points.

    Thin filaments in the *A* band are arranged in hexagonal display around thick filaments as in *B.* A longitudinal section through the plane represented by dotted lines in *B* would show two thin filaments between thick filaments. A plane of section parallel to the bottom of the figure would show only one thin filament between each pair of thick filaments (as in *A*). (After Huxley, Chap. 7 in *The Cell,* Vol. IV, Brachet and Mirsky, eds., New York, Academic Press, 1962.)

lated that these bridges, by repeatedly breaking contact with the thin filaments and reconnecting at sites distal to their central end, pull the central ends of the thin filaments and the Z bands closer together (Fig. 6–4). The process can be likened to two many-legged caterpillars, tail to tail, affixed to the two ends of the thick filaments, walking on movable treadmills—the thin filaments. In isometric contraction the bridges are assumed to be formed repeatedly at the same rather than

at sequential sites, maintaining tension between the two ends of the fiber. In other words, the caterpillars try to walk, but the treadmills are held fixed by opposing external forces tending to lengthen the sarcomere.

    It has long been known that the amount of isometric tension a muscle fiber can produce on contraction depends on the initial length of the fiber. The length-tension relationship is explained by the sliding-filament hypothesis, as shown in Figure

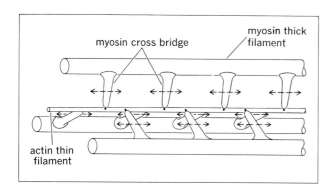

Figure 6–4. Diagram representing how cross bridges might cause sliding of thin filaments between thick filaments. (After Huxley, *Sci. Amer.,* Nov., 1958, *199,* 67–82.)

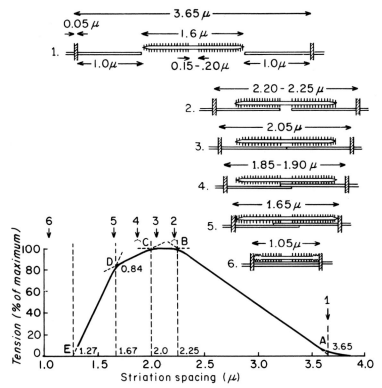

Figure 6–5. Length-tension curve of frog muscle fiber related to overlap of thick and thin filaments. See text for explanation. (After Gordon, Huxley, and Julian, *J. Physiol.* [*Lond.*], 1966, *184*, 170–192.)

6–5. The curve shows the relative tensions developed isometrically when a muscle fiber contracts at different initial sarcomere lengths. The insets diagram the relative positions of thick and thin filaments at different sarcomere lengths achieved by stretching of the muscle; the horizontal hatches represent bridges. When the muscle is stretched so that the sarcomere length is 3.65 μm, the thick and thin filaments do not overlap and bridges cannot be formed; contractile tension is near zero (point *A* on graph). As sarcomere length shortens progressively down to 2.25 μm, the overlap of filaments, and consequently the number of available bridge sites, increases progressively; contractile force increases linearly from *A* to *B*. Because the central portion (ca. 0.15 to 0.20 μm) of the thick filaments has no bridges, additional shortening of the sarcomere down to about 2.0 μm produces no further interaction between filaments; contractile tension remains constant (segment *BC* of curve). At still shorter lengths,

down to 1.65 μm, the ends of the thin filaments begin to overlap, interfering with the efficacy of the bridges; tension drops from *C* to *D*. At sarcomere spacings of 1.65 μm, the ends of the thick filaments butt against the Z bands, further limiting the efficiency of contraction; tension drops from *D* to *E*.

Chemical Composition of Muscle

Much effort has been expended in analyzing protein fractions chemically extracted from skeletal muscle in the hope of isolating the molecules responsible for contraction. Study of the structure and interactions of these molecules may one day reveal how the interfilamentous bridges form and break sequentially to cause sarcomere shortening. At present, this very active investigative field is in a state of perplexing flux, and molecular models of contraction are constantly being created and discarded. Although we still lack a totally satisfactory molecular model, some reasonably stable and well established facts may be summarized briefly. More detailed accounts can be found in the references at the end of this chapter.

Myosin and actin are the two major proteins in muscle. Two other proteins, troponin and tropomyosin, are present in smaller quantities but play a critical role in the contractile process.

Myosin is derived mainly, if not exclusively, from the thick filaments. As revealed by electron micrographs myosin molecules consist of a rodlike structure with two clubs at the end and a long tail. When appropriately treated *in vitro*, myosin molecules polymerize, producing strands with dimensions and configurations remarkably resembling those of the thick filaments. Significantly, myosin possesses adenosine triphosphatase (ATPase) activity, a property that provides the energy for muscle contraction. ATPase activity appears to be associated with the clubbed end of the molecule.

Actin, on the other hand, is derived from the thin filaments; it is more difficult to extract than is myosin, possibly because the thin filaments are tenaciously attached to the Z bands. Like myosin, it can be induced to polymerize, producing filaments that bear at least an encouraging resemblance to the thin filaments. Unlike myosin, actin does not possess ATPase activity. Although actin is quantitatively the major constituent of thin filaments, there is growing evidence that the thin filament *in vivo* also contains troponin and tropomyosin. A proposed model of the structure of a thin filament is illustrated in Figure 6–6. The actin portion, which constitutes the backbone of the thin filament, consists of two strands of spheres twisted together in a double helix, like a two-

stranded rope. The groove between the two strands is filled with tropomyosin, which has a fibrous molecular configuration; for those familiar with seamanship, the arrangement is reminiscent of worming that is set between the lays of a two-stranded rope. At approximately 400-Å intervals, globular troponin molecules are attached to the tropomyosin chain. Troponin will not bind to pure actin and requires tropomyosin as an intermediary.

When solutions of extracted myosin and actin-tropomyosin-troponin complex are mixed *in vitro* with calcium ions (Ca^{++}), magnesium ions (Mg^{++}), and ATP (the latter two substances bind to form a MgATP complex), ATP is split and the solution precipitates in a dense, contracted plug. Because ATP is also split to adenosine diphosphate (ADP) during muscle contraction, this phenomenon of "superprecipitation" has been looked upon as a test-tube model of the contractile process. Indeed electron micrographs of the superprecipitated material reveal cross bridges between the myosin threads and the actin-tropomyosin-troponin threads. Because the triggering of superprecipitation is quite sensitive to MgATP concentration, it is tempting to postulate that some mechanism of rapid variation of the concentration of either Mg^{++} or ATP might regulate the contraction-relaxation mechanism. However, calculations indicate that this would require far greater changes in concentration in these constituents than are actually observed during contraction.

It now seems clear for reasons to be described later that the controlling factor in the interaction of thick and thin filaments is the cyclic increase and decrease in sarcoplasmic concentration of ionic Ca^{++} during the processes of contraction and re-

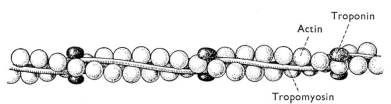

Figure 6–6. Molecular structure of actin-tropomyosin-troponin complex. (From Ebashi, Endo, and Ohtsuki, *Quart. Rev. Biophys.*, 1969, 2, 351–384.)

laxation. The following successive changes are currently believed to take place during the relaxation-contraction-relaxation sequence: At the outset the bridges are lacking because sarcoplasmic Ca^{++} concentration is low. Attached to the ATPase myosin clubs are ADP and inorganic phosphate, the products of reactions from previous cleavages; these reaction products are very slowly released from myosin, and their presence prevents the further splitting of ATP. When Ca^{++} ions are released into the sarcoplasm by mechanisms to be described later, they combine with troponin on the thin filaments, and this reaction stimulates the formation of bridges. Note that Ca^{++} only initiates the formation of bridges; its subsequent removal does not break the bridges. Once the bridges are formed, two processes occur: first, the energy from the original splitting of ATP changes the positions of the bridges so that they angle toward the center, pulling the thin filaments together and shortening the sarcomere; second, the liberation of the reaction products of ATP's splitting from myosin greatly accelerates, and ATPase activity is once more available for the splitting of ATP. ATP dissociates the actin and myosin, thus breaking the bridges. When ATP is absent, the bridges stay intact and the muscle remains stiffly contracted. This is what happens in *rigor mortis* of detective story fame. Once the bridges are detached, the cycle can be repeated as long as Ca^{++} is available in the sarcoplasm. Thus the cyclic variation in sarcoplasmic concentration of Ca^{++} plays the critical role in regulating the sequence. We turn now to the mechanisms governing the cyclic variations of sarcoplasmic Ca^{++} concentration.

Initiation of Contraction

The initial event in muscle contraction is depolarization of the muscle fiber membrane. This can be accomplished artificially by an electric shock. Just as in the axon, in the muscle the Hodgkin cycle is triggered by depolarization, generating an action potential that propagates by local-circuit current flow along the membrane. The conduction speed is only about 5 m/sec, much slower than in axons.

At particular sites along the muscle fiber the extracellular space of the membrane is continuous with a fine tubular system that penetrates the fiber transversely and winds tortuously between the myofibrils (Fig. 6–7). In frog muscle these *transverse tubules* are at the Z bands; in other species they occur at the junctions of the A and I bands. Since the transverse tubules are continuous with the extracellular space, it is presumed that the action potential invades them and thus penetrates deeply into the fiber. In their course through the fiber the transverse tubules approach closely, but are not continuous with, another tubular system that is longitudinally oriented and surrounds the myofibril. The *longitudinal tubules* form a closed system and are separated from both the sarcoplasm and extracellular fluid by continuous membrane; they can be visualized as a tubular, fenestrated bag surrounding the myofibril.

Where the longitudinal tubules come into close contact with the transverse tubules, the former expand to form bulbous *terminal cisternae*.

The transverse tubular system, together with the fenestrated central sac and the terminal cisternae, is known as the *sarcoplasmic reticulum*. In longitudinal sections of muscle the two cisternae and the transverse tubule between them form a characteristic picture known as the *triad* (Fig. 6–7). It is at the triad that the mechanical response is initiated by the action potential.

Electromechanical coupling is thought to occur as follows: In the resting state the sarcoplasmic concentration of Ca^{++} is extremely low, apparently because the longitudinal tubular system sequesters Ca^{++} into its interior by a highly efficient pumping mechanism. For contraction to occur, a supply of Ca^{++} in the sarcoplasm surrounding the filaments is essential. It is postulated that, as current flow generated by the action potential in the transverse tubules crosses the terminal cisternae of the longitudinal tubules, the properties of the cisternal membrane are so altered that Ca^{++} is released and diffuses into the sarcoplasm. The release of Ca^{++} into the sarcoplasm initiates the reactions leading to contraction. As the action potential wanes, the longitudinal tubular membrane

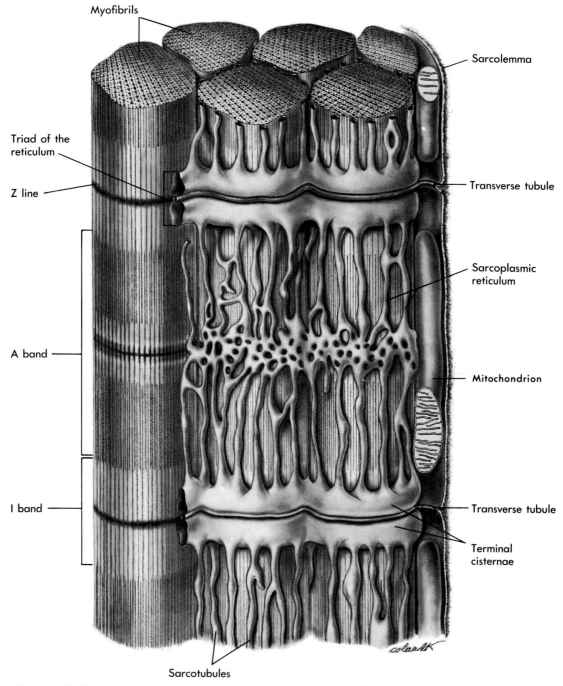

Myofibrils

Sarcolemma

Triad of the reticulum

Z line

Transverse tubule

A band

Sarcoplasmic reticulum

Mitochondrion

I band

Transverse tubule

Terminal cisternae

Sarcotubules

Figure 6–7. Muscle structure, showing relation of endoplasmic reticulum and of transverse tubular system to fibrils. (From Bloom and Fawcett, *A textbook of histology*, Philadelphia, W. B. Saunders Co., 1970.)

rapidly resequesters Ca++, ATP breaks the bridge coupling filaments, and the fiber relaxes.

The response to a single action potential is called a *muscle twitch*. Mechanical relaxation is not immediate; consequently the mechanical response considerably outlasts the membrane action potential and

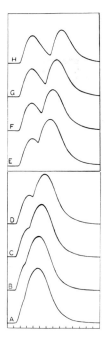

Figure 6–8. Summation of pairs of muscle twitches evoked by stimulation of the motor nerve at progressively shorter intervals. Time, below 20 msec. (After Cooper and Eccles, *J. Physiol. [Lond.]*, 1930, *69*, 377–385.)

its refractory period. A second action potential elicits a further contraction, and this is added onto the first, producing a greater tension—a phenomenon known as *summation* (Fig. 6–8). Generation of action potentials repetitively at high frequencies results in a smooth, sustained tension from two to four times greater than the twitch tension. The response of muscle to repetitive stimulation is called *tetanus*. Cardiac muscle cannot be tetanized because it has a singularly prolonged action potential and a refractory period approximating the duration of mechanical contraction.

In summary, although many details of the steps in muscle contraction remain conjectural, the following sequence of electromechanical coupling in muscle appears established:

Action potential of fiber membrane → action potential of transverse tubules of sarcoplasmic reticulum → current flow through cisternae of longitudinal tubular system → release of Ca⁺⁺ into sarcoplasm → binding of Ca⁺⁺ by troponin → sequential formation of bridges between thick and thin filaments and rapid release of ADP and inorganic phosphates from myosin →

sliding of thin filaments between thick filaments → dissociation by ATP of actin and myosin and breaking of bridges → continued formation and breaking of bridges in presence of Ca⁺⁺ → reabsorption of Ca⁺⁺ into sarcoplasmic reticulum → relaxation (lengthening) of fiber.

NEUROMUSCULAR TRANSMISSION

The End-Plate and Its Potential

The initiation of muscular contraction requires depolarization of the muscle fiber membrane such that the Hodgkin cycle is activated and an action potential is generated in the fiber membrane. Experimentally we accomplish this by passing a current outward across the fiber membrane. In nature, however, action potentials of muscle are generated by nerve impulses in motor nerve fibers at specialized sites, where they make contact with (but are not cytoplasmically continuous with) the muscle fibers, called either *motor end-plates* or *neuromuscular junctions*. At an endplate the message in the nerve must "jump the gap," or, more properly, the action potential of the nerve fiber must generate sufficient depolarization of the muscle fiber membrane to initiate a muscle action potential.

The structure of a motor end-plate is illustrated in Figure 6–9. Where the motor axon approaches the muscle fiber it loses its myelin sheath and splays out in a flattened plate. The plate is closely applied to the membrane of the muscle cell, the external surface being invested with Schwann cells, which separate it from extracellular space. In some species, *e.g.*, the frog, the ending lies in a gutter, or trough, in the muscle cell. The postjunctional membrane often shows specialized characteristics, such as repeated folding of the surface such that its area is considerably increased. The nerve terminal contains mitochondria and hundreds of spherical, membrane-bound structures, called *vesicles*. Sometimes one sees vesicles whose membranes are apparently fused with the surface membrane of the nerve terminal so that the vesicular lumen communicates with the narrow (200 to 500 Å) cleft

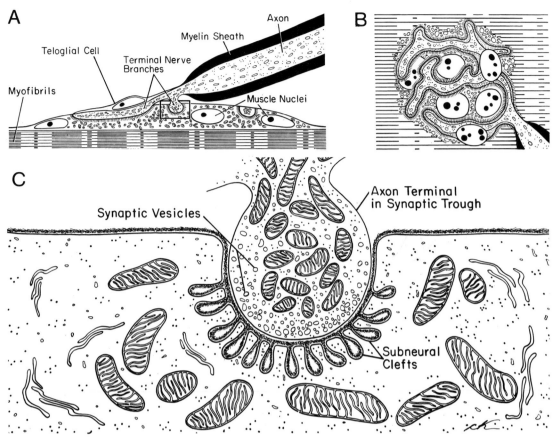

Figure 6–9. Schematic drawings of motor end-plates. *A* and *B,* Views from the side and from above, respectively. *C,* Enlarged view (as seen in electron micrographs) of the region outlined by the rectangle in *A.* (From Bloom and Fawcett, *A textbook of histology,* Philadelphia, W. B. Saunders Co., 1970.)

separating the nerve membrane from the muscle fiber membrane. This phenomenon is especially prominent in junctions poisoned with black widow spider venom, which appears to cause massive depletion of vesicles.

It is now established that the action potential of the nerve fiber propagates clear to the terminal and by mechanisms not completely understood triggers the release of acetylcholine (ACh), a stored chemical substance, from the vesicles into the junctional cleft.

The amount of ACh released depends, first, on the amplitude of the action potential. If the terminal is artificially depolarized so that the action potential is smaller than normal, a smaller quantity of ACh than normal is released. Conversely, an action potential in a hyperpolarized terminal is larger than normal and re-

leases a greater amount of ACh. Secondly, Ca^{++} is necessary for the release mechanism to operate. Depolarization increases Ca^{++} permeability of the terminal, and the influx of Ca^{++} somehow triggers release of ACh from the vesicles.

The released ACh, the neuromuscular transmitter, diffuses across the gap, attaches to specific receptive sites on the postjunctional membrane, and increases its permeability to both sodium (Na^+) and potassium (K^+) ions. Thus the influence of ACh is to drive the postjunctional muscle-membrane potential to a new value between the equilibrium potentials of K^+ (-97 mV) and Na^+ ($+66$ mV), *i.e.,* in a depolarizing direction. Measurements indicate that ACh drives the membrane potential toward a value (about 10 mV inside negative) between the equilibrium potentials of K^+ and Na^+. If ACh persisted in combination with the membrane receptors (we shall see that it does not), the membrane battery would be discharged almost completely because of the influx of Na$^+$ and the efflux of K$^+$.

The depolarization produced by a jet of released ACh following a motor-nerve action potential is called an *end-plate potential* (Fig. 6–10). The end-plate potential differs from an action potential in two important respects: (1) it is *local, i.e.,* nonpropagated, and diminishes in amplitude exponentially with distance from the end-plate (Fig. 6–10); and (2) it is graded rather than all-or-nothing, *i.e.,* its amplitude varies with the amount of ACh released. When a second nerve action potential is generated before the end-plate potential has dissipated, the two end-plate potentials sum, a phenomenon that is lacking in all-or-nothing action potentials.

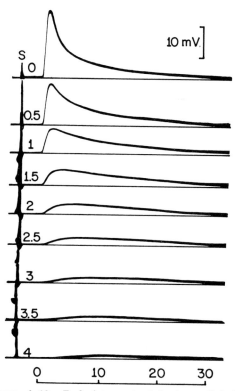

Figure 6–10. End-plate potentials intracellularly recorded from a curarized frog nerve-muscle preparation. Time, in milliseconds. Numbers on the left give the distance of the intracellular electrode from the end-plate. As distance increases, recorded potential becomes smaller and slower. (From Fatt and Katz, *J. Physiol.* [*Lond.*], 1951, *115,* 320–370.)

The function of the end-plate potential is to serve as a sink for current flow through the adjacent muscle cell membrane, depolarizing it to the threshold value required to initiate the Hodgkin cycle and an action potential, which then propagates along the fiber by local-circuit current flow. Normally the amount of ACh released by an action potential produces an end-plate potential of sufficient magnitude to ensure a triggered action potential. Consequently, neuromuscular transmission is normally obligatory: the muscle fiber always "does what it is told to do" by the motor nerve fiber.

The end-plate membrane differs from the remainder of the muscle membrane in several respects. First, it probably does not have the voltage-sensitive Hodgkin cycle and does not support all-or-nothing action potentials. Secondly, it is about 1000 times more sensitive to ACh than is nonjunctional muscle membrane. Although about only 10^{-17} mole of ACh is released by a nerve impulse, this is adequate to produce an end-plate potential sufficiently large to initiate an action potential.

When a muscle fiber is denervated, its sensitivity to ACh increases by as much as 100-fold over a period of 1 to 2 weeks—a phenomenon known as *denervation hypersensitivity.* Hypersensitivity is due not to increased end-plate sensitivity but rather to the development of multiple, highly sensitive sites in the nonjunctional membrane. When the muscle fiber is reinnervated, these ectopic receptor sites disappear and the fiber is once again controlled by the ACh sensitivity of the end-plate.

As hypersensitivity develops in denervated muscle, random twitches of individual hypersensitized muscle fibers, called *fibrillations,* begin to occur. Fibrillations represent twitches of muscle fibers from small quantities of ACh that normally are ineffective. Because fibrillations are asynchronous contractions of single muscle fibers, they are not readily visible through the skin, but they are detectable by electromyography (see Figure 6–14) and provide diagnostic clues to motor nerve damage.

Finally, the end-plate membrane is specialized by having concentrated on its surface an enzyme, acetylcholinesterase

(AChe), which catalyzes the hydrolysis of ACh to the relatively inert products choline and acetate. AChe limits the duration of ACh action on the end-plate by a factor of three and by so doing ensures that a nerve impulse will produce only one action potential in the muscle. A convenient way to think of these relations is to picture the postjunctional muscle membrane with two receptors for ACh: one receptor when combined with ACh increases permeability to Na^+ and K^+, leading to the end-plate potential; the other receptor is AChe. When combined with ACh it splits ACh, and, by mass action, promptly preempts more ACh from the "permeability receptor," thus curtailing the end-plate depolarization and limiting action potential generation.

Drugs and Synaptic Transmission

The mechanism of chemical transmission accounts for the action of a number of drugs, toxins, and chemicals, some of which are used clinically or are encountered in either disease or intoxication. These can be classified according to site and mechanism of action, as shown in Table 6–1.

Examples of agents in category Ia are local anesthetics that block the Hodgkin cycle and thus prevent the generation of action potentials; we have already discussed the blocking action of procaine on both the voltage-sensitive Na^+ and K^+ mechanisms and that of tetrodotoxin, tarichatoxin, and saxitoxin, which selectively block only the voltage-sensitive Na^+ channels (Chap. 5). When given systemically these agents block not only the nerve membrane but also the muscle membrane

and produce paralysis. They do not, however, block the ACh receptors of the end-plate, for ACh, locally applied to the poisoned end-plate membrane, still produces a depolarizing end-plate potential. This proves that the Na^+ and K^+ pores that are opened in end-plate membrane by ACh *are distinct* from those that are opened in nerve and muscle membrane by depolarization.

Another indication of the independence of chemically sensitive channels and voltage-sensitive channels derives from the observation that miniature end-plate potentials persist in the presence of tetrodotoxin. *Miniature end-plate potentials* are small, randomly occurring depolarizations having a time course similar to end-plate potentials that are recorded from the end-plate even when the nerve terminal is quiescent (Fig. 6–11). When the amplitudes of miniature end-plate potentials (mepps) are measured, the larger specimens are found to be multiples of the smallest. This has led to the concept of spontaneous quantal release of ACh in packets—perhaps vesiclefuls. Such quantal release of transmitter occurs randomly in resting junctions, giving rise to mepps.

Depolarization of the terminal by an action potential greatly accelerates and synchronizes the release of packets, or quanta, and produces an end-plate potential representing the summed effect of many quanta. Such massive, synchronous transmitter release is blocked by tetrodotoxin because the action potential is blocked, but the random, resting release of quanta continues unabated. In the poisoned preparation the influence of an action potential can be mimicked by a brief depolarizing pulse passed through the terminal; a full-blown end-plate potential

TABLE 6–1. Action of Drugs on Neuromuscular Function

I. Action on nerve.
    a. Alteration of excitability or conductivity.
    b. Alteration of ACh synthesis.
    c. Alteration of ACh release.
II. Action on postjunctional end-plate membrane.
    a. Alteration of ACh binding.
    b. Alteration of ACh destruction of AChe.
III. Action on muscle.
    a. Alteration of excitability or conductivity of muscle membrane.
    b. Alteration of contractile mechanism.

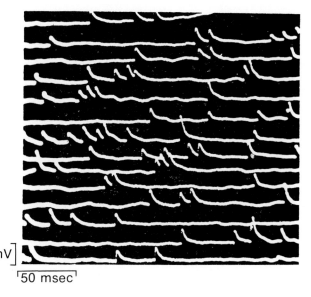

Figure 6–11. Spontaneous miniature end-plate potentials in resting frog nerve-muscle preparation. (From Fatt and Katz, *Nature*, 1950, *166*, 597–598.)

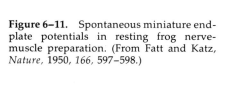

2mV

50 msec

results. Like natural transmitter release, such artificially induced transmitter release is Ca^{++}-dependent and is blocked by immersion of the preparation in a Ca^{++}-free external medium. This indicates that the channels that normally open to admit Ca^{++} during depolarization of the terminal are distinct from the voltage-sensitive Na^+ pores.

An agent that alters ACh synthesis (category Ib in Table 6–1) is hemicholinium. Synthesis of ACh occurs in nerve terminals and requires choline acetylase, an enzyme that is thought to be synthesized in the neuron soma and to migrate down the axon into the cytoplasm of the nerve terminal. In the presence of coenzyme A, acetate, choline, and ATP, ACh is formed. There are no known inhibitors of choline acetylase. Hemicholinium blocks ACh synthesis by embargo; it prevents entry of choline into the cell. The ACh content of terminals can be reduced to negligible levels by hemicholinium treatment followed by prolonged repetitive stimulation to deplete preformed stores.

An agent that prevents ACh release (type Ic in Table 6–1) is Mg^{++}; elevation of Mg^{++} concentration effectively blocks transmitter release and causes paralysis. Mg^{++} apparently competes with Ca^{++} for some receptor that must combine with Ca^{++} to initiate the transmitter-release mechanism. Increasing Ca^{++} promptly and effectively reverses the Mg^{++} block.

Administered parenterally, Mg^{++} also produces unconsciousness and respiratory arrest because, as we shall see later, the transmission from one nerve cell to another in the central nervous system involves release of a chemical transmitter, and this process, like release of the neuromuscular transmitter, is Ca^{++}-dependent.

Another agent that blocks transmitter release is the toxin of *Clostridium botulinum.* This normally harmless and ubiquitous organism becomes antisocial only when grown anaerobically; it then produces a toxin that is one of the most powerful poisons known. The conditions for toxin production are sometimes met in incompletely sterilized canned goods, and when such food is ingested, poisoning occurs. The signs and symptoms include nausea and vomiting, visual disturbances, and either weakness or paralysis of such severity that the outcome is usually fatal. Contrary to previous reports, botulinus toxin does not block axon terminals but rather blocks the ACh-release mechanism, possibly either by binding receptors normally activated by Ca^{++} ions or by preventing Ca^{++} entry during the action potential. The vesicles of poisoned terminals show no structural abnormality, the postjunctional membrane retains its sensitivity to ACh, and miniature end-plate potentials persist, although with diminished frequency.

From what has been said about Ca^{++} ions, alterations of serum Ca^{++} would be expected to alter neuromuscular transmission. In fact, the effects of alteration of serum Ca^{++} are complicated because Ca^{++} affects axon and muscle membranes as well as the transmitter-release mechanism. Lowering serum Ca^{++} increases the sensitivity of the Na^{++}-permeability mechanism of the Hodgkin cycle to voltage change; that is, as Ca^{++} is lowered, the amount of depolarization required to bring about a threshold alteration of Na^{++} permeability is reduced. When the ionized Ca^{++} level falls from the normal level of 6 or 6.5 mg/100 ml to about 4.3 mg/100 ml, both nerve and muscle membranes begin to discharge spontaneously, producing intermittent, severe muscle spasms.

The most commonly encountered effect of lowered serum Ca^{++} is, therefore, due to hyperexcitability of nerve (Ia in Table 6–1) and muscle membranes (categories Ia and IIIa in Table 6–1). The hyperexcitable state due to lowered Ca^{++} is known as *hypocalcemic tetany* (not to be confused with tetanus, which is due to intoxication with the toxin of the tetanus bacillus). Even in the absence of spontaneous spasms, lowered ionic Ca^{++} produces a condition termed as *latent tetany*, which can be detected by various diagnostic maneuvers that reveal the lowered thresholds of nerve and muscle membranes. One diagnostic sign is called *Chvostek's sign*. It is elicited by tapping the skin in front of the ear; the hyperexcitable facial nerve is caused to discharge by the mild (and normally ineffective) mechanical stimulus, producing a twitching of the facial musculature around the lips and nostrils. Another clue to latent tetany is *Trusseau's sign*, which is elicited by occluding the venous circulation of the arm with a sphygmomanometer cuff for 3 min; the anoxia produces discharge in hyperexcitable nerves of the arm, producing a spasmodic flexion of the wrist and metacarpophalangeal joints, extension of the phalangeal joints, and adduction of the thumb.

Tetany most commonly results from either parathyroid deficiency or vitamin D deficiency and is promptly relieved by injections of Ca^{++} salts. It may also occur in alkalosis, such as that produced by hyperventilation, because increasing the pH increases the binding of Ca^{++} by serum

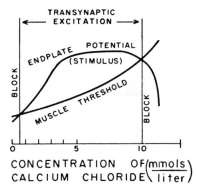

Figure 6–12. Relation of extracellular Ca^{++} concentration to transmitter release (size of end-plate potential) and to threshold of muscle membrane. (After Brink, *Pharmacol. Rev.*, 1954, 6, 243–298.)

protein and thus lowers ionized Ca^{++} concentration. At very low concentrations transmitter release from the terminal becomes inadequate to excite the muscle despite the low threshold. Increased Ca^{++} concentration restores transmitter release but eventually so raises the threshold that block occurs. The effects of Ca^{++} concentration on the transmitter-release mechanism and membrane excitability in the frog are diagrammed in Figure 6–12.

Several agents that alter ACh action on the end-plate membrane (type IIa in Table 6–1) may be mentioned. The most celebrated are curare, the Indian arrow-poison, and the clinically useful synthetic drug *d*-tubocurarine. Like ACh, curare and tubocurarine attach reversibly to the end-plate receptors, but unlike the ACh-receptor complex, the curare-receptor complex does not alter end-plate permeability. The curarized junction has a normal resting potential and is insensitive to ACh whether applied directly or released from an activated terminal. Thus the curarized subject is totally paralyzed and, without artificial respiratory support, may die of asphyxia from paralysis of the respiratory muscles. Tubocurarine is often used clinically in conjunction with anesthetics to facilitate muscle relaxation during surgery; artificial ventilation must of course be provided. Because the binding of receptors by curare is reversible, the drug is in time detoxified and excreted, and neuromuscular function then returns to normal. Paralysis from curare can also be reversed by administration of anticholinesterases (see later); these attach to the AChe receptor, and inactivation of AChe permits accumulation of ACh in concentrations sufficient to compete successfully with curare for receptor sites. Some animal toxins (from venomous toads and snakes) bind to the end-plate receptor irreversibly and cause a fatal paralysis that is not reversed by anticholinesterases.

Several other drugs compete with ACh for the end-plate receptor but cause paralysis by a different mechanism. Decamethonium bromide and succinylcholine are examples. Both mimic ACh; they attach reversibly to the postjunctional excitatory receptor, and the complex causes depolarization. Unlike ACh, however, the drugs are not destroyed by AChe and, therefore, cause a prolonged depolarization that may almost completely dissipate the end-plate membrane potential. Injection of these agents causes first fibrillary twitching as muscle fibers are depolarized to the threshold level, but excitation is rapidly succeeded by paralysis as membrane potential drops to lower levels because prolonged depolarization causes inactivation of Na^+ conductance in the adjacent muscle membrane (compare Figure 5–11C). Such drugs are known as *depolarizing blocking agents*. They produce a paralysis that is not antagonized by anticholinesterases. They are often used as adjuncts to general anesthetics to produce muscular relaxation. As with curare, recovery of function depends on detoxification and excretion of the drug. The resting membrane potential is then restored to normal levels by the Na^+-K^+ pump.

Agents that alter the destruction of ACh by AChe (category IIb in Table 6–1) are called *anticholinesterases;* the best known examples are physostigmine (eserine) and neostigmine. Inactivation of AChe by an anticholinesterase slows the dissociation of the ACh-receptor complex, permitting a more prolonged depolarization of the end-plate. The prolonged end-plate potential from a single nerve impulse may induce repetitive discharge of the muscle fiber. Certain other anticholinesterases, all being organic phosphate compounds, form an irreversible bond with AChe and therefore have a more lasting effect than do physo-

stigmine and neostigmine. The best known example is diisopropyl fluorophosphate (DFP), which was first studied in World War II as a "nerve gas." Poisoning with DFP causes first twitching and spasms, later paralysis when prolonged depolarization causes Na^+ conductance inactivation in the perijunctional muscle membrane. Death is asphyxial because of paralysis of the respiratory muscles. Several organic phosphate compounds having irreversible anticholinesterase action are used as insecticides and are occasional sources of accidental poisoning. Organic phosphates are especially dangerous because they can be absorbed in toxic quantities through the skin and also because their binding to AChe is extremely firm; the bond, however, can be broken by a treatment with an agent known as PAM (2-pyridine aldoxime methiodide).

Agents that alter muscle membrane excitability (category IIIa in Table 6–1) are the same as those that alter axon membrane excitability (Ia in Table 6–1). The mechanisms of excitability and conductivity are the same in muscle and nerve, and agents (procaine, tetrodotoxin, saxitoxin, etc.) that affect one similarly affect the other. A similar parallel can be drawn between transmitter release (electrosecretory coupling) and the mechanical response (electromechanical coupling). Elevated Mg^{++} concentration blocks both transmitter release and electromechanical coupling. Both blocks are reversed by administration of Ca^{++} salts.

THE MOTOR UNIT

Types of Motor Units

Most muscle fibers receive a single motor-nerve twig terminating at the end-plate. There are, however, many more muscle fibers in a given muscle than there are motor axons in the nerve supplying that muscle; it follows, therefore, that a number of muscle fibers are supplied by each axon in the nerve trunk. A motoneuron, its axon, and all the muscle fibers it supplies is called a *motor unit*. Since normally neuromuscular transmission at each fiber is so secure as to be obligatory, the discharge of a motoneuron causes contraction of all its subservient muscle fibers. Thus the motor unit determines the minimum quantum of normal muscular activity. The average size of motor units, as measured by determination of the innervation ratio (number of muscle fibers : number of motor axons), varies in different muscles according to their structure and function. The ratio is about 3:1 for the extraocular muscles, whereas the ratio is as high as 150:1 for some leg muscles. Muscles that execute small movements requiring fine gradations of contraction have smaller motor units than those that support either postural adjustments or grosser phasic shortenings.

It has long been known that muscles can be divided roughly into two types on the basis of gross appearance and speed of contraction, of which a convenient index is the twitch contraction time (from beginning to peak tension). Slow muscles (with contraction times of 35 msec or more) are dark red, whereas fast muscles (having contraction times less than 35 msec) are generally paler in appearance. A classic contrast is between the synergistic muscles of the calf of the leg: soleus is slow and red, whereas gastrocnemius is fast and pale.

Mysteriously, the contraction speed of a muscle seems to depend on its innervation. In newborn kittens soleus and gastrocnemius are equally slow, with contraction times of about 80 msec. During the first 4 weeks after birth both muscles become faster, and at 5 weeks gastrocnemius attains a stable, adult contraction time of about 20 msec; soleus once more becomes slower and finally stabilizes at a contraction time of about 70 to 75 msec. If in the newborn the nerves to the two muscles are severed and the central end of each is anastomosed to the stump of the other, soleus differentiates into a fast muscle and gastrocnemius into a muscle with a slower contraction time than normal. The mechanism of this trophic influence of nerve on muscle is unknown.

Recent studies of the properties of single motor units and of the histochemical characteristics of their muscle fibers have resulted in an extension of the old "fast and pale–red and slow" dichotomy. The muscle fibers composing soleus are all alike and will be called Type I fibers. They are characterized not only by slow contraction times but by relatively high oxidative metabolism (as measured by succinate dehydrogenase levels), high lipid metabolism, low glycogen stores, an extensive capillary supply, and low ATPase activity. The last characteristic is subject to some controversy, since the histochemical stain for ATPase activity is highly sensitive to pH and can yield contrary results at different pH values; nevertheless, for a fixed pH, Type I fibers are distinguished from Type II fibers. Type II fibers have the reverse of the characteristics enumerated above for Type I. Gastrocnemius, a pale, fast muscle, contains both Type I and Type II fibers, although the latter predominate. It also contains muscle fibers that are, in one or another respect, intermediate between Type I and Type II; in other words, a strict dichotomy into Type I and Type II fibers is probably an oversimplification. Nevertheless, recognition of the two extremes of what may well be a spectrum of muscle fiber types is useful, for it is becoming increasingly clear that the functional properties of muscle are closely related to the fiber types.

All of the constituent muscle fibers of a motor unit are of the same type, a finding that is in agreement with the trophic influence of nerve on muscle deduced from the crossed-innervation experiments described earlier. Motor units comprising Type I fibers produce less tension than those made of Type II fibers; they are smaller (i.e., have fewer muscle fibers). In the small, slow, Type I motor units the axons are smaller and less rapidly conducting than are those in the large, fast, Type II units. Type I units are more resistant to fatigue than are Type II units. As will be discussed in more detail in a later chapter, Type I units have low thresholds to reflex inputs and maintain tonic repetitive discharges, whereas Type II units tend to fire phasically in short bursts to intense reflex drives. As a first approximation it would thus seem that Type I units are admirably adapted biochemically and functionally to maintain the prolonged, repetitive discharge required in postural stances and to vary this discharge

TABLE 6–2. Properties of Mammalian Motor Units

Type I	Type II
High oxidative metabolism	Low oxidative metabolism
High lipid metabolism	Low lipid metabolism
Low glycogen stores	High glycogen stores
Low ATPase activity	High ATPase activity
Slow contraction time (>35 msec)	Fast contraction time (<35 msec)
Small size, low tension	Large size, high tension
Rich capillary supply	Sparse capillary supply
Innervation by small motoneurons and slowly conducting axons	Innervation by large motoneurons and rapidly conducting axons
Low reflex threshold	High reflex threshold
Tonic reflex discharge	Phasic reflex discharge
Minimal fatigability	Great fatigability

in accord with slight variations in input. On the other hand, Type II units are adapted for rapid, large phasic movements, as in "voluntary" behavior. The differences between the two types of units are summarized in Table 6–2.

Gradation of Muscle Contraction

In a contracting parallel-fibered muscle the total tension produced is the sum of the tensions of all the motor units acting. Therefore, one physiological means of increasing contractile tension is to increase the number of motor units active. However, reflex gradation of contractile tension is not a linear function of numbers of units active, because the reflex threshold is higher for the large motor units, innervated by large, rapidly conducting axons, than for the small units, innervated by slowly conducting axons. This means that low-level reflex drives recruit first the small units, producing relatively small-tension increments; increasing drives recruit the larger units, producing disproportionately large increments in tension. Thus gradation of contractile tension by motor unit recruitment occurs as an approximately exponential increase in tension.

The second determinant of tension gradation is the frequency of discharge of individual motoneurons. It has already been mentioned that muscle contractions can sum and that maximum tensions are produced by tetanic contractions in response to repetitive firing of motoneurons. The discharge frequency at which smooth, fused tetanus and maximal tension occurs is inversely related to contraction time, being less for slow soleus units (about 30 per second) than for fast gastrocnemius units (about 100 per second). As indicated by electromyographic recording from muscles with fine electrodes capable of detecting the activity of single motor units, the frequency of discharge increases from about 5 per second up to 50 per second as voluntary contraction increases from light effort to maximal. Although rates of 50 per second are insufficient to secure the full benefits of summation from fast muscles, gradation of discharge frequency nevertheless operates to effect a smoothly graded contraction. This is because voluntary muscular effort is sustained by the repetitive discharges of many motor units firing asynchronously, i.e., out of phase with one another.

The total tension at any time depends on the summed contractile tension of many units in various stages of contraction. Contraction is smooth and sustained even though individual units are responding with unfused twitches because as one unit relaxes another contracts and maintains the tension. Figure 6–13 illustrates diagrammatically how four asynchronously twitching units can collectively produce a sustained, relatively smooth tension; if more such units are summed, a perfectly smooth tension plateau results. Since the summed tension response depends on the number of units contracted at a given instant of time, increased frequency results in increased tension even in the frequency ranges below those required for fused tetanus.

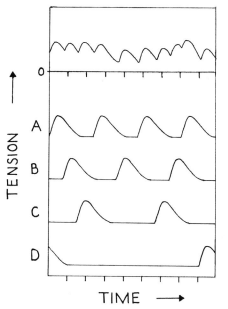

Figure 6–13. Summation (top record) of tensions developed by four motor units twitching asynchronously at different frequencies. Summed tension is relatively smooth and will be even smoother if other units are added. (From Ruch and Patton, eds., *Physiology and biophysics,* Philadelphia, W. B. Saunders Co., 1965.)

DISEASES OF THE MOTOR UNIT

As with drugs, so also diseases affecting the motor unit can be classified according to locus of attack, as shown in Table 6–3.

Altered Neuronal Excitability or Conduction

Diseases of type Ia (in Table 6–3) include those that attack motoneuron somata in the ventral horn, such as acute poliomyelitis, as well as those that attack the axons. The latter include traumatic severance of the axon and various periph-

eral neuropathies that block conduction; some of these attack primarily the myelin sheath and thus interfere with saltatory conduction. Since denervated muscle fibers are incapable of integrated activity, either weakness or paralysis results. However, muscular quiescence does not occur immediately, and the onset of motoneuron disease and peripheral neuropathies attacking motor axons is characterized by coarse involuntary twitchings of portions of the muscles, called *fasciculation* (Fig. 6–14*D*). Fasciculation is presumably due to spontaneous discharge of motoneurons irritated by the disease process. Since whole motor units rather than single fibers are involved, each discharge causes the entire cadre of muscle fibers in the unit to contract, producing a visible twitch. Fasciculation is distinguished from *fibrillation,* a condition in which single fibers twitching asynchronously produce movements too small to be detected through the skin (Fig. 6–14*C* and *E*).

As motoneurons die and their axons degenerate, denervation hypersensitivity develops and the sensitized fibers begin to fibrillate; thus as motoneuron disease develops, one often observes both fasciculation of motor units, irritated but still alive, and fibrillation of fibers sensitized by denervation. Fibrillation is detectable by electromyography, *i.e.,* by a recording of muscle action potentials through needle electrodes inserted into the muscle (Fig. 6–14). Fibrillary potentials are random and asynchronous and range from 10 to 200 μV in amplitude and from 1 to 2 msec in duration. Potentials produced by fasciculations are larger, ranging from 2 to 6 mV, and usually longer, ranging from 5 to 8 msec. As the disease progresses, denervated muscle fibers eventually lose their hypersensitivity, and unless rein-

TABLE 6–3. Neuromuscular Diseases

I. Diseases affecting motoneurons.
  a. Alteration of excitability or conduction.
  b. Alteration of transmitter release.
II. Diseases affecting postjunctional end-plate membrane.
  a. Alteration of end-plate sensitivity to ACh.
III. Diseases affecting the muscle.
  a. Alteration of excitability or conductivity of muscle membrane.
  b. Alteration of contractile mechanism.

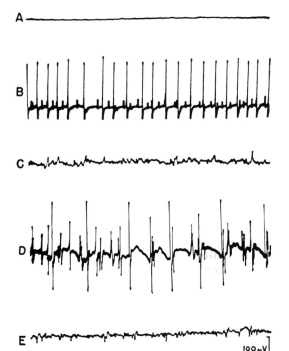

Figure 6–14. Normal and abnormal electromyograms recorded with needle electrodes inserted into various muscles in monkeys. *A,* From relaxed biceps muscle of normal monkey. *B,* Same as *A,* except taken during voluntary contraction of biceps; three motor units are distinguishable. *C,* Fibrillation in gastrocnemius muscle denervated 6 months previously. *D,* Fasciculation in relaxed triceps muscle of monkey during acute poliomyelitis (14 days after inoculation and 2 days after onset of paralysis). *E,* Fibrillation in gastrocnemius muscle in monkey 6 months after onset of paralytic poliomyelitis. (From Fulton, ed., *Textbook of physiology,* Philadelphia, W. B. Saunders Co., 1955.)

nervation occurs they undergo *atrophy; i.e.,* the myofibrils shrink in size and indeed may eventually be replaced by connective tissue.

In poliomyelitis the damage to motoneurons is spotty, and hence not all motor units of affected muscles atrophy. Often the remaining units appear increased in size ("giant motor units"). It is likely that giant motor units result from reinnervation of denervated muscle fibers by sprouts from intact motor axons, which insert into their squad of muscle fibers some adjacent muscle fibers denervated by the disease. Because of the trophic action of nerve on muscle fibers, all the muscle fibers of giant motor units are histochemically alike.

A major aim of rehabilitative medicine in either motoneuron disease or motor axon disease is to prevent atrophy. Direct electrical stimulation of the muscle, even in short daily bouts, reduces atrophy and fibrosis and either limits or prevents denervation hypersensitivity. If the axons have been interrupted but the motoneuron somata remain intact, the nerve fibers regenerate and may reestablish connection with the muscle fibers; when this occurs, denervation hypersensitivity disappears and function of the reinnervated fiber reverts to normal.

Defects of Transmitter Release

A classic example of defective transmitter release (type Ib in Table 6–3) is botulism, which we have already discussed. Another is the myasthenic syndrome, or "reverse myasthenia," a condition mysteriously associated with lung cancer and characterized by muscle weakness at the onset of exercise. With continuation of exercise the weakness diminishes, *i.e.,* the patient seems to "warm up" to maximum performance. This characteristic distinguishes the myasthenic syndrome from the classical *myasthenia gravis* (described later), in which muscle weakness intensifies with exercise. Recordings from muscle biopsies obtained from patients with inverse myasthenia indicate that the number and amplitude of miniature end-plate potentials are normal, suggesting that the vesicular content of transmitter is adequate and that the end-plate membrane sensitivity to ACh is unimpaired. However, the end-plate potential produced by a prejunctional action potential in the resting muscle is significantly smaller than normal and is often inadequate to generate a muscle action potential. This finding suggests that the number of vesicles released by the action potential is abnormally low.

The "warm-up" phenomenon is explained by the interaction of two opposing concomitants of iterative action of transmitter release: depression and facilitation. The former is due to transmitter depletion. Facilitation, an increasing efficiency of transmitter release with repetitive activity, may be partly due to posttetanic potentiation, although other factors probably operate. In normal muscles the interaction between depletion and facilitation tends to balance, and in any case it is not evident in gross function because each impulse liberates far more transmitter than is necessary to secure transmission. In the myasthenic syndrome the consequences of facilitation predominate because transmitter depletion is minimized by parsimonious release in the early stages of repetitive activity. Functional improvement appears as facilitation augments transmitter release to suprathreshold levels, and muscle fibers inadequately excited in the early stages are recruited into the squad of active fibers.

Decreased End-Plate Sensitivity

Examples of disorders of neuromuscular conduction due to toxic agents that bind the end-plate receptor of ACh include poisoning with curare and curarelike drugs. Such agents are often used as adjuncts to general anesthetics to provide maximal surgical relaxation. Certain snake venoms contain even more potent receptor binders, *e.g.*, cobra venom and α-bungarotoxin, derived from a poisonous Formosan snake. Although poisoning from these agents is uncommon in this country, they have been studied intensively because they provide valuable tools for investigation of the details of neuromuscular transmission in normal and disease states. For example, α-bungarotoxin, which binds irreversibly with the end-plate receptor protein for ACh, can be labeled with radioactive iodine, and muscle fibers incubated with labeled toxin can be examined by radioautographic techniques to locate the punctate sites of ACh receptors. In normal muscles the receptors are found only in the end-plate region, where radioautographs show a dense accumulation of black granules. In denervated muscles the black granules are found in great numbers in the extrajunctional regions of the fiber.

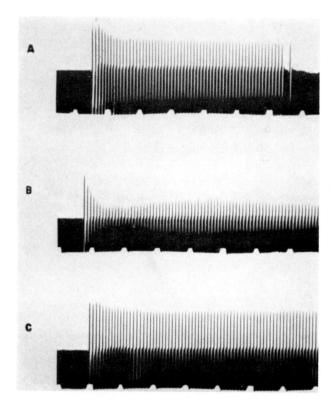

Figure 6–15. Muscle action potentials during repetitive stimulation of motor nerve in a patient with myasthenia gravis. The potentials are recorded from electrodes placed on the skin over the muscle so that each action potential represents the summed response of many individual motor units. Decline in amplitude therefore means that fewer muscle fibers are responding. *A,* Initial tetanus after rest. *B,* Second tetanus, 10 sec later. *C,* Third tetanus, 30 min after administration of prostigmine, an anticholinergic drug. Time at bottom of each record, 2 sec. (From Harvey and Masland, *Johns Hopk. Hosp., Bull.,* 1941, *69,* 1–13. © The Johns Hopkins University Press.)

The appearance of extrajunctional receptor sites corresponds temporally with the occurrence of denervation hypersensitivity and fibrillation, described earlier.

A relatively common neuromuscular disease recently shown to be associated with sparsity of junctional ACh receptors is *myasthenia gravis*. The disorder is characterized by a muscular weakness that progressively worsens with exercise to the point of near paralysis (Fig. 6–15). The patient often has normal strength on awakening in the morning but becomes progressively weaker as the day progresses. Some muscles (for example, the facial and extraocular muscles) are more vulnerable than others; a patient complaining of diplopia (double-vision) should always be suspected of myasthenia. Radioautographs of biopsied myasthenic muscles incubated with tagged α-bungarotoxin show a deficiency of end-plate ACh receptors. By refined biochemical treatment of α-bungarotoxin-bound receptors, the receptor protein can be isolated from tissues rich in ACh receptors; this protein injected into rabbits induces formation of antibodies against the protein, and the animals develop a syndrome muscle weakness resembling myasthenia gravis in the human.

Clinically, myasthenia gravis is treated effectively with anticholinesterase drugs (Prostigmin, or neostigmine), which potentiate the action of ACh. Indeed the diagnosis of myasthenia requires demonstration of an exercise-induced weakness that is reversed or ameliorated by anticholinesterase treatment.

Disturbances of Muscle Membrane Conduction

A disease of type IIIa (in Table 6–3) is myotonia, a condition in which voluntary effort produces an abnormally powerful and prolonged contraction. A patient releases any grasp on an object with great difficulty. In contrast to myasthenia, myotonia is most·pronounced after a period of rest; the patient's performance may improve from morning to evening. The disturbance appears to be due to an abnormally low threshold of the muscle fiber membrane so that it fires repetitively in response to the depolarization produced by ACh release (Fig. 6–16). That the muscle membrane is the site of the disturbances is indicated by the fact that direct electrical stimulation of denervated myotonic muscle causes prolonged repetitive firing and tetanic muscle contraction.

Studies of biopsied muscle from human patients and from a strain of goats that spontaneously develops the disease indi-

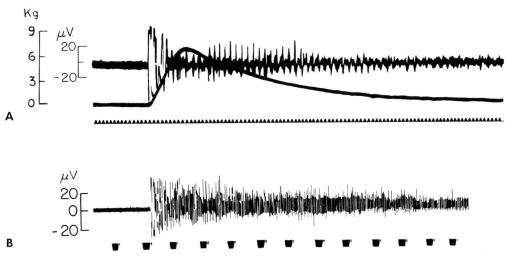

Figure 6–16. Electromyographic and tension recordings from the muscle of a myotonic goat. *A,* EMG and tension in response to a single maximal volley to motor nerve; time, 10 msec. *B,* EMG of denervated and curarized muscle of myotonic goat. Response elicited by mechanical tap on the muscle. (After Brown and Harvey, *Brain,* 1939, *62,* 341–363.)

cate that the muscle fiber membrane has an abnormally low permeability to Cl⁻ ions and thus an elevated resistance. Since $E = IR$, a transmembrane depolarizing current produces a larger voltage shift than normal when R is abnormally high; hence smaller than normal outward currents excite the myotonic muscle. The logical treatment for myotonia would be administration of a drug to restore Cl⁻ permeability to normal levels, but no such drug is known. Accordingly the treatment aims at elevating the threshold by systemic administration of local anesthetics (such as procaine), which block the voltage-sensitive Na⁺ and K⁺ channels of the Hodgkin cycle. Another agent that is effective for the same reasons is quinine.

Disturbances of the Contractile Mechanism

A disease affecting the contractile mechanism (type IIIb in Table 6–3) is progressive muscular dystrophy, in which the myofibrils undergo degeneration and disorganization. The disease strikes some fibers, leaving others intact, and the latter often undergo hypertrophy, producing a paradoxical state of weakness in muscles that are abnormally bulky.

Another condition affecting primarily the contractile mechanism is disuse atrophy, which may occur when a limb is immobilized in a plaster cast; the myofibrils of inactive muscles diminish in volume and are capable of less than normal tension development. A similar atrophy may occur when a muscle shortens abnormally, as happens after traumatic tenotomy; not only does the muscle become weak but it tends to become fixed at short length, a condition known as *contracture*. Denervated muscle fibers also atrophy, shorten, and develop contractures. Daily exercises to stretch such muscles alleviate the atrophy and contractures.

Still another disease affecting the contractile mechanism is McArdle's disease, in which exercise initiates painful muscle cramps. The shortened, cramped muscle shows little electromyographic activity; the cramp is therefore a contracture rather than a contraction, indicating a failure of

the contractile mechanism to relax. Such a failure might occur if Ca⁺⁺ were not promptly sequestered by the endoplasmic reticulum or if ATP were not available to break the bridge bonds. Analysis of muscle biopsy specimens from patients with McArdle's disease reveals a lack of phosphorylase, the enzyme that promotes breakdown of muscle glycogen to glucose-6-phosphate. Also, patients with the disease do not produce lactic acid on exercise, the acid being one of the end products of glycolysis. Since the glycolytic cycle is a major pathway for the synthesis of ATP, and since ATP is required both for breaking interfilamental bridges and for Ca⁺⁺ sequestration, it is tempting to postulate that a shortage of ATP is the immediate cause of the contracture. Surprisingly (and disappointingly), ATP levels seem to be near normal. Nevertheless, the knowledge of the specific enzyme deficit is a therapeutically useful datum; exercise tolerance in McArdle's disease is improved by administration of glucose, which can enter the glycolytic pathway beyond the phosphorylase step.

SMOOTH MUSCLE

Smooth muscle lacks the highly organized arrangement of contractile filaments that gives skeletal muscle its characteristic striated appearance. However, it has filaments similar to actin, and the actin will react with myosin of skeletal muscle to form actomyosin. It also contains troponin, tropomyosin, and myosin. The existence of thick filaments morphologically similar to those of skeletal muscle is controversial.

Smooth muscle is classified into two types: unitary (visceral) and multiunit. Unitary muscle is found mainly in visceral structures, *e.g.*, gut, uterus, and ureters, and it is characterized by "spontaneous" activity arising in pacemaker regions and spreading through the muscle mass almost as if it were a syncytium. Spontaneous activity does not depend on innervation, although neural influences may modulate and regulate pacemaker activity; in this respect unitary smooth muscle resembles cardiac muscle. Unitary muscle also contracts in response to stretch, and stretch-induced contraction is independent of innervation. Multiunit smooth muscle, exemplified by the pilomotor muscles, the nictitating membrane, the iris and ciliary muscles, and the larger blood vessels, responds only to neural impulses, and the basis of contraction is a motor unit, as in skeletal muscle. In electron micrographs unitary smooth muscle displays frequent "tight junctions" between adjacent muscle cells where the membranes appear to fuse. Tight junctions are believed to be areas of low electrical resistance permitting current flow from cell to cell. Multiunit muscles do not have tight junctions.

Smooth muscles are innervated by nerve fibers derived from the autonomic nervous system; some are innervated by both sympathetic and parasympathetic fibers, which may exert opposing actions on the muscle; others receive only a single supply. Discrete end-plates are lacking; nerve fibers run in grooves along smooth muscle cells, and vesicles occur in clusters. A single nerve fiber probably innervates several muscle fibers by these synapses *en passage*. Parasympathetic nerve fibers release norepinephrine. The effect of these transmitters varies from tissue to tissue and must be learned for individual effectors. For example, ACh inhibits and norepinephrine excites the cardiac pacemaker, but the effects are opposite on the smooth muscle of the gut. This emphasizes the dominance of the postjunctional receptor in determining transmitter action. It should also be noted that peripheral inhibition (*i.e.*, inhibition of effector cells) is possible with autonomic effector systems, in contradistinction to the exclusively excitatory effect of somatic motor fibers on skeletal muscle.

Finally, as in somatic motor endings, transmitter release from autonomic nerve endings supplying smooth muscle, heart muscle, and glands is Ca^{++}-dependent. Also, Ca^{++} is essential for the initiation of contraction in smooth muscle, although the means by which it is released and sequestered are not clear. Whatever the mechanism, it is more sluggish than that of the skeletal muscle, for the latency of contraction is 25 times longer. The duration of contraction is also much longer than in skeletal muscle, suggesting a slower sequestration process.

ADDITIONAL READING

General

Aidley, D. J. *The physiology of excitable cells.* Cambridge, Cambridge University Press, 1971, Chaps. 10–13.

Ebashi, S., Endo, M., and Ohtsuki, I. Control of muscle contraction. *Quart. Rev. Biophys.,* 1969, *2,* 351–384.

Wilkie, D. R. *Muscle.* London, Edward Arnold, Ltd., 1968.

Pathophysiology

Brody, I. A., Gerber, C. J., and Sidbury, J. B., Jr. Relaxing factor in McArdle's disease. *Neurology,* 1970, *20,* 555–558.

Brown, G. L., and Harvey, A. M. Congenital myotonia in the goat. *Brain,* 1939, *62,* 341–363.

Elmqvist, D. Neuromuscular transmission with special reference to myasthenia gravis. *Acta physiol. Scand.,* 1965, *64* (Suppl. 249), 1–34.

Layzer, R. B., and Rowland, L. P. Cramps. *New Engl. J. Med.,* 1971, *285,* 31–40.

Lipicky, R. J., Bryant, S. H., and Salmon, J. H. Cable parameters, sodium, potassium, chloride, and water content, and potassium efflux in isolated external intercostal muscle of normal volunteers and patients with myotonia congenita. *J. Clin. Invest.,* 1971, *50,* 2091–2103.

Mommaerts, W. F. H. M., Illingworth, B., Pearson, C. M., Guillory, R. J., and Seraydarian, K. A functional disorder of muscle associated with the absence of phosphorylase. *Proc. nat. Acad. Sci. (Wash.),* 1959, *45,* 791–797.

Rowland, L. P., Araki, S., and Carmel, P. Contracture in McArdle's disease. *Arch. Neurol.,* 1965, *13,* 541–544.

Rüdel, R., and Senges, J. Experimental myotonia in mammalian skeletal muscle: changes in membrane properties. *Pflügers Arch. ges. Physiol.,* 1972, *331,* 324–334.

CHAPTER 7

RECEPTORS

HARRY D. PATTON

GENERATOR POTENTIALS

SPECIFICITY OF RECEPTORS

MORPHOLOGICAL
DIFFERENTIATION OF
RECEPTORS

RECEPTORS AS
TRANSDUCERS

ADAPTATION IN
RECEPTORS:
   Velocity vs. Magnitude
    Signaling

PHASIC AND TONIC
RECEPTORS

MECHANISM OF
ADAPTATION

REPETITIVE FIRING OF
TONIC RECEPTORS

The foregoing chapters emphasize that the unique and distinctive property of excitable cells is their ability to respond to environmental changes by generating signals (action potentials) that can then propagate along their membranes to distant points. Action potentials transmitted over chains of neurons (by mechanisms discussed in the following chapter) are the coded language in which changes in the environment are signaled to the brain to make us aware of what is happening in the external world. Action potentials also constitute the messages that are transmitted from brain and spinal cord to muscles and glands, generating overt behavior. It is a basic axiom of physiology that everything we feel and everything we do is ultimately reducible to little puffs of sodium ion (Na^+) into, and little puffs of potassium ion (K^+) out of, myriads of nerve and muscle cells.

Chapter 5 emphasized that the underlying mechanism of generation of action potentials is the voltage-sensitive membrane permeability to Na^+ and to K^+ (Hodgkin cycle). To generate a signal in

an axon or in a muscle fiber, one need only depolarize the membrane by a threshold amount. The action potential, once generated, propagates itself by depolarizing adjacent regions of membrane (or nodes of Ranvier) without further dependence on the external stimulus that triggered the message. The *sine qua non* of neural action (and hence of awareness and behavioral response) is depolarization.

In the laboratory action potentials are most conveniently triggered by passage of an electrical current outward across the cell membrane to cause the requisite threshold depolarization. In nature, however, such stimuli are uncommon; intact animals respond to a variety of physical stimuli that are not in themselves electrical. Natural stimuli that produce action potentials and elicit both conscious awareness and behavioral responses are light (eye), mechanical deformation (ear, skin, muscles, tendons, joint capsules, vestibular apparatus), thermal changes (skin), and chemical changes (taste, smell).

Nonelectrical stimuli can generate action potentials because the terminals of dorsal root fibers ramifying in skin and deep structures have membranes specialized to depolarize to one or another kind of non-electrical natural stimulus. The depolarization causes outward current flow through the adjacent excitable membrane, triggers the Hodgkin cycle, and generates action potentials. These specialized terminals are called *receptors*, and the depolarization produced in them by the appropriate non-electrical stimulus is called a *generator potential*.*

GENERATOR POTENTIALS

The generator potential differs from the action potential in two important respects. First, it is purely *local* and incapable of propagation. Stated another way, the generator potential decrements rapidly with distance from the stimulated site, whereas the propagated action potential is of constant amplitude regardless of the distance between recording electrode and stimulus site. Secondly, the generator potential is *graded* in amplitude; *i.e.*, the amount of depolarization depends, through a considerable range, on the intensity of the stimulus. In contradistinction, the action potential is all-or-nothing in behavior, and its amplitude is independent of stimulus strength provided only that threshold is reached. In summary, the generator potential is stationary and graded; the action potential is propagated and all-or-nothing.

We have already seen that the peculiar properties of the action potential arise from the voltage sensitivity of the membrane permeability to Na^+ and K^+. Depolarization of the membrane to threshold so increases its Na^+ permeability that the influx of Na^+ swamps K^+ efflux and the membrane potential swings rapidly toward the Na^+ equilibrium potential, producing the rising limb of the action potential, the amplitude of which is independent of the stimulus. Obviously the smoothly graded

generator potential must depend upon some other mechanism. Another reason for believing that generator potentials and action potentials depend on different mechanisms is that the latter are readily blocked by the puffer-fish toxin, tetrodotoxin, whereas the former are little affected if at all. Tetrodotoxin-poisoned preparations are often employed when generator potentials need to be studied in isolation without the complication of superimposed action potentials.

Because the minute size of receptor terminals usually precludes accurate measurement of transmembrane potentials by intracellular recording, exploration of the mechanism of the generator potential is difficult. Because the generator potential is a depolarizing response, however, we can guess that an increase in Na^+ permeability is involved, for Na^+ is the major biological ion with an equilibrium potential on the "depolarized side" of the resting potential. It by no means follows that only Na^+ permeability is involved, for even if other ionic permeabilities, *e.g.*, chloride ion (Cl^-) and K^+, were increased, the membrane potential would seek a steady-state value somewhere between the equilibrium potentials of these ions.

In one invertebrate receptor that is sufficiently large to permit intracellular recording near the site of generator action, measurements suggest that the generator process moves the membrane potential toward a steady-state value of about 0 mV. One suggestion is that the generator mechanism causes a nonspecific leakiness of the membrane to Na^+, K^+, and Cl^-, a process that may be visualized as equivalent to opening pores, or leaks, in the receptor membrane that permit free passage of these ions. If enough such pores were created, the passive influx of Na^+ and Cl^- and passive efflux of K^+ would be expected to discharge the membrane voltage to zero. It is further postulated that the number of such pores opened is dependent on the strength of the stimulus. Since the greater the number of pores opened, the closer the membrane potential approaches the limiting steady-state value of zero, it follows that through the range from resting potential to zero, the amplitude of the generator potential is a function of stimu-

---

*There is one known clear exception to the rule that the generator potential is depolarizing: the retinal receptors (rods and cones) are hyperpolarized by light (see Chapter 16).

lus intensity. This is what is observed experimentally.

Although the relation between generator potential and stimulus intensity is direct, it is not linear. For a variety of receptors, generator potential amplitude is related to the log of stimulus intensity. Although there are reasons to expect deviations from linearity, the full explanation of the logarithmic relationship is not clear.

In summary, an appropriate natural stimulus applied to a receptor induces a graded depolarization of the receptor membrane. The current flows set up in adjacent membrane trigger the Hodgkin cycle and generate action potentials, which are all-or-nothing and propagated; this is illustrated diagrammatically in Figure 7–1. Because the generator potential obviously depends on an ionic mechanism quite different from that underlying the action potential, some physiologists have stoutly maintained that the two processes cannot be sustained by the same membrane and have distinguished between "electrically excitable" axon membrane and "nonelectrically excitable" receptor membrane. While it is obviously true that at the ultramicroscopic level exactly the same membrane locus cannot house both a Na^+-specific pore and a nonspecific pore, there is no reason why a patch of membrane might not vary sufficiently in molecular structure to permit close coexistence of different pores or channels.

For example, the exquisitely fine axon terminating in the Pacinian corpuscle, a mammalian mechanoreceptor, conducts action potentials to its tip, somewhat reluctantly and unreliably because of its small size and high internal resistance, but with sufficient clarity to demonstrate that the terminal membrane is capable of sustaining all-or-nothing threshold responses

as well as graded, local generator responses. Conversely, axons far removed from the site of normally occurring generator action respond to mechanical stimuli by graded depolarizations and conductance changes that are qualitatively similar to generator potentials of mechanoreceptors. Measurable mechanically elicited depolarizations of axons require greater displacements than do the terminals, presumably because axons have larger diameters than do terminals and hence require more displacement to stretch the membrane, a process thought to initiate the depolarization. For the Pacinian corpuscle, then, it does not seem necessary to postulate different kinds of membranes; the differences in behavior are satisfactorily explained solely on the basis of axon size. For other receptors it is less clear whether the same membrane can support both generator processes and all-or-nothing processes.

SPECIFICITY OF RECEPTORS

Although it has not been explicitly stated above, receptors are markedly selective in their responsiveness to physical stimuli. Specificity has been well documented in records taken from single axons while the receptors they supply are subjected to various kinds of stimuli. Such experiments demonstrate a striking lack of promiscuity in receptors; each responds most readily to one or another stimulus, while displaying relative indifference to other stimuli. For example, the Pacinian corpuscle is exquisitely sensitive to minute mechanical distortion (0.2 to 0.5 μm) but is not responsive to extreme thermal stimuli. Other receptors appear to be indifferent to mechanical stimuli but discharge readily to thermal stimuli above

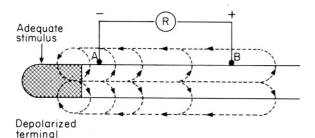

Adequate stimulus

Depolarized terminal

Figure 7–1. Diagram of receptor illustrating current flows in axon set up by generator depolarization in receptor terminal (*shaded*). Extracellular electrodes at *A* and *B* record generator potential. Note that current flow through axon membrane is outward, *i.e.*, depolarizing. (From Ruch and Patton, *Physiology and biophysics,* Philadelphia, W. B. Saunders Co., 1965.)

(warm receptors) or below (cold receptors) skin temperature. Even the nociceptors, endings that respond only to intense stimuli causing tissue damage, are often selectively sensitive; some respond to damaging mechanical stimuli (pinching, crushing) but not to damaging intensities of heat, cold, or irritating chemical agents.

The natural stimulus to which a receptor responds most readily is called the *adequate stimulus* for that receptor. It should be emphasized that the selectivity of receptors is relative; *i.e.*, the adequate stimulus is one to which the receptor responds most readily, not the only stimulus to which it will respond. A few receptors appear to have no clear adequate stimulus; cutaneous nociceptors innervated by unmyelinated afferent fibers appear to respond with equal ease to damaging thermal, mechanical, or chemical stimuli. Tissue damage, rather than the agent of cell destruction, appears to constitute the adequate stimulus. A chemical agent released from damaged cells has been postulated to be the common adequate stimulus for these seemingly indiscriminate receptors. Other nociceptors innervated by small myelinated fibers are much more selective and respond only to damaging mechanical stimuli.

The selectivity of receptors determines what events in the external world are transmitted to the central nervous system for interpretation. Many physical events in the external world, *e.g.*, ultraviolet and infrared radiations, or very low and very high frequencies of atmospheric oscillations beyond the auditory threshold, neither reach our attention nor generate behavior, because we do not have receptors to detect them. All impressions of the external world are filtered through selective receptors.

MORPHOLOGICAL DIFFERENTIATION OF RECEPTORS

Afferent terminals display a rich morphological variation, ranging from the highly specialized and distinctive photoreceptors of the retina and the distinctive hair cells of the cochlea to the spirals, coils, or branching anastomotic networks of receptors in skin, muscle, tendons, and viscera. Some receptors are encased in distinctive connective tissue capsules and are thus readily identifiable with the microscope.

It is natural to seek correlations between morphological and functional features of receptors. For many receptors the exercise is rewarding. There can be little doubt that the multibranched ending in tendons, called the Golgi tendon organ, is the terminal that responds to mechanical stretch of the tendon, and that the fine fibers surrounding the base of cutaneous hairs constitute the receptors that respond physiologically to displacement of hair. The behavioral characteristics of such receptors can be safely predicted from morphological inspection, and vice versa. However, for many receptors functional specificity is not clearly labeled morphologically. Hairy skin responds selectively to movement of hairs, mechanical distortion (touch, pressure), warmth, cold, and noxious stimuli but contains only two morphologically different receptor types—those around hair follicles and undifferentiated anastomotic unmyelinated networks. One can only conclude that some "look-alike" receptors are nonetheless functionally different. This is not to say that functional differences have no structural correlates. The significant structural differences underlying receptor specificity are almost certainly at the molecular level and, hence, are not detectable by conventional microscopy.

RECEPTORS AS TRANSDUCERS

In engineering parlance an instrument that converts one form of energy into another is called a *transducer*. A common example is the photocell; it converts a light signal into an electrical signal that can be used to ring bells, open doors, switch lights on or off, or to perform other bits of useful magic. The photocell has been refined so that its electrical output is a highly faithful analog of its photic input; *i.e.*, its output is linearly related to the intensity of, and reflects accurately the time course of, the light signal.

Receptors behave as transducers although, as will be discussed later, they differ in analog accuracy. For the moment we will consider the muscle-stretch receptor, one of the better analog transducers. This receptor consists of the unmyelinated terminal of an afferent axon wrapped helically around a small bundle of special muscle fibers. When the muscle fibers are stretched, the coils are distorted, and this produces a generator depolarization that varies in magnitude with amount of stretch. It has already been mentioned that the relation between stimulus (stretch) and output (depolarization) is logarithmic rather than linear, but otherwise the stretch receptor performs a function comparable to that of the photocell; *i.e.*, it converts one form of energy (muscle stretch) into another (electrical). If the stretch is imparted slowly, the output is a reasonably accurate analog of the input. Qualitatively other receptors behave similarly, transducing the adequate stimulus into an electrical depolarization.

The generator potential, being nonpropagated, is not *per se* capable of transmitting information to the central nervous system, but because it depolarizes the end-ing, it can generate action potentials that propagate centrally. It is these conducted signals that reach the brain and spinal cord.

Again resorting to engineering jargon, we can describe the generator potential as an amplitude-modulated output, *i.e.*, one that responds to variation of input magnitude by varying amplitude of output. Action potentials, however, are all-or-nothing events and cannot reflect variance of stimulus strength by changes in amplitude. The axon signals the magnitude of the generator potential by repetitive firing, the *frequency* of action potentials increasing as the amplitude of the generator potential increases. This is a frequency-modulated process. For a variety of receptors, subjected to slowly applied adequate stimuli, it has been found that frequency of firing varies linearly with the amplitude of the generator potential, which in turn is related to the log of the stimulus intensity. Thus, the process by which external events are converted into the language of the nervous system comprises two steps: an amplitude-modulated relation between stimulus and generator process and a frequency-modulated relation between generator potential and conducted action potentials.

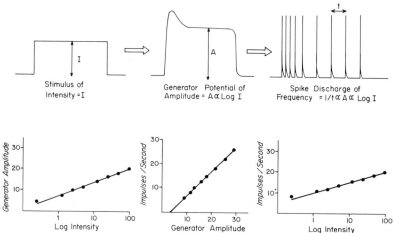

Figure 7–2. Diagram of steps in intensity coding in a tonic receptor. *Upper,* Stimulus produces generator potential shown here as it might be recorded in a receptor poisoned with tetrodotoxin for blockage of action potentials. In a normal receptor the generator potential induces repetitive firing; the figure on the right shows spikes that might be recorded from the axon at a distance from the receptor. *Lower,* Graphs relating stimulus intensity, generator potential amplitude, and action potential frequency in a photoreceptor. (From Ruch and Patton, *Physiology and biophysics,* Philadelphia, W. B. Saunders Co., 1965.)

The entire sequence is illustrated diagrammatically in the upper drawings of Figure 7–2. The time course of an adequate stimulus of intensity I is shown in the upper-left diagram. This produces a generator potential of amplitude A proportional to $log\ I$ (the overshoot of generator potential at the beginning will be discussed later). Normally, repetitive action potential spikes would be superimposed on the peak of the generator potential, but records of the sort shown can readily be obtained from receptors poisoned with tetrodotoxin, which blocks the Hodgkin regenerative mechanism but does not impair the generator mechanism. In the drawing on the right is illustrated what might be recorded from the axon of an unpoisoned preparation at a point too far central to the receptor for the generator potential to be recorded. Frequency of discharge is high during the initial period, then stabilizes at a value that is directly proportional to the amplitude of the generator potential, A, and to $log\ I$ of the adequate stimulus. The quantitative relationships between data obtained from a photoreceptor of a crab eye are portrayed in the graphs below.

ADAPTATION IN RECEPTORS:
Velocity vs. Magnitude Signaling

In Figure 7–2 the generator potential initially rises to a peak level and then subsides to a steady plateau value. To this extent, the generator potential is an imperfect analog of the square-wave stimulus. The figure on the right shows that the initial overshoot of the generator potential is faithfully reflected in the axon by a concurrent high-frequency discharge of action potentials that subsides to a steady frequency as the generator potential stabilizes.

The decrease in generator potential from peak to plateau during a prolonged stimulus is called *adaptation*. The same term is used to describe the decline of action potential frequency in the axon—a reasonable double usage since the latter change is a consequence of, and faithfully reflects, the adaptation of the generator potential. To measure the amount of adaptation of the generator potential, one measures from peak to plateau. To measure adaptation of action potential discharge, one measures decline of frequency from initial peak to stable plateau. The latter index of adaptation is the more commonly employed because action potentials are far easier to record than are generator potentials.

Thus far we have considered how receptors signal one characteristic of the adequate stimulus, *i.e.*, magnitude, or intensity. Another characteristic is velocity, or speed, of application of the stimulus. For example, with a stretch receptor, one can apply stretches of equal magnitude but at different rates, and he can examine how rate of stretch affects either the generator potential or the action potential frequency. Such experiments show that the rate of application of the stimulus has no significant effect on the plateau frequency but that it markedly affects the initial overshoot frequency. Stated another way, the amount of adaptation is a function of the velocity, but not of the magnitude, of the stimulus. This relationship is illustrated in Figure 7–3 for a joint capsule receptor that responds to passive flexion of the knee. The instantaneous frequencies of discharge are depicted when the knee was bent through an arc of 14 degrees at four different rates. For each the final plateau frequency was essentially the same, but the more rapid the movement, the greater the initial frequency. A similar relationship has been shown to obtain with a number of other receptor units.

It can be concluded then that receptors signal to the nervous system information about both the magnitude and velocity of the stimulus. How the nervous system uses the velocity information (if it does at all) is not clear. One can speculate, at least in an abstract way, how such information could be used in the programming of an appropriate motor response to an environmental change, the response being gauged to a predicted outcome derived from interpretation of rate of change. But speculations of this kind are not really very helpful without some concrete picture of how "frequency overshoots" regulate motor outputs.

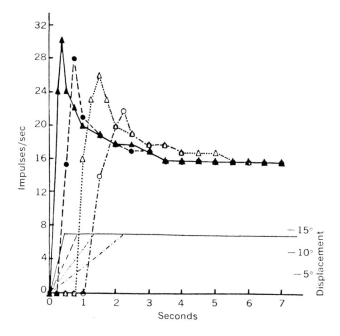

Figure 7–3. Graphs showing frequency of action potential discharge of a joint capsule receptor following moving the joint through an angle of 14 degrees (see lower graph). Four sets of data are shown, the rate of joint movement being variable. The plateau frequency is the same for all, but the initial frequency diminishes as speed of movement decreases in the following order: *filled triangles, filled circles, open triangles, open circles.* (From Boyd and Roberts, *J. Physiol.* [Lond.], 1953, *122,* 38–58.)

PHASIC AND TONIC RECEPTORS

Receptors vary widely in adaptation. So far we have considered only those receptors in which the process of adaptation leads to a stable, diminished generator potential and rate of firing. Such receptors are called *tonic receptors* because they fire continuously, or tonically, throughout the duration of the stimulus, the adaptive process modulating the frequency of discharge between two values, both of which are greater than zero. In other receptors the adaptive process is complete and the generator potential is a transient depolarization that rapidly wanes to zero even though the stimulus is maintained. Often cessation of the stimulus paradoxically leads to a new transient depolarization.

The axons of such receptors discharge one or two impulses at the onset of the stimulus and again one or two action potentials when the stimulus is removed but are silent in the interval between, even though the stimulus remains constant. Such receptors behave in "on-off" fashion and are called *phasic receptors* to emphasize their function in signaling transient rather than steady-state stimuli.*

Examples of phasic receptors are the Pacinian corpuscle and the hair receptor. Figure 7–4*A* shows the generator potentials elicited in a Pacinian corpuscle by a

---

*In older terminology, tonic and phasic receptors are often called *slowly adapting* and *rapidly adapting receptors.* Since the important distinction between the two is completeness, rather than speed, or adaptation, the terms *tonic* and *phasic* are preferred.

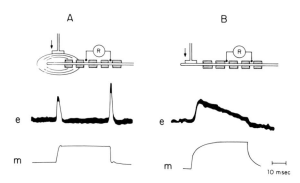

Figure 7–4. Generator potential in Pacinian corpuscle (*A*) before and (*B*) after removal of connective tissue capsule; *e,* generator potential; *m,* mechanical stimulus. Action potentials were blocked by drug treatment so that the generator potential could be recorded in isolation. (After Mendelson and Loewenstein, *Science,* 1964, *144,* 554–555.)

prolonged compression. Action potentials were blocked by appropriate drugs, otherwise one (or possibly two) action potentials would be superimposed on both the "on" and "off" generator potentials. Compare this behavior with that of the tonic receptor shown in Figure 7–2.

It is obvious that the generator potentials of phasic receptors are singularly poor analogs of the stimulus. Moreover, since the phasic receptor fires only when the stimulus is changing and not at all during unvaryingly maintained stimulation, it follows that the relationship between stimulus intensity and firing frequency described above for tonic receptors does not hold for phasic receptors. Indeed, such receptors fire repetitively only when the stimulus is oscillatory. In this circumstance the Pacinian corpuscle faithfully signals the *frequency* of the oscillatory stimulus through a range from approximately 40 to 1000 cycles per second. Intensity of the stimulus, however, determines the faithfulness of the entrainment. One-to-one following readily occurs with minimal displacements at 300 cycles per second, but reliable following with higher or lower frequencies requires more intense stimuli. It has been suggested that Pacinian corpuscles serve as seismoreceptors that are of biological value, not as earthquake detectors, but as signalers of the approach of a heavy-footed foe. In any case, it seems clear that the significance of firing frequency varies with different receptors.

MECHANISM OF ADAPTATION

At first thought one might suppose that the phenomenon of adaptation reveals some peculiar membrane property of the generator process. An alternative, however, is that adaptation may be either wholly or partly due to properties of tissues interposed between the stimulus and the receptor membrane.

The Pacinian corpuscle is an instance in point; the receptor terminal is encased in a complex, lamellated capsule through which the compressive force must be transmitted to distort the terminal. That such distortion is required to produce depolarization is indicated by experiments in which corpuscles were encased in a closed, fluid-filled chamber in which the pressure could be rapidly raised. In these circumstances the axon cannot be distorted, for the compressive force is uniformly distributed from all directions. Pressure elevations of 26-fold failed to produce a detectible generator potential, but outside the chamber asymmetrical pressure changes only $1/400$th of this produced clear depolarization. It seems that distortion of the ending from a roughly circular to a more nearly elliptical shape (thus increasing the circumference and stretching the membrane) is the adequate stimulus for the generator process. Since the distorting force must be transmitted to the sensitive terminal through the lamellated capsule, the physical properties of the latter may distort the force.

That this is indeed so is shown in Figure 7–4. On the left is shown the typical "on-off," adaptive response of an intact corpuscle to rapid compression. On the right the capsule has been carefully dissected away and a comparable compression applied to the naked ending, producing a generator potential that, although not a perfect analog of the stimulus, is nevertheless quite different from the "on-off" pattern in the intact preparation and resembles much more closely that of a tonic receptor. Thus it appears that the peculiar adaptive property of the Pacinian corpuscle is largely due to the physical properties of the capsule and is only partly due to intrinsic properties of the generator process.

A possible mechanism for the "on-off" behavior of the intact receptor is as follows. The lamellae of the capsule are filled with fluid, which moves sluggishly through the narrow interlaminar spaces. A force applied between two faces of the capsule is therefore initially transmitted directly to the terminal and flattens it, producing the "on response." Then, as the viscous fluid moves laterally, distending the elastic capsule at the sides, the pressure equalizes, the ending approaches its normal, nearly circular configuration, and the generator potential wanes. When the compressing force is removed, the elastic pressure from the sides due to distension of the capsule compresses the terminal from the sides, producing an "off-potential" until viscous movement of the fluid once again restores capsular shape and equalizes forces on the ending. It seems likely that the physical properties of transmitting tissues may play a similar role in determining the pattern of adaptation of other mechanoreceptors, whether tonic or phasic.

REPETITIVE FIRING OF TONIC RECEPTORS

In tonic receptors the second step of the transduction process is initiation of repetitive firing of the axon. As we have seen, the frequency of repetitive discharge of the axon is approximately directly proportional to the magnitude of the generator depolarization.

A simple explanation based on the recovery cycle of axons was first proposed by Adrian. In Chapter 5 it was pointed out that, for a brief time following the initiation of an action potential, the axon cannot be reexcited no matter how intense the stimulus; this is called the *absolute refractory period*. After the absolutely refractory period, the threshold returns to the resting level along an approximately exponential time course in accordance with the recovery of Na^+ activation; this period of elevated threshold is the *relatively refractory period*. The recovery curve following a single action potential at time zero is shown graphically in Figure 7–5.

Adrian's explanation was that if the generator potential depolarizes the axon to level x, a spike may be expected at time zero (x_1) and again at x_2 when the threshold has dropped along the curve to level x. The same process is repeated indefinitely as long as the generator potential maintains a depolarization at level x, and thus a regular sequence of spikes ($x_3 - x_4$) occurs. On the other hand, if the generator potential is smaller and depolarizes only to level y, the frequency of discharge is lower because a longer interval between each spike is required for the recovery process to reach the lower level, y.

This simple explanation of the mechanism of frequency-modulated signaling of stimulus intensity is attractive, but some discrepancies in the theory are immediately apparent. First, the theory predicts a nonlinear relationship between generator potential amplitude and action potential frequency rather than the linear relationship actually observed (see Figure 7–2). (Adrian did not have this information because generator potentials had not then been measured.) Secondly, in intracellular studies of repetitively discharging receptors, measurements of the membrane potential at which the spike is generated (firing level or threshold) indicate that the firing level increases only at relatively high intensities of stimulus and high frequencies of discharge. Through a considerable range of stimuli from moderate to low intensity, receptors discharge repetitively and regularly with no indication of elevated firing levels or thresholds. Hence something

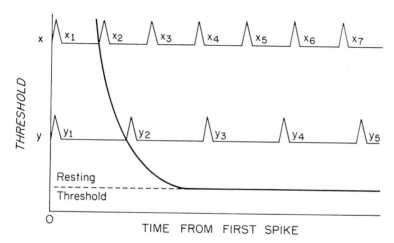

Figure 7–5. Diagram of Adrian's theory of repetitive firing of receptors. The curve shows the changes in threshold of an axon following generation of a single action potential at time zero. x_1 to x_7 show expected discharges if axon is subjected to a stable value, x. A lesser stable depolarization to y should produce action potentials y_1 to y_5 at a lower frequency.

other than the Adrian mechanism must be regulating repetitive firing through this range.

Intracellular records from receptors firing repetitively in response to invariant stimulation indicate that during each interspike interval the membrane depolarizes once again to the firing level and that the rate of depolarization is greater for strong stimuli than for weak ones. If the generator process consists of the creation of transmembrane channels through which Na^+, K^+, and Cl^- can pass freely and if the number of such pores or channels increases with stimulus intensity, it is easy to visualize why frequency increases with increasing intensity: a larger number of pores means that, after a spike, the membrane will be depolarized more rapidly to the firing level. With very intense stimuli the generator process may even curtail the postspike return of membrane potential to the resting level so that the interspike base line is closer to the firing level, a condition that further reduces the interspike interval required to depolarize to threshold. At very high intensities the depolarization process occurs so rapidly that it encroaches on the relatively refractory period; to this extent the Adrian mechanism participates in the frequency-intensity relationship.

ADDITIONAL READING

Goldman, D. E.   The transducer action of mechano-receptor membranes. *Cold Spr. Harb. Symp. quant. Biol.*, 1965, *30*, 59–68.

Gray, J. A. B.   Mechanical into electrical energy in certain mechanoreceptors. *Progr. Biophys.* 1959, *9*, 286–324.

Loewenstein, W. R.   Facets of a transducer process. *Cold Spr. Harb. Symp. quant. Biol.*, 1965, *30*, 29–43.

Patton, H. D.   Receptor mechanism. Chap. 4 in *Physiology and biophysics*, Ruch, T. C., and Patton, H. D., eds., Philadelphia, W. B. Saunders Co., 1965.

CHAPTER 8

SYNAPTIC TRANSMISSION

HARRY D. PATTON

THE QUESTION OF
ELECTRICAL SYNAPTIC
TRANSMISSION

CHEMICAL SYNAPTIC
TRANSMISSION

COMPARISON OF SYNAPTIC
AND NEUROMUSCULAR
TRANSMISSION

TRANSMISSION THROUGH
CHAINS OF NEURONS

TRANSMITTER STORAGE
AND RELEASE

POSTSYNAPTIC POTENTIALS

EXCITABILITY CHANGES
FOLLOWING SYNAPTIC
ACTION

THE INHIBITORY
TRANSMITTER

PRESYNAPTIC INHIBITION

In the foregoing chapter we discussed the mechanisms by which receptors signal to the central nervous system coded information about changes in the external world. These neural messages reach the spinal cord or brain via the dorsal roots or their cranial nerve counterparts. Before we become consciously aware of the external event, however, the information must be transmitted through the various ascending tracts of the spinal cord and brainstem to the cerebrum. Similarly, even the simplest adaptive motor response requires the transmission of information from receptors to the motoneurons controlling the muscles and glands. In this and the subsequent two chapters we will consider only the simplest adaptive motor responses, the spinal reflexes, leaving until later the more complicated mechanisms of sensation and "voluntary" motor behavior.

THE QUESTION OF ELECTRICAL SYNAPTIC TRANSMISSION

Transmission in the nervous system, unlike that in a telephone or telegraph system, does not employ continuous conductors; nerve impulses are relayed over chains of anatomically distinct neurons linked together by the apposition of the axon terminals of one cell to the dendrites or soma of another. These junctions are called *synapses.* Although the neuronal structure of the nervous system is universally accepted today, it was firmly established only as recently as the turn of the century, largely because of the monumental work of the Spanish neurohistologist Ramón y Cajal, who clearly demonstrated that each neuron is a separate cell, with no protoplasmic continuity at synaptic junctions. Today, when the "neuron doctrine" is so widely accepted that it is dismissed (as here) with a few brief words, it is amusing to read the passionately polemical literature of Cajal's day.

Since the synapse is a region of "contiguity, not continuity," where a narrow, but very real, gap separates the membranes of presynaptic and postsynaptic elements, it follows that the synapse is really a site of new impulse generation. Somehow the action potentials in the presynaptic terminals must generate a new action potential in the postsynaptic cell. Because conduction along the axon is accomplished by simple current flow, it is natural to guess that somehow current flow at the synaptic terminal depolarizes the postsynaptic cell. On further reflection, this "spark-plug" electrical theory of transmission is not easy to visualize. For example, the currents need to flow through two membranes, both the presynaptic and the postsynaptic, and since the intact membrane has a high electrical resistance, the likelihood of significant electrical coupling between the two elements is at best conjectural. The advent of intracellular recording made it possible to test this point directly, and the results of such experiments led to rejection of the electrical theory at least for studied mammalian synapses.

An exemplary experiment demonstrating the lack of significant electrical coupling between presynaptic and postsynaptic elements in a unique synaptic junction where both presynaptic and postsynaptic electrical activity can be recorded intracellularly at the site of synaptic transfer is shown in Figure 8–1. The upper trace in *B* shows the intracellularly recorded presynaptic action potential in the terminal; because the amplification was high, the peak of the spike was offscale. The lower trace shows the intracellular record from the postsynaptic element. During the presynaptic spike the membrane potential of the postsynaptic cell remained unaltered, indicating that no significant amount of current generated by the presynaptic spike had traversed the postsynaptic membrane. Indeed, it was not until the presynaptic spike had subsided and the membrane potential had returned to the resting level that the postsynaptic membrane began to depolarize. When this depolarization reached the threshold value, a postsynaptic action potential (its peak was also offscale) ensued.

The other two figures from the same experiment (*C* and *D*) show similar traces, except that they are frames taken during repetitive stimulation that fatigued the preparation, causing at first an increased synaptic delay between presynaptic and postsynaptic spikes, *C*, and subsequently failure of the postsynaptic depolarization to reach spike threshold in *D*. The initial,

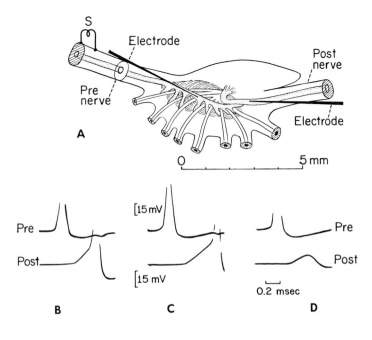

Figure 8–1. Intracellular records from presynaptic and postsynaptic elements in a simple invertebrate (squid) synapse. *A*, Diagram of stimulating and recording arrangement; synapse is axoaxonic. Both presynaptic and postsynaptic fibers are large, so that recording electrodes can be inserted to positions bracketing the synapse. *B*, Responses to single presynaptic shock through *S*. Postsynaptic spike arises from a slowly developing depolarization (EPSP), which begins only after presynaptic action potential has subsided. *C* and *D*, Single frames taken during a series of repetitive presynaptic stimuli, which "fatigue" the synapse, first decreasing the rate of rise of the EPSP and delaying the action potential in *C*, and later so decreasing EPSP that it fails to reach threshold in *D*. (*A*, After Bullock and Hagiwari, *J. gen. Physiol.*, 1957, *40*, 565–577. *C* and *D*, After Hagiwara and Tasaki, *J. Physiol.* [*Lond.*], 1958, *143*, 114–137.)

slow depolarization seen in isolation in *D* is called the *excitatory postsynaptic potential,* or EPSP; it will be discussed in more detail subsequently. For the moment, emphasis is placed on the virtual absence of electrical coupling across the synapse, a finding that conclusively eliminates the simple electrical hypothesis of synaptic transmission. In a few isolated instances intercellular coupling consistent with electrical transmission has been described in the mammalian nervous system, but most mammalian synapses appear to employ some other mechanism.

CHEMICAL SYNAPTIC TRANSMISSION

The alternative to the theory of electrical transmission is the *chemical hypothesis,* which postulates that the presynaptic action potential releases from the presynaptic terminals (or *synaptic knobs*) a pre-stored chemical transmitter agent. The transmitter then diffuses across the narrow (400-Å) synaptic cleft, attaches to postsynaptic receptor sites, and causes a change in permeability in the postsynaptic membrane, presumably by momentarily opening channels, or pores, permitting free exchange of ions. Assuming that these pores are nonselective and that they permit sodium (Na^+), potassium (K^+), and chloride (Cl^-) ions to pass freely along their electrochemical gradients, one would expect the membrane potential to seek a new steady-state value of approximately zero, *i.e.,* to move in a depolarizing direction. The EPSP is just such a potential; the synaptic delay (0.6 to 0.9 msec in mammals) is the time required for release, diffusion, and attachment of the transmitter to postsynaptic receptors.

The amplitude of the EPSP depends on the amount of transmitter released and consequently on the number of channels opened. If depolarization reaches threshold for the Hodgkin cycle, a postsynaptic spike is initiated, as in Figure 8–1*B*. Lesser amounts produce a subthreshold EPSP, as in Figure 8–1*D*, where repetitive stimulation either depleted presynaptic transmitter stores or in some way blocked the presynaptic receptors. During a sub-

threshold EPSP, the postsynaptic cell has a diminished electrical threshold; *i.e.,* it is easier to excite. The cell is said to be *facilitated,* and the process is called *facilitation.* The EPSP fades away in time as the transmitter is destroyed or diffuses away from the postsynaptic membrane through the synaptic gap.

COMPARISON OF SYNAPTIC AND NEUROMUSCULAR TRANSMISSION

The mechanism of synaptic transmission is reminiscent of neuromuscular transmission, where the chemical acetylcholine is released from motor nerve endings to produce the end-plate potential. Both the EPSP and the end-plate potential are *graded* processes, and their amplitudes depend on the amount of transmitter released. Both are local, *nonpropagated* responses and are recordable only at, or near, the site of transmitter action.

However, synaptic transmission differs from neuromuscular transmission in several important respects. First, whereas the neuromuscular transmitter is clearly acetylcholine, the central excitatory synaptic transmitter is not always acetylcholine. Neuropharmacological experiments suggest that there are several (perhaps many) central synaptic excitatory transmitters and that the agent varies with the synapse. Some likely candidates are various amino acids (glutamic, aspartic, cysteic), acetylcholine, and various catecholamines. At one synaptic site or another, these substances have been shown to mimic synaptic excitatory inputs when iontophoretically applied to the surface membranes of postsynaptic neurons. Detailed accounts of the complex field of synaptic pharmacology are to be found in the references listed at the end of this chapter.

Second, although the neuromuscular transmission system relies on a specific enzyme, acetylcholinesterase, to destroy the transmitter and limit the duration of the end-plate potential, most central synapses seem to rely on some other mechanism for breaking the transmitter receptor complex and returning the postsynaptic membrane potential to the resting level. In some synapses diffusion alone may account for the brief action of transmitter; in others reabsorption by the presynaptic terminal may limit its action.

Third, central synaptic transmission is far less secure than neuromuscular transmission. In normal circumstances neuromuscular transmission is obligatory, *i.e.*, the amount of transmitter liberated by a motor nerve impulse is always sufficient to produce an end-plate depolarization of threshold (or greater) magnitude. In central synapses subthreshold EPSP's and facilitation without discharge are common occurrences. This difference is partly related to an anatomical difference in the two junctions. At the neuromuscular junction, the relationship between nerve terminal and muscle fiber is usually one to one. In central synapses many presynaptic fibers converge on a single postsynaptic cell, encrusting its surface with synaptic knobs. The amount of transmitter released at each knob by a single impulse produces an EPSP of only 100 μV, which is far below threshold. Over a hundred individual knobs must be activated synchronously (or nearly so) to produce an EPSP of threshold magnitude in a spinal motoneuron. In other words, central synaptic transmission depends heavily on *summation* of action from many knobs, each releasing subliminal amounts of transmitter, whereas neuromuscular transmission depends on the massive release of a supraliminal quantity of transmitter from a single axon onto a single muscle fiber.

Finally, whereas the mammalian neuromuscular transmitter is always excitatory, some central presynaptic fibers liberate an inhibitory transmitter. The inhibitory transmitter makes the postsynaptic cell less excitable, *i.e.*, less easily discharged by excitatory fibers. This process, peculiar to central synapses, is called *inhibition*; it will be discussed in more detail below. For the moment you should merely register the fact that the behavior of a central neuron, *e.g.*, a spinal motoneuron, at any moment depends on the balance between its inputs from excitatory knobs and inhibitory knobs. The motoneuron is thus an integrator receiving "turn on" excitatory inputs and "turn off" inhibitory inputs from a variety of presynaptic channels. If

excitatory knobs dominate, their summed effects may depolarize the cell to threshold, and an action potential occurs.

Once generated, this action potential conducted through all of its branches ensures the obligatory contraction of all the constituent muscle fibers of the motor unit. If inhibitory knobs prevail, they prevent the summed EPSP's from reaching threshold, and the cell is quiescent. Since motoneurons are at all times subject to a variety of synaptic inputs, we may expect to find in a population of motoneurons a variety of states, ranging from active discharge through varying degrees of facilitation to deep depression of excitability. In the remainder of this chapter and in the chapters following we will discuss how this arrangement enables flexible and variable reflex adjustment to changing external conditions.

TRANSMISSION THROUGH CHAINS OF NEURONS

From the foregoing account it follows that transmission of messages through the nervous system involves mechanisms that are alternately electrical and chemical. In each individual neuron the electrical mechanism (Hodgkin cycle) is alone sufficient for generation and propagation of the message. At each point in the chain where one cell generates an action potential in another, release of a presynaptic chemical transmitter is required to initiate the requisite depolarization to trigger the Hodgkin cycle. This is true whether the postsynaptic element is a neurone, a skeletal or smooth muscle cell, or a glandular cell.

TRANSMITTER STORAGE AND RELEASE

We have already seen (Chap. 6) that in motor nerve endings the transmitter, acetylcholine, is manufactured and stored in discrete packets. It is reasonable to suppose that the tiny vesicles that jam the terminals (in electron micrographs) are packets of transmitter. In accordance with this hypothesis, those fractions of nerve muscle preparations obtained by density-gradient centrifugation that contain the synaptic vesicles have a high acetylcholine content. Synaptic knobs in the central nervous system are similarly characterized by the presence of round or ovoid vesicles, which are thought to be preformed packets of the appropriate transmitter, whatever it may be.

At both the neuromuscular junction and central synapses, a low-level, random release of transmitter occurs spontaneously in the absence of neural activity. An action potential in the terminal greatly accelerates the release rate of packets (vesicles?) of transmitter. At both sites the release mechanism requires calcium ion (Ca^{++}); probably the depolarization produced by the action potential increases Ca^{++} permeability of the terminal, and the resulting Ca^{++} influx, in some unknown way, triggers release of transmitter. Magnesium ions (Mg^{++}) block the release mechanism at both neuromuscular junction and central synapse, perhaps by competing with Ca^{++} for receptor sites essential to the release mechanism.

Finally, at both neuromuscular junction and central synapses, the amount of transmitter released appears to depend on the magnitude of the transient voltage shift induced by the action potential. Normally the action potential, being all-or-nothing, is of unvarying amplitude, but if the presynaptic fiber is hyperpolarized, the action potential is larger by the amount of the hyperpolarization, and the amount of transmitter released is dramatically increased. Hyperpolarization of terminals occurs following a period of high-frequency repetitive activity, presumably because such activity causes sufficient accumulation of intracellular sodium ions (Na^+) to elevate the concentration and stimulate increased Na^+ pumping. Relatively brief bouts of high-frequency presynaptic activity are followed by surprisingly prolonged periods (10 to 15 min) during which single action potentials release abnormally large quantities of transmitter. This phenomenon is called *posttetanic potentiation*. Later, we will describe situations in which presynaptic terminals are depolarized; then the amount of transmitter released by a nerve impulse is decreased (see Presynaptic Inhibition, below).

POSTSYNAPTIC POTENTIALS

We have already seen that the presynaptic release of excitatory transmitter induces, after a brief delay, a depolarizing response in the postsynaptic cell—the excitatory postsynaptic potential (EPSP). The EPSP resembles the generator potential of receptors and the end-plate potential in muscle in two ways; all three processes are *graded* and *nonpropagated*. One can thus be certain that the excitatory transmitter opens channels in the postsynaptic membrane that are distinct from the specific voltage-sensitive Na^+ channels responsible for the Hodgkin mechanism.

One way to explore the mechanism of the EPSP is to determine the steady-state value toward which the excitatory transmitter shifts the membrane. In some preparations this can be done by artificial adjustment of the membrane potential of the postsynaptic cell to varying levels by passage of current through the membrane with an intracellular electrode. One can then measure what influence the artificially adjusted "resting" membrane potential has on the shape and polarity of a synaptically evoked EPSP recorded through another intracellular electrode. The closer the membrane potential approaches the steady-state potential for the excitatory mechanism, the smaller should be the evoked EPSP. And if the membrane potential is artificially moved beyond this value the EPSP is expected to change polarity, for the transmitter should always shift the membrane potential toward the steady-state value, irrespective of the starting point.

Unfortunately, determination of the reversal level for the EPSP is fraught with numerous technical difficulties, partly because it is considerably removed from the resting potential so that rather large and potentially damaging artificial currents must be passed for the reversal level to be reached. Such experiments as have been performed suggest a reversal level near 0 mV. This is consistent with the hypothesis that the excitatory transmitter creates in the postsynaptic membrane nonspecific channels permitting Na^+, K^+, and Cl^- to pass more easily. It must be admitted, however, that this is more of a best guess than a clearly established fact.

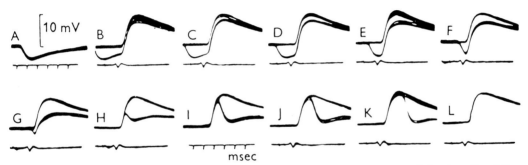

Figure 8–2. Postsynaptic potentials intracellularly recorded from a cat motoneuron following stimulation of inhibitory and excitatory presynaptic fibers. Upper traces (*A* to *F*) are intracellular recordings; lower traces (*G* to *L*) mark time of arrival of excitatory impulses (except in *A* and *I*, where time scales are substituted). *A*, IPSP resulting from inhibitory input; *L*, EPSP in the same cell after stimulation of excitatory presynaptic path. *B* to *K* show multiple superimposed traces, in half of which the excitatory fibers are stimulated in isolation. In the other half, inhibitory and excitatory fibers are stimulated in succession, the interval between the leading inhibitory stimulus and the excitatory stimulus gradually decreasing from *B* to *K*. The influence of the inhibitory process on the development of subsequent EPSP's can be seen by comparison of the two sets of records in each frame. (From Curtis and Eccles, *J. Physiol.* [*Lond.*], 1959, *145*, 529–546.)

The other response of mammalian neurons to presynaptic input occurs when inhibitory fibers are stimulated; this is called the *inhibitory postsynaptic potential*, or *IPSP*. A typical IPSP recorded in a mammalian motoneuron is shown in Figure 8–2*A*. Like the EPSP (Fig. 8–2*L*), the IPSP is a graded, nonpropagated response; it therefore reflects the transient establishment of ionic channels distinct from the voltage-sensitive Na$^+$ channels of the Hodgkin mechanism. It differs from the EPSP in polarity; at the normal resting potential for motoneurons, *viz.*, −70 mV, the IPSP is consistently a hyperpolarizing response; therefore, it must be the consequence of ionic channels distinct both from those underlying the action potential and from those underlying the EPSP.

Fortunately, it is easy to determine the reversal potential for the IPSP because it is close to the resting potential. When the postsynaptic cell is artificially hyperpolarized to various values from the resting level of −70 mV through −100 mV, the synaptically evoked IPSP first becomes smaller, and then at −80 mV it vanishes; at membrane potentials greater than −80 mV, the IPSP is a depolarizing rather than a hyperpolarizing response. This indicates that the inhibitory transmitter produces postsynaptic channels that drive the membrane potential toward a steady-state value of −80 mV.

Clearly the inhibitory channels are not Na$^+$ channels, for the Na$^+$ equilibrium potential of motoneurons is about +60 mV. The estimated K$^+$ equilibrium potential is about −90 mV, and Cl$^-$ is believed to be at equilibrium at the resting potential of −70 mV. The reversal level for the IPSP at −80 mV is thus midway between the equilibrium potentials of K$^+$ and Cl$^-$. Therefore, it is postulated that the inhibitory transmitter creates in the postsynaptic membrane channels that specifically permit easy transmembrane exchange of K$^+$ and Cl$^-$ ions. There is considerable additional support for this interpretation. The discriminatory selectivity of the inhibitory channels is based on size; K$^+$ and Cl$^-$ ions pass readily, whereas Na$^+$ ions are excluded because they have smaller hydrated sizes.

In summary, excitatory presynaptic action releases a synaptic transmitter that creates in the postsynaptic membrane channels permitting movement of Na$^+$, K$^+$, and Cl$^-$ along their respective electrochemical gradients. This moves the membrane potential toward zero, the magnitude of the change depending on the amount of transmitter liberated and the number of channels opened. If the depolarizing EPSP exceeds the threshold for triggering the Hodgkin cycle (about 10 mV depolarization), the postsynaptic cell discharges. Subthreshold EPSP's are accompanied by increased excitability (facilitation), which follows a time course similar to that of EPSP and fades to the resting level in 10 to 15 msec.

Inhibitory fibers, on the other hand, liberate a different transmitter (see below), which creates channels of low resistance specifically to the small ions K^+ and Cl^-. The membrane then seeks a steady-state level near -80 mV, which is midway between the equilibrium potentials of K^+ (-90 mV) and Cl^- (-70 mV). During this hyperpolarizing IPSP (10 to 15 msec) the excitability of the postsynaptic cell is decreased, for reasons that are discussed in the following section.

EXCITABILITY CHANGES FOLLOWING SYNAPTIC ACTION

One can test the excitability of motoneurons experimentally by passing currents from an intracellular microelectrode outward across the membrane. During an IPSP the amount of outward current required to depolarize the cell to threshold for the Hodgkin cycle increases. This increase is due partly to the hyperpolarization, which moves the membrane potential farther from the firing level. However, it is mainly due to the nature of the inhibitory process, which tends to "lock" the membrane potential near -80 mV and thus to oppose voltage shifts in the depolarizing direction. Because of this latter action an excitatory input produces less depolarization in an inhibited cell than in a resting cell. The intracellularly recorded interaction between EPSP's and IPSP's in a motoneuron is shown in Figure 8–2. When the inhibitory process precedes the peak of the EPSP, the latter is reduced in amplitude; when the IPS begins after the peak, the duration of the EPSP is drastically curtailed.

While the experiment shown in Figure 8–2 is a useful way to evaluate the interaction of excitatory and inhibitory processes, the experimental arrangement is unnatural in that the presynaptic action used to generate the processes is highly synchronous, i.e., the IPSP in A and the EPSP in L are the results of simultaneous stimulation of many inhibitory and excitatory fibers, respectively. In nature such synchronized inputs to motoneurons occur rarely if at all; normal presynaptic impulse traffic, both excitatory and inhibitory, is highly asynchronous, being generated by the repetitive firing of many receptors discharging at independently different frequencies, out of phase with one another. Thus normal motoneurons are subjected to a continuous higgledy-piggledy pitter-patter of both excitatory and inhibitory activity from myriads of synaptic knobs, each producing a far smaller effect than the massive, "cannonball" synchronous activity experimentally induced in Figure 8–2. The membrane potential (and excitability) of the cell is determined by the integrated balance of these inputs.

THE INHIBITORY TRANSMITTER

Because the underlying ionic mechanisms of the EPSP and the IPSP are so radically different, it is generally assumed that inhibitory knobs and excitatory knobs liberate different transmitters. Efforts to identify "the inhibitory transmitter" suggest that there may be several rather than one universal agent. At some synaptic junctions gamma-aminobutyric acid satisfactorily mimics the action of inhibitory impulses. On the other hand, for spinal motoneurons the amino acids glycine and alanine appear to be the candidates of choice. Students interested in synaptic transmitter pharmacology should consult more detailed accounts listed in the references.

Some drugs and chemical agents of clinical and toxicological importance owe their pharmacological notoriety to their abilities to alter the inhibitory process. For example, the analeptic alkaloid strychnine blocks the postsynaptic receptors for the inhibitory transmitter acting on spinal motoneurons. After strychnine administration, neither inhibitory volleys nor iontophoretic application of glycine to motoneurons produces the expected hyperpolarization and inhibition. Strychnine poisoning is characterized by severe convulsions, which are precipitated or exaggerated by any sudden stimulus, e.g., a loud noise, a flash of light, or a tap to the skin. The motoneurons, lacking the braking mechanism of inhibition, respond to synaptic inputs with abnormally intense repetitive discharge. The toxin of the tetanus bacillus, which causes lockjaw, also blocks inhibition but apparently by blocking release of the inhibitory transmitter. Tetanus toxin blocks synaptically evoked IPSP's but does not alter the hyperpolarization induced by applying glycine to motoneurons.

While in many instances the differences between excitatory and inhibitory synaptic actions are probably properly ascribable to differences in transmitters, it is equally possible that differences in postsynaptic receptor substances may sometimes determine the functional difference. For example, it has long been known that acetylcholine is excitatory at the neuromuscular junction but inhibitory in its action on the cardiac pacemaker. Recently it has been shown in an invertebrate preparation that a single presynaptic axon liberating acetylcholine at all of its endings induces EPSP's in some of its postsynaptic cells and IPSP's in others. Indeed in some cells receiving more than one knob from a single axon, both excitatory and inhibitory actions can be demonstrated; such variance seems to be due to local differences in postsynaptic receptor structure under different knobs derived from the same presynaptic axon.

PRESYNAPTIC INHIBITION

The inhibitory mechanism just described depends on a change in the postsynaptic cell induced by a transmitter liberated from presynaptic fibers; it is therefore known as *postsynaptic inhibition*. The hallmarks of postsynaptic inhibition are the following three postsynaptic changes: hyperpolarization (IPSP), decreased excitability (both to synaptic excitation and to artificially generated transmembrane current pulses), and decreased electrical resistance (due to increased permeability of the membrane to K^+ and Cl^-).

In another kind of inhibition the inhibitory input produces none of these changes in the postsynaptic cell but inhibits by reducing the amount of transmitter liberated from excitatory presynaptic endings and thus reducing to subthreshold levels the magnitude of the EPSP they produce. Inhibition that acts solely by reducing the effectiveness of excitatory presynaptic endings is called *presynaptic inhibition*. An example is illustrated in Figure 8–3. Note that the inhibitory input has no influence on either postsynaptic membrane potential or electrical excitability, but nevertheless occasions a reduction in the size of the EPSP induced by an excitatory input.

It has already been pointed out that hyperpolarization of synaptic endings increases the amount of transmitter liberated from the ending by an action potential. Conversely, if the terminal has a lower than normal resting potential when it is invaded by the action potential, the amount of transmitter released is less than normal. Accordingly it has been postulated that in presynaptic inhibition the inhibitory endings are actually excitatory knobs terminating, not on the postsynaptic cell, but on excitatory presynaptic endings. Synaptic knobs that seem to terminate on other synaptic knobs have been described by electron microscopists. It is postulated that activation of these knobs liberates a transmitter that produces a prolonged subthreshold depolarization of the knobs that are excitatory to the postsynaptic cell. When these excitatory terminals are depolarized, an action potential in them liberates onto the postsynaptic cell a subnormal quantity of transmitter, so that the ensuing EPSP is smaller than normal. Presynaptic inhibition thus acts by diminishing the efficacy of excitatory inputs to the postsynaptic cell.

Both presynaptic and postsynaptic inhibitory mechanisms may coexist at the same site. In general, however, the inhibitory action of dorsal root fibers on spinal motoneurons is predominantly postsynaptic. Presynaptic inhibition is more prominent at suprasegmental synaptic sites (*e.g.*, at the dorsal column nuclei, the thalamus, and the cerebral cortex).

The transmitter at presynaptic inhibitory endings is not known. Strychnine blocks postsynaptic inhibition but is strikingly ineffective in blocking presynaptic

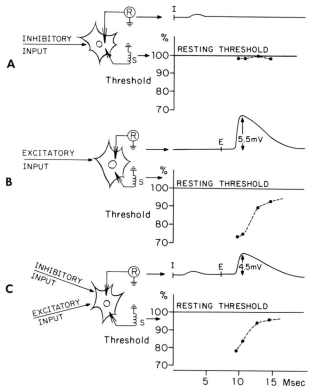

Figure 8–3. Distinctive features of presynaptic inhibition in a mammalian spinal cord. Two intracellular electrodes are inserted into the motoneuron, one (*R*) being used to record the transmembrane potential, the other (*S*) to pass stimulating currents outward through the membrane for measurements of electrical threshold of the cell.

A, Stimulation of the presynaptic inhibitory input in isolation fails to alter significantly either membrane potential or threshold of motoneuron. *B,* Stimulus to excitatory fibers in isolation at *E* causes EPSP of 5.5 mV and a 28 per cent decrease in threshold. *C,* Excitatory input at *E* is preceded by inhibitory stimulus at *I*. EPSP is reduced to 4.5 mV and threshold decrease is only 22 per cent. (From Ruch and Patton, *Physiology and biophysics,* Philadelphia, W. B. Saunders Co., 1965.)

inhibition, whereas the analeptic drug picrotoxin, even in subconvulsive doses, greatly reduces presynaptic, but not post-synaptic, inhibition. Conversely some general anesthetics, *e.g.,* barbiturates, potentiate presynaptic inhibition.

ADDITIONAL READING

Synaptic Physiology

Eccles, J. C. *The physiology of synapses.* Berlin, Springer-Verlag, 1964.

Eccles, J. C. *The physiology of nerve cells.* Baltimore, Johns Hopkins University Press, 1957.

Patton, H. D. Spinal reflexes and synaptic transmission. Chap. 6 in *Physiology and biophysics,* Ruch, T. C., and Patton, H. D., eds., Philadelphia, W. B. Saunders Co., 1965.

Synaptic Pharmacology

Cooper, J. R., Bloom, F. E., and Roth, R. H. *The biochemical basis of neuropharmacology.* New York, Oxford University Press, 1970.

Curtis, D. R. Central synaptic transmitters. Chap. 5 in *Basic mechanisms of the epilepsies,* Jasper, H., Ward, A. A., Jr., and Pope, A., eds., Boston, Little, Brown & Co., 1969.

McLennan, H. *Synaptic transmission.* Philadelphia, W. B. Saunders Co., 1970.

SPINAL REFLEX PATHWAYS

HARRY D. PATTON

In discussing the basic mechanisms of synaptic transmission in the foregoing chapter, we relied on experiments in which the activity of single neurons was intracellularly recorded during activation of various presynaptic pathways. Such experiments provide valuable insights into the intimate mechanisms of synaptic transmission. However, behavior is generated by the concerted activity of populations of neurons, and some important features of reflex function are best revealed by experiments that permit the activity of many cells to be recorded simultaneously.

EXTRACELLULAR MULTIUNIT RECORDING:
The Compound Action Potential

When a nerve trunk containing many axons is placed in contact with two record-

ing electrodes, as in Figure 9–1, and the nerve trunk is stimulated so that many of the constituent axons generate action potentials, a record is obtained that looks like the solid line on the right. When, as in diagram *1*, the action potentials have progressed as far as *A*, that point is negative to *B* since it is as yet quiescent, and the result is the rising phase of the solid line in the recording (arrow 1). In *2*, the active region has progressed to the right and depolarized both *A* and *B*, hence the recording device registers zero potential difference between the two points (arrow 2). In *3*, point *A* has repolarized, while *B* is still depolarized, so the recording instrument registers a swing in the opposite direction. The swing persists until the activity has progressed beyond *B* (to the right), when the recorder once again registers zero potential difference. The recorded activity is called a *compound action potential* because it reflects the compounded, or summed,

111

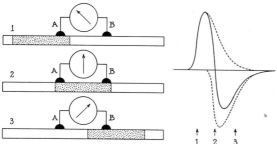

Figure 9–1. Diphasic extracellular recording of compound action potential in a nerve trunk containing many axons.

Left, Stippled area represents action potentials conducting from left to right at three instants of time in *1*, *2*, and *3*. In *1*, electrode *A* is negative to *B*; in *2*, *A* and *B* are equipotential; and in *3*, *B* is negative to *A*.

Right, Solid line is recorded diphasic action potential; *numbered arrows* indicate instantaneous differences in potential corresponding to the three stages of conduction at left. *Broken lines* represent electrical changes at each electrode; recorded potential is their algebraic sum. (From Ruch and Patton, *Physiology and biophysics,* Philadelphia, W. B. Saunders Co., 1965.)

effect of action potentials in many axons. When recorded as in Figure 9–1, the compound action potential is said to be *diphasically* recorded.

Diphasic recordings provide two pieces of information not immediately available from unitary intracellular records. First, a diphasic record clearly indicates that the underlying response is propagated. Secondly, it indicates the direction of propagation; for example, note that if the action potentials in Figure 9–1 proceeded from right to left (as shown they proceed from left to right), the polarity of the recording would be reversed.

Diphasic recording is, however, not often employed because usually one wishes to use the amplitude of the compound action potential as a measure of the number of active axons, and differential recording so distorts the record that potential amplitude is a poor gauge of the number of active axons. The nature of this distortion is indicated by the dotted traces in Figure 9–1. When the interelectrode distance is less than the wavelength of the action potentials, the changes under the two electrodes cancel one another and the resulting record is the algebraic sum of the actual potential changes. Since the region of an axon occupied at any one time by an action potential may be as much

as 5 to 6 cm, it is often difficult or impossible to make electrode placements that preclude cancellation and distortion.

One can avoid this difficulty by resorting to *monophasic recording,* as illustrated in Figure 9–2. The nerve trunk at *B* is crushed or otherwise damaged so that conduction is blocked. Because of the injury, point *B* is, in the resting state, negative to *A,* and an appropriate recording instrument registers a steady difference of potential, as shown in diagram *1.* When the compound action potential reaches *A,* as in *2,* the difference is obliterated. Thus, the change induced by the action potential is superimposed on the steady injury potential, and, since there is no conduction at *B,* the record is monophasic and cancellation is avoided. Monophasic (or "killed end") recording thus permits accurate registration of the compound action potential at *A.*

A recording of the compound action potential is mainly used as a gauge of the number and time of discharge of axons. In optimal circumstances the amplitude provides an approximate relative measure of the number of active axons, for the compound action potential represents the summed potentials arising from the active constituent axons and thus increases as additional axons are activated. There are

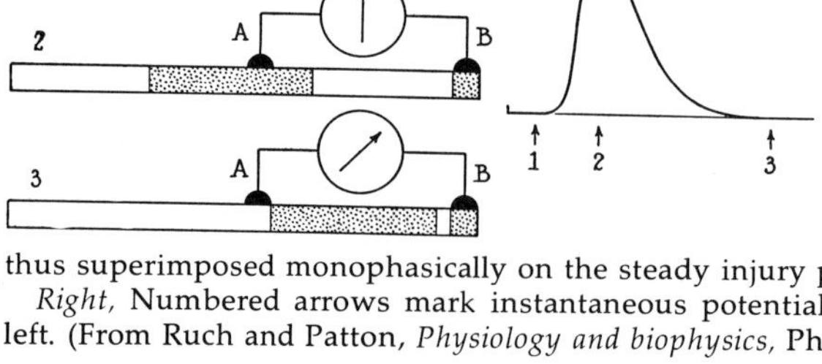

Figure 9–2. Monophasic extracellular recording of compound action potential from a nerve trunk containing many axons.

Left, Small stippled area under *B* indicates nerve trunk has been injured; consequently, a steady injury potential is recorded in *1, B* being negative to *A.* As action potential (*long stippled area*) progresses to *A* in *2, A* and *B* become equipotential. In *3,* action potential progresses beyond *A* (and shortly after is blocked) and *B* is once more negative to *A.* The action potential at *A* is thus superimposed monophasically on the steady injury potential.

Right, Numbered arrows mark instantaneous potentials recorded at three stages of conduction shown at left. (From Ruch and Patton, *Physiology and biophysics,* Philadelphia, W. B. Saunders Co., 1965.)

two limitations. First, although the transmembrane potential change during an action potential as measured with an intracellular electrode is at least approximately the same in all axons, the contribution of individual axons to an extracellularly recorded compound potential varies directly with axon diameter; *i.e.*, smaller axons contribute less than do larger ones. The error is minimized if one measures amplitudes of deflections resulting from axons of relatively uniform size. As we shall see, this requirement can often be satisfactorily approximated.

The second limitation is the requirement that the action potentials occur synchronously under the recording electrode. When different axons discharge at different times, their action potentials clearly will not sum but will be recorded as independent events separated in time. When discharges are asynchronous, areas under the tracing rather than amplitudes must be measured. Although this is feasible, it is tedious and time-consuming. A major factor causing asynchronous arrival of axon impulses at an electrode is the direct variation of conduction speed with axon diameter. In Chapter 5 we introduced a frequently used rule of thumb relating the conduction speed of myelinated mammalian axons to diameter, $S = 6D$, where S is the speed in meters per second and $D =$ the diameter (including myelin sheath) of axon. When the conduction distance between stimulating and recording electrodes is short, the com-

pound action potential is synchronous even in a mixed nerve trunk (containing fibers of different diameters). When the conduction distance is long, however, the compound potential becomes dispersed in time because the rapidly conducted action potentials of large axons arrive at the recording electrode earlier than do the slowly conducted contributions of small axons. Such a compound action potential is recorded as a series of elevations representing the activities in fibers of differing diameters (Fig. 9–3). The amplitude of each elevation depends on the numbers of active fibers of given size ranges, the amplitudes of individual constituent spikes (inversely related to diameter), and the synchrony of discharges.

Fiber size determines not only conduction velocity and spike amplitude (extracellularly recorded) but also threshold to externally applied electrical stimuli. The amount of transmembrane depolarization required to trigger the Hodgkin cycle does not vary significantly with fiber size, but the ease with which one can accomplish the requisite depolarization by passing current between two extracellularly placed electrodes is directly related to fiber diameter; *i.e.*, large fibers have lower thresholds than do small fibers. The reason is not hard to understand. For current from extracellular electrodes to alter membrane potential, it must flow in through the membrane at the anode and out at the cathode, where it causes depolarization. That part of the current flow that follows the low-

Figure 9–3. Compound action potential of saphenous nerve of cat recorded 3.5 cm from stimulus site. The two elevations, α and δ, represent the summed activity of fiber groups of different diameters and conduction speeds. Compare with the diameter spectrum of myelinated afferent axons in Figure 9–4. (Courtesy of Dr. H. S. Gasser.)

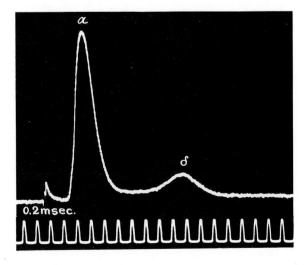

resistance extracellular pathway between the external electrodes has no effect on membrane potential, or excitability. Since a large axon has a lower resistance to longitudinal internal current flow than does a small axon, more current pursues the effective internal path in large axons and hence a smaller shock is required to force current against the internal resistance and produce the requisite transmembrane depolarization. Size-related differences in threshold to externally applied currents are thus not reflections of either differing membrane properties or intrinsic thresholds but rather are consequences of the external location of the electrodes. To this extent relation between size and threshold is an artifact, but it is nevertheless a convenient artifact for the experimentalist because, by careful adjustment of stimulus, he can excite large fibers to the exclusion of small ones. As stimulus strength to a nerve trunk is gradually increased, the population of excited fibers increases in accordance with the size principle, each increment in stimulus recruiting successively smaller axons.

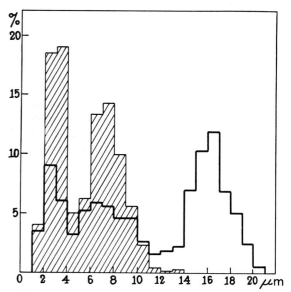

Figure 9–4. Histogram showing diameters of myelinated afferent fibers measured from cross sections of nerve trunks stained with osmic acid. *Heavy line,* diameters of afferent fibers in deep nerve trunk de-efferented by appropriate ventral root section. *Thin line and hatched area,* diameters of fibers in a cutaneous nerve. (From Ruch and Patton, *Physiology and biophysics,* Philadelphia, W. B. Saunders Co., 1965.)

HISTOLOGICAL COMPOSITION OF NERVE TRUNKS

Functionally the constituent nerve fibers of mixed peripheral nerve trunks are divided into afferent and efferent categories. The fiber compositions of these two functional components can be separately determined in nerves de-efferented by sectioning of the appropriate ventral roots and permitting the motor fibers to degenerate or in deafferented nerves in which dorsal root section degenerates the afferent fibers.

Morphologically peripheral nerve fibers, whether afferent or efferent, are divided into myelinated and unmyelinated categories. Myelinated fibers are usually viewed in sections stained with osmic acid since it selectively stains the myelin sheath black, producing in cross sections a black doughnut, the hole of which is the unstained central axon. Silver stains impregnate axis cylinders and hence reveal both myelinated and unmyelinated components.

The small (less than 1 μm in diameter), unmyelinated axons outnumber by three to four times the large (1 to 21 μm), myelinated axons among the afferent fibers. Unmyelinated motor axons are less frequent; they are all autonomic fibers supplying smooth muscle and glandular tissue.

In the diameter histogram of Figure 9–4 are compared the myelinated afferent fiber compositions of a cutaneous nerve trunk (*shaded*) and a deep nerve trunk (*unshaded, thick line*). Note that in each the diameter spectrum displays clear peaks, fibers of certain diameter being more numerous than others. The spectrum for the cutaneous nerve displays two clusters of myelinated fibers, one ranging from about 6 to 14 μm and the other from 1 to 6 μm. Other cutaneous nerve trunks show a similar distribution of diameters, except that the upper limit of the larger fibers may sometimes be as large as 17 or 18 μm. The large fibers (6 to 18 μm in diameter) are called cutaneous *alpha* fibers; the small (1 to 6 μm) are called cutaneous *delta* fibers. The more numerous unmyelinated

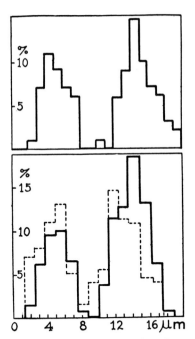

Figure 9–5. Diameter spectrum of myelinated efferent fibers. *Upper,* Data from a ventral root. *Lower,* Data from gastrocnemius nerve deafferented by degenerative dorsal root section.

Solid line, data from a section taken 50 mm from muscle; *dotted line,* from a section 8 mm from muscle. Shift of spectrum to left close to the muscle reflects branching of axons, the branches being smaller than parent axons. (From Ruch and Patton, *Physiology and biophysics,* W. B. Saunders Co., 1965.)

fibers (less than 1 μm) (not shown in the graph because it was prepared from measurements of axons in an osmic acid–stained nerve) are called *C fibers.*

The deep nerve trunk has a trimodal distribution of afferent fiber diameters. The largest fibers (12 to 21 μm) are called *Group I,* the intermediate cluster (6 to 12 μm) *Group II,* and the small myelinated group (1 to 6 μm) *Group III.* Deep nerve trunks also contain unmyelinated fibers, called either *Group IV* or *C fibers.*

The diameter distribution of myelinated efferent fibers in a deafferented mixed nerve is shown in Figure 9–5. The distribution is strikingly bimodal; the large fibers (8 to 20 μm) are called *alpha motor fibers* and the small fibers (1 to 7 μm) are called *gamma motor fibers.* Unmyelinated fibers, comprising sympathetic axons, are not shown.

SIMPLE SPINAL REFLEX PATTERNS

Many of the largest afferent fibers in deep nerve trunks, the Group I fibers, after entering the spinal cord through the dorsal roots, plunge uninterruptedly through the spinal gray matter and make direct synaptic contacts with motoneurons. The reflex path thus formed is called the *monosynaptic reflex,* or the *two-neuron arc.* Because the afferent fibers are large and rapidly conducting and because only one synaptic delay is incurred, the earliest discharge over the ventral root following a dorsal root volley is that ascribable to the monosynaptic reflex (see *a* in trace *E* of Figure 9–6). Both because the afferent fibers are reasonably homogeneous in diameter and because the number of synaptic relays is minimal, the ventral root compound action potential is synchronous and the number of motoneurons discharged monosynaptically can be satisfactorily gauged by measurement of the amplitude of the early reflex discharge.

Following the monosynaptic discharge, labeled *a* in Figure 9–6, trace *E,* is a prolonged asynchronous discharge of motoneurons, labeled *b.* This late discharge becomes more prominent as the stimulus strength is increased (*F* to *I*) and incorporates into the afferent volley more of the smaller-diameter fibers. The later discharges are mediated over *polysynaptic* channels, in which one or more intraspinal neurons, called *interneurons,* are intercalated between primary afferent fibers and the motoneurons. Interneurons contribute to the asynchrony of discharge because they are often arranged in circuits, which greatly prolong the bombardment of motoneurons even after the impulses in the primary afferent fibers have died out. These circuits are diagrammed in Figure 9–7. Such behavior is called reflex *after-discharge.*

The records of Figure 9–6 suggest that large-diameter afferent axons make monosynaptic connections, whereas smaller axons contribute only to polysynaptic reflex pathways. Since the largest afferent axons, the Group I fibers, are found only in deep nerves (*cf.* Fig. 9–4), one might

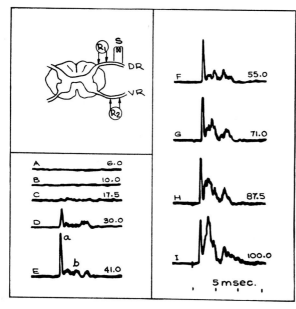

Figure 9–6. Reflex discharges elicited by dorsal root shocks of varying intensity. Single shocks of varying intensity were delivered to the dorsal root (*DR*) at *S*. Electrodes R_1 recorded dorsal root compound action potential; electrodes R_2 on ventral root (*VR*) recorded resultant reflex discharge. Traces *A* to *I* show reflex discharges at R_2 as shock strength was progressively increased. Numbers above traces, computed from R_1 recording, indicate number of afferent fibers excited expressed as a percentage of total fiber content of dorsal root. In *E*, *a* is the monosynaptic discharge and *b* the polysynaptic discharge. (After Lloyd, J. Neurophysiol., 1943, *6*, 111–120.)

guess that they are the source of the monosynaptic arc. The guess is easily verified. If the experiment of Figure 9–6 is repeated but with the stimulus applied, not to the dorsal root, but rather to the cut central end of a deep nerve trunk, a pure monosynaptic discharge is recorded from the ventral root, provided that the stimulus is kept sufficiently weak to excite only the large, low-threshold, Group I afferent fibers (Fig. 9–8*A*). When the stimulus to

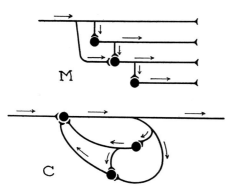

Figure 9–7. Two kinds of spinal interneuronal circuits that prolong delivery of impulses to motoneurons. *M*, Multiple-chain arrangement, in which variable numbers of synaptic delays cause staggered delivery of impulses at the terminals on the right. *C*, Closed-chain circuit, in which interneurons excited by afferent fiber at right can be reexcited through feedback paths. This is also called a *reverberating interneuronal chain*. (From Ruch and Patton, *Physiology and biophysics,* Philadelphia, W. B. Saunders Co., 1965.)

the deep nerve is increased to intensities capable of exciting Group II fibers or the Group III and Group IV (or C) fibers, the synchronous monosynaptic ventral root discharge is followed by the characteristic asynchronous polysynaptic discharge. That cutaneous afferent axons make no monosynaptic connections is indicated by experiments in which the central end of a cut cutaneous nerve trunk is stimulated; regardless of stimulus strength the only ventral root discharge is the delayed asynchronous pattern characteristic of polysynaptic pathways (Fig. 9–8 *B*). We conclude, therefore, that the monosynaptic reflex arc is fed exclusively by *Group I afferent fibers (12 to 21 μm), found only in deep mixed nerve trunks. Polysynaptic connections are made by smaller afferent axons of muscle nerves (Groups II, III, and IV) and all cutaneous afferent axons (alpha, delta, and C).*

Having identified the afferent limbs of the monosynaptic and polysynaptic channels, we turn next to the efferent distributions of these two kinds of reflex discharges to muscles. To do this, we record the reflex discharge, not from the ventral root, but from the nerve trunks carrying motor axons to the various muscles of the limbs. When the stimulus is applied to cutaneous, or small-diameter, deep afferent axons of the leg, the resultant polysynaptic discharge is found widely distributed in motor axons supplying ipsilateral *flexor muscles.* In the opposite leg,

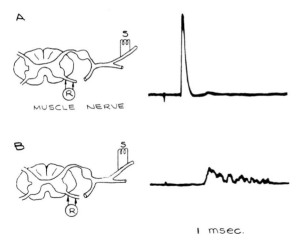

A

MUSCLE NERVE

B

| 1 msec. |

CUTANEOUS NERVE

Figure 9–8. Ventral root reflex discharges elicited by stimulation of the central end of a severed muscle nerve, *A,* and by similar stimulation of a cutaneous nerve trunk, *B.* In *A* the stimulus is barely strong enough to excite all the Group I fibers and a few Group II fibers, so a slight polysynaptic discharge is seen following the prominent monosynaptic spike. With weaker stimuli adequate only for Group I afferent axons, the discharge is purely monosynaptic. In contrast, stimulation of a cutaneous trunk elicits only a polysynaptic discharge, as in *B,* regardless of the strength of stimulus. (From Ruch and Patton, *Physiology and biophysics,* Philadelphia, W. B. Saunders Co., 1965.)

polysynaptic discharges occupy axons supplying *extensor* muscles.

On the other hand, when the stimulus is applied exclusively to Group I afferent fibers of muscle nerves, the efferent discharge is confined to axons supplying the muscle from which the afferent volley came. For example, stimulating Group I afferent fibers in the soleus nerve monosynaptically discharges only those motoneurons whose axons innervate the soleus muscle. Thus, the monosynaptic reflex arc is a highly focused system in contradistinction to the polysynaptic arcs, which diffusely activate ipsilateral flexor motoneurons and contralateral extensor motoneurons, whose cell bodies are located in relatively widely separated segments of the spinal cord. The introduction of interneurons into the arc thus serves not only to make motoneuron discharge prolonged and asynchronous, but also to diffuse the input into motoneuron populations located at different levels of the spinal cord and even into some on the opposite side.

In summary, then, the monosynaptic

arc is fed exclusively by the large Group I afferent fibers, found only in muscle nerves, and these discharge only those motoneurons whose efferent axons traverse the nerve trunk from which the afferent volley arises. The polysynaptic arcs are fed by smaller afferent axons of muscle nerves and by all cutaneous afferent axons, and they discharge ipsilateral flexor and contralateral extensor motoneurons.

DIVERGENCE AND CONVERGENCE: Fractionation of Postsynaptic Populations

Before discussing further the characteristics of monosynaptic and polysynaptic reflexes, we must digress momentarily to consider in detail two important anatomical features that have thus far been mentioned only in passing. The first describes the fate of individual primary afferent fibers on entering the spinal cord. Each fiber divides and subdivides, producing many terminal branches, which supply synaptic knobs to many postsynaptic neurons. This is called the *principle of divergence.* Because of divergence, no one dorsal root fiber contributes enough synaptic knobs to any one postsynaptic cell to secure its discharge, although each contributes to the innervation of many postsynaptic cells.

The second anatomical feature describes the innervation pattern from the postsynaptic side. Each postsynaptic cell receives synaptic knobs from many individual parent presynaptic fibers. This is called the *principle of convergence.* No one synaptic knob is capable of generating an EPSP of threshold amplitude; motoneuron discharge requires nearly synchronous activation of knobs arising from as many as 100 to 200 presynaptic fibers converging upon it.

The important point to glean from the foregoing paragraph is that synaptic transmission is not a simple cell-to-cell relay, as is often represented in diagrams. Rather, each postsynaptic cell receives information from many presynaptic inputs, and each presynaptic fiber provides synaptic knobs to many postsynaptic cells. Indeed, attempting to draw a realistic diagram is a frustrating exercise doomed to produce a confusing array of chicken tracks almost as complicated as the spinal cord itself!

Without using diagrams, then, visualize a population of postsynaptic cells receiving a volley of impulses from a number of presynaptic fibers; for simplicity assume that all the fibers are excitatory and that the knobs are synchronously activated. Some cells in the population receive enough synaptic knobs from the activated fibers to reach threshold; *i.e.*, in these cells the ensuing EPSP's depolarize them sufficiently to trigger the Hodgkin cycle and to elicit an action potential. Cells thus discharged are said to be in the *discharge zone* of the reflex. Other cells in the population receive some synaptic knobs from the activated fibers but too few to produce a discharge; these cells are occupied by subliminal EPSP's, which cause for some 12 to 15 msec a gradually waning increase of excitability corresponding to the time course of the EPSP. These cells, "nudged but not captured" by the presynaptic volley, are said to be the *subliminal fringe.*

An afferent volley of impulses thus creates, in the pool of postsynaptic cells it serves, two identifiable subpopulations— the discharge zone and the subliminal fringe. An afferent volley, no matter how large, never discharges the entire motoneuron population. The afferent volley "fractionates" the postsynaptic population.

If the number of presynaptic fibers activated is increased, some of the cells previously in the subliminal fringe are recruited into the discharge zone because the additional activated knobs now suffice to bring them to threshold. At the same time, the subliminal fringe grows because postsynaptic cells not receiving any knobs from fibers activated by the weak volley receive knobs from the fibers added to the volley by the stronger stimulus. Irrespective of the volley size, it always exerts on its postsynaptic pool a greater influence than is evidenced by the discharge zone alone; in addition it puts a cadre of postsynaptic cells in its subliminal fringe "on the alert," at least for some 12 to 15 msec.

With this in mind, we can attempt to visualize what happens in a pool, or population, of postsynaptic cells receiving normal afferent inputs from receptors. Some of these active fibers liberate excitatory

transmitter, others inhibitory transmitter, and impulses arrive at the knobs in a highly asynchronous pattern, each producing small (100 μV or less) EPSP's, either excitatory or inhibitory depending on the transmitter released. The membrane potential of each postsynaptic cell at any moment is determined by the summed influences of impulses arriving at that moment and over the previous 12 to 15 msec. In these circumstances, the composition of the discharge and subliminal populations may change with slight changes of input, and the responsibility for maintaining the motoneuron discharge underlying a reflex contraction of a muscle may rotate. Moreover, a shift in the input so that inhibitory fibers predominate may silence the population and thus relax a contracted muscle.

DETECTION OF FACILITATION AND INHIBITION

The features just described will be touched on again in the subsequent chapter when reflexly induced behavior in intact preparations is considered. For the moment, attention is directed specifically at the implications of convergence and divergence for experiments in which the central reflex connections of different afferent fibers are explored. Thus far we have relied exclusively on experiments in which *discharges* of ventral roots or of peripheral nerves are measured after synchronous activation of afferent fibers of different sizes and sources. Such experiments measure only the *discharge subpopulation* but provide no information concerning either subliminally excitatory or inhibitory influences of afferent fibers on postsynaptic cells.

To detect such actions we employ what is known as the *conditioning-testing technique.* We use a known excitatory input as the test volley and adjust its intensity so that a moderate discharge is produced, as measured by the size of the compound action potential of the ventral root. Then we gauge the influence of other afferent sources by setting up in them a conditioning volley that precedes the test volley by less than 15 msec. If the antecedent, conditioning volley is inhibitory, the number of motoneurons responding to the test volley is decreased and the ventral root compound potential is diminished. If the conditioning volley is subliminally excitatory, the test volley discharges a greater number of motoneurons than expected, and a larger (or facilitated) test response is recorded from the ventral root.

Facilitation is detectable only if the conditioning and testing fibers have some common elements in their respective subliminal fringes. If the conditioning volley has a discharge zone of its own, its subliminal effects can be gauged by simultaneous stimulation of the conditioning and testing pathways. If the resultant ventral root response is greater than the sums of the responses to stimulation of the two paths in isolation, we can conclude that the two volleys have in their respective subliminal fringes some common postsynaptic elements, and that these common elements are recruited into the discharge zone when both paths are activated.

Finally, it may be noted that by slightly modifying the conditioning-testing technique one can measure the time courses of excitatory and inhibitory influences. The only requirement is to vary the interval between conditioning and test volleys and to use the size of the test response as a measure of the amount of either facilitation or depression persisting at each interval of time following the conditioning volley. Conditioning volleys that make monosynaptic connections produce excitability changes with time courses that mimic reasonably closely the time courses of decay of unitary IPSP's and EPSP's because the conditioning volleys reach the motoneurons without the temporal dispersion caused by interneurons. Polysynaptic facilitation and inhibition curves have greater durations and latencies of onset and show peaks and remissions reflecting the reverberation of impulses through self-reexciting interneuronal circuits (see Figure 9–7).

FACILITATION AND INHIBITION IN SPINAL REFLEXES

Using the conditioning-testing technique, we can now proceed to examine in more detail the central connections of afferent fibers underlying monosynaptic and polysynaptic reflexes.

We have already seen that Group I afferent fibers monosynaptically discharge only their homonymous motoneurons, i.e., only the motoneurons supplying the muscle from which the afferent volley originates. Using the conditioning-testing technique, however, we can show that other motoneurons do receive *heteronymous* input from these same afferent fibers. These heteronymous connections, however, are far from promiscuous; they occur only between the afferent and efferent elements supplying muscles *acting at the same joint*. For example, Group I fibers from soleus (an ankle extensor) make no connections with motoneurons supplying either the quadriceps (a knee extensor) or the hamstring muscles (knee flexors), but they do make connections with motoneurons supplying other muscles acting at the ankle. The Group I fibers are the snobs of the afferent community, talking only to family members; family membership is determined by action at the same joint. Moreover, the kind of synaptic action varies with the kind of action the motoneurons exert upon the joint. Motoneurons that innervate synergistic muscles, i.e., muscles that act at the same joint and in the same way, have facilitatory (subliminally excitatory) monosynaptic interconnections with their respective Group I fibers. Motoneurons that innervate antagonistic muscles receive inhibitory interconnections from their respective Group I fibers.

An example will clarify this precise ordering of Group I reflex connections. Group I afferent fibers arising from gastrocnemius (ankle extensor) muscle make excitatory connections with the homonymous gastrocnemius motoneurons, some of which may be fired (discharge zone) and others merely facilitated (subliminal fringe). In addition, these same fibers make monosynaptic excitatory connections with motoneurons supplying soleus, a synergistic ankle extensor, but these connections are sparse so that the heteronymous synergistic motoneurons supplying soleus are only in the subliminal fringe. Finally, the influence of gastrocnemius Group I volleys on moto-

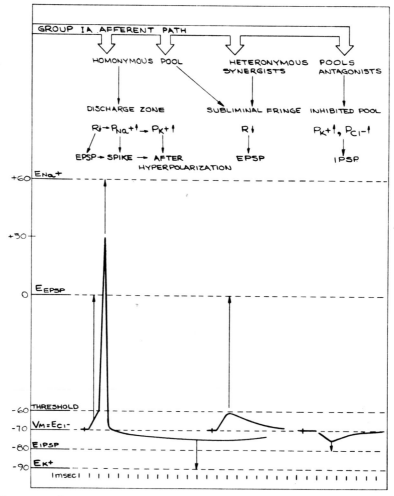

Figure 9–9. Summary of monosynaptic reflex connections and events. *Upper,* Functional connections of Group I afferent fibers and the changes in permeability that they exert on motoneurons; *R,* membrane resistance; *P,* permeability.

Lower, Intracellularly recorded responses and reversal potentials toward which each process tends to drive the membrane potential, as indicated by the arrows. *Vm,* resting membrane potential; E_{Na+}, E_{K+}, and E_{Cl-}, equilibrium potentials for the indicated ions: E_{IPSP} and E_{EPSP}, reversal potentials for IPSP and EPSP. (From Ruch and Patton, *Physiology and biophysics,* Philadelphia, W. B. Saunders Co., 1965.)

neurons supplying tibialis anterior, an antagonistic ankle flexor, is inhibitory. This completes the listing of connections of these afferent fibers: excitatory to homonymous motoneurons, subliminally excitatory to synergistic heteronymous motoneurons, and inhibitory to heteronymous antagonistic motoneurons. These relations are summarized and related to the material in Chapter 8 in Figure 9–9.

There is some reason to believe that whereas the excitatory paths are monosynaptic, the Group I inhibitory pathway is disynaptic; *i.e.,* it contains a single interneuron. This means that if a synchronous Group I afferent volley arrives at the spinal cord, its inhibitory influence on antagonistic motoneurons lags by approximately 0.5 to 1.0 msec (one synaptic delay) the onset of its excitatory influence on the homonymous and synergistic motoneurons. This delay can be detected in inhibitory curves derived from the conditioning-testing procedure; maximum inhibition occurs 0.5 msec after the arrival of the inhibitory impulses at the cord.

However, since normal inputs to motoneurons are highly asynchronous, the difference is of little significance; the putative inhibitory interneuron is more celebrated as a source of polemics between impassioned investigators than as a significant factor in spinal reflex regulation.

Next we consider the polysynaptic reflexes. It has already been pointed out that the smaller afferent fibers make rather diffuse polysynaptic excitatory connections with ipsilateral motoneurons supplying flexor muscles acting at all joints of the ipsilateral limb. On the contralateral side the excitatory connections are to extensor motoneurons. The conditioning-testing procedure permits us to determine that these same fibers inhibit the ipsilateral extensor motoneurons and the contralateral flexor motoneurons. As mentioned above, the time course of polysynaptic inhibition is prolonged and irregular in intensity, reflecting the role of interneurons in prolonging the delivery of impulses to the motoneurons beyond the duration of the primary afferent input.

THE LAW OF RECIPROCAL INNERVATION

Dissimilar as the monosynaptic and polysynaptic paths are, there is an important similarity in the pattern of their connections. In either instance *a volley of impulses that excites the motoneurons supplying a particular muscle also inhibits the motoneurons supplying antagonistic muscles.* This is called the *law of reciprocal innervation.* In the instance of the monosynaptic reflex, the excitatory connections are limited to the homonymous motoneurons, and inhibitory knobs are restricted to the motoneurons directly supplying antagonistic muscles. In the instance of the polysynaptic path, the excitatory connections are more diffuse, involving all the ipsilateral flexor and contralateral extensor motoneurons. Accordingly, the inhibitory connections are similarly diffuse, involving all the motoneurons supplying the antagonistic ipsilateral extensor and contralateral flexor muscles.

The utility of reciprocal innervation is intuitively clear: an input that generates muscle contraction by exciting the motoneurons at the same time "turns off" the motoneurons supplying opposing muscles. Thus, there are no conflicts in the command messages issuing from the spinal cord to the subservient muscles. Reciprocal innervation is not confined to the few reflex paths we have discussed; indeed, it appears to be a common principle of synaptic interrelation and occurs repeatedly in the nervous system.

ADDITIONAL READING

Laporte, Y., and Lloyd, D. P. C. Nature and significance of the reflex connections established by large afferent fibers of muscular origin. *Amer. J. Physiol.,* 1952, *169,* 609–621.

Lloyd, D. P. C. Neuron patterns controlling transmission of ipsilateral hind limb reflexes in cat. *J. Neurophysiol.,* 1943, 6:293–315.

Patton, H. D. Special properties of nerve trunks and tracts. Chap. 3 in *Physiology and biophysics,* Ruch, T. C., and Patton, H. D., eds., Philadelphia, W. B. Saunders Co., 1965.

Patton, H. D. Spinal reflexes and synaptic transmission. Chap. 6 in *Physiology and biophysics,* Ruch, T. C., and Patton, H. D., eds., Philadelphia, W. B. Saunders Co., 1965.

CHAPTER 10

REFLEX BEHAVIORAL PATTERNS

HARRY D. PATTON

Thus far we have dealt with reflex paths as functional anatomical thoroughfares through the spinal cord, with little concern for their respective roles in regulating behavior in the intact animal. In this chapter we will describe some simple behavioral patterns elicited by natural stimuli to the hind limbs of an animal in which the spinal cord has been transected above the lumbosacral segments that give rise to the spinal dorsal and ventral root supplies to the legs. In such a "spinal" preparation only the segmental reflex arcs remain intact in the decentralized spinal cord stump, a condition that assures that the observed behavior is not obligatorily dependent on neural connections with higher levels of the nervous system. Moreover, complete anesthesia prevails below the level of the transection, so that the investigator can with clear conscience freely employ even noxious stimuli without resorting to the use of anesthetic agents, which would depress the nervous system and alter behavior. Finally, having identified the various reflex behavioral patterns, we will attempt to assign them to the various pathways already described.

In man and apes, acute transection of the spinal cord results in severe depression of reflex transmission in the isolated segments below the transection, known as *spinal shock*. Spinal shock may last for a week or more and is so extreme that reflex responses, even to such intense stimuli as cutaneous burns, are completely obliterated. Primates are so dependent on the facilitatory inputs to the spinal cord from suprasegmental structures that their acute withdrawal paralyzes the intact segmental mechanisms. In time spinal shock wears off, for causes that are even more mysterious and obscure than those underlying the condition itself. One suggestion is that degeneration of descending fibers induces hypersensitivity of the spinal motoneurons and interneurons to transmitters in much the same way that denervated muscle develops numerous new receptors to acetylcholine, so that transmitters released from intact segmental reflex terminal knobs become more effective. An alternative hypothesis is that degeneration of some terminals stimulates the sprouting of new synaptic knobs from the segmental afferents, comparable to the sprouting of remaining intact fibers to reinnervate partially denervated muscle fibers (see Chapter 6).

In the cat and dog, spinal shock is far less prominent; apparently, in lower forms the motoneurons are less dependent on cerebral influence. Indeed, in the cat immediately after spinal transection, one can elicit several reflexes that in man are for a time held in complete abeyance by spinal shock.

THE FLEXION–CROSSED EXTENSION REFLEX

If a noxious stimulus is applied to the skin or deep structures of the leg in a "spinal" cat, a characteristic reflex adjustment occurs. (A noxious stimulus is one that either causes or threatens to cause tissue damage, *e.g.,* pinching, cutting, burning, or application of irritant chemicals.) The reflex movement is flexion of the stimulated limb, occasioned by contraction of the flexor muscles acting at all joints. The limb withdraws from the irritating stimulus; the reflex is said to be *nocifensive* (*i.e.,* defensive).

Palpation of the limb muscles indicates that the extensor muscles relax, whereas the flexor muscles contract, a finding suggesting that the extensor motoneurons are inhibited. Inhibition of extensor motoneurons is even more clearly demonstrated in electromyograms of extensor muscles; motor unit discharge ceases during reflex withdrawal. Such behavior accords with *the law of reciprocal innervation* (Chap. 9). In addition to ipsilateral flexion, extension of the contralateral leg is induced by noxious stimulation, a consequence of excita-

tion of extensor motoneurons and inhibition of flexor motoneurons in the contralateral ventral horn. This behavioral pattern is called the *crossed extension reflex*; it is best thought of not as a separate reflex but as a crossed component of the ipsilateral flexion reflex.

Sherrington first pointed out that the flexion reflex serves a protective, or nocifensor, function because the extremity is withdrawn from a damaging stimulus and thus injury is either curtailed or prevented. The crossed extension component of the reflex enables the opposite limb to bear the weight of the body while the ipsilateral limb forsakes its postural duty in self-defense. Thus the flexion–crossed extension pattern is a simple, automatically wired-in mechanism that provides the animal with a primitive "first-line" defense mechanism against injury without resultant postural collapse.

Although the flexion reflex is in a sense stereotyped and inflexible, it nevertheless varies somewhat in accord with the location of the noxious stimulus on the limb. This variance reflects mainly the intensity, timing, and sequence of activation of motoneurons supplying different flexor muscles, which in turn alter the speed, direction, and sequencing of the withdrawal movement in a way that is appropriate to provide protection from variously located stimuli. Such "local sign" permits appropriate withdrawal movements to protect against such variable threats as, for example, those occasioned by a burn to the dorsum of the foot and by stepping on a tack.

The pattern of the flexion–crossed extension reflex is immediately reminiscent of that of the polysynaptic pathways described in the preceding chapter. In addition, there is good evidence that many small myelinated afferent fibers (Group III and cutaneous delta) and unmyelinated fibers (C and Group IV), all of which feed polysynaptic arcs, terminate peripherally in receptors that respond selectively to noxious or damaging stimuli. For these reasons, it is widely accepted that the polysynaptic arcs fed by small myelinated and unmyelinated afferent fibers constitute the functional anatomical substrate of the flexion–crossed extension reflex.

The behavioral significance of the poly-synaptic paths fed by the large alpha cutaneous and Group II deep afferent fibers is a mystery. The former supply cutaneous tactile receptors, and the latter terminate in the secondary endings of muscle spindles. Since these receptors are clearly selectively activated by quite innocuous stimuli, they do not qualify for a role in the behavioral nocifensor flexion reflex. It has been suggested that they play a role in the bilateral alternating pattern of the flexion component of stepping, but the arguments are controversial, and the alpha cutaneous and Group II paths must be labeled as arcs without a clearly established behavioral correlate.

THE TENDON JERK

Another reflex that is easily elicited in the spinal animal is the tendon jerk. The stimulus is a brief tap on a muscle tendon to impart a brief stretch to the muscle. The reflex response is a brief twitch contraction of the stretched muscle. The reflex can be elicited in any muscle, and the reflex contraction is always confined to the stretched muscle. Electromyographic recording indicates that motor unit discharge in direct antagonists of the stretched muscle ceases during the tendon jerk, a sign that their motoneurons are inhibited. The reflex latency is singularly brief (19 to 24 msec for quadriceps in man), and there is no afterdischarge. All these considerations suggest that the tendon jerk is mediated by the monosynaptic arcs fed by the large Group I afferent fibers of muscle nerves. This suggestion was conclusively proved by Lloyd, who showed that the central delay of the tendon jerk is too brief to allow more than one synaptic delay.

The behavioral utility of the tendon jerk is not immediately apparent, since it is not easy to appreciate the biological value of a twitch contraction in a briefly stretched muscle. In fact, the tendon jerk is quasi-artifactual because of the unnaturally brief and sudden stimulus used to elicit it. Such a sudden, transient stretch excites many stretch receptors in the muscle simultaneously and generates in their axons a brief, synchronous volley of action potentials. These action potentials are conducted centrally by fibers of reasonably homogeneous diameters; therefore, they suffer little temporal dispersion and arrive at the motoneurons at about the same time. The motoneurons, momentarily flooded by a massive release of transmitter, discharge synchronously, and the resultant efferent volley causes a twitch contraction of the muscle.

With the possible exception of the repeated transient stretches that muscles undergo when we perform acrobatic antics on a pogo stick, they are never exposed to the kind of transient stretch occasioned by the neurologist's rubber tomahawk. Normally, stretching of muscle results from gravitational forces, which, as we stand erect, tend to buckle the joints and thus to stretch the muscles holding the limb extended. Such stretches are sustained rather than transient; unlike a tendon tap, they induce in the muscle stretch receptors a sustained, repetitive firing of impulses. The firing frequency of each receptor is determined jointly by the magnitude of stretch and its threshold, and so the excited receptors fire out of phase with one another. Accordingly, the input to the motoneuron pool is a sustained, asynchronous pitter-patter of excitatory impulses. The motoneuron discharge is similarly sustained and asynchronous, and so the resulting contraction is smooth and sustained, in striking contrast to the transient and biologically futile twitch of the tendon jerk.

Viewed in this way, the monosynaptic stretch reflex is revealed as the functional mechanism for standing upright. The tendency of gravitational forces to lengthen the antigravity extensor muscles is counterbalanced by the development of reflex contractile tension of the stretched muscle. If the stretching force is increased, as by sudden placement of a load on the shoulders, the stretch receptors fire at greater rates, driving the motoneurons at greater rates and increasing the contractile tension to balance the increased stretching load.

The stretch reflex thus provides a mechanism for maintaining the upright position under a variety of load conditions without requiring "conscious" effort to adjust. The tendon jerk is a phasic by-product of the reflex, seen only when an unnaturally brief and transient stretch is applied. As such, the tendon jerk *per se* has no biological value. It, however, provides an exceedingly useful indicator of moto-neuron excitability and of the integrity of reflex pathways in neurological patients. It should be remembered, however, that the synchronous spinal input evoked by tendon tap is a powerful stimulus to moto-neurons, and for this reason it may fail to reveal a moderate depression of reflex mechanisms. The careful neurologist al-ways tests reflex excitability in muscles not only by tapping the tendon but also by deliberately flexing and extending the appropriate joints; thus, he gauges the resistance of the muscles to both brief and sustained stretches.

The recognition of the significance of the tonic stretch reflex (or myotatic reflex), of which the tendon jerk is a phasic mani-festation, is mainly attributable to the studies of Sir Charles Sherrington during the late years of the last century. We will now trace the major steps in Sherrington's analysis to clarify and expand the sum-mary description just given.

DECEREBRATE RIGIDITY

Whereas the tendon jerk is easily elicited in the acute spinal preparation, the tonic stretch reflex is best studied in the decere-brate preparation. This is an animal in which the brainstem has been transected between the superior and inferior colliculi, and the cerebral hemispheres, basal ganglia, thalamus, and hypothalamus have been removed. By any standard, decere-bration is a radical neurosurgical proce-dure, but it is compatible with life because it leaves intact the medulla, in which the vital processes of respiration and main-tenance of blood pressure are integrated.

A striking feature of the decerebrate preparation, once the anesthetic (usually ether) employed during the operation has worn off, is its curiously rigid posture. All four extremities protrude in rigid exten-sion, and efforts of the observer to flex the limbs meet with resistance because the ex-tensor muscles contract vigorously when stretched. Although the decerebrate prep-aration neither rights itself nor stands voluntarily, the extensor posture is ade-quate to support the weight of the body. Once propped up and balanced, the decerebrate cat stands rigidly at attention. Postural changes are not confined to the limb musculature; the head is held erect, the jaw is rigidly clamped shut, and the tail stands erect, like the flagstaff of a yacht. Sherrington noted that the decerebrate posture is subserved by those muscles which, in the upright animal, resist the gravitational tendency of joints to collapse. He labeled the decerebrate posture as an exaggerated caricature of standing.

That the hyperactivity is confined to antigravity muscles is further substantiated by a study of the pattern of decerebrate rigidity in different species. In man a state similar to (but not identical with) decere-brate rigidity is a commonly encountered sequela of an apoplectic stroke due to either hemorrhage or infarction in the internal capsule. The immediate conse-quence of this vascular catastrophe (to be discussed in more detail in later chapters) is flaccid paralysis of the contralateral mus-culature, but in time this is replaced by hyperactive tendon jerks and a postural stance in which the leg is extended but the arm adducted at shoulder and flexed at elbow and wrist. Since man is bipedal, the antigravity muscles in the arm are not ex-tensors but rather the anatomical flexors of elbow and wrist. When decerebration is performed in the sloth, whose customary posture is hanging belly up from tree branches, the rigidity in all four extremi-ties is found in flexor muscles, for in the sloth's upside-down world the flexors are the antigravity muscles.

Sherrington postulated that decerebrate rigidity is due to an exaggeration, or hy-perexcitability, of the spinal reflex under-lying standing. We need not now explore in detail why decerebration increases stretch reflexes except to say that the sec-tion interrupts suprasegmental pathways that in the intact animal inhibit the spinal stretch reflex mechanism and obscure some of its properties; the subject of re-flex exaltation by release from inhibition is discussed in subsequent chapters dealing with spasticity in man. For the moment we will use the decerebrate cat as the ideal preparation in which to study the spinal stretch reflex at its liveliest.

Sherrington proved his hypothesis that decerebrate rigidity depends on segmental afferent input by showing that rigidity in the hind limb is promptly replaced by flaccid compliant paralysis when the lumbosacral dorsal roots are cut. He next attempted to locate the responsible receptors. Neither removal nor anesthetization of the skin of legs and feet altered the rigidity; hence the receptors are not cutaneous. Anesthetization of tendon and joint capsules was similarly ineffective in abolishing rigidity; therefore, these structures are not the sites of the responsible receptors. But when the tendon of a muscle was cut and pulled to stretch the muscle, active resistance was encountered. Taken collectively, these observations led Sherrington to postulate that the responsible receptors are muscle-length detectors lying either in the muscle or tendon and that their adequate stimulus is stretch, or lengthening, of the muscle.

To test this hypothesis Sherrington used an ingenious device known as the "fall table" (Fig. 10–1). The table top could be either raised or lowered when the aperture in the piston in the oil-filled dashpot was opened. The speed of descent of the elevated top was regulated by variation of the size of the aperture. The leg of an experimental animal was fixed to a stand on the table, and the cut tendon of the quadriceps muscle (an antigravity knee extensor) was attached to a tension-recording device (myograph) mounted on a support independent of the movable table top. When the aperture was opened, the table top dropped smoothly and stretched the muscle by an amount measured with another recorder. In this way it was possible to record the force developed in the muscle when it was extended at a known rate by a known amount.

Records obtained from an antigravity muscle of a decerebrate cat when it was stretched 8 mm in 1 sec are shown in Figure 10–2. The dotted line (T) shows the displacement of the table top (muscle stretch); the solid line (M) records the force developed. Part of this force was due to the viscoelastic properties of the muscle, which are unrelated to reflex contraction. The irrelevant passive viscoelastic component can be measured separately by

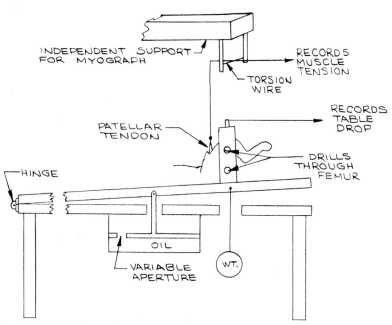

Figure 10–1. "Fall table" similar to that used by Sherrington to demonstrate the stretch reflex. (From Ruch and Patton, *Physiology and biophysics*, Philadelphia, W. B. Saunders Co., 1965.)

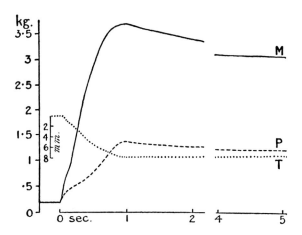

Figure 10–2. Stretch, or myotatic, reflex of the cat demonstrated with a "fall table." *M,* tension developed in innervated quadriceps muscle; *T,* relative elevation of table, which was dropped 8 mm; *P,* passive elastic tension developed by similar stretch after denervation of the muscle. Tension difference (*M − P*) represents active reflex tension. (From Liddell and Sherrington, *Proc. roy. Soc.,* 1924, *B96,* 212–242.)

repetition of the stretching procedure after denervation of the muscle; the dashed line (*P*) shows the tension in the paralyzed muscle. The difference between curves *M* and *P* therefore gives a measure of the force developed in the muscle by reflex contraction.

One can use the fall-table technique to demonstrate other features of the stretch reflex that follow logically from what has been said of the functional anatomy of reflex paths. For example, if, while an extensor muscle is stretched, an ipsilateral cutaneous nerve trunk is electrically stimulated, the tension drops promptly to the level of tension in the denervated muscle; the ipsilateral extensor neurons are inhibited by polysynaptic arcs fed by cutaneous fibers. Stretch reflex tension also drops when an antagonistic flexor muscle is concurrently stretched, for antagonistic muscles are reciprocally linked by their respective Group I afferent fibers.

It should be noted that the stretches imparted to muscles by the fall table are sustained and hence mimic the normal stretches elicited by gravitational forces much more closely than do the transient stretches induced by tendon taps. The input from stretch receptors is repetitive and asynchronous, and the motoneuron discharge is similarly repetitive and asynchronous; thus the reflex contraction is smooth and sustained.

In decerebrate preparations sustained stretch reflexes can be elicited by the fall-table technique only in antigravity muscles. Stretching a flexor muscle produces only a feeble and poorly sustained phasic contraction. The difference in response between extensor and flexor muscles is not a reflection of any difference in the peripheral reflex machinery of the two classes of muscles; flexor muscles are as richly endowed with stretch receptors and Group I fibers as extensor muscles. Moreover, phasic contractions to tendon tap (called "pluck" reflexes) can be evoked in flexor muscles even in decerebrate preparations in which sustained stretches fail to produce tonic stretch reflexes (a good demonstration, incidentally, of the immensely greater potency of synchronous inputs compared to asynchronous inputs). It seems likely, therefore, that the difference is either mainly or wholly due to decerebration; *i.e.,* the release from suprasegmental inhibition unequally favors the extensor reflexes.

STRETCH RECEPTORS OF MUSCLE AND TENDON

The receptors in muscles and tendons that respond tonically to stretch are of two kinds: Golgi tendon organs and muscle spindles. A Golgi tendon organ is illustrated in Figure 10–3. The afferent fibers that end in these receptors are large myelinated axons of Group I size (12 to 20 μm), and they lose their myelin as they penetrate the connective tissue sheath surrounding a bundle of tendon fibers and break up into a complex network closely investing the tendon fibrils. These receptors are most numerous at the mus-

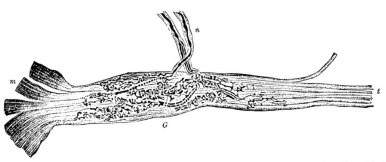

Figure 10–3. A Golgi tendon organ. At left, muscle fibers (m) end in tendon bundles (t) that extend to the right near the junction of muscle and tendon. Two nerve fibers (n) pass to the tendon and branch profusely between and around the tendon bundles, forming the end organ (G). (From Creed *et al., Reflex activity of the spinal cord,* London, Oxford University Press, 1932.)

culotendinous junction, but they also occur on the tendinous ends of muscle fibers that do not extend the full length of the muscle and that attach to the perimysium of adjacent muscle fibers. In fact even the tendinous ends of muscle spindles (see later) are often supplied with Golgi tendon endings. For this reason Golgi tendon organs are not completely eliminated by anesthetization of the tendon of the whole muscle. The tendon endings are displaced by the stretching of the tendon fibers and the displacement produces in them a tonic generator potential and repetitive discharge.

The muscle spindle is more complex (Fig. 10–4). It lies in the muscle belly and consists of seven or eight specialized muscle fibers, called *intrafusal fibers,* enclosed in a spindle-shaped connective tissue capsule. The tendinous ends of the intrafusal fibers project beyond the capsule and attach either to the muscle tendon or to the perimysium of adjacent regular, or *extrafusal,* muscle fibers, so that extension of the muscle stretches the spindle and its enclosed intrafusal fibers. The intrafusal fibers are striated at the two extremities but not in the central region; therefore, it is believed that the central region is noncontractile. The two striated poles receive small (2 to 7 μm in diameter) motor fibers, called either *gamma or fusimotor fibers.* The central noncontractile region is supplied with two kinds of afferent endings. One is supplied by Group I myelinated axons (12 to 20 μm); on penetrating the capsule they lose their myelin and form helical coils around the intrafusal fibers. They

are called either *primary or annulospiral endings.* The other receptor is supplied by Group II myelinated axons (6 to 12 μm). These also lose their myelin and terminate on either side of the annulospiral endings. They are called *secondary endings,* or, because their configuration suggested to some imaginative histologist a floral display, *flower-spray endings.* Both annulospiral and flower-spray endings are depolarized by stretching of the spindle, presumably by distortion of their delicate endings. Both are tonic receptors that discharge impulses repetitively during sustained stretch, the frequency of discharge varying with magnitude of stretch.

One can also excite both spindle endings by holding the muscle length fixed and stimulating the small fusimotor fibers supplying the two contractile extremities. Because these fibers are few and feeble, they produce no readily detectable tension in the muscle; but contraction of the poles stretches the central, noncontractile part of the intrafusal fibers, and the resulting distortion of the endings causes discharge. The role of fusimotor fibers will be discussed in more detail later.

SERIES AND PARALLEL ARRANGEMENT OF RECEPTORS

There are thus three stretch-sensitive elements in muscles and tendons. The flower spray endings can be eliminated as the source of the stretch reflex because they are innervated by Group II fibers, and these fibers make only polysynaptic

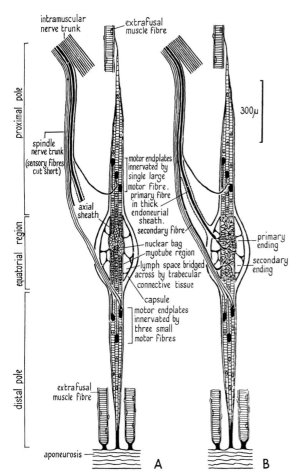

intramuscular
nerve trunk

extrafusal
muscle fibre

300μ

proximal pole

spindle
nerve trunk
(sensory fibres
cut short)

axial
sheath

motor endplates
innervated by
single large
motor fibre.
primary fibre
in thick
endoneurial
sheath.
secondary fibre

nuclear bag
myotube region
lymph space bridged
across by trabecular
connective tissue

capsule

motor endplates
innervated by
three small
motor fibres

primary
ending

secondary
ending

equatorial region

distal pole

extrafusal
muscle fibre

aponeurosis

A   **B**

Figure 10–4. The muscle spindle and its nerves. *A* shows only the motor fibers (fusimotor fibers) innervating the intrafusal fibers; *B* shows in addition the afferent fibers and their termination in the equatorial, or "nuclear-bag," region. (From Barker, *Quart. J. micr. Sci.*, 1948, *89,* 143–186.)

connections, whereas the stretch reflex is clearly monosynaptic. Choosing between the annulospiral spindle ending and the Golgi tendon organ is harder because both are innervated by Group I fibers.

A significant difference between spindle endings and tendon endings is illustrated in Figure 10–5. Spindle endings are situated in *parallel* with the extrafusal muscle fibers and therefore share with them the burden of passive stretch and fire, as shown. But if the extrafusal fibers contract, the spindles become slack, and discharge ceases. By contrast, the tendon organs are arranged in *series* with the con-

tractile elements of the muscle. Passive stretch, insofar as it elongates tendons, causes them to discharge as shown. But, if the tendon ends are fixed and the muscle contracts, the tendon organs are further distorted and the discharge is increased, not terminated as in the case of the spindle discharge. One can therefore distinguish spindle receptors from tendon receptors by their behavior during muscle contraction; the former pause and the latter accelerate. This difference in behavior during muscle contraction is the basis for dividing Group I afferent fibers into two subclasses: Group IA, supplying spindle endings, and Group IB, supplying tendon organs.

Another difference between the two receptors is that spindle endings have lower thresholds to passive stretch than do Golgi tendon organs. The discrepancy is due not to differences in sensitivity of the two endings but rather to differences in the physical properties of muscle and tendon. For both spindle and tendon organ the adequate stimulus is mechanical displacement of the sensitive terminals. Passive elongation of the tendon-muscle complex occurs mainly at the expense of the muscle, because of its high compliance relative to that of the tendon; *i.e.,* a stretch occasions much greater distortion of spindle endings than of tendon endings. When the tendon ends are fixed and the muscle contracts, the resulting shortening must perforce be at the expense of tendon length, and in these conditions tendon organs fire at relatively low tensions. Consequently, spindles are poor tension detectors and sensitive length detectors, whereas tendon organs are the opposite.

We now address ourselves to two further questions: (1) Which of the two receptors subserves the stretch reflex, and (2) what is the function of the other?

THE SILENT PERIOD OF THE TENDON JERK AND CLONUS

Fulton and Pi Suñer first pointed out that the parallel arrangement of muscle spindles and contractile elements (extrafusal fibers) provides an explanation of some distinctive features of the tendon

MUSCLE STRETCHED   MUSCLE CONTRACTED

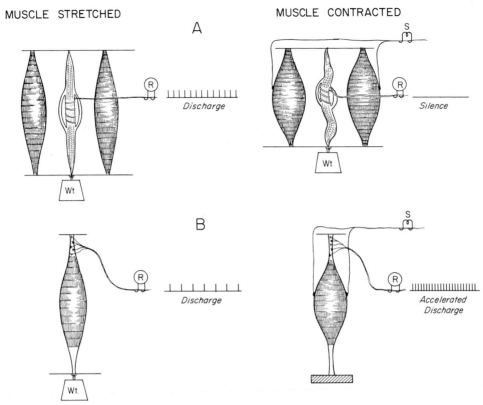

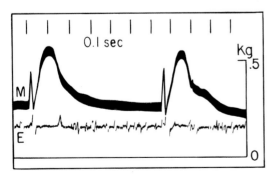

Figure 10–5. Relation of muscle spindles and tendon organs to muscle fibers. *A,* Spindle is arranged "in parallel" with muscle fibers so that muscle contraction slackens tension on spindle. *B,* Tendon organ is arranged "in series" with muscle fibers so that both passive and active contraction of muscle cause receptor to discharge. (From Ruch and Patton, *Physiology and biophysics,* Philadelphia, W. B. Saunders Co., 1965.)

jerk in both normal and spastic subjects and deduced that the annulospiral endings subserve the stretch reflex.

If, as in Figure 10–6, a muscle is moderately stretched, an asynchronous moto-

Figure 10–6. Recording of tension (*M*) and electromyogram (*E*) during tendon jerk in gastrocnemius muscle of decerebrate cat. Time, 100 msec. (After Creed *et al., Reflex activity of the spinal cord,* London, Oxford University Press, 1932.)

neuron discharge can be recorded by electromyographic electrodes placed over the muscle. If the tendon of the lightly stretched muscle is now sharply tapped, a synchronous discharge of motor units occurs, and this initiates a twitch. During the rising phase of the twitch the electromyogram becomes flat, an indication that during contraction the motoneurons cease to discharge. This "silent period" in the electromyogram persists throughout the development of reflex tension and is broken by a somewhat less prominent synchronous discharge when the twitch contraction is about half dissipated in relaxation. The resumption of motor unit discharge is often accompanied by a discernible hump, called the *myotatic appendage,* on the falling phase of the tension record (*second trace* in Figure 10–6).

In the spastic subject, the tension record displays a repeating series of myotatic appendages, so that the reflex response

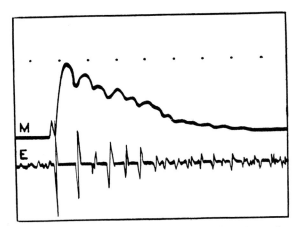

Figure 10–7. Clonus. Electrical (*E*) and mechanical (*M*) records of quadriceps muscle. A slight stretch previously applied produced a tonic reflex discharge in the muscle, as indicated by the asynchronous waves in *E*. A tap on the tendon, indicated by the first sharp deflection in *M*, elicited a brisk jerk reflex followed by a typical clonic discharge, evident in both *M* and *E*. Time (above), 100 msec. (After Denny-Brown, *Proc. roy. Soc.* 1929, *B104*, 252–301.)

to tendon tap is an oscillatory series of twitch contractions, each being grafted onto the tail of the preceding twitch (Fig. 10–7). The electromyogram reveals that each mechanical twitch is preceded by a synchronous motoneuron discharge and that each contractile response induces a silent period in the discharge. This oscillatory phenomenon is called *clonus*. Although a myotatic appendage, or hump, is often observed in the tension records of normal subjects, sustained clonus is a pathological sign and betokens hyperactivity of the stretch reflex mechanism.

Fulton and Pi Suñer proposed that the silent period, the myotatic appendage, and clonus are all understandable if the muscle spindles are the receptors responsible for the stretch reflex. Because the spindles are arranged in parallel with the contractile elements, they become slack when the muscle contracts, and cessation of afferent input silences the motoneurons. Motoneuron silence in turn leads to muscular relaxation, and this once more stretches the spindles so that they discharge again, reflexly initiating the myotatic appendage. In the spastic subject the stretch reflex mechanism is abnormally sensitive, and the process may be repeated indefinitely, each contraction turning off spindles (and

hence the motoneurons), and each resulting relaxation turning them on again—hence the phenomenon of clonus.

It should be noted that in Fulton and Pi Suñer's model the critical event underlying the oscillatory behavior in clonus is withdrawal of afferent input during contraction and restitution of that input during muscular relaxation. There is little doubt that the peculiar properties of the spindle receptors are partly responsible for clonus, but other observations persuasively suggest the participation of additional factors. For example, Denny-Brown discovered that a tendon tap causes electromyographic silence not only in the tapped muscle but also in others, even in some which act at remote joints. Such "joint-jumping" silencing of motoneurons cannot be due to withdrawal of input from spindle receptors because the axons supplying annulospiral endings make central connections only with the motoneurons supplying muscles acting (either synergistically or antagonistically) around a single joint. It can only be concluded that the electromyographic silence of motoneurons supplying remote muscles is due to an inhibitory input arising from the stretched muscle. Once such stretch-evoked inhibition is conceded, the possibility that the silent period in the stretched muscle is at least partly due to inhibition must also be acknowledged. In fact, there is good evidence, to be described in the following section, that such is the case and that the source of the inhibitory input is the Golgi tendon organ and the Group IB afferent fibers.

AUTOGENIC INHIBITION AND THE CLASP-KNIFE REFLEX

An attempt to flex the knee of either a decerebrate cat or of a spastic human meets with resistance because the hyperactive stretch reflex opposes the lengthening of the antigravity knee extensor muscles. If the examiner persists in bending the knee the resistance at first mounts further but then suddenly melts at an advanced point in the traverse, and the limb flexes readily. The behavior of the limb reminded Sherrington of that of a spring-loaded jackknife, so he called it the *clasp-knife reflex*. Electromyographic records show that during forced flexion of the joint, the stretched muscle displays mounting motor unit discharge until the clasp-knife reflex occurs, at which time discharge abruptly ceases; that is, the clasp-knife reflex brings into abeyance the motoneuron discharge driven by the spindles.

We noted earlier that because tendon organs are located on the relatively noncompliant tendons, they are less sensitive to passive stretch than are the spindles located in the bellies of the more compliant muscles. On the other hand, tendon organs are quite sensitive to muscle contraction when it occurs against an extending force, for in these circumstances even the stiff tendon fibrils are stretched. This explains why the clasp-knife reflex manifests itself after the stretch reflex has built up considerable contractile tension in the stretched muscle.

Sherrington postulated that the clasp-knife reflex protects the muscles and tendons from overload. Within limits reflex contractile tension in a muscle increases with increasing stretch, so that joints do not bend and upright posture is automatically maintained even with variation in the load. But carried to extremes, continued contraction against overwhelming stretching forces could lead to devastating tensions that could tear tendon and muscle. Sherrington postulated that the mounting discharge from tendon organs as contractile tension increases prevents this catastrophe; in the interests of tissue preservation the emergent clasp-knife reflex prudently quells the valiant but immoderate neural mechanism for upright posture when tension reaches ominous levels.

Laporte and Lloyd studied the synaptic connections of IB afferent fibers by electrophysiological methods and established that their reflex pathway is disynaptic; *i.e.*, it contains one interneuron between the IB fiber and motoneuron. They also found that the reciprocal connections of the clasp-knife reflex path are the functional reverse of those underlying the stretch, or myotatic, reflex. That is, IB fibers from a muscle establish disynaptic inhibitory connections with the motoneurons supplying that muscle and with those supplying synergists, but the fibers make disynaptic facilitatory connections with motoneurons supplying antagonistic muscles. For this reason, they rechristened the clasp-knife reflex the *inverse myotatic reflex*. An exception to the inverse relationship is that IB fibers from a given muscle make disynaptic inhibitory connections with some motoneurons supplying muscles acting at other joints; these connections presumably account for the silent period observed by Denny-Brown in remote muscles during a tendon jerk. The behavioral significance of such "joint-jumping" inhibition is unclear.

THE FUSIMOTOR SYSTEM

We have already noted that the two contractile poles of the intrafusal fibers receive motor fibers, called gamma, or fusimotor, fibers. Fusimotor fibers constitute a distinct cluster in the diameter spectrum of motor fibers, ranging from 2 to 7 μm, as compared to 8 to 20 μm for the alpha motor fibers that supply the regular extrafusal motor fibers (Fig. 10–8). Because of their small size, fusimotor fibers are excited only by electrical stimuli in excess of that required to excite all the alpha fibers.

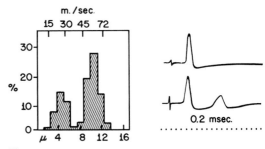

Figure 10–8. Diameter spectrum and compound action potential of motor fibers supplying soleus. *Left,* Note distinct bimodal distribution of fiber diameters. Velocity spectrum shown on upper ordinates.

Right, Upper trace, Compound action potential elicited by stimulus just maximal for large-diameter, rapidly conducting fibers. *Lower trace,* Stronger stimulus elicited a second deflection ascribable to activity in the small, slowly conducting fibers. (Histologic data after Eccles and Sherrington, *Proc. roy. Soc.,* 1930, *B106,* 326–357; electrical data after Kuffler et al., *J. Neurophysiol.,* 1951, *14,* 29–54.)

When the stimulus is increased beyond alpha intensity, the tension developed by the muscle shows no further increments, although the fusimotor fibers (which numerically constitute about one third of all motor fibers) are added to the volley. The reason is that the contraction of the tiny intrafusal muscle fibers resulting from fusimotor activation develops too little tension to add measurably to that produced by the more powerful extrafusal fibers. It is thus clear that the functional significance of the fusimotor system must be something other than development of tension between the two ends of the muscle.

Because fusimotor fibers cause the two contractile poles of the intrafusal fibers to contract, they alter the tension of the equatorial, noncontractile part of the muscle spindles, on which the annulospiral coils and the secondary endings lie. Indeed, intense fusimotor activity can initiate spindle discharge that, playing on the alpha motoneurons, may reflexly cause extrafusal contraction (Fig. 10–9). Short of this, fusimotor discharge by tautening of the spindle reduces the amount of passive stretch required to initiate spindle discharge; i.e., the fusimotor system biases the sensitivity of the spindle to stretch. This is one example of an efferent system originating in the central nervous system that, by varying the sensitivity of a peripheral receptor, modulates the afferent input into the central nervous system. Other examples will be encountered later.

Given such a system, one is tempted to postulate for it various roles in explaining some of the many puzzling features of motor behavior not readily accounted for by the isolated spinal stretch reflex arc; for example, the interplay between postural stances and phasic movement. The stretch reflex, as described by Sherrington, adequately accounts for the stereotype of stable upright posture but not for rapid alterations of posture that occur, for example, when the standing human subject "voluntarily" executes a kick or leg flexion. Even in different static postures the simple stretch reflex sometimes fails to account for the position of the limbs; for example, a seated human subject maintains flexion of the knee (which stretches the extensor quadriceps), whereas an unmodulated

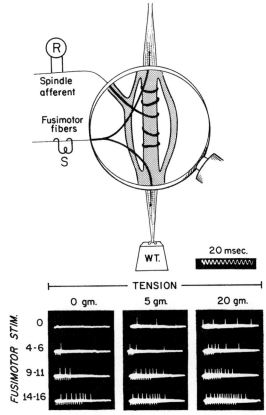

Figure 10–9. Effects of tension and fusimotor stimulation on discharge rate of spindle ending. Upward deflections in traces are action potentials of a single isolated spindle afferent fiber. Small deflections below the base line in some records are shock artifacts produced by stimulating fusimotor fibers. Note that discharge rate depends on both passive tension and fusimotor activity. (After Kuffler *et al.*, *J. Neurophysiol.*, 1951, 14, 29–54.)

stretch reflex would order awkward extension of the leg at right angles to the chair, a state indeed approximated in the spastic patient.

Modulation of the stretch reflex stereotype might be accomplished by excitatory or inhibitory synaptic action directly on alpha motoneurons, rendering them more or less excitable and thus more or less accessible to input from stretch receptors. Alternatively, synaptically mediated variation of fusimotor activity, by alteration of receptor sensitivity, might vary the amount of IA drive to the alpha motoneurons for a given muscle length and thus alter reflex response. Finally, variation of combinations of fusimotor and alpha motoneuron modulation might operate to vary behavior. Unfortunately, the choice between these alternatives cannot be made until more is known of the synaptic drives to both alpha motoneurons and fusimotor neurons in various states, and this is singularly difficult to achieve, especially for the small fusimotoneurons.

However, certain features of fusimotoneuron discharge can be documented. First, in spinal animals it has been shown that fusimotoneurons are subject to a number of inputs, all polysynaptic, fed by dorsal root afferent fibers. They are especially sensitive (but not exclusively so) to cutaneous inputs; their firing patterns markedly change in response to light tactile stimulation. Strikingly they seem to receive few, if any, inputs from IA fibers. No clear-cut functional anatomical pattern between input and output is immediately evident, except that, roughly speaking, fusimotor arcs tend to mimic the pattern of the flexion reflex. A cutaneous stimulus to the limb often excites ipsilateral fusimotoneurons supplying spindles in flexor muscles and reciprocally inhibits those supplying spindles in extensor muscles. The opposite pattern is often observed on the contralateral side. There are, however, exceptions to this crude generalization.

In addition to segmental inputs, many descending pathways originating in supra-segmental structures alter fusimotor activity; these include motor cortex, pyramidal tract, reticular formation, red nucleus, basal ganglia, thalamus, and cerebellum. Again the pattern of synaptic action is complex, variable, and incompletely worked out. In general, however, it can be said that descending pathways that influence fusimotor neurons also synaptically alter alpha motoneuron behavior. It therefore seems unlikely that there are pathways that exert their effects exclusively on one or the other of the two kinds of motoneurons, although there may be quantitative differences.

Another consistent finding is that fusimotor neurons are more sensitive to synaptic inputs than are alpha motoneurons. This appears to be a consequence of the smaller size of fusimotor neurons. In Chapter 6 it was pointed out that motor units innervated by small motoneurons respond to synaptic drives more readily

than do those supplied by large motoneurons. The "size principle" carries over to the even smaller fusimotoneurons. Intracellular recordings show that small cells present relatively high resistances to the passage of currents through the microelectrode; in other words, the voltage drop (current × resistance) for a given current is greater in a small cell than in a large cell. For a given transmembrane current the small cell is depolarized more and hence is brought to threshold with smaller inputs. With increasing synaptic drives, the first spinal elements to discharge are the fusimotor neurons, followed in turn by the small alpha motoneurons, and finally by the larger phasic motoneurons, supplying large numbers of muscle fibers.

Further confusion has been added to an already perplexing subject by the finding that fusimotor fibers are of two kinds, called *static* and *dynamic*. It has already been mentioned (Chap. 7) that many receptors signal to the nervous system both the velocity (phasic, or dynamic, response) and the magnitude (static response) of the applied stimulus. This is true of the annulospiral endings (innervated by Group IA fibers); they show a prominent overshoot of discharge frequency proportional to the rate of stretching as well as a sustained plateau of discharge frequency related to the magnitude, but independent of the rate, of the stretch. The secondary endings (Group II fibers) are far less sensitive to velocity; their phasic, or dynamic, responses are either small or absent. It is likely that phasic, or dynamic, behavior is due to differences in the viscosity or compliance of the nonreceptive portions of the fiber relative to the equatorial region where the receptor ending terminates. If the annulospiral ending lies on a relatively compliant part of the fiber, a sudden extension will momentarily distort the compliant region more than the viscous poles, causing an initially high discharge frequency.

A mechanical analog of a system sensitive to velocity is illustrated in Figure 10–10. Adaptation to rapid extension occurs as the viscous ends sluggishly elongate, reducing the stretch on the central region with consequent decline of the discharge frequency to a stable plateau. On the other

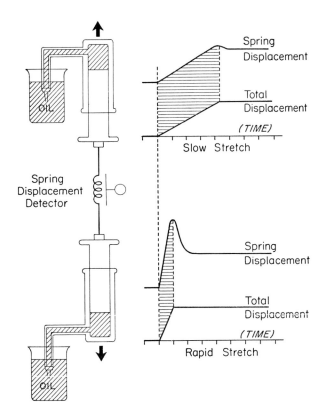

Figure 10–10. Physical model mimicking the velocity-sensitive dynamic, or phasic, response of the primary ending of the muscle spindle. The two oil-filled syringes provide a viscous resistance to extension and are analogies of the two poles of the intrafusal fiber. The displacement detector (primary endings) is on a nonviscous, elastic portion of the system. Diagrams show the response to two different rates of extension.

hand, if the terminal lay on an intrafusal fiber that has relatively uniform structure and viscosity along its length, it would be less sensitive to velocity, although it would retain its sensitivity to magnitude of stretch.

Histologically, intrafusal fibers are of two types, called *nuclear-bag* and *nuclear-*

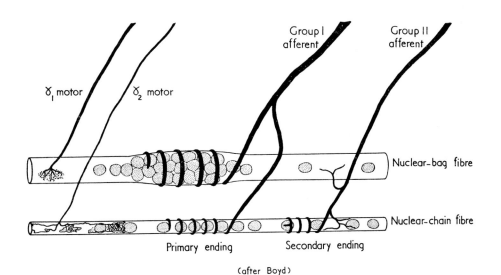

(after Boyd)

Figure 10–11. Primary and secondary endings on nuclear-bag and nuclear-chain fibers. Whether the fusimotor, or gamma, fibers innervating the two kinds of fusimotor fibers are of different sizes, as shown, is controversial. (From Mathews, *Physiol. Rev.*, 1964, 44, 219–288.)

chain fibers (Fig. 10–11). In both, only the distal, or polar, regions contain contractile fibrils, the central region being occupied by a bulbous collection of nuclei (nuclear bag) or a row of nuclei (nuclear chain). It is easy to imagine that these central regions are less viscous than the contractile poles. Annulospiral endings wrap around the central (presumably nonviscous) region of both types of fibers (see Figure 10–10); they are therefore positioned to give dynamic as well as static responses. Secondary endings are largely confined to nuclear-chain fibers and are positioned on the parts of the fiber presumed to be more viscous; hence they would not be expected to be velocity-sensitive.

The two types of fusimotor fibers differentially affect the dynamic and static responses of annulospiral endings; the static fibers increase the static responses of both primary and secondary endings, whereas the dynamic fibers increase only the dynamic response of primary endings. Perhaps the static fibers innervate only the nuclear-chain fibers, and the dynamic fibers innervate only the bag fibers, but the evidence on this point is inconclusive. Recent intracellular recordings from intrafusal muscle fibers indicate that dynamic fibers elicit only junctional potentials and never conducted spikes in the muscle fibers. These junctional potentials are not accompanied by overall contraction of the fiber but presumably by a local contracture-like state that might be expected to increase the stiffness of the fiber. Such an increase of viscosity in the polar regions could well account for the exaggeration of the dynamic response of primary endings. Static fibers may (but do not always) generate all-or-nothing spikes in intrafusal fibers and cause detectable shortening.

RENSHAW INTERNEURONS AND RECURRENT INHIBITION

One further feature of spinal reflex arcs is the phenomenon of recurrent inhibition. Cajal noted that the axons of motoneurons near their origins often give off collateral branches that turn upward into the gray matter. Renshaw found that antidromic stimulation of the ventral root synaptically elicits a high-frequency burst of impulses in small neurons in the ventral horn. Since these elements are wholly contained within the gray matter, they are properly classed as interneurons and are called, for their discoverer, Renshaw interneurons.

Eccles and associates established that the axons of Renshaw interneurons play back upon local motoneurons and exert upon them an inhibitory action. It follows that when a motoneuron is synaptically driven to discharge impulses into the ventral root, the recurrent collaterals excite the Renshaw cells and thus inhibit the local motoneurons. The "negative feedback" of the Renshaw circuit thus limits the discharge of motoneurons. Probably the inhibitory Renshaw neurons also receive inputs other than the recurrent collaterals. Renshaw inhibition is undoubtedly another factor (in addition to autogenic inhibition and withdrawal of spindle input) contributing to the silent period of the tendon jerk. Numerous theories concerning the functional role of Renshaw inhibition have been proposed, but these will not be discussed here.

SUMMARY

Some of the segmental inputs to alpha motoneurons that have been discussed are illustrated diagrammatically in Figure 10–12. For simplicity only an extensor motoneuron is depicted; a flexor motoneuron could be similarly depicted, except that the influence of the cutaneous afferents and the small-diameter (less than 12 mm) deep afferents would be reversed. The figure depicts only the segmental afferent fibers; descending paths from suprasegmental structures are not shown. The membrane potential of the motoneuron is thus at all times the integrated summation of multiple influences converging upon it from both segmental and suprasegmental levels. This is what Sherrington meant when he dubbed the motoneuron "the final common path."

Tension in a muscle depends not on a single motoneuron but on the behavior of the population of motoneurons supplying its constituent fibers. We must therefore try to imagine a population, or pool, of

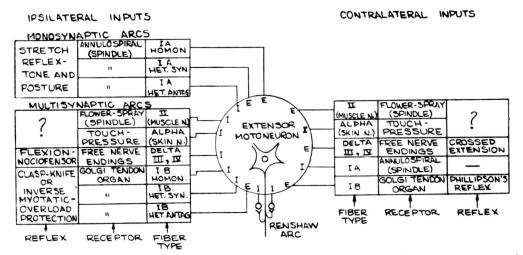

Figure 10–12. Segmental afferent inputs converging on a typical motoneuron supplying an extensor muscle. The influence of each input is indicated as excitatory (*E*) or inhibitory (*I*). (From Ruch and Patton, *Physiology and biophysics,* Philadelphia, W. B. Saunders Co., 1965.)

motoneurons rather than the single representative of Figure 10–12. At any moment some of these motoneurons are in the discharge zone and others in the subliminal fringe. A slight change in input in the excitatory direction produces a very striking change in discharge by recruiting into the discharge zone some units in the subliminal fringe whose membrane potentials are already hovering near the threshold level. Conversely, a shift toward inhibition reduces the size of the discharge zone by depressing the firing of those elements that were previously excited to just above threshold. The important point to recognize is that the behavior of the muscle depends on the population response and that small shifts in the input can effect

relatively large quantitative changes in the output.

To carry the argument further, we might try to visualize a number of motoneuron populations supplying different muscles, recalling that motor behavior depends on the integrated activity of many muscles. With variations of timing and intensity of contraction of muscles, an infinite variety of movement patterns, or postural stances, are possible, even though each afferent pathway exerts upon its postsynaptic motoneurons stereotyped action. It is this feature of synaptic organization that makes the spinal cord a flexible and responsive director of behavior even though the individual components are relatively immutable.

ADDITIONAL READING

Henneman, E. Organization of the spinal cord. Chap. 74 in *Medical physiology,* Mountcastle, V. B., ed., St. Louis, The C. V. Mosby Co., 1968.

Henneman, E. Spinal reflexes and the control of movement. Chap. 75 in *Medical physiology,* Mountcastle, V. B., ed., St. Louis, The C. V. Mosby Co., 1968.

Patton, H. D. Reflex regulation of movement and posture. Chap. 7 in *Physiology and biophysics,* Ruch, T. C., and Patton, H. D., eds., Philadelphia, W. B. Saunders Co., 1965.

Matthews, P. B. C. Muscle spindles and their motor control. *Physiol. Rev.,* 1964, *44,* 219–288.

CHAPTER 11

THE AUTONOMIC NERVOUS SYSTEM

JOHN W. SUNDSTEN

THE VISCERAL MOTOR
SYSTEM CONTRASTED
WITH THE SOMATIC
MOTOR SYSTEM

GENERAL ORGANIZATION
OF THE AUTONOMIC
NERVOUS SYSTEM

PERIPHERAL DISTRIBUTION
OF AUTONOMIC FIBERS

THE SYMPATHETIC CHAIN
(TRUNK)

THE PARASYMPATHETIC
FIBERS

THE AUTONOMIC GANGLIA

NEURAL TRANSMITTER
SUBSTANCES

AUTONOMIC REFLEXES
AND FUNCTIONS

The autonomic nervous system (ANS) is the part of the peripheral nervous system that regulates smooth muscle, cardiac muscle, and glands; it is thus a *visceral motor system.* The visceral reflexes that constitute autonomic functioning occur automatically; there is no conscious sensation of the events taking place. Hence, traditionally the autonomic nervous system has been thought of as an *involuntary* system that makes appropriate adjustments in the visceral effectors to keep the internal environment constant. This tendency in an organism to maintain a steady state is called *homeostasis.*

The term *involuntary* is perhaps too restrictive because to a certain extent one can voluntarily alter portions of the system. For example, accommodation for near vision by converging the eyes also involves changes in the smooth muscles controlling lens and pupil size, and sexual activity certainly includes a variety of autonomic changes. Furthermore, there is increasing

evidence that man as well as experimental animals can be trained through conditioning techniques to have partial control over the cardiovascular and gastrointestinal systems. For example, some patients with essential hypertension have been trained through instrumental conditioning (biofeedback) to lower their systolic blood pressure, at least under laboratory conditions. However, neither the therapeutic benefit of this nor the mechanism by which it occurs has yet been established.

The efferent pathways to visceral structures are for the most part well established; less well established are the components of the central nervous system that are essential for the smooth and appropriate operation of the autonomic reflexes. Such components reside in many sites of the neuraxis besides the spinal cord: parts of the cerebral cortex, hypothalamus, brain stem, and probably also cerebellum. Descending pathways (many and for the most part indirect) associated with these

138

structures can clearly influence the autonomic effectors. The *hypothalamus* is the major integrative region of the central nervous system that affects autonomic functioning; it has sometimes been referred to as the *head ganglion* of the autonomic nervous system. A brief example of how the hypothalamus affects a spinal cord reflex involving visceral effectors is described in the paragraph that follows.

Consider the vasomotor reflex response to cold stimulus. Exposure to peripheral cold results in reflex cutaneous vasoconstriction (operating at a spinal level), which prevents the loss of heat from the surface of the body. However, if one exercises in the cold (*e.g.*, skis), the body produces *excess* heat. As the temperature of the blood rises, the temperature detectors in the hypothalamus that are responsive to heat are activated; and they, in turn, through connections to descending pathways (finally, the reticulospinal tracts), *inhibit* the spinal cord's vasoconstrictor reflex. This allows the cutaneous vessels to dilate, and heat is given off in spite of the demand made by the peripheral cold stimulus.

The preceding example illustrates that reflexes involving visceral effectors are subject to control by the more rostral parts of the central nervous system, just as reflexes involving somatic musculature are.

THE VISCERAL MOTOR SYSTEM CONTRASTED WITH THE SOMATIC MOTOR SYSTEM

There are several major differences in innervation between visceral and somatic structures, some of which are illustrated in Figure 11–1. First, the effectors controlled by the autonomic nervous system are the *smooth muscles, exocrine gland tissue,* and *specialized cardiac tissue,* whereas those controlled by the somatic motor system are the skeletal muscles. Further, the efferent pathway to the visceral structures is a *two-neuron chain,* composed of *preganglionic* and *postganglionic* neurons, with a synapse interposed in an *autonomic ganglion* located peripherally, whereas the efferent pathway to the somatic structures is a single motoneuron. The cell body of the preganglionic

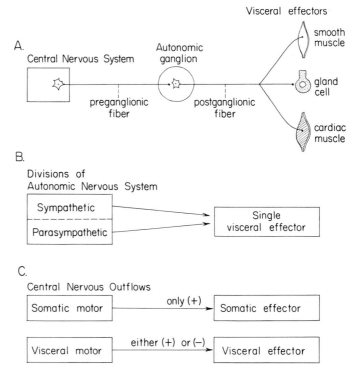

Figure 11–1. General principles of autonomic innervation. *A,* Overview of the innervation of visceral effectors. *B,* Dual innervation of visceral effector. *C,* Contrast between somatic motor outflows and visceral motor outflows.

neuron is located in the central nervous system, and that of the postganglionic neuron is in the ganglion. The distribution of the autonomic nerves is also more complex than that of the somatic nerves because visceral effectors are distributed more widely than somatic effectors, and the autonomic centers giving rise to the first neuron in the two-neuron chain are restricted within the central nervous system to certain areas in the spinal cord and brainstem. Functionally, too, control over the visceral effectors differs from that over the somatic effectors; for the most part dual processes of facilitation and inhibition operate at the effector level in the former, whereas only facilitation operates in the latter. Recall that stimulation of somatic motor nerves causes only contraction in skeletal muscle; in contrast, stimulation of visceral motor nerves may cause either contraction*or* relaxation in smooth muscle, depending on the visceral structure in question.

GENERAL ORGANIZATION OF THE AUTONOMIC NERVOUS SYSTEM

The autonomic nervous system has two anatomically separate components, the *sympathetic* and *parasympathetic.* These arise from different portions of the central nervous system (Fig. 11–2) and have different means of distribution to visceral struc-

tures (Figs. 11–3 and 11–4). The sympathetic (or thoracolumbar) division originates from preganglionic neurons in the *intermediolateral gray column* of the spinal cord. This column of cells is positioned, as its name implies, between the posterior and anterior gray and extends from the first thoracic cord segment to the second lumbar. The parasympathetic (or craniosacral) division arises from preganglionic neurons located in certain brainstem nuclei associated with cranial nerves (Edinger-Westphal nucleus [III], salivatory nuclei [VII and IX], and dorsal motor nucleus of the vagus [X]) and in sacral segments (S2 to S4) of the spinal cord. In other words, the sympathetic outflow is entirely from the spinal cord, whereas the parasympathetic outflow is partially from the brainstem and partially from the spinal cord. The preganglionic parasympathetic cell bodies occupy an intermediate position in the sacral cord, as the sympathetic ones do in the thoracic cord, but they do not form a clearly visible intermediolateral column of cells.

Fibers descending in the reticulospinal tracts in the lateral white matter (Fig. 11–5) enable the more rostral parts of the central nervous system to influence the preganglionic outflow of the autonomic nervous system. These fibers end on interneurons in the intermediate gray matter. The sympathetic intermediolateral gray has a segmental organization, as prevails elsewhere in the central nervous system;

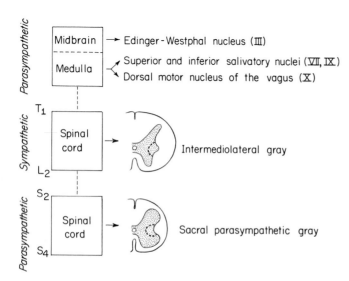

Figure 11–2. The sympathetic and parasympathetic divisions of the autonomic nervous system. The locations of preganglionic cell bodies for the sympathetic and sacral parasympathetic divisions are shown in cross sections of the spinal cord. The nuclei and associated cranial nerves for the cranial parasympathetic division are listed.

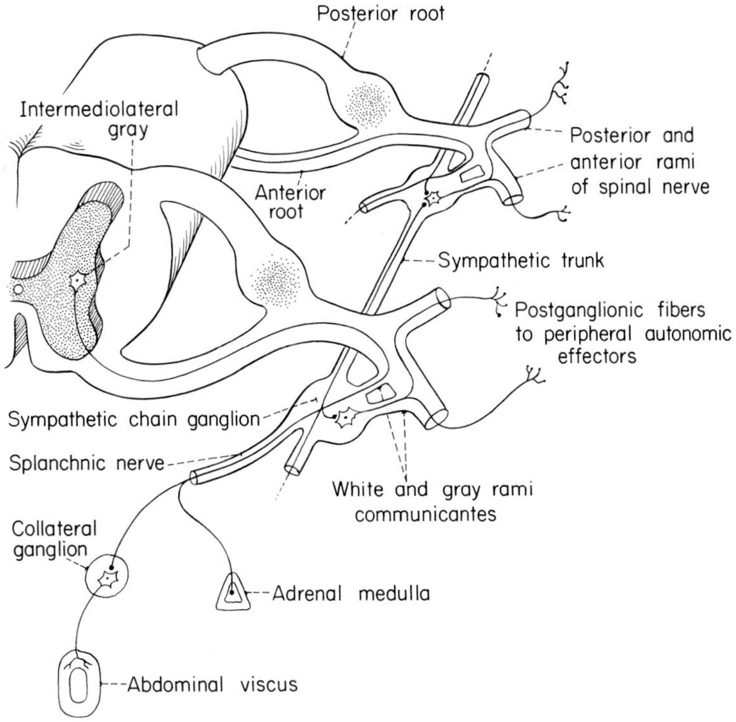

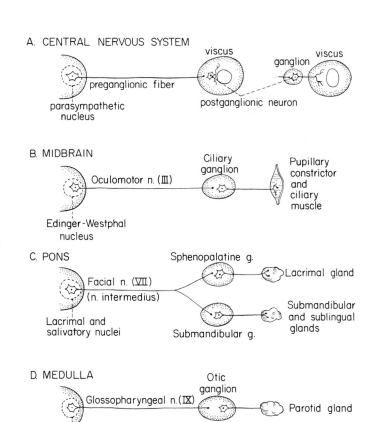

Figure 11–3. The origin of and routes taken by the sympathetic preganglionic and postganglionic fibers..

Figure 11–4. Parasympathetic innervation. *A*, General plan (most appropriate for vagal and sacral outflows). *B*, Oculomotor nerve. *C*, Facial nerve. *D*, Glossopharyngeal nerve.

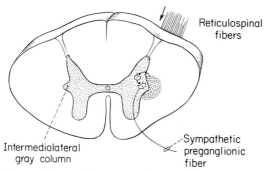

Figure 11–5. Illustration of reticulospinal fibers descending in the lateral white column. One fiber is shown terminating on an interneuron that synapses in the intermediolateral gray column.

this is illustrated schematically in Figure 11–6. For clarity, only selected areas of the body are shown in relation to (1) the vasomotor outflow and (2) the innervation of certain structures. The essential point to note is that the entire column of preganglionic cells is arranged so that the more rostral parts of the body are represented in the upper thoracic cord segments and the caudal regions in the lower thoracic and lumbar cord segments. The parcellation also makes it possible for different parts of the autonomic outflow to function separately when required even though there is a tendency for the sympathetic system to discharge as a unit (see later in this chapter).

The topographical organization of the

intermediolateral column and the fibers descending to it has its clinical corollaries. For example, transection of the spinal cord below T6 would severely impair vasomotor and sudomotor (sweat glands) functioning in the lower extremities but not in the upper extremities. Transection above T5 would affect autonomic effectors in the upper limb, face, and heart as well. Also, damage to the brainstem can result in autonomic disturbances. In a lesion of the lateral medullary plate (see Chapter 29), Horner's syndrome, with miosis (small pupil), ptosis (drooping eyelid), and anhidrosis (decreased facial sweating), may be present because of interruption of the sympathetic pathway descending to the preganglionic outflow.

PERIPHERAL DISTRIBUTION OF AUTONOMIC FIBERS

Both the sympathetic and parasympathetic divisions of the autonomic nervous system have preganglionic fibers, autonomic ganglia, and postganglionic fibers, but they use different anatomical routes to innervate any given organ. Each division of the autonomic nervous system has separate nerves, and their respective autonomic ganglion cell groupings are located differently. This is not surprising, since the autonomic outflows originate in sites rang-

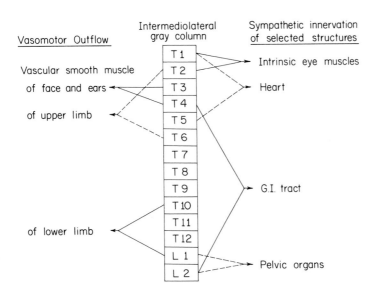

Figure 11–6. The rostral-to-caudal topographical arrangement of the sympathetic outflow from cord segments T1 to L2. Examples of the vasomotor outflow are shown at the left, and of the general sympathetic outflow to some selected structures at the right.

ing from the midbrain to the sacral spinal cord. The nerves that are distributed to the body cavities are the *vagus* and *pelvic splanchnic* nerves for the parasympathetic system and the *thoracic* and *lumbar splanchnic* nerves for the sympathetic system. The parasympathetic supply to the thoracic cavity and most of the abdominal cavity is by the *vagus nerve* (from the medulla), and that to the pelvic organs is by the *pelvic splanchnic nerves* (from the sacral cord). The sympathetic supply to the thoracic viscera is directly via the *sympathetic trunk,* that to the abdominal organs is via the *thoracic splanchnic nerves,* and that to the pelvic structures is via the *lumbar splanchnic nerves.*

The parasympathetic fibers to the smooth muscles and the glands in the head course with cranial nerves, the oculo- motor, facial, and glossopharyngeal nerves. The sympathetic supply to the head leaves the superior cervical ganglion of the sym- pathetic trunk and then travels with branches of the internal and external caro- tid arteries. The autonomic fibers are very small, only a micrometer or less, and these commonly travel with larger nerve trunks and vessels.

The autonomic effectors of body wall and extremities have a sympathetic supply but no parasympathetic supply. Sympa- thetic nerves reach smooth muscles and glands via available peripheral nerves and blood vessels after leaving the sympathetic trunk.

This brief outline may seem rather com- plex but can be understood clearly (see Table 11–1) if the principles underlying each of the outflows are looked at. The sympathetic system will be dealt with first.

Figure 11–3 is a schematic view of a cross section of the sympathetic system through the thoracic spinal cord, with attached roots, rami, and sympathetic ganglia. The entire preganglionic outflow leaves the cord between T1 and L2 via the anterior roots and reaches the chain ganglia via the *white rami communicantes,* attached to the anterior ramus of the spinal nerve. One of three events occurs in the chain ganglia: (1) the preganglionic fiber may synapse in the ganglion it first enters, or (2) it may ascend or descend to other chain ganglia before synapsing, or (3) it may pass through to synapse in a *collateral ganglion.* Postganglionic neurons return to the spinal nerve from the chain ganglia via the *gray rami communicantes* and are thence dis- tributed to smooth muscles and glands peripherally in the body wall and extrem- ities. The postganglionic fibers may leave the nerves at any time and travel instead with larger blood vessels and then smaller ones; for example, the sympathetic inner- vation to the head is by way of branches of the carotid arteries. The *thoracic viscera* are innervated by many small sympathetic postganglionic fibers that form specific organ plexuses, for example, the cardiac, pulmonary, and esophageal plexuses. These fibers come directly from thoracic and cervical chain ganglia, again often travelling with blood vessels.

The innervation of the *abdominal viscera* is somewhat more complex because the postganglionic fibers arise from *collateral ganglia* instead of from the chain ganglia. The collateral ganglia (*e.g.,* coeliac and su- perior mesenteric ganglia) are situated in plexuses of fibers usually clumped around the branches of the abdominal aorta; the *thoracic splanchnic* nerves carry pregan- glionic fibers to them. Postganglionic fibers easily reach the nearby organs by travelling with their arterial supplies. The adrenal medulla is peculiar in that it has no postganglionic supply; it receives pre- ganglionic sympathetic fibers directly from the thoracic splanchnic nerves. It has no parasympathetic supply. Whereas the chromaffin cells that make up the adrenal medulla are derived from the same neural crest cells that form autonomic ganglion cells, they have differentiated into en- docrine cells that secrete adrenalin instead of into neurons.

The *pelvic viscera* also receive a post- ganglionic sympathetic supply from col- lateral ganglia, the *inferior mesenteric gan- glion* and ganglia in the continuous *hypogas- tric* and *pelvic plexuses.* The *lumbar splanchnic nerves* carry the preganglionic fibers to the inferior mesenteric ganglion. From there, the postganglionic fibers travel in the *hypo- gastric plexus* to reach specific organ plexuses in the pelvic cavity. Both the sympathetic and parasympathetic supplies to specific structures are listed in Table 11–1.

TABLE 11–1.   Summary of the Innervation and Function of Major Autonomic Effectors

	Preganglionic Neuron	Postganglionic Neuron	Function
HEAD STRUCTURES			
Eye: Pupillary and Ciliary Muscles			
Sympathetic	Cord segments T1 to T2.	Superior cervical ganglion.	Pupillary dilation (mydriasis); accommodation for far vision.
Parasympathetic	Edinger-Westphal nucleus (oculomotor nerve — III).	Ciliary ganglion.	Pupillary constriction (miosis); accommodation for near vision.
Lacrimal Gland			
Sympathetic	Cord segments T1 to T2.	Superior cervical ganglion.	Vasoconstriction.
Parasympathetic	Lacrimal part of superior salivatory nucleus (facial nerve — VII).	Sphenopalatine ganglion.	Tear secretion and vasodilation.
Parotid, Submandibular, and Sublingual Salivary Glands			
Sympathetic	Upper thoracic cord segments.	Superior cervical ganglion.	Salivary secretion (mucous-low enzyme); vasoconstriction.
Parasympathetic			
Parotid gland	Inferior salivatory nucleus (glossopharyngeal nerve — IX)	Otic ganglion.	Salivary secretion (watery-high enzyme); vasodilation.
Submandibular and sublingual glands	Superior salivatory nucleus (facial nerve — VII).	Submandibular ganglion.	Same as above.
THORACIC VISCERA			
Heart			
Sympathetic	Cord segments T1 to T4.	Upper thoracic to superior cervical chain ganglia.	Acceleration of heart rate and force of contraction; coronary vasodilation.
Parasympathetic	Dorsal motor nucleus (vagus nerve — X).	Cardiac plexus.	Deceleration of heart rate and force of contraction; coronary vasoconstriction.
Esophagus			
Sympathetic	Thoracic cord segments.	Thoracic and cervical chain ganglia.	Vasoconstriction.
Parasympathetic	Dorsal motor nucleus (vagus nerve — X).	Intramural plexuses.	Peristalsis and secretion.

THE SYMPATHETIC CHAIN (TRUNK)

The sympathetic chain of ganglia with interconnecting fibers forms a trunk that extends from close to the base of the skull in the neck to the coccyx. It is placed bilaterally alongside the vertebral bodies (for which reason it is also called a *paravertebral chain*) and caudally joins in the midline at the *coccygeal ganglion*, or *ganglion impar* (Fig. 11–7). In the embryo a sympathetic paravertebral ganglion is present for each spinal cord segment, but in the adult many of these have fused to form larger ganglia. This is most apparent in the neck region, where there are only three ganglia: the *inferior cervical*, which is fused with the first thoracic, forming the *stellate ganglion;* the *middle cervical ganglion;* and the *superior cervical ganglion.* The last is the cranialmost of the sympathetic ganglia and is also the largest, having formed from the four rostral cervical sympathetic primordia. It is

TABLE 11–1. **Summary of the Innervation and Function of Major Autonomic Effectors**
(Continued)

	Preganglionic Neuron	Postganglionic Neuron	Function
THORACIC VISCERA *(Continued)*			
Lungs			
Sympathetic	Cord segments T2 to T6.	Thoracic chain ganglia.	Bronchial dilation.
Parasympathetic	Dorsal motor nucleus (vagus nerve – X).	Pulmonary plexus.	Bronchial constriction.
ABDOMINAL VISCERA			
Stomach and Intestine			
Sympathetic	Cord segments T5 to T12 (thoracic splanchnic nerves).	Coeliac and superior mesenteric ganglia.	Inhibition of peristalsis and secretion; sphincter contraction.
Parasympathetic	Dorsal motor nucleus (vagus nerve – X).	Intramural plexuses.	Peristalsis and secretion.
Adrenal Medulla			
Sympathetic	Cord segments T8 to T11 (thoracic splanchnic nerves).	The adrenomedullary cells are derived from neural crests but have no dendrites nor axons. They are endocrine cells.	Secretion of epinephrine and norepinephrine directly into the blood.
Parasympathetic (none)			
Descending Colon			
Sympathetic	Cord segments T12 to L2 (lumbar splanchnic nerves).	Inferior mesenteric ganglion.	Inhibition of peristalsis and secretion; vasoconstriction.
Parasympathetic	Cord segments S2 to S4 (pelvic splanchnic nerves).	Intramural plexuses.	Peristalsis and secretion.
PELVIC VISCERA			
Sigmoid Colon, Rectum and Anus, Bladder, Gonads and Associated Ducts and Organs, and Erectile Tissue			
Sympathetic	Cord segments T12 to L2 (lumbar splanchnic nerves).	Inferior mesenteric ganglion (hypogastric nerves).	Inhibition of peristalsis and secretion; anal and bladder sphincter contraction; vasoconstriction; ejaculation.
Parasympathetic	Cord segments S2 to S4 (pelvic splanchnic nerves)	Intramural or specific organ plexuses.	Peristalsis and secretion; bladder detrusor muscle contraction; penile and clitoral erection.

embedded in the carotid sheath. All of the sympathetic postganglionic innervation to the head comes from this ganglion, *e.g.,* pupillary dilation, facial sweating, and vasoconstriction.

Since the entire preganglionic outflow is only between the first thoracic cord segment and the second lumbar cord segment, the question arises about the course taken by the preganglionic fibers to reach the cervical ganglia and the lower lumbar and sacral ganglia. The answer is that pre-

ganglionic fibers simply ascend or descend through the sympathetic chain until they reach the appropriate ganglion, where they then synapse on the ganglion cells that form the postganglionic neurons (Fig. 11–7).

It should now be clear why there are no *white rami communicantes* other than those associated with the spinal cord outflow T1 to L2; *i.e.,* there are only *gray rami communicantes* attaching the cervical chain ganglia and the remaining lumbar and

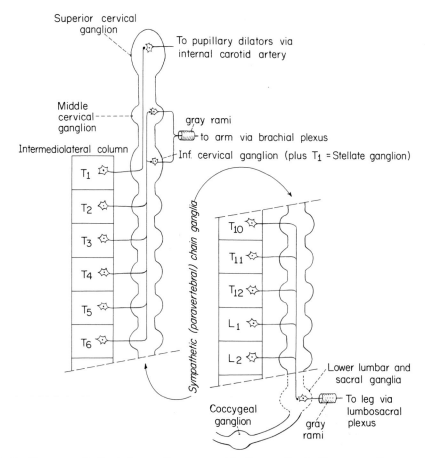

Figure 11–7. The sympathetic chain ganglia on one side. Preganglionic fibers ascending to cervical ganglia to innervate the pupil and arm and descending to lumbar and sacral ganglia to innervate the leg are also shown.

sacral chain ganglia to spinal nerves or blood vessels. For instance: Nerves innervating the arm arise from spinal cord segments C5 to T1, but the vasomotor (sudomotor and pilomotor also) outflow to the arm arises from cord segments T2 to T6. Thus, the preganglionic fibers must ascend through the sympathetic chain to the stellate and middle cervical ganglia, where they synapse. The postganglionic fibers via the *gray rami communicantes* can then easily join the nearby brachial plexus (and subclavian artery), which has the C5 to T1 root fibers in it, for distribution to the arm. Similarly, lower lumbar and sacral chain ganglia are attached to the origins of the lumbosacral plexus only by gray rami, which provide a route for postganglionic fibers to the spinal nerves (or blood vessels) ultimately reaching the lower extremity.

THE PARASYMPATHETIC FIBERS

The parasympathetic outflow is easier to understand since there are well-defined nerves associated with both its cranial and sacral components. In summary, the nerves with parasympathetic components are the oculomotor (III), facial (VII), glossopharyngeal (IX), vagus (X), and pelvic splanchnic (S2 to S4) nerves.

In general, the parasympathetic preganglionic fibers are much longer than the postganglionic fibers since the parasympathetic ganglion cells are grouped either close to the structure to be innervated or within its wall (Fig. 11–4). The latter principle is illustrated very well by the major parasympathetic nerve, the vagus nerve, which wanders through the neck, thoracic and abdominal cavities, supplying preganglionic fibers to postganglionic neurons in the walls of the viscera. The postganglionic ganglion cells are on or within the wall of the visceral structure itself. In the gastrointestinal system, the ganglion cells are found in the *myenteric* and *submucosal plexuses*. In the heart, the clusters of postganglionic ganglion cells are found in the epicardium of the atrium and in the interatrial wall. Similarly, the pelvic splanchnic nerves carry the preganglionic fibers (S2 to S4) to the pelvic cavity (see the example of bladder innervation in Figure 11–11). The ganglion cells giving rise to the postganglionic fibers are usually embedded in the plexuses found in relation to the walls of the different pelvic viscera.

The remaining cranial nerves with parasympathetic components (III, VII, IX) have well-defined ganglia associated with the visceral effector organs innervated. These are summarized in Figure 11–4: (1) the oculomotor nerve and ciliary ganglion, innervating the intrinsic eye muscles; (2) the facial nerve (intermedius portion) and sphenopalatine and submandibular ganglia, innervating the lacrimal gland, and the submandibular and sublingual salivary glands; and (3) the glossopharyngeal nerve and otic ganglion, innervating the parotid salivary gland.

THE AUTONOMIC GANGLIA

The autonomic ganglia can be divided into two structurally similar groups, the *sympathetic ganglia* and the *parasympathetic ganglia*. It should be clear from the information already given that the sympathetic ganglia are located as either chain ganglia or collateral ganglia (paravertebral or prevertebral in position, respectively). The parasympathetic ganglia are either terminal unnamed ganglia associated with the vagus nerve or the sacral outflow that are located within the wall of the structure innervated, or named ganglia attached to the other cranial nerves with parasympathetic components, as shown in Figure 11–4.

The autonomic ganglion cells are multipolar and receive sympathetic input of an *en passage* type; that is, the preganglionic fibers wind around the dendritic processes,

making multiple synaptic contacts. When an autonomic ganglion is denervated by removal of the preganglionic fibers coming to it and time is allowed for degenerative processes to take place, about 20 per cent of the synaptic contacts remain intact. It is thought that these come from interneurons and/or from recurrent collaterals of other ganglion cells. The morphology of the synapses in autonomic ganglia is similar to that found in the central nervous system; but, in addition to the membrane thickenings and the small, clear vesicles (*cholinergic* — see later), larger vesicles are apparent, some granulated. The role of the larger, granulated vesicles in preganglionic fiber endings has not been satisfactorily worked out, but similar ones in postganglionic endings contain the catecholamine neurotransmitters. The presence of interneurons and collaterals in autonomic ganglia suggests that their role is more than a single relay of information from preganglionic cell to postganglionic cell. It is likely that the ganglia themselves can carry out some integrative functions. In this respect it is significant that inhibitory postsynaptic potentials have been recorded from some mammalian sympathetic ganglion cells.

The axonal processes of the sympathetic ganglion cells, the postganglionic fibers, are unmyelinated and small (1 μm or less) and innervate the visceral effector directly. These fibers typically show beaded swellings in their terminal parts. Such thickenings contain synaptic vesicles with dense cores, which are readily identified by fluorescence microscopy. The dense core granules contain the transmitter substance *norepinephrine (noradrenalin)*. The relationship between postganglionic fibers and smooth muscle effector cells is somewhat simpler than that found in skeletal neuromuscular junctions. The terminal axon is bare, and most commonly the junctional gap between terminal axon swellings and the effector cell membranes is much greater than that in skeletal muscles (up to several thousand angstroms in some tissues). Thus, the transmitter substance has a greater diffusion distance, a difference that is reflected in a relatively long junctional delay of about 10 msec or more between postganglionic fiber and neuroeffector. Also, the action of the neurotransmitter is more prolonged, probably because of its slower degradation; in cholinergic endings acetylcholinesterase (AChe) rapidly removes the acetylcholine (ACh).

NEURAL TRANSMITTER SUBSTANCES

The terms *adrenergic* and *cholinergic* are used to indicate whether an autonomic neuron uses *norepinephrine (noradrenalin)* or *acetylcholine* as its transmitter substance. Since *all* preganglionic fibers, sympathetic and parasympathetic, release acetylcholine, transmission in all autonomic ganglia can be referred to as *cholinergic*. (Recall, however, that large core vesicles are present in some synapses.) Similarly, *all* postganglionic parasympathetic neurons are cholinergic. The postganglionic sympathetic neurons are mainly *adrenergic*; two exceptions are the postganglionic sympathetic cholinergic fibers to sweat glands and to blood vessels in skeletal muscle.

Blood vessels in skeletal muscle also have adrenergic constrictor fibers; the cholinergic ones actively cause vessels to dilate. The adrenal medullary cells are also adrenergic. Their main secretion is epinephrine (adrenalin), although they also release noradrenalin. The former is used in various metabolic pathways.

Many investigators have worked on the peripheral paths of the autonomic nervous system over the past 50 years to elucidate the chemical nature of neural transmission. In the early part of the century it was known that practically all organs contain amines, particularly norepinephrine (NE), and that this store is dependent on an intact nerve supply. For example, in experiments it was found that (1) cutting of adrenergic nerves caused a depletion of the norepinephrine in the organ, and (2) subsequent regeneration of the nerves reestablished norepinephrine content. Further, extracts of nerves to organs with a rich sympathetic supply, such as the spleen and vas deferens, were found to behave

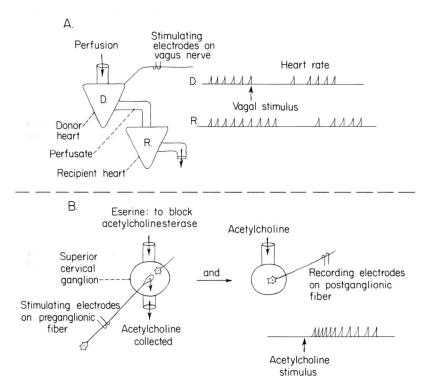

Figure 11–8. The classic demonstrations of chemical transmission in autonomic ganglia. *A*, Otto Loewi's experiment on the heart. *B*, Feldberg and Gaddum's experiment on the sympathetic ganglion. See text for details. (*A*, After Bain, *Quart. J. exp. Physiol.*, 22, 269–274, 1932. *B*, After Feldberg and Gaddum, *J. Physiol.* [*Lond.*], 81, 305–319, 1934.)

like norepinephrine. In part through the efforts of von Euler and coworkers (see Nobel Address in *Science, 173,* 202–206, 1971), norepinephrine was eventually identified as the transmitter substance found in postganglionic sympathetic nerves and was shown to be bound to subcellular particles, probably the dense core vesicles that are visible by electron microscopy.

Chemical transmission at a visceral organ level was first demonstrated by Otto Loewi in 1922 in a classic experiment that purportedly first occurred to him in a dream. Vagal nerve stimulation was known to inhibit heart rate, and since this inhibition outlasts the stimulation, Loewi proposed that a humoral mediator released by the nerve is responsible. His experimental test is illustrated in Figure 11–8*A.* A donor heart (*D*) was perfused, and the effluent was given to a recipient heart (*R*). Subsequently, electrical stimulation of the vagus nerve to the donor heart was applied, and it resulted in the expected cessation of heartbeat. The new finding was that the recipient heart, connected only by the perfusate channel, also stopped beating. Loewi thus established that the vagal stimulation released a chemical agent. He named the substance "vagusstoff" (now known to be *acetylcholine*) after the vagus nerve.

Chemical transmission in *sympathetic ganglia* was demonstrated by Feldberg and Gaddum 10 years later by the following experiment (Fig. 11–8*B*). Since the superior cervical ganglion was already known to contain acetylcholine (ACh), Feldberg and Gaddum proposed that preganglionic stimulation should release it. Feldberg had previously shown that after stimulation of the splanchnic nerve, ACh can be collected and assayed from the adrenal gland, providing the destruction of ACh is prevented by suitable pharmacological blockade with eserine. He and Gaddum then demonstrated that when the superior cervical ganglion is perfused with eserine, electrical stimulation of its preganglionic fibers will cause ACh to appear in the effluent collected. In addition, they showed that action potentials can be recorded from the postganglionic fibers (without stimulation of the pre-

ganglionic fibers) by perfusion of the ganglion with ACh. These pioneer experiments paved the way for acceptance of the cholinergic nature of transmission through the autonomic ganglia.

AUTONOMIC REFLEXES AND FUNCTIONS

Most of the motor functioning of the autonomic nervous system—the contraction of, or secretion by, visceral effectors—does not reach the conscious level. For example, at any given moment we are not aware of either the size of the pupil or the status of the cardiovascular, respiratory, gastrointestinal, or genitourinary systems. Rather, autonomic reflexes maintain the internal environment in a condition appropriate to the many demands put on the body, whether for action or repair, just as the reflexes involving somatic effectors do. Although the afferents from the viscera serve primarily reflex functions, some also provide sensory information concerning the conditions of bladder or bowel fullness, thirst, hunger, and sexual arousal.

Of particular clinical importance are afferents from visceral structures that evoke sensations of pain when stimulated. Visceral pain fibers are small and are either unmyelinated or thinly myelinated, as all the visceral afferents are. In the periphery they meander around blood vessels, and in the body cavities they are also prominent in the muscular walls of the hollow organs. The adequate stimulus for activation of the pain fiber is excessive distention of the organ wall. Normally the mucosa associated with the viscera is insensitive to pain, but in hyperemic or inflammatory conditions it becomes a site for the origin of pain.

The afferent fibers from body cavities travel mainly with the nerves of the sympathetic division of the autonomic nervous system, and those from the periphery with the somatic nerves (Fig. 11–9). The afferents from thoracic and abdominal viscera pass through the sympathetic chain ganglia without synapsing and reach the spinal nerves via the *white rami communicantes.* Their cell bodies are located in the dorsal

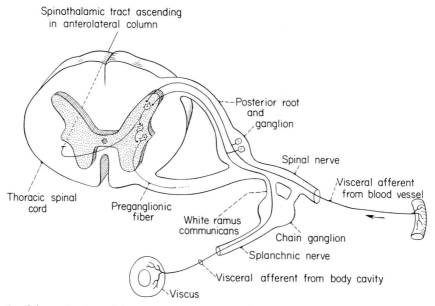

Figure 11–9. Schematic view of the course taken by a visceral afferent fiber from the abdominal cavity and of the course taken by one from a peripheral blood vessel. The ascending visceral pain pathway and a reflex connection are shown in the spinal cord section.

root ganglia intermixed with those of the somatic afferents.

The ascending pathway for visceral pain is in the anterolateral column of the spinal cord (Fig. 11–9). It is intermixed with the spinothalamic fibers carrying somatic pain but is positioned more medially, encroaching on the propriospinal path (see also Figure 13–7). It is probably a multisynaptic path that relays in the reticular formation. Note that the transection of the anterolateral column for the relief of intractable visceral pain must extend to the gray matter to be effective.

The vagus nerve also carries some visceral pain fibers, but only from the upper portions of the esophagus and trachea; most of the vagal afferents convey mechanoreceptor input for reflex activities. Pain fibers from the pelvic organs travel in the pelvic splanchnic (*parasympathetic*) nerves. In addition, *somatic nerves* may carry "visceral" pain from certain areas lining the body cavities, for example, the parietal peritoneum and parietal pleura, which are structures that are innervated by segmental nerves (see Chapter 14). The cell bodies of the visceral afferents in cranial nerves VII, IX, and X, *e.g.*, taste afferents, are in the ganglia

associated with those nerves: facial nerve, geniculate ganglion; glossopharyngeal nerve, inferior (petrosal) ganglion; and vagus nerve, inferior (nodose) ganglion.

Both the visceral afferents and visceral efferents are components of visceral reflexes that are responsible for maintaining the constancy of the internal environment. Somatic afferents can also affect visceral efferents, and visceral afferents can affect somatic efferents. Thus, all reflexes can be categorized as either *viscerovisceral*, or *viscerosomatic*, or *somatovisceral*, or *somatosomatic*, depending upon the source of the afferent and the type of effector (Table 11–2).

An example of a viscerovisceral reflex, the *carotid sinus reflex*, is illustrated in Figure 11–10. As blood pressure increases, the walls of the carotid sinus are distended and the afferent endings located there are stimulated. The visceral afferent input to the CNS is via the glossopharyngeal nerve, which is attached to the medulla. In the medulla these primary afferents terminate in the *nucleus solitarius*, from which connections are made with two different sets of neurons in the tegmentum at this level. One set affects the vagus nerve, and the other affects the sympathetic outflow via

TABLE 11–2. Categories of Reflexes with Examples

Reflex Category	Adequate Stimulus	Response
Visceroviseral	Carotid sinus distention.	Decreased heart rate.
Viscerosomatic	Ruptured appendix.	Abdominal cramping.
Somatovisceral	Peripheral cold.	Vasoconstriction.
Somatosomatic	Muscle spindle stretch.	Knee jerk.

the reticulospinal path descending to the spinal cord. The appropriate interneurons scattered in the medulla activate the *dorsal motor nucleus* of the vagus and thus cause vagal inhibition of heart rate. Simultaneously, *reticulospinal fibers* are stimulated, and they inhibit, through interneurons in the spinal cord, the preganglionic sympathetic outflow to the heart and cutaneous arterioles. The decrease in impulse traffic over the peripheral sympathetic system allows the heart to slow passively and, along with the active vagal inhibition, causes a decrease in heart rate and force of contraction. This decrease, combined with the decrease in peripheral vascular resistance brought on by passive vasodilation, results in a decrease in blood pressure, and the initial increase is countered. As tension lessens in the carotid sinus, there is less

impulse traffic in the visceral afferents, and the blood pressure increases again. Such changes in blood pressure cycle about a mean value or set point are determined by the CNS. Under appropriate conditions (*e.g.*, fear, excitement), the set point can be changed by autonomic centers in the forebrain, notably the hypothalamus and cingulate cortex, parts of the limbic system.

There are two features of autonomic nervous system functioning that are often expressed as *general rules*. The first is that the sympathetic and parasympathetic components cooperate to maintain a constant internal environment in the face of a changing external environment. Within this context, the sympathetic system is brought into widespread activity under emergency conditions, such as physical

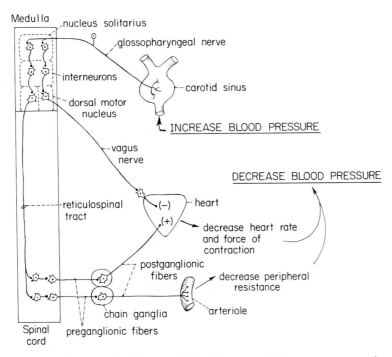

Figure 11–10. The carotid sinus reflex. Increase in blood pressure initiates a sequence of events that results in a decrease in blood pressure (see text).

exercise, fear, rage, and other stressful situations, which call for widespread adjustments in, for example, the cardiovascular system. Heart rate, cardiac output, and blood pressure increase as various visceral and peripheral vascular beds are shut down, so that more blood is shunted to the vital organs, such as the liver, brain, and muscles. On the other hand, the parasympathetic system subserves "local" protective functions that are aimed at maintaining and restoring bodily reserves. For example, the parasympathetic system protects the retina from excessive light by constricting the pupil, promotes the digestion and assimilation of food by increasing the motility and secretions of the digestive tract, and empties the bladder and rectum.

The second rule pertains to the *dual innervation* of visceral effectors; the sympathetic and parasympathetic components generally have antagonistic functions on a given structure. The size of the pupil is determined by the antagonistic effects of the autonomic supply to the pupillary muscles. The sympathetic nerves innervate the pupillary dilators, and the parasympathetic nerves (oculomotor) the pupillary constrictors. Horner's syndrome illustrates this. If the cervical sympathetic chain on one side is damaged, the pupil is smaller (resulting in miosis) on that side because of the unapposed action of the constrictor muscles. Note that ipsilateral facial dryness because of the lack of innervation of the sweat glands and facial warmth and redness because of vasodilation are also present.

Another example of dual innervation is that of the smooth muscles and secretory cells of viscera in the thoracic and abdominal cavities. In contrast to the effect on the pupil, here the antagonism is on the same effector cell. The bronchial musculature is relaxed by sympathetic discharge and constricted by parasympathetic discharge. Bronchial secretion is decreased by sympathetic discharge and increased by parasympathetic discharge. Such reciprocal effects also occur in the gut; stomach motility and secretion are increased by parasympathetic (vagus nerve) activity and decreased by sympathetic (thoracic splanchnic nerve) activity. However, the gut sphincters are relaxed by

vagal nerve stimulation and contracted by splanchnic nerve stimulation. Similarly, heart rate is decreased by vagal stimulation and increased by sympathetic stimulation. The innervation of the bladder is illustrated in Figure 11–11.

These examples (see also Table 11–1) illustrate the general rule, but many tissues do not function under such a delicate balance between the two systems. The muscles of the ciliary apparatus in the eye, which account for our ability to focus on near objects (accommodation), are supplied *mainly* by parasympathetic fibers from the ciliary ganglion; sweat glands, the smooth muscles associated with skin hairs, and cutaneous blood vessels receive *only* a sympathetic nerve supply; the adrenal gland receives *only* a sympathetic (preganglionic) nerve supply; the detrusor muscle of the bladder receives *only* a parasympathetic supply. Furthermore, dual innervation need not always be antagonistic. The erectile tissue of the penis receives a vasodilator supply from *both* the pelvic splanchnic and the sympathetic nerves, which are activated under appropriate conditions of sexual excitement.

The *inhibitory process*, whether sympathetic or parasympathetic, is another characteristic factor of the autonomic nervous system; inhibition takes place at the periphery in addition to within the central nervous system. For example, the heart is slowed by vagal stimulation because of an inhibitory action of the cholinergic postganglionic neurons on the cardiac neuroeffector tissue (*i.e.*, the sinoatrial node, which is the pacemaker), and the spontaneous activity of bronchial muscle and intestinal muscle is inhibited because of the hyperpolarizing action of the norepinephrine released from the postganglionic sympathetic endings. Note also that there are sympathetic cholinergic fibers that actively dilate blood vessels in skeletal muscles by inhibitory means. These instances illustrate direct inhibition of an effector tissue. The more general instance of the inhibition of smooth muscle in the peripheral arterioles is indirect, similar to that found in the relaxation of skeletal muscle. That is, the vasodilatory process results as a passive phenomenon brought about by a decrease in impulse

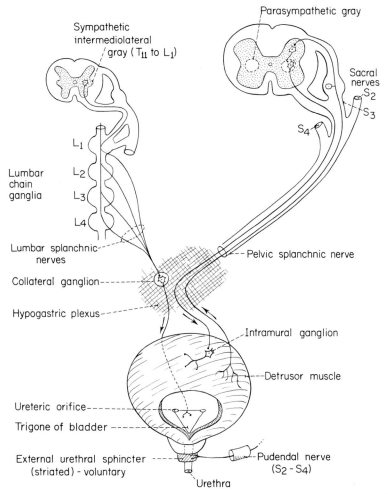

Figure 11–11. Innervation of the bladder. The sympathetic fibers innervate blood vessels of the bladder wall and the ureteral muscles that extend into the *bladder trigone*. The parasympathetic fibers affect only the *detrusor muscle* of the bladder. Bladder fullness is signaled to the central nervous system by the afferent fibers from the bladder wall. They travel in the pelvic nerve as shown, and in the spinal cord are found in the posterior columns. Pain fibers follow mainly the parasympathetic route and to a less extent, the lumbar splanchnic nerves. In the spinal cord they travel in the anterolateral columns. Note that in anterolateral cordotomy for the relief of intractable bladder pain, the sense of bladder fullness is not impaired because the afferents in the posterior columns are still intact.

Voluntary urination begins when intra-abdominal pressure increases and the external sphincter relaxes by the effect of descending influences from the cerebrum on the spinal cord somatic motor outflows. Contraction of the detrusor muscle empties the bladder. Micturition does not involve the sympathetic system. However, note that in ejaculation the sympathetic fibers cause contraction of the trigone musculature, thus preventing backflow of semen into the bladder. In spinal cord injuries that sever the long tract systems ascending to, and descending from, higher centers in the brain, the detrusor muscle can empty the bladder automatically through spinal reflex action.

traffic in the sympathetic effector nerves. The inhibitory process has taken place in the spinal cord, not actively at the effector, as in the other examples previously cited.

The demands causing increased activity of the autonomic nervous system are not always those characterized either by *emergency* or by *restorative* states. The autonomic nervous system is always operating in less dramatic terms, in concert with the descending systems regulating skeletal muscles (overt behavior) and the ascending systems regulating the sleep-wakefulness continuum (consciousness). The normal alert state is characterized by (1) a widespread but not fully active sympathetic discharge maintaining cardiovascular function; (2) an adequate level of activity in descending tracts influencing the alpha and gamma motoneurons so that muscle tone is appropriate for postural changes and movement; and (3) sufficient midbrain-thalamocortical "arousal" to bring about the electroencephalographic desynchronization found in the alert, waking state. This has been called the *ergotropic* state. The reciprocal condition has been called the *trophotropic* state. It is characterized by (1) parasympathetic dominance, (2) decreased muscle tone, and (3) cortical electrical synchronization representative of the relaxed condition. Obviously, we cycle imperceptively between these extremes, spending more or less time in either of the states, according to

our individual physiology and patterns of behavior. The point to be stressed is that the autonomic nervous system is always functioning *pari passu* with the rest of the nervous system, although we are not generally aware of it. Note, however, that good arguments have been made to support the theory that modern life is more akin to battlefield situations, where "fight or flight" decisions prevail, than to pastoral swings between ergotropic and trophotropic states. Psychosomatic disease is commonplace. An integral part of the etiology of "executive ulcers," "hypertension," and "tension headaches" is either the overfunctioning or underfunctioning of some component of the autonomic nervous system, along with increased activity in the somatic musculature.

ADDITIONAL READING

Axelrod, J. Noradrenaline: Fate and control of its biosynthesis. *Science,* 1971, *173,* 598–606.

Bennett, M. R. *Autonomic neuromuscular transmission.* Cambridge, Cambridge University Press, 1972.

Euler, U. S. von Adrenergic neurotransmitter functions. *Science,* 1971, *173,* 202–206.

Patton, H. D. The autonomic nervous system.

Chap. 10 in *Physiology and biophysics,* Ruch, T. C., and Patton, H. D., eds., Philadelphia, W. B. Saunders Co., 1965.

Pick, J. *The autonomic nervous system: Morphological, comparative, clinical, and surgical aspects.* Philadelphia, J. B. Lippincott Co., 1970.

Skok, V. I. *Physiology of autonomic ganglia.* Tokyo, I. Shoin Ltd., 1973.

CHAPTER 12

INTRODUCTION TO SENSORY PHYSIOLOGY

HARRY D. PATTON

SENSORY VERSUS MOTOR RESPONSES

Basic Considerations and Definitions

MEASUREMENTS OF SENSATION

PARAMETERS OF SENSATION

Quality or Modality
Intensity
Localization
Duration and Temporal Patterns of Stimuli
Affect

MECHANISMS OF NEURAL CODING

Coding of Modality Discrimination
Coding of Intensity Discrimination
Coding of Localization
Coding of Duration and Temporal Patterns of Stimuli
Coding of Affect

SENSORY VERSUS MOTOR RESPONSES

Upon entering the spinal cord, a dorsal root fiber bifurcates, sending one branch rostrally and one caudally (Fig. 12–1). Usually the rostral branch is the longer; for some of the medium-sized myelinated afferent fibers the rostral branch runs through the dorsal columns uninterruptedly from the site of entry all the way to the dorsal column nuclei, where it terminates on secondary neurons. Both rostral and caudal branches of small myelinated and unmyelinated fibers are relatively short and proceed only one or two segments before terminating on secondary neurons in the posterior gray matter. In addition to the two longitudinally running (rostrocaudal) primary branches, each fiber, whether large or small, gives off a variable number of secondary, collateral branches (reflexomotor collaterals), which penetrate vertically (dorsoventrally) through the gray matter to make connections either with interneurons or, in the case of the largest primary afferent fibers, with motoneurons in the anterior horn (Fig. 12–1).

The foregoing is a brief resume of basic neuroanatomical facts already covered; they are reviewed here to emphasize that nerve impulse traffic originating in receptors is relayed, upon entering the central nervous system (CNS), over two kinds of neuron chains. One, fed by the reflexomotor collaterals, leads to a *motor response* and is the segmental reflex system already dealt with in Chapters 9 and 10. The other comprises ascending neural chains fed by the rostral branches of afferent fibers; *some* of those chains relay information from receptors to the higher

155

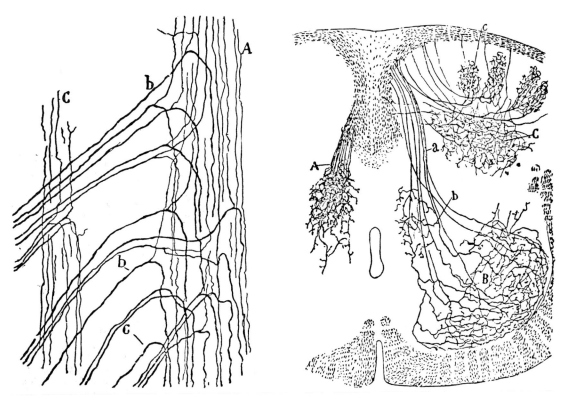

Figure 12–1. Intramedullary course of dorsal root fibers. *Left*, Longitudinal view from above. Fibers of both medial (*A*) and lateral (*C*) divisions of the root bifurcate into ascending (upward) and descending (downward) rami. *Right*, Cross section showing reflexomotor collaterals branching off at right angles from ascending and descending rami. (From Cajal, S. R.: Histologie du système nerveux de l'homme et des vertébrés, Madrid, Consejo Superior de Investigaciones Cientificas Instituto Ramón y Cajal, 1952.)

neural centers subserving sensation and perception. The organismic response to activation of these ascending chains is a *sensory response*, a "conscious" psychological event. This chapter and those following deal with the physiological mechanisms of sensation and perception and with the sensory consequences of injury to the nervous system.

Basic Considerations and Definitions

Establishment of two basic facts will simplify the discussion. First, although it is pedagogically expedient to distinguish between reflex motor responses and sensory responses, the two are not mutually exclusive. Indeed, one and the same primary afferent fiber may feed information into reflex channels and into ascending sensory channels. Thus the pathways

now to be considered are not entirely new but rather are continuations, or extensions, of afferent paths already described.

A simple example will clarify the roles of the motor and sensory chains in integrated behavior. When one steps on a tack, nociceptors are excited, and impulses are generated in the small myelinated and unmyelinated fibers innervating them. Such inputs feed polysynaptic reflex channels, exciting ipsilateral flexor motoneurons and inhibiting ipsilateral extensor motoneurons, and the foot is consequently withdrawn from the harmful stimulus (Chap. 10). In addition, crossed connections excite extensor motoneurons and inhibit flexor motoneurons on the contralateral side, and the resulting crossed extension provides one-legged support for the body during protective withdrawal of the injured limb. While these motor adjustments are being executed, signals are racing rostrally along the ascending pathways to arouse a sensation of pain, which alerts the organism to the unfriendly element of his environment—in this instance, the tack. Thus alerted, he initiates more involved and purposive defensive actions, *e.g.*, swearing, plucking the tack from the skin, rubbing the wound, applying medicaments. The spinal reflex mechanism is a relatively crude automatic first line of defense; its major virtue is speed. The belated arrival of information at the centers for perception allows deliberate evaluation and elaborate motor response.

A second point deserving emphasis is that although all sensory fibers are afferent fibers, not all afferent fibers are sensory. When we call a fiber or a tract *sensory*, we mean that its messages contribute to *conscious awareness* of one or another facet of external events. Only those afferent fibers that connect with ascending systems leading to the thalamus and sensory cortex are sensory; other afferent fibers subserve purely reflex functions without sensory concomitants. For example, the afferent fibers innervating the baroreceptors of carotid and aortic sinuses provide information important in reflex adjustments of circulation, but these are "unconscious" adjustments because none of the information is fed into ascending thalamocortical systems. Nor is demonstration that afferent information is fed into ascending spinal pathways sufficient proof that the information is "sensory."

For example, the rostrally directed branches of the lumbosacral Group I afferent fibers supplying annulospiral and Golgi tendon endings in leg muscles converge on cells in Clarke's column; their axons course rostrally in the dorsal spinocerebellar tract to the cerebellum. Although parts of the cerebellum send projections to the thalamus, those portions receiving input relayed from muscle and tendon receptors of the leg do not, for selective stimulation of Group I fibers from the leg elicits no activity in either thalamus or cortex. This part of the ascending proprioceptive afferent system from the leg thus appears not to be a non-sensory, long intersegmental reflex system. The problem of distinguishing between reflex afferents and sensory fibers and tracts is an important part of neurophysiology and clinical neurology. The neurologist daily faces the problem of localizing lesions underlying *sensory losses*, a problem that requires distinction between sensory and reflexomotor afferent paths. It is, therefore, important to use the words "sensory" and "afferent" discriminatingly.

MEASUREMENTS OF SENSATION

Sensations are subjective phenomena and are therefore more difficult to study and to evaluate than are motor responses, which can readily be measured quantitatively and objectively. Until recently, most studies of sensation were conducted on man because verbal reports were deemed necessary. However, the rapidly developing field of experimental psychology has provided behavioral techniques that permit reliable quantitative studies of sensory function in experimental animals. The trick is to establish a "language" in which a specific question can be put to the animal and in which he can signal an unambiguous answer.

For example, a hungry animal can be trained to press a lever when a light comes on to release a bit of food. Prompt lever manipulation following onset of the light signal is taken as evidence that the animal "senses" the light; it is simple then for the investigator to vary the intensity of the light signal and thus to evaluate the animal's visual threshold. In a refinement, developed by Blough, the animal is trained to press one lever, A, for food when the light is on, and another lever, B, to intensify the light signal when it drops below visual threshold. Lever A not only releases a food reward but dims the light incrementally, so that after a number of rewarded presses, the signal falls below the animal's threshold, and it must then resort to lever B to increase the light signal incrementally. The visual threshold is decisively bracketed between the intensities at which the animal oscillates from one lever to another. Using colored lights, one can measure the spectral visibility curves of an experimental animal with an accuracy and reliability rivaling, if not exceeding, those of similar measurements in man. Using variations of these procedures, the behaviorist can similarly evaluate other sensory functions in experimental animals. The advantage is that testing can be carried out before and after controlled neurosurgical lesions, the extent of which can be checked at autopsy.

Another field that contributes to sensory studies, particularly in man, is psychophysics. *Psychophysics* is a branch of psychology that aims at quantitative scaling of sensation. The psychophysicist asks his subject not "How intense is the light?" but "How intense is your visual sensation?" He then attempts to relate quantitatively the physical intensity to the subjective intensity. Obviously, the trick again is to devise a quantitative language, or scale, for subjective events. There are a number of approaches to this complicated problem, most of which are beyond the scope of the present discussion, but a couple of simple examples will illustrate the methodology behind them.

The first method, time-honored and traditional, measures the difference limen, or "just noticeable difference" (j.n.d.). The test subject is presented with a reference stimulus and is asked to choose from a continuum of other stimuli the one that is just distinguishable, *i.e.,* the one that produces a sensation just detectably greater or less than that produced by the reference. Such measurements were first carried out by Weber over 100 years ago on the discrimination between weights that the subject hefted. Weber found that the magnitude of the difference increment, or j.n.d., varied directly with the magnitude of the reference weight (I) and that the ratio of the j.n.d. to the reference weight was constant:

$$\frac{\text{j.n.d.}}{I} = k$$

This is known as *Weber's law,* and the Weber ratio for weights (k) was found to be 1:30. This means that with a 30-g reference, 29- and 31-g weights are distinguishable, but with a 60-g reference, discrimination is no better than 58 and 62 g, weights falling between these values all producing indistinguishable sensations. The j.n.d. is thus a measure of error, and

Weber found that the absolute magnitude of error increases as intensity increases.

Some years later Fechner repeated some of Weber's experiments and further subjected the results to a theoretical treatment, which caused considerable controversy. Fechner assumed that the detectable psychological increment (ΔS) was a minute sensory unit and proportional to the Weber ratio: $k\Delta S = \Delta I/I$ (where $\Delta I =$ the j.n.d. and I, the reference), or $\Delta S/\Delta I = 1/kI$. He then assumed that $\Delta S/\Delta I$ were true limiting values and that $dS/dI = 1/kI$. Integration yields the following relation, known as *Fechner's law*:

$$S = a \log I + b$$

where a and b are constants. *Fechner's law thus states that the magnitude of the sensation is directly proportional to the log of the physical stimulus.* Fechner's mathematical legerdemain has been much discussed and criticized and some of his assumptions are undoubtedly questionable.

Measurement of the j.n.d. is in effect a measure of sensory error, *i.e.,* of the range of sensory ambiguity. When psychophysical data are collected in other ways, the results are somewhat different. In the method of magnitude scaling the subject is presented with a reference stimulus and a series of other stimuli greater or less than the reference. He is then asked to assign magnitude numbers to each stimulus, assuming the reference to be ranked as a certain number, for example, 10. Ranked magnitude opinions of this sort are surprisingly reliable, judged either from data obtained from the same subject tested at different times or from data obtained from different subjects tested in the same way.

When the ratings are plotted against the physical intensities, the resulting curves are best fitted by the equation

$$S = kI^n$$

when k and n are constants. Such a power function, first proposed by Stevens, is a straight line when plotted on a log-log scale, the slope of the line being the exponent n ($\log S = n \log I$), whereas the relationship proposed by Fechner is linear on a semilog plot. For many sensory functions the difference between the two fits is small through the physiological range of intensities, but the relationship is of some interest because the parameter of neural action underlying intensity discrimination must bear a similar quantitative relationship to physical intensity. The matter will be discussed further subsequently.

PARAMETERS OF SENSATION

Sensory experience is not a unified neural event but is compounded of several parameters, or aspects, which, although usually fused in consciousness, are neurophysiologically independent and which may be dissociated or differentially affected by neural lesions. The easiest way to appreciate the compound nature of sensory experience is to consider the kinds of information that a sensation provides about the external world. Consider, for example, the sensation in a blindfolded subject aroused by a pin prick to the dorsum of the left hand. What deductions can be made about what has happened to him? Even without visual clues a normal subject can distinguish on the basis of his sensations: (1) the kind or quality of the stimulus, (2) the intensity of the stimulus, (3) the location of the stimulus, (4) the duration and temporal pattern of the stimulus, and (5) the affective content of the stimulus.

Quality or Modality

Quality discrimination is probably the most elementary kind of sensory discrimination. There is something unique about the conscious experience elicited by a pin prick that distinguishes it clearly and unambiguously from the conscious experiences elicited by other kinds of stimuli, such as a light touch with a wisp of cotton, displacement of a joint, or thermal stimulation of the skin. Indeed, the close one-to-one relation between sensation and stimulus is reflected semantically in our use of the same word to indicate both events; *e.g.*, a touch stimulus arouses a touch sensation. This is unfortunate, for it tends to obscure the fact that there are two distinctive events, a physical one in the skin

and a psychic one in the brain. Since quality of sensation is so distinctive, we deduce that there must be something uniquely different about the *neural messages* underlying different sensations. In other words, information about quality must somehow be coded in the neural messages. It is the job of neurophysiology to crack this code.

Intensity

We have already mentioned that normal subjects can gauge the intensity of a physical stimulus with considerable accuracy and that this ability depends on a measurable quantitative relationship between the physical and psychological events. Again, it follows that there must be something distinctively different about the *neural messages* underlying the conscious sensation aroused by a gentle pin prick and that elicited by a more intense jab. Another task of neurophysiology is to determine how information about intensity is coded in neural messages.

Localization

The normal human subject can localize with considerable accuracy the locus of the pin prick. Acuity of localization can be tested simply by having the blindfolded subject point with his finger to the site of stimulation. The capacity to localize cutaneous stimuli is called *topognosis*, and loss of this function is called *atopognosis*.

In addition to tests of topognoses, several tests of perceptual function that depend partly or wholly on localizing acuity are commonly employed by neurologists. (A *perception* is a conscious process involving either a *learned* combination of sensory modalities or a discrimination depending heavily on a learned comparison of sensations. Recognition of spatial and temporal patterns of stimulation are perceptions.) One such test is measurement of the two-point threshold. *Two-point threshold* is defined as the smallest distance between two simultaneously applied punctate stimuli that can be recognized as two rather than as only one. Two-point threshold is an

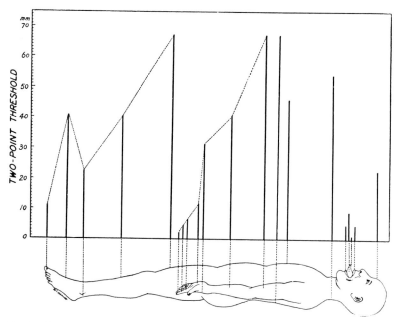

Figure 12–2. Regional variation in tactile two-point threshold in man. (From Ruch and Patton, eds., *Physiology and biophysics,* Philadelphia, W. B. Saunders Co., 1965.)

estimate of error in localization and is a kind of "just noticeable difference" threshold. Figure 12–2 shows that the two-point threshold varies regionally, being smallest on the fingers, toes, and tongue and quite large on the axial parts of the body. Although this is usually ascribed to presumed differences in innervation density, other factors may be involved. Recent experiences with a prosthetic device for the blind in which a television camera activates a grid of pegs pressed against the skin of the back indicate that subjects can, with training, learn to recognize visual patterns thus transduced into cutaneous pressure patterns with an accuracy that is surprising in view of the crude two-point discrimination (7 cm) on the back. Two-point acuity depends in part on practice and training.

A second perceptual test involving localization is the *figure-writing test (graphesthesia).* A digit from 0 to 9 is traced lightly on the blindfolded subject's skin. Recognition of the digit clearly depends on the subject's ability to discriminate the spatial pattern of stimulation. Graphesthesia improves with practice. A reading device for the blind projects an alphabet onto the skin of the fingers by air jets. With training, subjects

attain reading speeds of up to 30 words a minute.

Another test of perceptual function is that for *stereognosis,* the ability to recognize the shape, or spatial pattern, of cutaneous stimulation. As we shall see later, astereognosis may occur in neurological patients who have little or no defect in modality discrimination; such patients are aware of an object in the hand but are unable to identify it.

Finally, a test that often reveals unilateral disturbances of localization requires recognition of *simultaneously applied bilateral stimuli.* When homologous points on the two sides of the body are stimulated (*e.g.,* touched or tapped), normal subjects are of course aware of both stimuli and can readily distinguish between unilateral and bilateral stimulation. In neurological patients who have suffered unilateral damage to sensory pathways, however, simultaneous bilateral stimuli are felt on only one side (the side ipsilateral to the lesion). This phenomenon is called *extinction.* The defect occurs even in patients who readily recognize either stimulus when it is applied in isolation. Even with eyes open the patient does not feel the stimulus on his "bad" side—"I know you touched me on both sides because I saw you, but I felt it on only one side." Extinction of one of two simultaneous stimuli bilaterally applied is a delicate test of perceptual function and often reveals a defect not obvious from other tests.

Just as quality and intensity must be coded in neural messages, so also must localization. That is to say, there must be distinctive differences in the neural messages set up by stimuli applied to different parts of the body.

Duration and Temporal Patterns of Stimuli

Onset and cessation of stimuli are promptly recognized; the lag (reaction time) is satisfactorily accounted for by conduction time. Reaction time measurements (*e.g.*, depressing a key to signal onset and cessation of a sensation) include afferent and efferent components. In a monkey, the reaction time to a visual stimulus can be shortened from 30 to 40 msec if an electrical stimulus to the visual cortex is substituted for the visual stimulus; the latency of electrical responses of visual cortex to retinal stimulation with light is of the same order.

The ability to recognize varying temporal patterns of stimulation (*e.g.*, flutter, or vibration) is often tested in neurological examinations with a vibrating tuning fork pressed against the skin. The ability to recognize vibrations is called *pallesthesia*. Again, it may be assumed that the neural message underlying perception of vibration must contain some variable that reflects the temporal pattern of the stimulus.

Affect

A final parameter of perception is affect, *i.e.*, the pleasantness or unpleasantness of a stimulus. Some perceptions are pleasant (*e.g.*, warmth, sexual sensations), some unpleasant (*e.g.*, pain, cold), while others are neutral (*e.g.*, sense of position, touch). Again, it may be presumed that the messages underlying these different percep-

tions must somehow be fundamentally different.

In summary, sensory messages contain in coded form information about "whatness," "muchness," "whereness," "longness," and "goodness" of stimuli arising in the external world.

MECHANISMS OF NEURAL CODING

The neural messages generated by stimulation of receptors are action potentials, and so the codes for sensory data must correspond to variables of action potentials. A priori, two general ways (not necessarily mutually exclusive) by which coding might occur seem plausible; these may be termed *pattern coding* and *place coding*. In pattern coding, each signaled piece of information is envisioned as being represented as a distinctive temporal pattern of cell discharge in sensory receiving areas. Pattern coding is economical in the sense that each transmission line can be used (on different occasions) to signal different kinds of information; the only limitation is the number of distinctive patterns. The Morse code is a simple example of pattern coding.

In place coding, on the other hand, it is postulated that discharge of a unique set of centrally located neurons underlies each discriminable sensory event. A typewriter is place-coded; no matter how it is activated, the *e* key, for example, will produce only *e* and *e* can be produced only by activation of the *e* key. Place coding is more prodigal of elements and transmission lines than pattern coding because each line carries only one kind of information; any cross talk between lines is inadmissible. For example, if modality is postulated to be place-coded, one must demonstrate for each modality "private" paths from the periphery to the central receiving centers; if in transmission messages elicited by different stimuli converge on common elements, the message becomes ambiguous.

We can now discuss what is known (or guessed) about the mechanisms of coding underlying the various parameters of sensation. In the case of pattern-coded components, we will consider the ancillary question of the nature of the patterns and, in place coding, the question of the identity and location of the specific sensory cells.

Coding of Modality Discrimination

The mechanism for modality discrimination is probably the most controversial and least securely established of all the mechanisms for the sensory parameters. The traditional view is that modality is place-coded, and we can trace the origin of this notion.

It has been stressed that a place-coded mechanism requires "private paths" from the periphery to the receiving center. In the case of modality discrimination, this means that some pathways must be found that are modality-specific throughout. In Chapter 7 we emphasized that most receptors respond selectively to a specific kind of physical energy. Even the nociceptors, once thought to be promiscuously sensitive to any kind of damaging stimulus, appear to be somewhat selective, for Perl and Burgess find some nociceptors that respond to intense mechanical stimuli (pinching, crushing) but not to damaging extremes of heat or cold nor to irritating chemical agents. Thus, in the primary element, the necessary (but not sufficient) condition of modality specificity appears to be well established. However, maintenance of purity becomes increasingly less probable with increasing synaptic relays, since the principle of convergence, which operates at each relay site, encourages mixture of inputs. Indeed, Wall, after careful sampling of secondary neurons in the dorsal horn, was unable to find enough selectively sensitive specimens to support a place-coding hypothesis and, by exclusion, favored pattern coding of modality. It should be remembered, however, that theory does not require that all pathways be modality-specific; existence of some specific paths suffices, and in fact there is no way to know how many activated specific central cells might suffice to establish a unique sensory experience.

Recently, Burgess and Perl have re-investigated the properties of cells in the dorsal horn and have found convincing evidence for modality specificity of secondary neurons. Even the projection of many nociceptors appears to be, at least in part, onto selected secondary neurons, a finding of considerable importance since Wall was especially critical of place-coding theories of pain. Burgess and Perl found dorsal horn elements fed exclusively by small myelinated afferent fibers (delta fibers) that are excited selectively by damagingly intense mechanical cutaneous stimuli. Also in ascending tracts of the cord and in relay sites in the medulla, thalamus, and cortex, fibers and cells are found that appear to respond selectively to one or another kind of peripheral stimulus. In the sensory cortex and in the thalamus modality-specific cells that respond selectively to deflections of hairs, light indentation of skin, or joint movement can be identified. Modality-specific cortical units responding to thermal and noxious stimuli have not been convincingly demonstrated, although in anesthetized animals posterior thalamic units responding to noxious stimuli have been reported; the special case of pain sensation will be discussed in more detail later. At present, we can conclude that, for most modalities, there appears to be satisfactory evidence for the existence of some private pathways.

Demonstration of modality-specific afferent pathways is a necessary, but not sufficient, condition for the validation of the place-coding theory. An independent, testable consequence of the theory is that the specificity of the sensory response should be independent of the kind of physical stimulus that causes the specific central cells to discharge. That this is true for cutaneous senses was first noted in the 19th century by Müller, who formulated his findings as the *law of specific nerve energies.* Müller's "law" states that the quality of sensory experience depends on *which* receptors are excited, not on *how* they are excited. Müller found that punctate cutaneous sites that yield cold sensations to cold stimuli also yield cold sensations to warm stimuli—the phenomenon of "paradoxical cold." The important determinant of sensory uniqueness is thus *which* pathway is excited, not *how* it is excited. This is exactly what is expected if the ascending pathways are simply excitatory lines to the specific place-coded receiving areas.

For certain of the special senses, the evidence for place coding is even stronger. Electrical stimulation of cells in the visual cortical receiving area in conscious human patients produces sensations of flashing lights, and similar stimulation in the auditory receiving cortex produces auditory hallucinations. In these instances, the ascending pathways are bypassed and hence can play no role in determining the identity of the sensory response. It was the concept of place coding of modality that prompted DuBois Reymond's whimsical prediction that if the auditory pathways were connected to the visual cortex and the optic pathways to the auditory cortex, we would see thunder and hear lightning!

Assuming, then, that modality is place-coded, we proceed to the more difficult question of locating the specific cells whose discharge is the physical correlate of modality recognition. One approach is the one just cited, namely, to search for centrally located cells, the stimulation of which will produce a specific sensory response. For vision and audition, this is easily accomplished. The cutaneous modalities, however, do not have private macroscopic receiving areas but project haphazardly to common thalamic and cortical sites, so that separate areas related to the several cutaneous sensory modalities are not easily identified. Stimulation in the somatosensory cortex produces a tingling sensation in which the separate modalities are not recognized. Another approach is to attempt to abolish modality discrimination by destroying central neuron populations. For vision, once again this method yields a decisive answer, for destruction of the visual cortex in the occipital lobe produces in man complete and irreversible blindness. It seems reasonable to conclude, therefore, that the cells in the visual cortex or those in the lateral geniculate body (the thalamic nucleus projecting to the visual cortex) are the cells whose discharge underlies conscious sensation of vision. (The geniculate body is included as a possible site because it undergoes retrograde degeneration when the visual cortex is removed, so that a lesion of the cortex is at once also a lesion of the thalamus.

Also, because the visual cortex sends corticofugal projection fibers to the lateral geniculate nucleus, electrical stimulation of the visual cortex causes relayed discharge of geniculate cells.) But vision is the only sensory modality so decisively abolished by cortical destruction. Lesions of the somatosensory cortex in man (causing retrograde degeneration of the posteroventral thalamic nucleus, which receives the major ascending pathways carrying somatosensory information) do not produce serious permanent loss of ability to distinguish sensory modalities. As we shall see, such lesions impair other parameters of somatic sensation, but modality discrimination is disturbed either little or not at all. It appears then that the specific cells for distinguishing or "sensing" cutaneous modalities lie at some more caudal site in the brain. The exact location is unknown.

Coding of Intensity Discrimination

There is a time-honored notion that intensity discrimination is pattern-coded. One of the best-established properties of tonic receptors is their ability to vary frequency of firing as a function of intensity of stimulation (Chap. 7). Moreover, for many receptors, the frequency of discharge through the range in which frequency varies with intensity appears to be related to the log of the stimulus, and this relationship in the heyday of the Weber-Fechner formulation was deemed by many to be a satisfying correlation between psychophysical and physiological measurements. Unfortunately, the behavior of the primary elements tells us little about coding of intensity unless frequencies set by primary elements are relayed faithfully over each of the elements of the ascending synaptically linked chain. Mountcastle finds that the frequency of firing of cortical cells responding repetitively to joint displacement fits a power function (*i.e.*, a log-log relationship) better than a semilog function of joint position and cites his results as vindication of Stevens' psychophysical measures. Actually, the difference between a semilog and a log-log function is not great through the critical range, and the argument may be a tempest in a teapot. Nevertheless, it does seem likely that frequency is the neuronal code for intensity discrimination for modalities mediated by tonic receptors. The additional correlate of intensity is the number of units activated, so that an ability to meter the number of discharges per unit of time may determine perception of intensity.

For modalities served by phasic receptors, frequency is not the major determinant of intensity. A disturbing fact is that the majority of cells in sensory cortex and thalamus that respond to cutaneous stimulation (movement of hairs, light touch, and so forth) do so in a phasic, "on-off" fashion. The only measurable changes in such units when stimulus intensity increases are decreased latency and a limited increase in number of spikes per discharge. Such changes no doubt alter the population pattern of discharge in a complex way, and such collective pattern codes may underlie intensity discrimination.

There is evidence that cortical and thalamic cells play an important part in determining intensity discriminations, for appropriate cortical ablations produce serious impairment of these functions in both man and chimpanzees.

Coding of Localization

The ability to localize a stimulus is thought to depend on place coding. One of the most striking features of the ascending sensory pathways is their topographical organization. A *topographically organized system* is one in which at each level those elements receiving input from a body surface region are spatially collected together and occupy a predictable position with respect to elements receiving input from neighboring areas on the body surface. In a topographically organized system information from the body surface is projected onto the higher receiving centers in an organized fashion. The basis for a crude kind of topographical projection has already been described anatomically in terms of segmental entry of dorsal root fibers into the spinal cord; the resultant representation of dermatomes in tracts and central nuclei is preserved in the laminar structure of the tracts.

One can demonstrate topographical

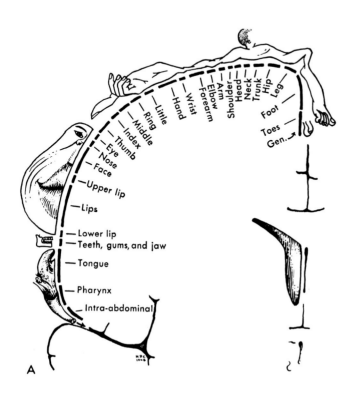

Figure 12–3. Diagram of representation of body surface in postcentral gyrus as mapped by punctate electrical stimulation of the exposed cortex in human subjects. Figurine depicts the relative areas of representation of different body areas. (From Penfield and Rasmussen, *The cerebral cortex of man*, New York, Macmillan & Co., 1952.)

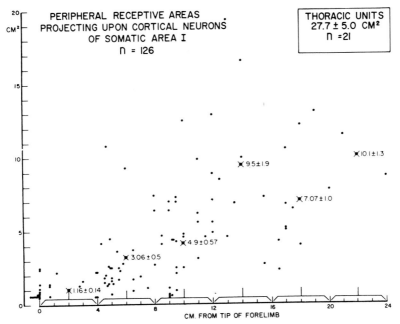

Figure 12–4. Relation between size and location of receptive fields of somatosensory cortical neurons responding to stimulation of the contralateral forelimb in the cat. Dots represent data from individual cells; crosses mark means of fields grouped into classes by 4-cm distances from toes. Units receiving input from the thorax were offscale on the ordinate; the mean and standard error for these units is given in the box at the upper right. (From Mountcastle, *J. Neurophysiol.*, 1957, 20, 408–434.)

organization functionally by mapping the electrical responses of the sensory cortex to exploratory stimulation of the contralateral body surface. Such studies readily reveal relatively distinct cortical receiving areas for stimuli applied to the leg, arm, and face. More careful exploration reveals continuous but overlapping representation of individual dermatomes in the postcentral gyrus.

Another method is to chart the body areas to which human subjects localize sensations aroused by punctate electrical stimulation of the sensory cortex. Such maps (Fig. 12–3), obtained from neurosurgical patients with craniotomies performed under local anesthesia, agree well with those obtained by the evoked potential method in monkeys and chimpanzees. Thus, the functional and anatomical substrate of dermatomal localization is easily demonstrated.

Such methods, however, are inadequate to reveal an organization suitable to explain the fine spatial discriminations of two-point threshold and graphesthesia. To gain some idea of how these discrimina-

tions might be coded, we need to consider the receptive fields of single neurons. By the receptive field of a cortical cell responding to cutaneous stimulation (for example), we mean the spatial extent of the cutaneous surface wherein stimulation will cause that neuron to discharge. Mountcastle has made a thorough study of the receptive fields of cortical cells in the somatosensory receiving area and finds that field size varies from a few square millimeters to several square centimeters and that receptive field size varies with its location, being smallest for units receiving input from the distal parts of the limbs and greatest for those having fields on the trunk (Fig. 12–4). There is thus an inverse relation between field sizes and sensory acuity, as might be expected if localization is place-coded. The discharge of a cell having a receptive field of 3 mm² has in it the information that the stimulus fell somewhere within this small area, whereas the discharge of a cell with a larger receptive field signals a correspondingly less precise localization of the stimulus.

Two other factors make signaling of localization more precise. The first is overlap of receptive fields of different cortical units. For example, simultaneous discharge of two cells having a limited region of overlap of receptive fields signals stimulation within the region of overlap and, hence, provides localizing information that is more discrete than in the discharge of either unit alone. If within a cortical focus there are many units with small overlapping fields, distinctive signaling of considerable resolution is theoretically possible.

A second factor increasing the acuity of cutaneous localization is the phenomenon of *lateral inhibition.* If a stimulus is applied just outside the receptive field of a cortical unit, that element not only fails to discharge but its responsiveness to excitatory stimuli applied within the receptive field is diminished. Stated another way, a stimulus applied to a spot on the skin causes discharge of cortical cells whose receptive fields include this spot, but it also inhibits the discharge of units having receptive fields in adjacent skin. In the case of two-point threshold, such a mechanism could serve to sharpen the cortical boundaries of discharging units and increase the contrast between the two regions of high activity corresponding to the cortical foci for the two cutaneous points.

That cells in the cortex, the thalamus, or both are essential for localization is well established by the observation that human subjects who have suffered lesions of the sensory cortex have as their major sensory and perceptual deficit great difficulty in discriminating the spatial aspects of stimulation. Indeed, this appears to be the major sensory function of the thalamus and cortex; modality discrimination remains intact and intensity discrimination, although impaired, is usually not abolished following a lesion of either the sensory cortex or the thalamus. Such patients are thus by no means anesthetic, but characteristically their two-point thresholds are increased; they have difficulty in pointing accurately to a stimulated site (atopognosis) and suffer severe impairment of graphesthesia and stereognosis. *Whereas "whatness" appears to depend little on the cortex and "how muchness" only partly, "whereness" depends heavily on the thalamus and cortex.*

The foregoing description is best documented for those modalities that are mediated by the fibers in the dorsal column–medial lemniscal system. The mechanism of localization of anterolateral column ("spinothalamic") modalities and especially of pain, presents special problems and is reserved for discussion later (Chap. 14).

Coding of Duration and of Temporal Patterns of Stimuli

Judgments concerning onset and cessation of stimuli are presumably correlated with onset and cessation of firing of some set of central neurons. Such discrimination is thus thought to be pattern-coded. However, the mechanism, little studied, must vary with modality. For example, for those modalities that discharge central cells in a phasic, "on-off" fashion, the signal is ambiguously the same for the two events. Even those cortical cells that are driven tonically show considerable adaptation of firing pattern, so that the analog of duration is not perfectly coded by repetitive firing.

A special problem of temporal pattern recognition is the appreciation of oscillatory cutaneous stimuli, such as are produced by holding a vibrating object (such as a tuning fork) on the skin. There appear to be two kinds of peripheral receptors that signal to the central nervous system information about such stimuli. Both are phasic receptors and, hence, provide only distorted information about steady, maintained mechanical distortion of the skin. Subjected to vibratory stimuli, however, these receptors generate repetitive discharges, one spike being associated with each cycle of oscillation. Messages generated in such receptors contain information concerning the temporal frequency of the mechanical oscillation; they differ from other receptors in which frequency of discharge is correlated with intensity of stimulus.

One of the two vibration-sensitive receptors produces such stimulus-locked, entrained discharges for frequencies from 5 to 50 Hz; above and below these frequencies the threshold (measured in terms of required magnitude of skin deformation) rises sharply. This low-frequency receptor is located in glabrous (nonhairy) skin. The other receptor has a lower threshold but entrains faithfully only to higher frequencies, from 50 cps to greater than 300 cps; it is located subcutaneously and is presumed to be the Pacinian corpuscle (Chap. 7).

Measurements of thresholds for sensations of flutter (5 to 50 cps) and vibration (greater than 50 cps) as a function of frequency are best fitted on log-log plots by two straight lines having different slopes and intersecting at about 40 to 50 cps (Fig. 12–5). Iontophoretic anesthetization of the superficial skin elevates thresholds to flutter sensations without affecting vibratory sensation. It thus seems that recognition of temporal patterns of stimulation depends on two specific receptors with frequency-dependent sensitivities that permit entrainment of nerve impulses through ranges of frequency. More recently, Mountcastle and his colleagues

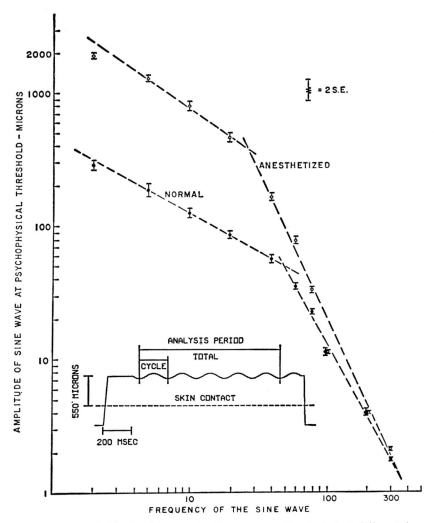

Figure 12–5. Human thresholds for flutter and vibration sensation tested at different frequencies. Inset shows diagrammatically the wave form of the stimulus; sine wave oscillations were superimposed on a base line indentation (550 μm) of the skin of the thenar eminence. Threshold for recognition of oscillation depends on frequency. The lower curve was from normal skin; the upper curve, from skin iontophoretically anesthetized with cocaine. Anesthetic has little effect on thresholds for frequencies above about 50 cps (vibration) but severely impairs recognition of oscillations below 50 cps (flutter). The latter sensation is ascribed to cutaneous receptors, whereas vibration is probably mediated by subcutaneous receptors (Pacinian corpuscles). (From Mountcastle *et al., Science,* 1967, *155,* 597–600.)

have found cells in the somatosensory cortex and thalamus of monkey that behave as though they were being driven by one or the other of these two frequency-sensitive receptors and that develop rhythmic entrained discharges during cutaneous stimulation with the appropriate frequency.

If the proposed mechanism for flutter-vibration perception is correct, it is an instance in which *both* place coding and pattern coding are employed: place coding because specific cells in sensory receiving areas are involved and pattern coding because the prerequisite for recognition of vibration is spike entrainment in these cells.

Coding of Affect

That affect is a separable component of certain sensory modalities is indicated by the finding that neural lesions or drugs may selectively abolish affect without seriously impairing modality recognition. For example, lesions interrupting the fiber tracts connecting the prefrontal cerebral cortex with subcortical centers relieve the suffering of patients with intractable pain, although the pain as a recognizable sensation persists. The patient continues to hurt, but the pain doesn't bother him. Morphine has a similar effect; it limits the agony of pain without altering the pain threshold.

When electrodes are permanently implanted in selected cortical and subcortical sites in experimental animals and are connected through a lever switch to a stimulating circuit, the animals constantly press the lever as if they derived intense satisfaction from the brain stimulus. So powerful is the satisfaction from such self-stimulation that it can be used effectively as a reward in a training situation and the animal quickly learns to carry out relatively complex tasks to acquire his "electrical martini." Conversely, at other electrode emplacement sites electrical stimulation appears to be unpleasant; animals quickly learn complex tricks to avoid or to discontinue such stimuli. There thus appear to be separate brain sites, stimulation of which elicits strong affective states, positive or negative, depending on location.

Comparable sites have also been stimulated in conscious humans. Stimulation of "positive" sites produces a feeling of abstract pleasure unrelated to any particular sensation, whereas stimulation at negative sites produces a feeling of displeasure similarly divorced from specific sensation. The effective regions are mostly in the hypothalamus, midthalamus, and rhinencephalon, structures to be described later (Chaps. 26 and 27). For the moment, it suffices to note the existence of central neuronal groups, activity of which is associated with pleasure, and others that signal negative affect. A plausible hypothesis is that sensations having positive affect (*e.g.*, satiety, sexual sensations) have strong connections with the "pleasure" neurons and that those having negative affect (pain, cold, hunger) feed collaterals to the "displeasure" system. If this is so, affect is a place-coded parameter of selected sensory modalities. Interestingly, those modalities having strong affect (pain, thermal sensation, sexual sensation) reach the brainstem via the anterolateral spinal ascending system, whereas the dorsal column system mediates sensory modalities (*e.g.*, limb position) that are affectively bland.

ADDITIONAL READING

Mountcastle, V. B. Sensory receptors and neural encoding: introduction to sensory processes, in *Medical physiology*, Mountcastle, V. B., ed., St. Louis, The C. V. Mosby Co., 1974.

Ruch, T. C. Somatic sensation, in *Physiology and biophysics.* Chap. 14 in Ruch, T. C., and Patton, H. D.,

eds., Philadelphia, W. B. Saunders Co., 1965.

Stevens, S. S. Sensory power functions and neural events, in *Handbook of sensory physiology: principles of receptor physiology*, Loewenstein, W. R., ed., New York, Springer-Verlag, 1971.

CHAPTER 13

SOMATIC SENSATION AND ITS DISTURBANCES

HARRY D. PATTON

SENSORY DISSOCIATIONS

In the preceding chapter, sensory experience was analyzed into a number of constituent components, or parameters. Such analysis may seem arbitrary and conjectural, but the concept of the compound nature of sensation is extremely useful clinically; indeed, it derives largely from observations on human patients.

Disease of the nervous system rarely abolishes all parameters of sensation uniformly. Commonly one or more parameters are deranged, and others are left either intact or less disturbed. The nature of the disturbance and the geographical pattern of sensory defect on the body surface are important clues to the location and sometimes to the type of neural lesion. Therefore, in performing a diagnostic sensory examination the neurologist must *note carefully both which sensory functions remain intact and which are lost.*

A sensory disturbance in which one or more sensory parameters are disturbed more than others is called a *dissociation of sensory parameters*, or simply a *sensory dissociation*. The four most commonly encountered dissociations are discussed below.

Dissociation of Modalities

One or more sensory modalities (*e.g.,* pain and temperature) are selectively lost, but others remain unimpaired (*e.g.,* touch, position, and vibratory sensation). Modality dissociations are most likely to occur when a lesion (*e.g.,* a tumor) affects parts of the nervous system where pathways mediating different modalities are spatially separated so that one tract may be interrupted but not the other. The common finding of modality dissociations, particularly in association with lesions of the spinal cord,

169

is one of the main reasons for assuming that modality is place-coded rather than pattern-coded.

Topographical Dissociation

After a neural lesion, sensation is usually disturbed over part of the body surface but is intact elsewhere. Accurate mapping of the boundaries between normally sentient and either hypesthetic or hypalgesic* skin areas is important, for the geometrical pattern of sensory disturbance varies with the location and type of lesion.

Dissociation of Levels of Sensation

In neurological patients a recognition of quality often remains intact, but discriminations of the spatial and temporal qualities of the stimulus are impaired. Stated otherwise, sensation is intact, but perception is blunted. Thus a patient may recognize a light touch with a wisp of cotton but have difficulty in localizing the stimulus. Other perceptual functions, such as graphesthesia, stereognosis, recognition of two-point stimuli and of simultaneously applied bilateral stimuli, may also suffer even though the sensory modalities underlying these discriminations appear intact.

Dissociation of Affect

In this dissociation sensory modalities normally having a strong affective component become colorless and lacking in affect, although awareness of stimulation and recognition of modality remain intact. Thus a patient, although aware of pain sensations, may report that they are no longer unpleasant and disturbing; he hurts but does not "suffer." The tranquility produced by certain narcotic drugs, notably morphine, is mainly due to selective suppression of affective reactions to pain without serious defect in recognition of pain as a distinctive sensory modality.

Hypesthesia is reduced tactile sensibility; *hypalgesia* is reduced pain sensitivity.

Conversely, in some neurologic diseases, affect may be heightened or exaggerated, and this alteration may affect sensations having both negative (*e.g.*, pain) and positive (*e.g.*, warmth) affect.

PERIPHERAL NERVE LESIONS

It has already been emphasized that each afferent nerve fiber in a peripheral nerve trunk terminates distally in a receptor that is, within broad limits, selectively sensitive to one or another kind of stimulus. Consequently, each afferent axon signals to the central nervous system information about only one kind of peripheral event; *i.e.*, each is a modality-specific conduit.

Since the afferent nerve fibers in a trunk differ from one another in diameter (and hence conduction velocity) and in the presence or absence of a myelin sheath, physiologists and neurologists have long been intrigued by the possibility that these morphological differences might be correlated with specific sensory function. The question can be explored by painstaking dissection of single fibers and determination of both their conduction speeds (from which diameter can be estimated) and their functional specificity. However, before one can assert that such correlations are relevant to sensation, he must demonstrate that the identified peripheral fibers feed into ascending systems reaching suprasegmental sensory structures (thalamus, sensory cortex) to distinguish them from simple nonsensory segmental (or intersegmental) reflex afferent fibers. This latter requirement is especially difficult to achieve, for as sensory information is relayed centrally over successive neurons, the complicated patterns of divergence and convergence make it easy for the investigator to lose his way.

The cherished dream of correlating afferent fiber diameter with sensory function has been only partly realized. The largest myelinated afferent fibers of deep nerve trunks — 12 to 20 μm in diameter and known as Group I fibers — are the clearly established parents of stretch-sensitive elements in muscle and tendons. They constitute the afferent limb of the

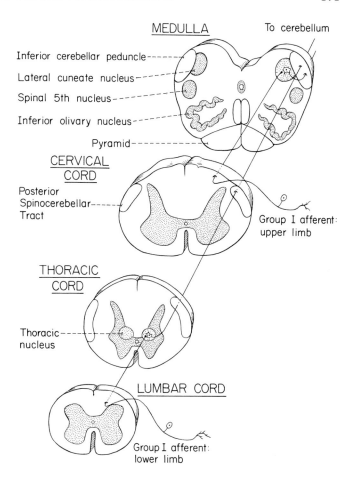

MEDULLA

To cerebellum

Inferior cerebellar peduncle

Lateral cuneate nucleus

Spinal 5th nucleus

Inferior olivary nucleus

Pyramid

CERVICAL CORD

Posterior Spinocerebellar Tract

Group I afferent: upper limb

THORACIC CORD

Thoracic nucleus

LUMBAR CORD

Group I afferent: lower limb

Figure 13–1. Major ascending pathway from afferents in the upper and lower limbs to the cerebellum.

stretch reflex and the inverse myotatic reflex, respectively. The central projections of these fibers terminate several segments rostral to their entry sites, on the cells of Clarke's column on the medial aspect of the dorsal horn; these cells in turn send axons in the dorsal spinocerebellar tract (dorsolateral white column) to the cerebellum (Fig. 13–1) and appear to have no sensory function. Group I fibers do, however, appear to have a weak projection to the cortex, for weak stimulation of a deep nerve adequate only for the large Group I fibers produces a small evoked cortical potential, the significance of which is unclear. Certainly signals from the muscle spindle and the Golgi tendon organ are inadequate for position sense, because appreciation of joint position and movement in the fingers is abolished by local anesthesia of the joint capsules, a procedure that spares the muscle and tendon receptors.

A variety of cutaneous mechanoreceptors with discharge properties suitable for signaling information concerning deformation of the skin (touch and pressure) have been described. Some are associated with hairs; others are found in hairless (glabrous) skin. There is good evidence both from gross cortical potential studies and from single cortical cell recording that these mechanoreceptors have a rich projection to the thalamus and cortex. It is not necessary to describe here in detail the distinctive properties of the numerous, different cutaneous mechanoreceptors; it is sufficient to say that as a group they are innervated by fibers ranging from the largest (about 18 μm) to the smallest (less than 1 μm, the unmyelinated C fibers). In other words, "touch-pressure" information is relayed by fibers that span the entire diameter spectrum of the cutaneous nerve trunk.

On the other hand, noxious (pain?) and

thermal stimuli excite receptors that are served by small myelinated fibers (delta fibers, 1 to 6 μm in diameter) and by unmyelinated C fibers (less than 1 μm thick), a relationship that has been convincingly established by single-fiber recording. Among the delta population are found a significant number of units that respond only to strong *noxious mechanical* stimulation (cutting, pinching) of skin or subcutaneous structures; such units are surprisingly insensitive to noxious heating and cooling and to application of chemical irritants (acid, bradykinin). The C-fiber population contains considerable numbers of such high-threshold mechanoreceptors but also many units that respond in "polymodal" fashion not only to noxious mechanical stimuli but also to noxious thermal and chemical stimuli. These polymodal nociceptors also show an interesting property of sensitization. Once they have been excited by a noxious stimulus, their thresholds to subsequently applied stimuli are diminished, and they then respond to relatively mild stimuli. This behavior is reminiscent of the hyperalgesia that develops in injured skin, for example, the heightened sensitivity of sunburned or bruised skin. Other experiments have revealed in the marginal region of the dorsal horn secondary neurons that are fed exclusively by myelinated high-threshold mechanoreceptors and others that seem to be driven both by the polymodal C-fiber elements and by myelinated high-threshold mechanoreceptors.

In addition to nociceptors, the delta- and C-fiber populations contain elements responsive to innocuous thermal stimuli, and the secondary elements fed selectively by these thermoreceptors are found in the marginal region of the dorsal horn. Finally, many fibers activated by low-threshold mechanoreceptors are found in both the myelinated delta- and the unmyelinated C-fiber populations.

In summary, then, cutaneous mechanoreceptors relaying information relative to mechanical deformation of skin (touch and pressure?) utilize fibers that span the full range of fiber diameters, but nociceptors and thermoreceptors utilize only the small myelinated delta fibers and the unmyelinated C fibers.

Because C fibers conduct at speeds of less than 1 m/sec and the largest delta fibers at 30 m/sec, nociceptive messages traversing long conduction pathways (*e.g.,* from the tip of the finger or of the toe) become temporally dispersed, so that the more rapidly conducted signals reach the brain sooner than the messages generated in the more sluggish C fibers. One can readily demonstrate the sensory consequences of this dispersion by the simple experiment of holding the tip of his finger or toe momentarily against a hot light bulb or a lighted cigarette. The sensory consequence is *double pain,* a momentary sharp, pricking pain that rises to a crescendo and then subsides (fast, or first, pain), followed by a second, duller, aching sensation (slow, or second, pain). Fast pain is conducted over delta fibers and slow pain over C fibers. If the same stimulus is applied to more proximal parts of the arm or leg, the conduction path is decreased and the degree of dispersion decreases just as the lead of a fast over a slow runner becomes less as the track is shortened. Correspondingly, the interval between the onset of fast and slow pain becomes less, and for stimulus sites more proximal than the forearm, the two components can no longer be distinguished.

Clinically, the importance of the correlation between fiber size and sensory function, imperfect though it is, is that certain injuries and diseases (peripheral neuropathies) sometimes selectively affect fibers according to diameter. Hence, insofar as diameter and function are correlated a modality dissociation may result. For example, pressure blocks large fibers more readily than small ones and causes disproportionately severe impairment of touch, pressure, position sense, and vibration, with little impairment of pain and thermal sensation. When pressure block progresses until the smallest myelinated fibers cease conducting, leaving only the C fibers operant, fast, pricking pain disappears and only the aching sensation of slow pain remains. Characteristically, slow pain is poorly localized, a feature that will be discussed later. Slow pain is also peculiarly unpleasant; *i.e.,* it has high affect (hyperpathia). In contradistinction to pressure block, cutaneous nerve block by a local anesthetic is more effective against small fibers than large fibers and produces a modality dissociation that is the reverse of that found during the development of pressure block.

Similarly, peripheral neuropathies of toxic, nutritional, or infective origin may show some selective predilection for fibers of different sizes and can thus cause modality dissociations. Pernicious anemia, which results from a deficiency of vitamin B_{12}, causes both degeneration of spinal tracts (subacute combined degeneration) and peripheral neuropathy, the latter being principally injurious to myelinated fibers. Arsenic poisoning also causes a peripheral neuropathy affecting mainly myelinated fibers. In both pernicious anemia and arsenic poisoning, touch-pressure, vibration, and position sense are

severely affected; pain and thermal sensation, less so. The peripheral neuropathy associated with alcoholism and deficiency of vitamin B_1 (beriberi), on the other hand, selects small fibers and produces a modality dissociation that is the reverse of the foregoing.

Although peripheral neuropathies can produce modality dissociations, these are usually less clear than those accompanying lesions of the spinal cord in which the fiber tracts mediating different sensory modalities are spatially separated from one another so that complete selective destruction of one tract can occur with complete sparing of the other. Complete interruption of a cutaneous nerve trunk cannot (with a qualification to be described presently) produce a dissociation of modality, for the fibers mediating all sensory modali-

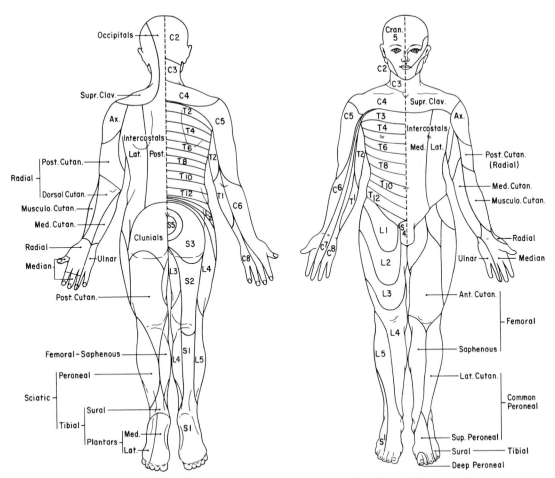

Figuge 13–2. Dermatome map and cutaneous nerve distribution in man.

ties from the skin supplied by the nerve are severed. The outstanding sign of a severed cutaneous nerve is the topographical dissociation that it causes. Each peripheral nerve trunk has a distribution on the body surface that is predictable (within limits). The area of skin supplied by a cutaneous nerve is called a *peripheral nerve field*. On the arms and legs, these have irregular configurations that recognizably differ from the orderly bandlike pattern of the dermatomes to be described later (see Figure 13–2).

At first thought, one might suppose that interruption of a cutaneous nerve trunk would produce complete anesthesia throughout the cutaneous area supplied by that trunk. In fact, this is not so because there is extensive overlap in the distributions of the cutaneous trunks (not shown in Figure 13–2). Consequently, the area of total anesthesia is much smaller than the full area of distribution of the interrupted nerve; indeed, in some skin areas in which overlap is most extensive (trunk), loss of a small nerve trunk causes total anesthesia nowhere but rather results in an irregularly bounded area of diminished sensory acuity that insidiously shades into skin of normal sensitivity. With interruption of larger nerve trunks, anesthesia occurs in what is called the *autonomous zone of the nerve trunk, i.e.,* the skin area supplied by, and only by, that trunk. Surrounding the anesthetic autonomous zone is a marginal zone in which sensory acuity is diminished but not abolished. Interestingly, the contours of the anesthetic zone begin to shrink within a few days after nerve section. Recovery is far too rapid to be accounted for by regeneration of fibers across the cut, although such regeneration does contribute to the much slower final recovery. The early shrinkage of the anesthetic zone is due to an ingrowth of nerve fibers from adjacent intact nerve fibers derived from trunks other than the severed one. What triggers this sprouting of fibers and endings into the denervated autonomous zone is unknown; perhaps the degenerating terminal fibers release some chemical agent that provokes growth of intact fibers in adjacent regions.

It was earlier stated that complete section of a cutaneous nerve produces no modality dissociation because the lesion is not selective and interrupts all fibers. This statement is not quite true, for immediately surrounding the anesthetic autonomous zone is found an intermediate zone in which only pain can be elicited; this zone shades into the marginal zone, in which all modalities can be elicited, although sensitivity is diminished. The marginal zone in turn shades into normally sensitive skin. The modality dissociation in the intermediate zone comes about because pain fibers of adjacent trunks overlap more extensively than do the fibers mediating other modalities. The pain elicited from the intermediate zone where other modalities are lacking resembles in two ways the pain sensitivity remaining after myelinated fibers have been blocked by pressure. First, it has a peculiarly unpleasant aching quality (hyperpathia); and, secondly, it is diffuse and poorly localized. The defective localization of pain when it is elicited in isolation will be discussed later.

In summary, the major distinguishing feature of peripheral nerve lesions is the kind of topographical dissociation produced. In addition, certain peripheral neuropathies that selectively attack fibers according to size may produce a modality dissociation, but the dissociation is usually relative rather than absolute.

DORSAL ROOT LESIONS

The primary afferent fibers of the peripheral nerve trunks are collected together in the dorsal roots, whence, after traversing the dorsal root ganglia that contain their cell bodies, they enter the spinal cord. The dorsal roots are sites of central confluence of afferent fibers arriving from the various peripheral nerve trunks. In the thoracic cord, this confluence is accomplished by a relatively straightforward joining of segmental trunks, the so-called dorsal and ventral rami uniting. In the lumbosacral and cervicothoracic cord, the confluence is complicated by the lumbosacral and brachial plexuses, the multiple interconnections of which make possible an extensive reshuffling of fibers. Because of the interchange of fibers via the rami of the plexuses, afferent fibers that were fellow travelers in a peripheral nerve trunk may become separated and enter the cord through different dorsal roots.

For example, in Figure 13–2, consider the skin area on the anteromedial surface of the thigh supplied by the anterior cutaneous branch of the femoral nerve (left leg). Those fibers supplying the skin of the knee eventually enter the cord through the L4 dorsal root (along with fibers reaching the plexus from the saphenous branch of the femoral nerve). But fibers supplying the more proximal parts of the anterior cutaneous field are separated in the plexus, so that some enter dorsal roots L3, L2, and L1. The partition of fibers is not helter-skelter but orderly, so that the area of skin supplied by a dorsal root is continuous and is characterized by a regular border that is recognizably different from the polygonal configuration of the peripheral nerve field.

The area of skin supplied by a single dorsal root is called a *dermatome*, which means a slice of skin. The slicelike configuration of the dermatomes is a reflection of the segmental organization of the nervous system. Consider the embryo as a slightly curled cylinder resembling a Polish sausage. Each segmental nerve supplies a circumferential band of skin, which might be demarcated by two horizontal slices through the sausage. In the torso this bandlike arrangement persists in the adult, and the dermatomes of the two sides are regular horizontal strips of skin meeting at the middorsum and curving down slightly to join again in the midventral plane. In the limbs the pattern is disturbed. As the embryonic limb buds develop, they carry with them the overlying bands of skin and their accompanying nerves; torsion of the limbs distorts, but does not obliterate, the segmental pattern.

It is important for the physician to have a clear concept of dermatomes because they determine the patterns of *topographical dissociation* that follow dorsal root lesions; these patterns are often distinguishably different from the peripheral nerve fields. Moreover, as we shall see presently, the fibers that are gathered together in the dorsal roots remain in spatial conjunction in spinal paths and in their central projections, so that a dermatomal topographical organization persists all the way from dorsal root to sensory cortex. Accordingly, lesions of the central nervous system that interrupt ascending sensory paths produce sensory defects that have a topographical distribution on the body surface characterized by dermatomal borders. Mapping of the borders provides valuable information about the location of a lesion and may be an essential guide to the neurosurgeon who wishes to intervene. Some examples will be presented shortly.

Dermatome charts often differ somewhat one from the other. The variance is due to several factors. First, the composition of roots, although generally following an orderly pattern, is subject to some individual variation. Second, dermatomes, like peripheral nerve fields, overlap extensively, so that some areas of skin are innervated by as many as three dorsal roots. Overlap makes accurate representation of dermatomes on a single figurine impossible. Compiled maps are thus compromises, and different compilers make different compromises. Third, most dermatome maps are pieced together from data collected from patients with naturally occurring lesions or diseases, rather than from controlled, experimentally induced lesions of the kind one can produce in animals.

Finally, some variance is traceable to the choice of methodology of mapping. Probably the most reliable method of mapping dermatomes is the method of *remaining sensibility*, first attempted by Sherrington in monkeys and later applied to human patients by the German neurosurgeon O. Foerster. Because of the extensive overlap of dermatomes, mapping of the cutaneous area affected by section of a single dorsal root is difficult. Sherrington, therefore, chose a reverse procedure; he cut three or four dorsal roots above and three or four roots below the one for which he wished to map the dermatome. The sensory consequence of this procedure is an island of sensitivity surrounded above and below by a sea of anesthesia. The island of remaining sensitivity can be mapped with relative ease and accuracy. As just mentioned, Foerster applied this method to human patients clinically selected for therapeutic dorsal rhizotomy (dorsal root section). For reasons not clearly stated, Foerster apparently believed not only that this drastic surgical procedure was justified but also that sparing one intermediate root in a series of seven would not jeopardize the clinical results!* In any event, Foerster's experiments produced what is probably the best and the most widely used dermatome map in man. Dermatome charts obtained by methods other than that of remaining sensibility include maps of the area of cutaneous vasodilation produced by antidromic stimulation of dorsal roots (Foerster), or of the areas of cutaneous eruption in herpes zoster (Head), or of hypesthesia in patients with ruptured intervertebral discs (Keegan and Garnett). In general, these methods are less reliable than that of remaining sensitivity and yield results only partially in accord with Foerster's data.

For most purposes the physician need not remember every detail of the dermatome charts, but he should learn a few landmarks. Figure 13–3 presents a useful figurine of some key boundaries. With man in the unusual (and undignified) quadripedal posture and with his lower leg laterally rotated, the bands in the limbs are easier to visualize. A line passing just rostral to the ear marks the upper boundary of C2 (C1 is lacking because in man there is no dorsal root for C1). A line cutting the posterior aspect of the arm marks T1; one through the groin, L1; and another through the derrière, S3 (the remaining sacral dermatomes are concentric perianal circles like the circles around the bull's eye of a target). Two additional land marks, the nipple at T4 and the umbilicus at about T10, are also useful to remember.

Like peripheral nerve fibers, dorsal root fibers mediating different modalities are intermixed, so that modality dissociations are not common in dorsal root lesions.

---

*To quote directly from Foerster's 1933 article: "I need not discuss here the circumstances under which such a selected procedure may be undertaken."

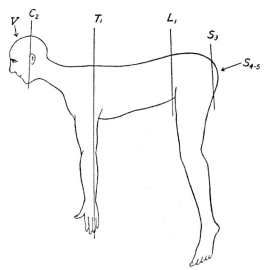

Figure 13–3. Some major dermatomal landmarks in man. (After Monrad-Krohn, *The clinical examination of the nervous system,* 3rd ed., London, H. K. Lewis, 1926.)

However, some diseases attacking dorsal roots may selectively attack fibers according to size and hence cause some dissociation of modalities. In *tabes dorsalis*, a form of syphilis in which the spirochaete sets up housekeeping in the dorsal root ganglia, the larger myelinated fibers suffer disproportionately. Accordingly, the sensations most prominently affected are touch-pressure, proprioceptive, and vibratory sensation. Position sense is especially severely impaired, and severe ataxia—errors of force, rate, range, and direction of movement due to loss of sensory input from the joints—is striking, particularly when the patient is deprived of visual cues about limb position. The gait of the blindfolded tabetic is awkward and stumbling, although he walks satisfactorily when he watches his feet. Thermal sensation and pain remain intact; the latter has the characteristic unpleasant quality and long latency of C-fiber pain.

The most reliable cue to dorsal root disease is the topographical dissociation which is dermatomal in distribution. A classic example is herpes zoster (shingles), a virus infection of the dorsal root ganglia. The disease is characterized by hyperalgesia and pain confined to the dermatome supplied by the infected root; sometimes several adjacent ganglia are involved. After a few days, there appears in the affected dermatome a vesicular rash that often "paints" on the skin the borders of the dermatome with artistic resolution. Head used such eruptions to map the dermatomes. In some instances, the rash involves only part of the hyperalgesic dermatome; some of the differences between Head's maps and those of Foerster are probably ascribable to the variability of the extent of herpetic eruptions.

Another common affliction of dorsal roots results from rupture of intervertebral ligaments and extrusion of the nucleus pulposus into the intervertebral canal. Rupture may occur at any vertebral level but is most common in the lumbosacral region, where back strain due to the lifting of heavy objects is particularly prone to cause damage to the discs and the intervertebral ligaments. Figure 13–4 shows that the cord ends at the level between vertebrae L1 and L2 and that the roots (both dorsal and ventral) destined to exit at more caudally located interspaces run up and down the vertebral canal for several vertebral segments to reach their appropriate foramens.

For example, the L5 dorsal root enters the canal between L5 and S1 vertebrae but joins the cord at the level of the T12-to-L1 interspace. The canal from L1 and L2 vertebrae down to the sacral vertebrae is thus occupied only (but fully) by roots. (This, incidentally, is why spinal taps are done below L1; the slippery roots are less likely to be punctured by an inserted needle than the firmer and more rigidly fixed cord.) When the nucleus pulposus is extruded into the crowded canal, it compresses and irritates the roots. The result is pain that the patient feels as if it were originating from the *dermatomes supplied by these roots.* If the condition is uncorrected, irreversible root damage occurs and muscle weakness results (because of loss of ventral root fibers), as well as hypesthesia and numbness in the affected dermatomes (damage to dorsal root fibers). Keegan and Garnett charted the dermatomes by mapping the areas of hypesthesia. The treatment of ruptured discs is surgical, *i.e.,*

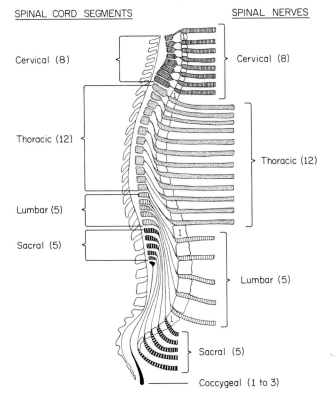

SPINAL CORD SEGMENTS SPINAL NERVES

Cervical (8)   Cervical (8)

Thoracic (12)   Thoracic (12)

Lumbar (5)   Lumbar (5)

Sacral (5)   Sacral (5)

Coccygeal (1 to 3)

Figure 13–4. Diagram of spinal cord, spinal roots, and vertebrae. Roots C1 to C7 exit above the corresponding vertebrae. Root C8 emerges between vertebrae C7 and T1. From T1 to S5 each root is assigned the number of the vertebra caudal to its exit point. (After Haymaker and Woodhall, *Peripheral nerve injuries: principles of diagnosis,* Philadelphia, W. B. Saunders Co., 1945.)

laminectomy and removal of the extruded particles. Careful sensory mapping is thus important to the neurosurgeon since it guides him about where to intervene.

The pain produced by a ruptured disc has an important bearing on the question of sensory localization. Although the site of irritation is at the root within the vertebral canal, the patient feels the pain in the leg; such pain is said to be *projected*. Projection of pain is an error of localization in which the sensation caused by irritation of a sensory path at some point *central to the receptors is interpreted as coming from the peripheral receptive field of that path*. The phenomenon of projection suggests that sensory localization is a learned discrimination and that sensory signals in central pathways, no matter where they originate, are interpreted in accordance with our learned image of the body surface and our past experiences, in which visual cues provide association between stimulus locus and sensory experience.

Projection is not a unique characteristic of root pain. A common example involving a peripheral nerve is the sensation caused by a blow on the "crazy bone" which is felt in the ulnar nerve distribution in the hand. An even more dramatic example is phantom limb pain, which often occurs in amputees. Abortive regenerative sprouts of the severed nerves in the stump cause the formation of a highly sensitive ball of fibers (neuroma), stimulation of which projects pain. The pain is felt as if it were coming from the limb that is no longer there!

SPINAL SENSORY PATHWAYS

On entering the spinal cord, fibers of different sizes and functions begin to be sorted out and segregated. The larger myelinated fibers penetrate the cord dorsum more medially than do the small myelinated and the unmyelinated fibers. This separation of medial and lateral divisions is more prominent in some roots than in others and probably receives undue emphasis in textbooks. The larger fibers of the medial division give off perpendicularly directed collateral branches, which form synaptic connections with interneurons or motoneurons (or both); their centrally directed branches make up the dorsal columns.

It has already been mentioned that the largest myelinated (Group I) fibers from the lumbosacral segments traverse the dorsal columns for only a few segments before terminating on the cells of Clarke's column. They, in turn, spawn the axons that make up the dorsal spinocerebellar tract (see Figure 13–1), which seems to have no sensory function. However, many of the medium-sized myelinated fibers remain in the ipsilateral dorsal column all the way to the gracile and cuneate nuclei at the junction between medulla and cervical cord, where they form connections with secondary neurons in these nuclei (Fig. 13–5). In their course throughout the dorsal columns, these long, central extensions of the primary afferent fibers maintain an orderly topographical relationship that appears to be determined by simple engineering convenience. Progressively from caudal to rostral, each added dorsal root contributes fibers to the dorsal columns, and these push medially the fibers already contributed to the tract by the more caudal dorsal roots.

The dorsal columns thus become laminated with the contributions of the more caudal segments situated medially. In functional terms the dorsal columns are laminated in dermatomal representation. In the rostral part of the cord, so many fibers accumulate that the dorsal column becomes two tracts: a medially situated fasciculus gracilis, containing fibers from sacral and lumbar roots, and a lateral fasciculus cuneatus, containing the fibers from thoracic and cervical segments. The tracts end in the gracilis and cuneate nuclei, which bear to each other the same spatial relationship that their respective tracts do, the gracile nucleus being medial to the cuneate nucleus. Lateral to the cuneate nucleus is the lateral cuneate nucleus, which receives the Group I afferents from the upper extremity and projects to the cerebellum; it is thus the homolog of Clarke's column and, like it, seems to have no sensory function (see Figure 13–1).

The lamination of the dorsal columns enables lesions to produce sensory defects

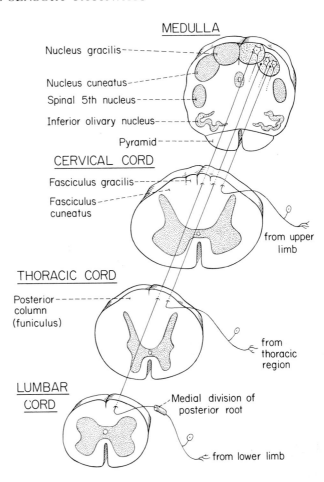

MEDULLA

Nucleus gracilis

Nucleus cuneatus

Spinal 5th nucleus

Inferior olivary nucleus

Pyramid

CERVICAL CORD

Fasciculus gracilis

Fasciculus cuneatus

from upper limb

Figure 13–5. Topographic organization of the medium-sized fibers in the posterior columns. The gracile and cuneate axons (*dotted*) in their further course cross the midline to form the medial lemniscus (see Figure 13–8).

THORACIC CORD

Posterior column (funiculus)

from thoracic region

LUMBAR CORD

Medial division of posterior root

from lower limb

in some dermatomes while sparing others. For example, a laterally situated tumor in the cervical region may press against the fasciculus cuneatus and cause sensory disturbances in the arm without disturbance of the leg. Or a medially situated tumor, even at the cervical level, may damage the fasciculus gracilis selectively, causing sensory disturbances in lumbosacral dermatomes sparing the arm. In such instances, accurate localization of the lesion may require diagnostic procedures ancillary to neurological examination.

Although the dorsal columns are large, well-defined anatomical entities, their sensory function is surprisingly controversial, and recent experimental results cast some doubt on the accounts commonly found in neurology texts. The latter accounts are deduced mainly from analysis of sensory disturbances produced by naturally occurring lesions affecting the dorsal columns. Unfortunately, such le-

sions are rarely discrete and usually include structures and pathways other than the dorsal columns. For example, tabes dorsalis does indeed cause a massive degeneration of the fibers in the dorsal columns that can be readily detected by stains of degenerating myelin. This is not surprising, since many of the dorsal root neurons affected by tabes unquestionably project through the dorsal columns. However, tabetic lesions undoubtedly destroy many other dorsal root neurons that have shorter intramedullary courses and that form synapses with secondary neurons whose axons do not traverse the dorsal column. Being secondary neurons, these axons do not degenerate and hence do not stain. Which of the sensory defects of tabes are ascribable to loss of the demonstrably degenerated dorsal column fibers and which to the occult interruption of polysynaptic ascending paths is not easy to decide.

Another commonly studied lesion that affects, but is not confined to, the dorsal column is traumatic lateral hemisection of the spinal cord such as that caused by a parasagittal bullet or stab wound. The resulting neurological disturbance is called the *Brown-Séquard syndrome*. Because the dorsal columns are uncrossed in their trajectory through the cord (in contradistinction to the anterolateral pathways, which cross the cord within a few segments of the root entry — see later), it is often assumed that the *ipsilateral* sensory defects in the Brown-Séquard syndrome are due to dorsal column section. The ipsilateral sensory consequences of lateral hemisection of the cord include loss of vibratory sensibility, sense of movement (kinesthesia) and position of joints, and impairment of touch with retention of pain and temperature sensation — a clear-cut *dissociation of modalities*. The deficits are all caudal to the level of transection, and the upper border has a dermatomal configuration — a *dermatomal topographical dissociation*. Touch and pressure are not lost; recognition and discrimination of light touch persist, although the threshold may be elevated. However, the ability to discriminate spatial aspects of tactile stimuli is ipsilaterally impaired in patients with the Brown-Séquard syndrome. Thus, two-point threshold is increased; localization, stereognosis, graphesthesia, and appreciation of simultaneously applied bilateral tactile stimuli are severely impaired or lost — a *dissociation of levels of sensation*. It can be concluded that the information required for localizing tactile stimuli reaches the brainstem exclusively via uncrossed tracts (dorsal columns?), whereas some of the fibers relaying information needed to recognize light touch as a distinct modality project into crossed spinal paths (spinothalamic?).

Another way to analyze the functions of the dorsal columns is to sample with microelectrodes single fibers in the rostral tracts or cells in the gracile and cuneate nuclei during natural stimulation of the ipsilateral body surface. Such studies indicate that dorsal columns and dorsal column nuclei contain only elements that respond to mechanical deformation of the skin or to movement of the limbs; no elements responding selectively to noxious or to thermal stimuli are found. Cutaneous mechanosensitive elements of the dorsal columns include units phasically discharged by displacement of hairs or by light touch of hairless skin. Others respond rhythmically to vibratory stimuli and presumably provide the sensory input for pallesthesia. Units responding to joint movement are found in both the cervical dorsal columns and in the dorsal column nuclei; these elements respond phasically and perhaps provide the neural cue for appreciation of joint movement but probably not for position. Tonic elements that vary their frequency of firing in accordance with fixed position of joints are found in the dorsal roots, but their rostral extensions appear to leave the dorsal columns after a few segments, for they cannot be backfired antidromically by cervical dorsal column stimuli. The pathway over which information signaling joint position reaches thalamus and sensory cortex is not clear.

Recordings from secondary neurons in the gracile and cuneate nuclei reveal some characteristics of the sensory projection system that bear on the mechanism of localization. Each secondary neuron responding to tactile stimuli has a distinctly circumscribed receptive field, *i.e.*, an area of skin from which it receives excitatory input. The size of the receptive field is related to its location; it is smaller for the apical portions of the limbs (*i.e.*, hands and feet) than for the more proximally located fields on arm, thigh, and trunk, a relationship similar to the regional variation of two-point discrimination (see Figure 12–2). The receptive fields of secondary elements in the dorsal column nuclei are about 10 times larger than those of primary elements in the dorsal root or dorsal column; the increase presumably reflects the consequences of convergence of primary onto secondary neurons. This means that the discharge of a secondary neuron has in it only one tenth of the localizing information that a primary element has; *i.e.*, relay reduces spatial resolution. For example, the discharge of a secondary neuron with a receptive field of 10 cm^2 carries information only that the stimulus was somewhere in that 10-cm^2 patch of skin, whereas a primary element with a receptive field of

1 cm² signals a much more precise localization.

Several factors mitigate the sloppiness attending convergent relay of information. First, as emphasized previously, localization is not a single-unit function but is probably determined by the spatial pattern of excitation of populations of cells. The discharge of two elements having overlapping receptive fields narrows the localization to the region of overlap. Secondly, in the dorsal column nuclei, the phenomenon of lateral inhibition increases the resolution of two-point discrimination; each stimulus depresses the cells weakly excited by the other. A third feature of transmission across the dorsal column nuclei that undoubtedly influences in a complex way the localizing information of the relayed message is modulation of transmission by corticofugal systems, i.e., by systems of fibers arising in cerebral cortex and descending the brainstem to reach the dorsal column nuclei. One such system of fibers travels with the pyramidal tract, a prominent descending path to be described later. These fibers facilitate transmission across the dorsal column nuclei; the receptive field of a cuneate neuron is markedly increased by electrical stimulation of the pyramidal tract. Other fibers reaching the nuclei both through the pyramid and other (extrapyramidal) paths inhibit transmission through the nucleus and tend to restrict receptive fields. This means that transmission through the dorsal column nuclei is not a simple process of relay and that the brain is not a captive audience for every stray event that occurs at the periphery. Rather, how much information enters the portals of consciousness depends in part on the influence of these gating circuits originating in cerebral cortex or brainstem nuclei. The size and configuration of the receptive field of a cuneate neuron in an intact waking animal vary, depending on the corticofugal influences. The critical question of how the modulating corticofugal systems are driven and regulated remains unanswered; it is intriguing to speculate that their activity may somehow underline the variations of sensory experience and acuity with attention or alertness.

So far we have considered the spinal course and function of the larger myelinated primary afferent fibers of the medial division of the dorsal roots. Tracing the small myelinated and unmyelinated fibers of the lateral division is even more formidable, for small fibers are both more difficult to record from and harder to trace anatomically; the degenerating myelin stains are useless in tracing the C fibers, although in dorsal roots these are three to four times more numerous than are the myelinated fibers. The classic description of the fate of the fibers of the lateral division is that they enter the posterolateral fasciculus (tract of Lissauer) at the tip of the dorsal horn, run with it for two or three segments, and terminate on the small cells in the substantia gelatinosa (Fig. 13–6). These cells are said to send their axons across the cord directly or to make synaptic contact with tertiary neurons that cross the cord in the ventral white commissure just below the central canal and then ascend the spinal cord in the contralateral anterolateral white column. Some of these fibers constitute the spinothalamic tract, but they are inextricably mixed in the anterolateral column with a generous number of fibers that reach no higher than the reticular substance of the brainstem (spinobulbar and spinotectal fibers), as well as with the propriospinal fibers, which link one segment of the cord with another, more rostrally placed segment (Fig. 13–7).

The foregoing account is beyond doubt oversimplified. What is clear is that the small fibers of the lateral division run rostrally several segments before terminating. It has already been mentioned that some fibers bearing information from nociceptors and thermoreceptors terminate in the marginal region of the dorsal horn on cells that are probably the secondary neurons of the pain and thermosensory pathways (Fig. 13–6, inset). Some of these cells are the origins of the crossing fibers that make up the spinothalamic and spinobulbar system of the anterolateral column, for they can be antidromically fired by stimulation of the contralateral cervical anterolateral column or of the contralateral thalamus. Other antidromically fired cells lie deeper in the gray matter and are probably tertiary neurons.

The role of the substantia gelatinosa is

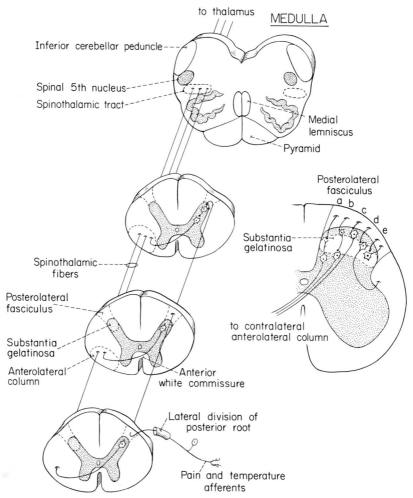

Figure 13–6. Origin and course of the spinothalamic tract. The inset at the right illustrates connections made by cells possibly giving rise to the anterolateral column fibers (*a, b, c*). Note that the cells of the substantia gelatinosa feed back into the white matter, either the posterolateral fasciculus (*e*) or the propriospinal bundle (*d*).

puzzling. The dendrites of its small cells (from which no one has yet successfully recorded action potentials) apparently receive synaptic knobs from primary fibers, but their axons connect with other cells of the substantia gelatinosa. Some of these axons traverse the tract of Lissauer to terminate on cells of the substantia gelatinosa at a more rostral segment (75 per cent of Lissauer's tract is composed of such axons). The substantia gelatinosa thus appears to be mainly a closed system projecting onto itself. Some axons of cells in the substantia gelatinosa do connect with dendrites of larger cells situated more deeply in the

dorsal horn; the axons of these cells disappear into the dorsolateral white matter for destinations unknown. In short, the substantia gelatinosa is a mystery.

In summary, what seems to be well established is that the small myelinated and unmyelinated fibers presumably mediating pain and temperature sensation have short ascending rami that terminate, after traversing two or three segments, on cells of the marginal zone. These cells project either directly or through interneurons through the ventral white commissure to the contralateral anterolateral column. Some of these axons are thus secondary;

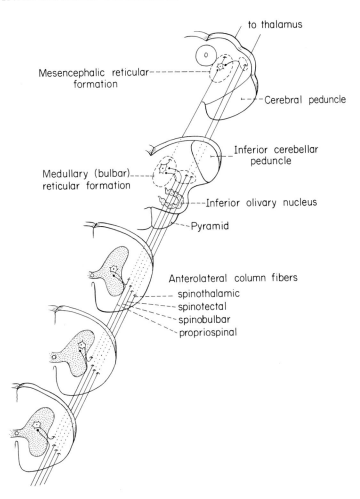

Figure 13–7. The component fibers of the anterolateral column. Note that only part of these ascending fibers reach the thalamus directly.

to thalamus

Mesencephalic reticular formation

Cerebral peduncle

Inferior cerebellar peduncle

Medullary (bulbar) reticular formation

Inferior olivary nucleus

Pyramid

Anterolateral column fibers
spinothalamic
spinotectal
spinobulbar
propriospinal

others are either tertiary neurons or of higher order. Those that travel all the way to the somatosensory "relay" nucleus of the thalamus (nucleus ventralis posterolateralis) are properly termed spinothalamic tract fibers (Figs. 13–7 and 13–8); others terminate in the midline nuclei of the thalamus. Still others terminate in the reticular formation of the bulb (spinobulbar fibers) or of the mesencephalon (spinotectal fibers), whence after repeated synaptic interruptions they eventually project to the mesencephalic reticular formation and the posterior thalamus. Still other anterolateral column fibers terminate in the spinal cord at more rostral levels — propriospinal fibers. It should be emphasized that spinothalamic, spinobulbar, and propriospinal fibers are so commingled in their course through the cord that there is no way to destroy the various components selectively. Accord-

ingly, in this account, the loose term *anterolateral column* is used, the more specific terms *spinothalamic* and *spinobulbar tracts* being reserved for those few situations in which anatomical knowledge merits such distinctive usage.

The anterolateral column, like the dorsal column, is topographically laminated, and again the organization is dermatomal and apparently a consequence of engineering convenience. Because the tracts are crossed, the dermatomal arrangement is the reverse of that found in the uncrossed dorsal columns. In progressing rostrally along the cord, each bundle is successively displaced laterally by new bundles added from more rostral segments. Consequently, in the cervical anterolateral column the caudal segments are represented superficially (laterally) and the rostral segments deeply (medially). Compression from a lat-

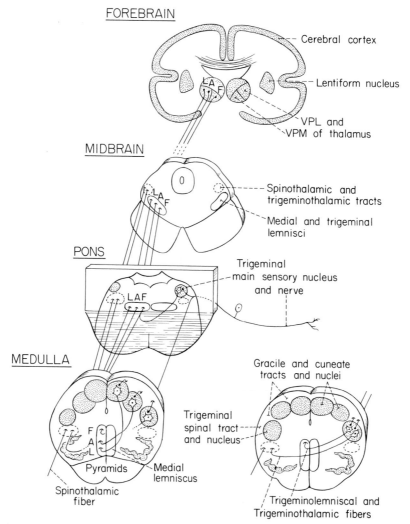

Figure 13–8.   Sensory paths ascending through the brainstem. *VPM*, nucleus ventralis posteromedialis; *VPL*, nucleus ventralis posterolateralis. Note that the trigeminal input feeds into both the medial lemniscus (trigeminal lemniscus) and spinothalamic (trigeminothalamic) systems. The topographical arrangement of fibers in the medial lemniscal system is also indicated: leg (*L*), arm (*A*), and face (*F*). A portion of the trigeminal system is shown in the section of medulla at the lower right. Pain input ascends in *trigeminothalamic* fibers that have crossed and traveled with the spinothalamic fibers. Touch input is relayed to cells whose axons cross and form a *trigeminolemniscal* portion of the medial lemniscus. Note that the ascending fibers carrying different sensory modalities (pain versus touch) are intermingled as they enter the thalamus, but the topographical relationship of leg, arm, and face (lateral to medial) is maintained. (Refer to Figure 13–11 for summary.)

erally situated cervical tumor thus causes sensory disturbances first in the contralateral leg. Similarly, a unilateral superficial anterolateral cordotomy (see later) results in analgesia and athermesthesia on the opposite side of the body in dermatomal segments far inferior to the level of the section, the discrepancy between the level of the lesion and that of the sensory border depending on the depth of the cut.

What sensory modalities are mediated by the anterolateral column system? Fortunately, we do not have to depend wholly on capricious pathologic states to provide lesions of this system, for there is a proper medical indication for its controlled surgical interruption. Because an intact anterolateral column is required for pain sensation, neurosurgeons often perform what is known as *anterolateral cordotomy* for relief of intractable pain (for example, in inoperable carcinoma). The procedure consists of cutting through the entire ventral quadrant (usually bilaterally), the dentate ligament being used as the upper border (the pyramidal tract, a motor path, lies just dorsal to the dentate ligament!). Examination of a patient who has sustained unilateral anterolateral cordotomy reveals several sensory changes, as discussed in the following three paragraphs.

First, contralateral loss of pain and temperature sensation below the level of the lesion can be expected. The upper border of the analgesic region (if the section extends to the midline) is dermatomal in contour and lies two or three segments below the level of the section; this is because the pain and temperature fibers travel two or three segments in the ipsilateral cord before terminating on secondary neurons. Parenthetically, it can now be mentioned that lateral hemisection of the cord obviously destroys the anterolateral column as well as the dorsal columns. Accordingly, the Brown-Séquard syndrome is characterized not only by the ipsilateral disturbances of tactile, joint, and vibratory sensibility already described but also by *contralateral* analgesia and thermesthesia. In other words, the Brown-Séquard syndrome is characterized by a double-reversed dissociation of modalities on the two sides of the body. In addition, because of interruption of descending motor paths (to be discussed later), lateral hemisection causes *ipsilateral* paralysis.

Second, loss of sensation of orgasm results if the cordotomy is bilateral. The operation does not interfere with erection or ejaculation, but the sensory experiences associated with these phenomena are irreversibly obliterated.

Third, loss of sensations of tickle and itch in the affected contralateral dermatomes occurs. The receptors for these annoying sensations are probably similar to those mediating pain (naked, undifferentiated nerve terminals) and, like the information from nociceptors, tickle and itch utilize the crossed anterolateral system. In this connection, it is interesting to recall that the modalities mediated by the anterolateral columns thus far enumerated — pain, thermal sensation, sexual sensations,

and tickle — are all modalities more or less heavily colored by affect. That is, they not only provide information concerning events in the external world but also arouse conscious reactions of pleasure or displeasure with the course and nature of these events. This is in contrast to the coldly and precisely informative nature of the sensory information relayed over the ipsilateral pathways (dorsal columns?). Perhaps the affective components of anterolateral column modalities are a special function of the spinobulbar fibers or the fibers that project to midline and posterior thalamic groups. The reticular formation and nonrelay portions of the thalamus are "hot spots" for positively and negatively reinforcing phenomena revealed in self-stimulation experiments. Unfortunately, there is no way to test this intriguing hypothesis because the components of the anterolateral column are not separable.

Anterolateral cordotomy produces no detectable alteration of tactile sensibility. However, it has already been mentioned that in the Brown-Séquard syndrome the *recognition* of tactile stimuli remains intact although the ability to *localize* touch is seriously impaired. The ipsilateral retention of modality discrimination of touch after hemisection of the cord clearly forces the conclusion that some tactile information employs a crossed path, and the anterolateral system, being the best known candidate, is believed to mediate some tactile sensation. The deduction is reinforced by the well-demonstrated presence among the peripheral delta- and C-fiber populations (the peripheral inputs to the anterolateral system) of elements that respond to movement of hairs or mild mechanical deformation of skin.

Because the tactile sensations presumably mediated by the anterolateral system are imprecisely localized, it is often said that the dorsal columns mediate "fine touch" and the anterolateral system, "crude touch." These are objectionable terms because they imply that there are two qualitative kinds of touch, an implication that is by no means justified. Indeed, qualitatively the touch sensations of a patient with the Brown-Séquard syndrome do not seem to differ from those of the normal subject or of a patient surviving an anterolateral cordotomy; the difference is that the Brown-Séquard patient cannot tell *where* he is touched. It will be argued below that this is so because the tactile projections through the ipsilateral (dorsal column–medial lemniscus?) system maintain a relatively rigid spatial organization, each element having a restricted, discrete receptive field. Although lateral inhibition can be demonstrated for secondary elements of the anterolateral system and although corticofugal modulation probably is also operative, the anterolateral system seems nevertheless to be spatially "sloppy," with central neurons having very large receptive fields. The consequences and significance of this sloppiness will be discussed in more detail later.

The functional identity of the crossed pain-temperature pathway as revealed by studies of anterolateral cordotomy patients and the Brown-Séquard syndrome serves to explain the symptom complex of a neurological disease, syringomyelia. In syringomyelia cystic swellings develop in isolated parts of the central canal of the spinal cord. The axons crossing in the ventral white commissure to reach the opposite anterolateral column are vulnerable to compression by the cyst or syrinx. The result is *bilateral* loss of pain and temperature sensibility in the dermatomes feeding the decussating neurons. Because the disease develops insidiously and because modalities are dissociated, with touch being left intact, the patient may be unaware of his disease and sustain injuries in the analgesic region (*e.g.*, cigarette burns of the fingers) before suspecting that something is wrong. As the disease progresses, the symptomatology becomes more complex, for other spinal structures (dorsal columns, ventral horn) may eventually become involved.

In summary, lesions of the spinal cord are particularly likely to cause modality dissociations because the spatial segregation of modality-specific fibers makes possible selective interruption of one pathway along with absolute or relative sparing of others.

BRAINSTEM PATHWAYS

The axons arising from the cells of the dorsal column nuclei decussate and make up the medial lemniscus at the junction between medulla and spinal cord (Fig. 13–8). In crossing, the fibers maintain a strict topographical organization; and in the crossed tract, which lines itself up vertically near the midline and perched atop the pyramidal tract, the fibers from rostral segments (cuneate nucleus) are dorsal to those from the more caudal segments (gracile nucleus). The topographical arrangement is thus represented by a figurine standing upright on the pyramids. (As we shall see presently, secondary fibers from the trigeminal nuclei are added to the tract most dorsally and complete the figurine by adding the face.) More rostrally in the pons, the vertical orientation of the medial lemniscus gives way to a horizontal one, the ventrally placed fibers (leg representation) swinging laterally. At the same time, the lemniscal fibers and the brainstem extension of the anterolateral system (the spinal lemniscus) approach one another and in the mesencephalon become so intermingled that they can no longer be clearly differentiated as they run rostrally to terminate together in the nucleus ventralis posterolateralis (VPL) of the thalamus.

The decussation of the fibers that form the medial lemniscus has a twofold significance for clinical neurology. First, it brings to an end the clear-cut segregation of pathways according to modality that characterizes the arrangement in the spinal cord from root to bulb. Accordingly, the likelihood of dissociation of modalities is less for brainstem lesions than for cord lesions. Secondly, the horizontal topographical arrangement, opposite in cord for anterolateral and dorsal column systems, is brought into accord; medial lemniscal and spinal lemniscal (spinothalamic) fibers entering the thalamus together are arranged so that in both the caudal segments (leg) are represented laterally, intermediate segments (trunk) in the middle, and rostral (arm) segments, medially (Fig. 13–9). Finally, the secondary trigeminal pathways subserving somatic sensation from the face terminate most medially in the nucleus ventralis posteromedialis.

Several cues for distinguishing cord and brainstem lesions may be mentioned.

(1) Clear-cut modality dissociation suggests a cord lesion.

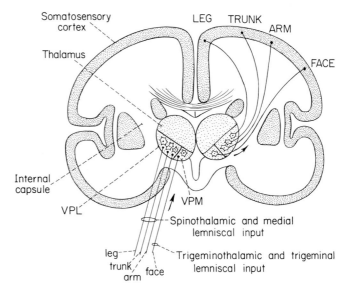

Figure 13–9. Schematic frontal section through the forebrain, showing the topographical organization of the ascending sensory input to the thalamus and the output to somatosensory cortex. *VPM,* nucleus ventralis posteromedialis; *VPL,* nucleus ventralis posterolateralis.

(2) Sensory disturbances of the face indicate a brainstem (or a high-cord) lesion.

(3) Brainstem lesions causing sensory disturbances usually damage adjacent motor systems; impairment of motor functions mediated by cranial nerves indicate a supraspinal lesion.

TRIGEMINAL PATHWAYS

Somatic sensation from the face is mediated by the three branches of the trigeminal (fifth cranial) nerve—the ophthalmic, maxillary, and mandibular divisions. Figures 13–2 and 13–10 show the areas of distribution of these branches. The cell bodies (with the notable exception of the large myelinated Group I fibers supplying the muscle spindles in the muscles of mastication) lie in the semilunar, or Gasserian, ganglion, which is a homolog of the dorsal root ganglia. The secondary neurons of the trigeminal system lie in a continuous column of gray matter, extending from the C2 segment to the mesencephalon (Fig. 13–10). Although they are continuous, different portions of this column have different names (and probably different functions). The caudal part is the spinal nucleus of cranial nerve V; along its lateral edge runs a tract of finely myelinated and unmyelinated fibers (the spinal tract of cranial nerve V), which may be considered

a homolog of the tract of Lissauer. Ninety per cent of its fibers are less than 4 μm in diameter. The tract consists of branches of primary afferent fibers descending to connect with cells in the spinal nucleus, which resembles and is continuous with the substantia gelatinosa. The most caudal part of the nucleus receives fibers from the ophthalmic division; the maxillary and mandibular divisions terminate in successively more proximal portions. The spinal nucleus is supposed to mediate pain and temperature sensibility from the face, and this supposition is the basis of a surgical procedure, trigeminal tractotomy, designed to relieve the pain of trigeminal neuralgia, or tic douloureux (see Chapter 4). The operation is similar to anterolateral cordotomy, except that the section is of intramedullary primary afferent fibers, whereas in cordotomy the tract fibers of higher order neurons are interrupted. In many cases trigeminal tractotomy is effective; it produces ipsilateral analgesia and thermesthesia in the face and leaves touch intact or only moderately impaired, *i.e.,* a dissociation of modalities. It is this dissociation that makes tractotomy preferable to either peripheral nerve section or avulsion of the Gasserian ganglion. The latter procedure, of course, causes loss of all sensory modalities and ulceration of the cornea is a complication, for the loss of the blink reflex leads to painless but destructive corneal damage.

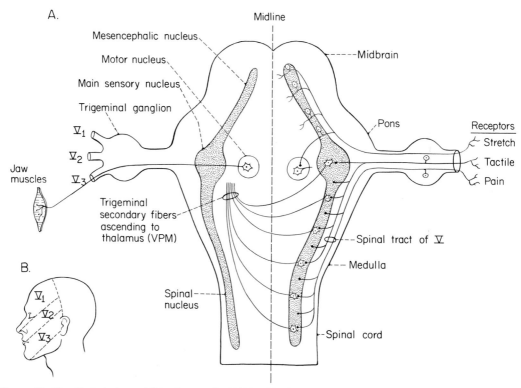

Figure 13–10. Dorsal view of the trigeminal nuclear complex, the primary afferent fibers to it from the face, and its output to the thalamus. The dermatomal distribution of the trigeminal nerve is shown in the inset at the left. Divisions of the trigeminal nerve: V_1, ophthalmic; V_2, maxillary; and V_3, mandibular. *VPM*, nucleus ventralis posteromedialis.

The intermediate portion of the trigeminal nucleus, called the *main sensory nucleus of V*, is thought to be the relay station for tactile impulses from the face. Single-unit recording from this nucleus and from the spinal nucleus confirms some separation of tactile and nociceptive regions, but there is considerable overlap, and the separation is not as complete as was originally believed. The most rostral portion of the trigeminal complex, the *mesencephalic nucleus of V*, contains pseudounipolar cells similar to dorsal root ganglion neurons. These cells are exceptional in that they seem to be primary neurons with their cell bodies within the central nervous system rather than in a ganglion. Peripherally, they are thought to supply the stretch receptors of the muscles of mastication and possibly of the extraocular muscles; short-latency responses are recorded in the mesencephalic nucleus when the jaw and eye muscles are stretched.

The central branch of these cells terminates in the motor nucleus of cranial nerve V (which lies medial to the main sensory nucleus), completing a monosynaptic stretch reflex arc for jaw muscles comparable to the monosynaptic stretch reflex arc for limb muscles. Others connect with motoneurons of nerves III, IV, and VI and thus create a similar arc for eye muscles.

The fibers from the trigeminal nuclear complex that reach the thalamus travel through the brainstem in three separate paths. Those that originate in the more caudal part of the spinal nucleus become incorporated into the spinothalamic system. Fibers from the more rostral part of the spinal nucleus and the main sensory nucleus join the medial lemniscus; they accumulate in its dorsal part and then lie medial to the limb and trunk representation as the lemniscus rotates in the pons. These two systems, sometimes called the *trigeminothalamic tract* and the *trigeminal lemniscus*, respectively, form collectively a crossed ventral secondary ascending trigeminal system. The medial lemniscus moves laterally in the pons, and in the midbrain its *trigeminal lemniscal* components mingle with the trigeminothalamic fibers that are situated laterally. The whole trigeminal ascending system then enters the ventralis posteromedialis nucleus of the thalamus. Fibers conveying trigeminal input also enter the reticular formation, analogous to the propriospinal and spinobulbar systems from the spinal cord. This pathway forms a multisynaptic ascending trigeminal system located dorsally in the tegmentum; it provides for an alternate means of conveying sensory input from the face to the thalamus. The major sensory paths from the posterior roots and the trigeminal nerve to the cerebral cortex are summarized in Figure 13–11.

In the rostral medulla, the crossed fibers of the spinothalamic and trigeminothalamic systems lie close to the ipsilateral spinal trigeminal tract (primary afferents) in the dorsolateral part of the bulb. Vascular lesions in this area cause bilateral impairment of pain and thermal sensation in the face and contralateral impairment of pain and thermal and tactile sensibility in the trunk and extremities, a highly distinctive topographical and modality dissociation.

The lateral position of the crossed pain fibers is exploited in *mesencephalic tractotomy*, a surgical procedure employed for the relief of intractable pain. Section of the fibers produces analgesia over the contralateral limbs, trunk, and head.

THALAMUS AND CORTEX

The highest reaches of the classic sensory pathways are the thalamic nuclei and the cerebral cortical areas to which they project (Fig. 13–12 and Table 13–1). The so-called thalamic relay nuclei, *i.e.*, those that receive ascending input from ascending pathways and project to the cerebral cortex, are so intimately connected with the cortex that there is little profit in at-

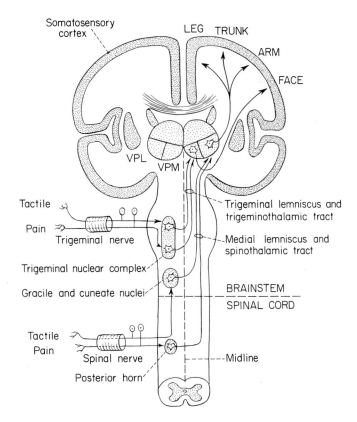

Figure 13–11. Summary of major afferent pathways for tactile and pain input to thalamus and cortex. *VPM*, nucleus ventralis posteromedialis; *VPL*, nucleus ventralis posterolateralis. (Refer to Figure 13–8.)

TABLE 13–1.   Major Thalamic Nuclei, Their Inputs and Cortical Projection Sites

Input Category	Input Tract	Thalamic Nucleus	Cortical Projection*
Somatosensory	Medial lemniscus and spinothalamic tract (spinal lemniscus): from body.	Ventralis posterior—VP (posterior ventral): into its lateral part—VPL.	Parietal cortex: postcentral gyrus (3, 1, 2).
	Trigeminal lemniscus: from head.	Ventralis posterior—VP: into its medial part—VPM.	As above.
Visual	Optic tract.	Lateral geniculate—LG.	Occipital cortex: along calcarine fissure on lingual and cuneate gyri (17)—striate cortex.
Auditory	Brachium of inferior colliculus.	Medial geniculate—MG.	Temporal cortex: transverse temporal gyri (41).
Olfactory	None.	None.	Frontal and temporal prepyriform cortex.
Cerebellar	Superior cerebellar peduncle (brachium conjunctivum).	Ventralis lateralis—VL (lateral ventral).	Frontal cortex: precentral gyrus (4) and anteriorly.
Striatal (basal ganglia)	Thalamic fasciculus.	Ventralis lateralis and ventralis anterior—VA (anterior ventral).	Frontal cortex: across the three frontal gyri posteriorly (6, 8).
Hypothalamic	Mammillothalamic tract.	Anterior nuclear complex.	Cingulate gyrus anteriorly (24).
	Periventricular fiber system.	Medialis dorsalis—MD (dorsal medial).	Frontal cortex: anterior to areas 6 and 8 ("prefrontal" cortex).
"Association" thalamic nuclei: usually considered to receive only from other thalamic nuclei (but there is evidence that the geniculates also project to the pulvinar, and sometimes the medialis dorsalis nucleus is placed in this category).		Lateralis dorsalis—LD (dorsal lateral).	Cingulate gyrus posteriorly (23).
		Lateralis posterior—LP (posterior lateral).	Parietal cortex: superior parietal lobule (5, 7).
		Pulvinar.	Parieto-occipito-temporal association cortex.

*Brodmann areas are shown in parentheses.

tempting to sort out the relative sensory functions of each.

The sensory "relay" nuclei are the nuclei ventralis posterolateralis (body) and ventralis posteromedialis (face) for somatic and visceral sensation and the lateral and medial geniculate bodies for vision and audition, respectively. The nucleus ventralis lateralis receives the brachium conjunctivum from the cerebellum and projects to the precentral cortex, but its role in sensation is not clear.

The other relay nuclei are (see Figure 13–12 and Table 13–1): nucleus ventralis anterior (receives from the basal ganglia), nucleus medialis dorsalis, and nucleus anterior (receives from the hypothalamus). Note that either the Latin names for thalamic nuclei, or their abbreviations, or their Anglicized versions are in common use. Thus, *ventralis posterolateralis, VPL,* and *posterolateral ventral* all refer to the same nucleus.

Thalamic neurons that project to the sensory cortex undergo irreversible retrograde degeneration after a cortical lesion; the cell bodies disappear and are replaced by glia. Indeed this is the classic anatomical technique for mapping thalamocortical projections. Thus a lesion of the cortex is at the same time a lesion of the thalamus, and one cannot readily decide whether a resulting sensory deficit is due to extirpation of cortex or to degeneration of the thalamus. Similarly, a thalamic lesion deafferents the cortical area to which the destroyed cells project; again, assignment of responsibility for sensory deficit is equivocal. Finally, each thalamic area projecting to the cortex receives corticothalamic fibers from the area to which it projects; consequently, electrical stimulation of the cortex excites both the cortex and the thalamus, an arrangement that clouds the interpretation of sensory consequences of stimulation of either cortex or thalamus.

It has already been pointed out that spinal and medial lemniscal and trigeminal ascending pathways become increasingly mingled as they approach the midbrain and that they terminate together in the posteroventral thalamus (Fig. 13–9). Although the fibers from the spinal lemniscus terminate somewhat more caudally than

A. LATERAL VIEW OF HEMISPHERE

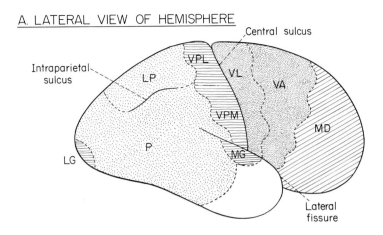

B. MEDIAL VIEW OF HEMISPHERE

Figure 13–12. Thalamic nuclei and their cerebral cortical projection sites. *A* and *B,* The right cerebral hemisphere; the dotted lines represent approximate projection boundaries that cut across different cortical gyri. *C,* The right thalamus and representative frontal sections (*a* to *d*) through it. The thalamic nuclei and their projection areas are shaded according to categories as follows: somatosensory and special sensory, *horizontal shading*; cerebellar and striatal, *dense stippling*; hypothalamic, *oblique shading*; and "association," *light stippling.*

Thalamic nuclei: *A,* anterior; *CM,* centromedian; *LD,* lateralis dorsalis; *LG,* lateral geniculate; *LP,* lateralis posterior; *MD,* medialis dorsalis; *MG,* medial geniculate; *P,* pulvinar; *VA,* ventralis anterior; *VL,* ventralis lateralis; *VPL,* ventralis posterolateralis; *VPM,* ventralis posteromedialis.

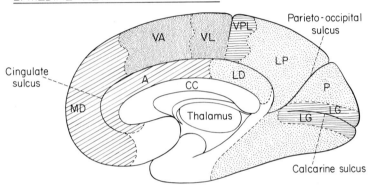

C. DORSOLATERAL VIEW OF THALAMUS

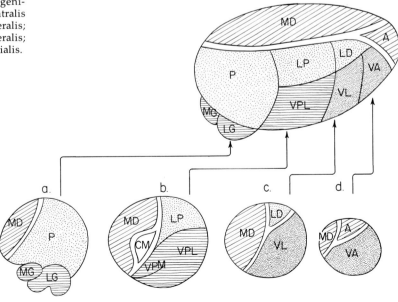

those of the medial lemniscus, the admixture is so great that the likelihood of selective damage with a resulting modality dissociation is minimal. Consequently, lesions of the thalamus or cortex do not cause modality dissociations.

Although modalities are mixed, the topographical organization remains intact. Exploration of the posteroventral thalamus with recording electrodes during stimulation of the body surface reveals an orderly array of dermatomal representation; the caudal segments are arranged laterally in the nucleus ventralis posterolateralis (VPL), the rostral segments more medially in the VPL, and the face most medially in the nucleus ventralis posteromedialis (VPM). The spatial order is maintained in the thalamocortical projection to the primary sensory cortex in the postcentral gyrus. This can be readily mapped by "gross" recordings from an electrode placed on the pial surface of the postcentral gyrus; tactile stimulation of the appropriate contralateral body site yields a large positive-negative potential fluctuation ("primary cortical potential") that is mainly due to summed synaptic potentials of cortical cells. Careful electrical mapping reveals that caudal segments (leg) are represented medially in the cortex mainly on the mesial surface within the longitudinal fissure. Trunk, arm, and face follow in orderly array, passing from medial to lateral, from longitudinal fissure to lateral (Sylvian) fissure. There is considerable overlap of the dermatomal representation thus crudely mapped, but the order is quite evident. The area of cortex devoted to individual dermatomes is unequal; those dermatomes in which sensory discrimination is most acute have disproportionately large cortical representation. For example, the fingers, lips, tongue, and toes have large cortical receiving zones, whereas the representation of the trunk is relatively minuscule.

Careful mapping reveals that the body surface is twice represented in the postcentral gyrus. The projection just described is known as somatosensory receiving area I. Laterally, buried within the fold of the Sylvian fissure is somatosensory area II. This area is somatotopically organized also; the representation is a mirror image of area I, *i.e.,* face, arm, leg. Somatosensory area II receives input from both sides of the body, whereas area I responds only to contralateral stimuli. The significance of this double representation is controversial; in the monkey and in man, the second receiving area is smaller and less prominent than in the cat.

Electrical stimulation of the postcentral cortex in conscious human patients substantiates the organization of thalamocortical organization revealed by anatomical (degeneration) and electrophysiological mapping. The skull can be opened under local anesthesia and electrical stimuli applied directly to the exposed brain; the patient is asked to report the nature and location of induced sensations. Neurosurgeons often employ this procedure to locate epileptogenic sites for extirpation. Such induced sensations are usually described as having a tingling or prickling quality rather than a clear tactile or thermal characterization. This accords with the admixture of modalities in the thalamus and cortex, so that an electrical stimulus excites, willy-nilly, cells receiving from different peripheral receptors. Sometimes electrical stimulation of the cortex evokes sensations of movement of a joint, a finding that suggests that joint sensation has a prominent thalamocortical representation. Significantly, stimulation of the sensory cortex is painless, and unpleasant or noxious sensations are not reported; this finding will be discussed subsequently.

Although the patient cannot accurately describe the quality of cortically induced sensations in terms of individual cutaneous modalities, he consistently localizes the sensation on the body surface with precision and accuracy (Fig. 12–3). Such localization is another example of the principle of projection and suggests that the significance of the precise topographical organization of sensory cortex and of the discrete receptive fields of its constituent cells is to provide the functional and anatomical substrate for place coding of localization. This conclusion is further substantiated by the sensory consequences of thalamocortical lesions, which as previously emphasized, do not cause anesthesia or prominent disturbances of discrimination of modalities but rather cause serious and irreversible impairment of the capacity to recognize the spatial aspects of stimuli.

The discussion thus far has been perhaps unduly focused on the classic sensory pathways that feed the relay nuclei of the thalamus and on the thalamic projections to the primary sensory cortex of the postcentral gyrus. This biased emphasis is partly because the classic pathways, being simpler and less confounded by multiple synaptic interruptions (each of which multiplies the investigator's chance of "losing his way"), have been most thoroughly studied. Cortical sites other than the postcentral gyrus clearly receive input from the periphery via thalamic nuclei other than the classic relay nuclei. For example, the so-called association cortex of the posterior parietal lobe (areas 5 and 7 of Brodmann) shows primary evoked potentials in response to tactile stimulation of the body surface, but these responses differ from those of the postcentral gyrus in that they lack any clear topographical organization. Also, individual cells in association cortex, unlike those in the postcentral cortex, show little modality specificity and often respond not only to different somatosensory stimuli but also to visual and auditory inputs. It is for this reason that the term *association cortex* is used, for presumably such cells are involved in complex functions relating several sensory modalities. The thalamic input to posterior parietal cortex is via the pulvinar and the lateralis posterior nucleus (Fig. 13–12 and Table 13–1), which do not receive direct connections from auditory, visual, or somatosensory pathways but which possibly receive branches from neurons in the relay nuclei of these modalities. The pulvinar and lateralis posterior nucleus thus seem to be alternate routes to the cortex and are likely sites of convergence of signals from different modalities. The lateralis dorsalis nucleus is also an association nucleus and projects to the medial aspect of the parietal lobe, as well as to the posterior part of the cingulate gyrus.

Lesions of the posterior parietal lobe in the dominant hemisphere (see Chapter 25) produce complex disturbances of perception. The patient, although clearly neither blind nor anesthetic, seems to be inattentive to events, visual or somatosensory, occurring in that portion of the external world contralateral to the lesion. For example, the patient may shave only the "good" side of his face or comb only the "good" side of the head, or in other ways seemingly ignore the half of the body contralateral to his lesion. If the patient is asked to draw a face, the result often has only one eye and one ear, the omission being in the patient's defective visual field. The defect is clearly not due to blindness since the patient can, upon request, trace accurately the outlines of his drawing with his finger, but he seems incapable of detecting any defect in his drawing. Yet when the same drawing is reversed as a mirror image so that the blank areas fall within his "good" visual field, he promptly fills in the missing parts. Localization of, and attention to, cutaneous stimuli is similarly impaired contralateral to the lesion. Often noxious stimuli on the "bad" side are perceived as especially unpleasant and evoke exaggerated affective reactions, such as tears, shrieks, and entreaties to the examiner not to repeat the stimulus. Yet if noxious stimuli are simultaneously applied bilaterally to homologous skin areas, the patient is aware only of the stimulus on the good side and reacts normally. Extinction blocks the hyperpathic overresponse. Finally, posterior parietal lesions near the parietotemporal junction may cause an aphasia of the receptive type (see Chapter 25).

ADDITIONAL READING

Libet, B. Electrical stimulation of cortex in human subjects, and conscious sensory aspects. Chap. 19 in *Handbook of sensory physiology, II. Somatosensory system*, Iggo, A., ed., New York, Springer-Verlag, 1973.

Mountcastle, V. B. Neural mechanisms in somesthesia. Chap. 10 in *Medical physiology*, Mountcastle, V. B., ed., St. Louis, The C. V. Mosby Co., 1974.

Ruch, T. C. Neural basis of somatic sensation. Chap. 15 in *Physiology and biophysics*, Ruch, T. C., and Patton, H. D., eds., Philadelphia, W. B. Saunders Co., 1965.

Semmes, J. Somesthetic effects of damage to the central nervous system. Chap. 18 in *Handbook of physiology, II. Somatosensory system*, Iggo, A., ed., New York, Springer-Verlag, 1973.

CHAPTER 14

VISCERAL SENSATION AND REFERRED PAIN

HARRY D. PATTON

VISCERAL AND
PSEUDOVISCERAL SENSORY
PATHS

REFERRED PAIN

MECHANISM OF REFERRED
PAIN

LOCALIZATION OF PAIN

VISCERAL AND PSEUDOVISCERAL SENSORY PATHS

We have thus far considered only those sensory modalities that are mediated by receptors located in skin, muscles, tendons, and joints (somatic sensation). This chapter deals with visceral sensation.

By strict definition, *visceral sensation* refers to sensation arising from the hollow structures of the thorax, abdomen, and pelvis, but the term is often used loosely to include sensations mediated by receptors located in the linings of the body cavity (the pleura, peritoneum, and mesentery) and those in the diaphragm; a better term for these sensations is *pseudovisceral sensations*. True visceral sensations are distinguished anatomically from somatic sensations in that they are conducted by peripheral afferent fibers that reach the nervous system via visceral nerve trunks in company with autonomic efferent fibers supplying the smooth muscle and glandular structures of the viscera. Pseudovisceral sensory fibers supplying the pleura, peri-

toneum, mesentery, and diaphragm, like those subserving deep somatic sensation, enter the dorsal roots through deep nerve trunks and the ventral ramus of the dorsal root.

Visceral sensations can be conveniently classified as (1) organic sensations and (2) visceral pain. *Organic sensations* are those sensory modalities that signal a bodily need and generally lead to behavior that satisfies that need. Examples are (1) hunger sensations, (2) thirst, (3) sexual sensations, (4) nausea, (5) sensations of bladder and bowel fullness. For the most part, organic sensations are mediated by afferent fibers that reach the nervous system in the company of parasympathetic efferent fibers; the afferent fibers often have their cell bodies in the ganglia of cranial nerves (vagus, glossopharyngeal) that contribute to the cranial division of the parasympathetic nervous system. The organic sensations will not be dealt with in this chapter.

Visceral pain, a modality of obvious clinical importance, is mediated by small

194

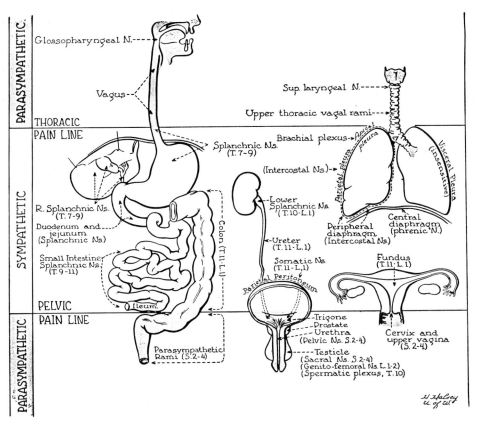

Figure 14–1. Pain innervation of visceral structures. Afferent fibers mediating pain from extreme proximal and distal visceral structures travel with parasympathetic trunks; most of the viscera receive pain afferents from sympathetic nerve trunks. (From Ruch and Patton, eds., *Physiology and biophysics*, Philadelphia, W. B. Saunders Co., 1965.)

medullated and unmyelinated fibers that reach the nervous system mainly in company with sympathetic efferent fibers, although pain from some pelvic structures and the esophagus are exceptions to this rule (Fig. 14–1). Centrally the fibers traverse the sympathetic ganglion chain but promptly find their way through the white ramus communicans into the mixed nerve trunks and thence into the dorsal root ganglia, wherein their cell bodies lie in company with somatosensory neurons. There is thus nothing unique or peculiar about visceral pain afferents save for their peripheral course. The latter, however, is of practical significance to the neurosurgeon, who sometimes interrupts these fibers for relief of visceral pain. He may accomplish this for a given organ, *e.g.*, the kidney, by stripping the arteries supplying the organ, because sympathetic efferent

fibers and the visceral sensory fibers are distributed to the viscera over plexuses that follow the arteries.

Alternatively, a broader deafferentation is accomplished by extirpation of the sympathetic ganglion chain. Fortunately, sympathetic efferent fibers have limited significance for survival, so that periarterial stripping and sympathetic ganglionectomy are both tolerable surgical procedures. A final alternative for surgical relief of visceral pain is anterolateral cordotomy, for in their central projections, visceral pain fibers follow the same course as do somatic pain fibers.

REFERRED PAIN

A peculiarity (but, as we will see, not a unique peculiarity) of visceral pain is that it is often referred; that is, it feels as though it were coming not from the viscera but from the body surface. Reference of pain is thus an error in localization, but the error is systematic rather than random, for the reference *is always to the dermatomes innervated by the same dorsal roots that supply the irritated visceral structure.* For example, the pain fibers supplying the myocardium originate in dorsal root ganglia T1 to T5, and the pain associated with myocardial infarction or an anginal attack characteristically feels as though it were coming from the corresponding dermatomes, the anterior chest wall to below the nipple (T5) and down the medial aspect of the arm (T1 to T2). Referred pain should be clearly distinguished from projected pain, previously described. Both are errors or confusions in localizing the source of painful stimulation. Projected pain is induced by irritation of pathways or nerve trunks but is erroneously ascribed to the stimulation of the peripheral receptors, whereas referred pain is caused by irritation of receptors, but the receptors are erroneously located in the skin rather than in the viscera.

Although the phenomenon of reference is a striking feature of visceral pain, not all visceral pain is referred. The patient with angina or a coronary infarction reports, in addition to the superficial pain in chest and arm, a deeper, poorly localized ache in the general vicinity of the heart. This is presumably unreferred visceral pain.

Finally, it should be emphasized that referred pain is not unique to visceral structures but may also occur with pseudovisceral pain, which is mediated by somatic afferent fibers. Diaphragmatic pain is an example. The pain fibers supplying the central region of the diaphragm traverse the phrenic nerve, which derives from spinal segments C3 and C4. Irritation of the central diaphragm (*e.g.*, by a subphrenic abscess) is commonly referred to the C3 to C4 dermatomes in the neck and the shoulder. Portions of the pericardium and of the biliary tract are also supplied by pain afferents from the phrenic nerve; pain of biliary colic may be referred to the shoulder. A particularly dramatic instance of referred pain occurs in gynecological practice after a procedure known as Rubin's test. This test is designed to establish patency of the Fallopian tubes by the forcing of CO_2 through the cervix, uterus, and tubes. If the tubes are patent, a bubble of gas escapes the fimbria into the peritoneal cavity. When the patient is in the horizontal position, this causes no discomfort, but as soon as she stands, the bubble floats upward in the peritoneal cavity and comes to rest below the diaphragm. For some reason, this elicits pain, and the pain is referred to the shoulder. The pain subsides as the gas bubble is dissolved (this is why the rapidly absorbed CO_2 is used rather than air).

Like true visceral pain, some pseudovisceral pain may be unreferred. For example, pain induced by probing of the parietal peritoneum or pleura is unreferred and accurately localized.

Frequently, irritation in the abdominal cavity is compounded of confusing and shifting mixtures of referred and unreferred pain of both the visceral and pseudovisceral types. In the early stages of acute appendicitis, pain referred to the midline in the umbilical region is dominant, but as inflammation spreads to the parietal peritoneum, the pain shifts to a sharply localized position in the right lower quadrant (McBurney's point). The pain from a renal calculus in the upper ureter is often referred to the testicle, but as it passes down the ureter, the localization may move to the back and then to the groin.

In summary, then, referred pain may be either visceral or somatic (pseudovisceral). The essential condition for reference appears to be a stimulus site located where other sensory cues (*e.g.*, vision) for localization are either lacking or ambiguous, a point which will be further developed presently.

MECHANISM OF REFERRED PAIN

There are two general theories for the mechanism of referred pain. Both postulate that the basic confusion arises from convergence of visceral (or pseudovisceral) afferent fibers and of cutaneous somatic afferent fibers on higher order neurons in the pain pathway. Selzer and Spencer identified in the dorsal horn unitary elements that receive input from small afferent fibers in both cutaneous and visceral nerve trunks. Discharge of such an element therefore signals ambiguously that a stimulus has occurred at either a visceral or a cutaneous site but carries no information about which one of the alternatives is correct.

The *convergence-facilitation*, or *irritable focus*, theory postulates that the visceral afferents are unable to discharge the secondary neurons but are capable of lowering their thresholds so that they discharge in response to smaller cutaneous inputs than usual. According to this theory, the pain is felt in the cutaneous site because that is where the impulses originate; the visceral irritation only facilitates their transmission across the first relay. The theory implies the existence of a tonic "spontaneous" discharge of cutaneous nociceptors that in the absence of visceral input fails to be transmitted to the secondary neurons; sampling of single cutaneous nociceptive fibers does not bear this out. Attempts to test the hypothesis by anesthetization of the dermatome of reference are ambiguous, because in some instances it diminishes the pain; in others it is ineffective.

The *convergence-projection* theory avoids the unlikely assumption of tonic activity of cutaneous pain afferents and ascribes the error in referred pain to a learned interpretation of the ambiguous signals in secondary neurons. It has been emphasized that visceral and pseudovisceral pain differ from cutaneous pain in that the subject usually has no secondary cues (*e.g.*, visual, tactile) to location of the noxious stimulus. Such cues provide the basis for a learned image of the relation between spatial aspects of cutaneous stimuli and a particular sensation. The convergence-projection theory maintains that the ambiguous signals in secondary neurons are interpreted in terms of a learned concept of the body surface, based almost entirely on a cutaneous curriculum. In other words, the pain is felt at a site learned by multiple cues to be associated with the sensation.

Several observations seem to bear out this notion. During World War II, pilot trainees often complained of pain in filled teeth at high altitudes. At first this phenomenon was erroneously ascribed to expansion of air pockets in incompletely filled cavities. Further study revealed that the causative irritation was expansion of air in the maxillary sinuses; mechanical irritation of the sinus mucosa with a probe produced dental pain identical with that caused by decompression. Significantly, pain was always referred to filled teeth. Accordingly, a controlled study was carried out. Two groups of pilots were subjected to dental repair, half under local anesthesia and half without anesthesia. Subsequent studies of pain produced by decompression revealed a significant difference. Subjects who had had painless dental repair reported accurately localized pain over the zygoma. Subjects who were alumni of the Spartan School of Dentistry felt pain in the previously abused teeth.

In other words, habit-bound, rational man tends to interpret ambiguous pain signals as emanating from a previously hurt site, the location of which he has learned from dolorous past experience. The wise dental practitioner is well aware of this propensity and makes careful examination before extracting a tooth incriminated by a suffering patient. Often the offending tooth is remote from the filled or previously infected tooth that the patient incorrectly identifies as the source of pain.

LOCALIZATION OF PAIN

It has been argued that localization of a sensory stimulus is place-coded and highly dependent on integrity of cerebral cortex. For touch, this argument has already been documented. Throughout the tactile pathways in the spinal cord, through the thalamus to the sensory cortex, spatial organization is preserved, and each cell has a relatively small and discrete receptive field. The mixing influence of convergence is tempered by lateral inhibition and by corticofugal modulation. Stimulation of cortex evokes precisely localized (or projected) sensations, and ablation of sensory cortex, which leaves modality discrimination intact, works havoc with localization of tactile stimuli. Indeed, the functional significance of the cortical representation of touch seems to be mainly, if not exclusively, related to spatial discrimination.

For pain (and for other modalities mediated by the anterolateral column system), the situation seems to be different. First, although cortical lesions produce defects in localization of pain equaling the aberrations of tactual topognosis, single-unit analysis reveals few cortical elements responding selectively to noxious stimuli. Secondly, electrical stimulation of sensory cortex elicits bland sensations lacking any clear component of pain. Single-unit explorations of sensory cortex and posteroventral thalamus reveal many cells responding to tactile stimuli and joint movement, but cells responding selectively to noxious stimuli are conspicuously sparse or absent. Indeed, there seems to be little evidence that pain information reaches the sensory cortex. Unitary explorations downstream to the cortex in the posterior thalamus and reticular formation reveal cells that appear to respond mainly to intense stimuli of the kind that cause pain. But the receptive fields of these cells are immense—sometimes including both sides of the body and all four extremities! The discharge of such cells contains information that is adequate to signal no more than "I have been hurt somewhere." The sensory content of anterolateral column messages seems to be singularly devoid of spatial information.

How then to account for disturbances of pain localization following cortical lesions, if pain does not project to the cortex? Or, how to account for the precision of normal cutaneous pain localization when the central cells have such outrageously large receptive fields? A logical guess is that localization of pain depends on the simultaneous stimulation of sensory modalities other than pain, modalities that have spatially organized pathways to the cortex, comprising neurons with discrete receptive fields. Since nociceptors have high thresholds, they are rarely selectively excited, and it seems likely that the incidental stimulation of receptors having spatially organized projections to the thalamus and cortex provides the cues for precise localization of pain. In other words, the cues for localization of pain seem to be mediated by fibers that signal modalities other than pain (*e.g.*, touch).

If this interpretation is correct, it follows that excitation of nociceptors in isolation should produce poorly localized pain. Several examples may be cited. The pain in the intermediate zone following a peripheral nerve lesion (where only pain can be elicited) is diffuse and poorly localized. Similarly, the pain induced by a noxious stimulus to a limb in which ischemia has blocked all but the C fibers of peripheral nerves is diffuse. Tooth pain, which probably results from selective excitation of nociceptors, is notoriously poorly localized. And finally, visceral (and pseudovisceral) pain, which involves only nociceptors or other receptors projecting through the anterolateral column system, gives rise to sensations that are, by habit, erroneously referred to skin regions supplied by afferents having spatially organized trajectories.

ADDITIONAL READING

Ruch, T. C. Pathophysiology of pain. Chap. 16 in *Physiology and biophysics*, Ruch, T. C., and Patton, H. D., eds., Philadelphia, W. B. Saunders Co., 1965.

CHAPTER 15

PHYSIOLOGICAL OPTICS

HARRY D. PATTON

LENSES

IMAGE FORMATION BY
LENSES

THE REFRACTIVE
MECHANISM OF THE EYE

ACCOMMODATION

OTHER PUPILLARY
REFLEXES

REFRACTIVE ERRORS AND
THEIR CORRECTION

APPENDIX:
The Lens Equation

In Chapter 7 it was pointed out that physical stimuli are often materially altered by transmission through non-neural tissues intervening between the external world and the receptor. This feature of the transduction process is nowhere more clearly exemplified than in the special senses in which the most elaborate mechanisms for presenting the physical stimulus to the receptors have evolved. In this chapter we consider the alterations that light rays undergo in their journey between the cornea and the retina. The structures bringing about these changes can be likened, with some accuracy, to the various elements of a photographic camera, the eye having counterparts of a camera lens with variable focus, a variable aperture (iris), and a light-sensitive receptive surface (the retina). The simple parallel between photography and vision breaks down once light strikes the retina; the camera has no counterpart for the complex neural events underlying visual perception. In the present chapter we will consider only the relatively simple optical events that focus light rays on the retina.

LENSES

Light from a point source spreads in the surrounding medium as a wave disturbance, the advancing front of which can be represented at successive intervals by a series of concentric spheres (Fig. 15–1). At any point on the wave-front the direction of propagation is at right angles to the front; these directions are designated *rays* of light. At sites near the point source, the wave-front is markedly curved and the rays are radially divergent. As the distance increases, the circumference of the front so increases that a segment of the spherical wave-front approximates a plane surface; the rays are then virtually parallel. For practical purposes, light reaching the eye from a point source 21 feet (6 meters) away can be considered to be composed of parallel rays. When the luminous point is on the horizontal axis of the eye, the parallel rays enter the eye perpendicular to its vertical axis; if they proceeded unaltered to the retina, multiple images of the point source would be formed. For a single image of the point to be formed, the

199

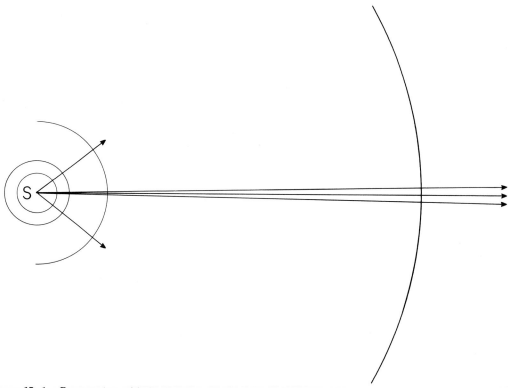

Figure 15–1. Propagation of light from a point source, S. The wave-front at any point is represented as a sphere with its center at S. Rays are at right angles to the wave-front. At distant sites a segment of the wave-front approaches a plane, and the rays become nearly parallel.

parallel rays must be reassembled and brought to a point focus. This requires a lens system, the basic principles of which are briefly reviewed here. More detailed accounts can be found in standard physics texts.

The magic of a lens depends on its ability to "bend" or change the direction of light rays passing through it; this property is called *refraction*. Refraction, in turn, results from the physical fact that the speed of light varies with the medium in which it travels. In general, the denser the medium, the slower the speed of transmission. Thus the speed of light progressively diminishes in passing from a vacuum to air, to water, to oil, to glass. The capacity of a medium to impede light waves is measured by its index of refraction (n_{med}), defined as the ratio between the speed of light in air (v_{air}) to that in the specified medium (v_{med}):

$$n_{med} = v_{air}/v_{med}$$

The index of refraction of a vacuum is thus less than 1.0. The index of refraction of water is 1.333, and the indices for various oils, mineral crystals, glass and plastics are all more than 1.0, ranging up to 2.4 for diamonds. Measurements of the speed of light transmission are difficult to achieve, and there are simpler indirect ways to measure refractive indices; but, no matter how measured, the index of refraction of a material depends on the material's ability to alter the speed of light waves entering it from another medium.

Figure 15–2A depicts a photic wave-front in air emanating from a distant source and passing through a plate of glass whose plane is parallel to the wave-front, *i.e.*, perpendicular to the rays. In passing from air to glass, the wave is slowed, but when it emerges again into air on the other side, its speed is restored. In this circumstance the direction of the rays is unaltered, and unless elaborate measure-

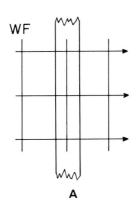
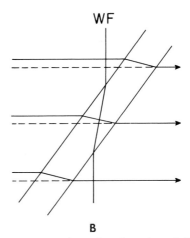

Figure 15–2. Passage of a wave-front of light from a distant source through a glass plate. *A,* The parallel rays are perpendicular to the plate; emerging rays are not deviated. *B,* Rays strike the plate obliquely. In the glass the wave-front (*WF*) is impeded, and rays are bent toward the perpendicular. Emerging rays are bent away from the perpendicular; they are displaced but not deviated in direction.

ments are made, we cannot detect that the interposed glass plate has affected transmission at all. *Light rays perpendicular to a plane refractile surface are not altered in direction.*

When, however, the wave-front approaches the glass obliquely, as in Figure 15–2*B,* that portion of the front within the glass moves more slowly than that portion in air, and there is an angle between the airborne and glassborne portions of the front. *The direction of the rays is shifted toward the perpendicular to the surface.* Of course, as the wave enters air again on the opposite side, the emergent rays are bent back away from the perpendicular and assume a direction parallel to, but displaced

from, that on the entry side. *Light rays passing obliquely through a refractile medium with a plane surface are displaced but not changed in direction.* Such a system cannot serve as a focusing lens; the emergent rays remain parallel because rays "bent" on entering the glass are "unbent" as they reenter air; what is accomplished on one side is undone on the other.

A way to prevent this compensatory effect is to construct the two surfaces of the refractile material with opposite slopes, so that entrant rays and emergent rays are bent in the same direction, as in a simple prism (Fig. 15–3*A*). Rays entering the prism are bent toward the perpendicular of the front face (*i.e.,* downward), and

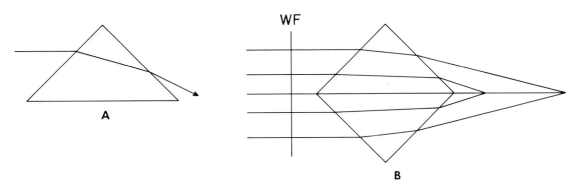

Figure 15–3. Refraction by prisms. *A,* Light ray striking the prism perpendicular to its altitude is bent downward on entering the glass and again on emerging into the air. *B,* Two prisms are placed base to base. Light rays entering near the apices focus farther behind the prisms than do those entering near the bases.

emergent rays are bent away from the perpendicular of the back face (also downward). If now two prisms are joined together base to base (Figure 15–3B), rays passing through the upper half are bent downward and those traversing the lower half are bent upward, and the projections of these rays intersect on the right at a focal point.

Although the introduction of oppositely oriented surfaces obviates the problem of compensatory bending of rays on the two sides, it still fails to focus all the parallel rays, because each incident ray makes the same angle with the surface and accordingly is bent by the same amount. Therefore, the intersection points of the emergent rays vary with their entry sites, those entering near the apices being focused farther behind the prisms than those entering closer to the apposed bases; a prism produces dispersion rather than focus. What is required is a geometrical surface that will bend the apical incident rays proportionately more than those entering the center of the lens. A satisfactory approximation to this condition is accomplished by making the two surfaces spherical, so that the angle of the perpendicular is continuously variable from periphery to center (Fig. 15–4A). The angle of incidence of parallel rays is then also continuously variable, and since the angle of refraction is related to the angle of incidence, peripheral rays are bent more than central rays, and all focus sharply at the same point behind the lens. Such a biconvex

lens, because it makes parallel rays converge to a point focus, is called a *converging* lens. It is also possible to construct a biconcave lens, in which the emergent rays are bent away from the center; such a lens is called a *diverging* lens, and it produces no real focus of emergent rays (Fig. 15–4B).

There are two defects in a simple biconvex converging lens; both arise because a simple spherical surface only approximates the ideal geometrical configuration for focusing. The approximation worsens as the entry sites move from the center to the periphery of the lens, where the change in the angle of incidence per increment of distance from the equator of the lens departs significantly from linear proportionality. Rays entering at the edges of the lens are bent disproportionately more than those traversing more central regions and consequently are focused at points closer to the back of the lens (Fig. 15–5A). This defect is termed *spherical aberration*, and it accounts for the expense of wide-angle camera lenses in which specially ground surfaces or compensatory mechanisms must be employed to provide fine focus of marginal rays. If one can afford to waste some light, a simpler and easier way to counter spherical aberration is to block out the aberrant peripheral parts of the lens with a diaphragm, so that only the reasonably satisfactory central portion of the lens is employed (Fig. 15–5B). As we shall see, this is the mechanism employed in the eye, where the iris serves as a diaphragm.

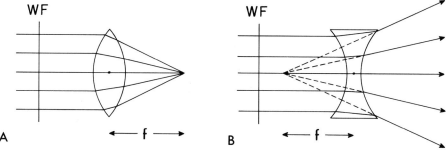

Figure 15–4. Action of lenses on parallel rays of light. The focal distance (*f*) depends on the index of refraction of the lens and on the radius of curvature of its surface. *A*, Biconvex or converging lens. *B*, Biconcave lens, causing divergence of emerging rays, which do not form real focus. Extrapolation of emerging rays to their point of convergence in front of the lens defines the virtual focus.

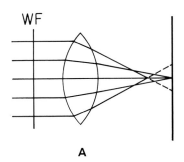
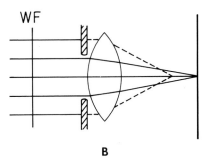

Figure 15–5. Spherical aberration and its correction with a diaphragm. *A,* Because a spherical surface does not change the angle of incidence in direct proportion to distance from the lens equator, marginal rays are refracted too much and focus closer to the lens than do central rays. *B,* Blurring is diminished by exclusion of the marginal rays with a diaphragm.

The other defect of spherical lenses is called *chromatic aberration* and arises because short wavelengths are impeded and hence are bent more than long wavelengths; this means that violet and red rays come to different focuses, producing a spectral blur. Chromatic aberration is exaggerated by changes in the lens that increase the amount of refraction because the spectral discrepancies are thus magnified. It follows that the peripheral rays, which are bent more than the central rays, are most likely to suffer from chromatic aberration. Again a diaphragm ameliorates the defect.

Since the function of a lens is to bend light rays, the power of a lens is a measure of its ability to perform this function. There are two obvious ways to increase lens power: (1) by using materials of greater indices of refraction and (2) by decreasing the radius of curvature of the lens; a fat lens is more powerful than a skinny one. The first expedient is obviously limited by availability of materials, and the second is limited by burgeoning problems of spherical and chromatic aberration. Since more powerful lenses bend light rays more, the convergence occurs closer to the lens back than in a weaker (less curved) lens. Measurement of the focal length (*f*), *i.e.,* the distance from lens center to the principal focus where the emergent rays converge, is thus a simple way to measure power. Since focal length and lens power are inversely related, power is defined as the reciprocal of the focal length; *i.e.,* $P = 1/f$. The unit of power is the *diopter,* defined as the power of a lens with a focal length of 1 m. For example, a lens with a focal length of 0.5 m has a power of 1/0.5, or 2, diopters.

A biconcave lens does not focus rays behind the lens because the emerging rays diverge, but a focal distance can be defined by extrapolation of the divergent rays back to a convergence point in front of the lens (Fig. 15–4*B*). To a viewer on the back side of the lens a parallel-rayed light source appears to emanate from this virtual principal focus. The power of a diverging lens is measured in negative diopters. In practice, the easiest way to measure the power of a diverging lens is to match it with a converging lens whose refraction is just abolished when combined with the diverging lens; a converging lens of 0.5 diopter, for example, is neutralized by a diverging lens of −0.5 diopter.

IMAGE FORMATION BY LENSES

Thus far attention has been confined to the refraction of parallel light rays arising from a distant point source on the principal axis of the lens, *i.e.,* on the line passing through the lens center. We now consider the formation of the image of an extended object (rather than a single point) by converging lenses (Fig. 15–6). Only one point on the object lies on the principal axis; the other points emanate parallel rays, some of which strike the curved surface of the lens obliquely. To describe the course of these rays we need to define the

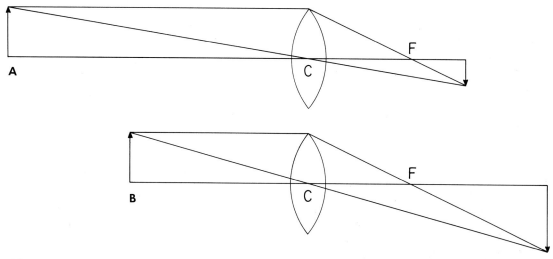

Figure 15–6. Formation of images of extended objects by a biconvex lens. Each point of the image is formed by the intersection of the deviated rays passing through F with undeviated rays passing through C. In A the object is far from the lens, in B closer. The image in B is larger and farther back than in A because the slope of the ray passing through C is greater in B.

optical center (C) as a point in the lens through which light rays pass without deviation, irrespective of their angles of incidence. We have already seen that the parallel ray passing through the principal axis is undeviated, so the optical center must lie along its traverse. Rays striking the lens obliquely from above or below and intersecting the perpendicular in the middle of the lens are also undeviated, because on entry they are bent downward and on emerging they are bent upward; the compensatory feature of the biconvex surface does not apply to these oblique rays. The emergent ray is slightly displaced, but with thin lenses this displacement is negligible. This means that we can always draw a ray from a point on an object through the optical center as a straight line, whether it enters the lens perpendicularly or obliquely. We can draw another ray from the same point parallel to the principal axis of the lens; this ray is refracted and passes through the principal focus. Where the undeviated ray and the refracted ray intersect is the image of the point. Obviously, a series of such lines could be drawn emanating from different points on the object and terminating as different points of the image, and thus the image of the entire object can be constructed. The image as constructed is inverted.

The slope of the deviated ray emerging from the lens is independent of the distance of the object from the lens and is determined only by the invariant principal focus. However, the slope of the undeviated line passing through the optical center becomes steeper as the object approaches the lens, and consequently the intersection of the two rays (*i.e.*, the image) moves farther behind the lens. The size of the image is also increased (Fig. 15–6). The quantitative relation between object distance *(o)*, image distance *(i)*, and focal distance *(f)* is given by the lens equation: $1/f = 1/i + 1/o$. The precise derivation of this equation is complex and can be found in physics texts; a simplified approximate derivation is given in the appendix of this chapter. Substituting some values for *o* in the equation illustrates how image distance varies with object distance. For example, if $o = \infty$, $1/f = 1/i$ and $i = f$; that is, the image is formed at the principal focus. The size of the image relative to the object is given by i/o, or $i/\infty = 0$. This is merely a repetition of what has already been established; parallel rays from an infinitely distant source all converge at the principal focus, so that the image size is infinitely small.

If the object is brought closer to the front of the lens, for example to a distance equal to $2f$, $1/f = 1/2f + 1/i$, or $1/i = 1/f - 1/2f$, and $i = 2f$. The image size is $i/2f = 2f/2f = 1$. Moving the object from ∞ to $2f$ thus moves the image back from f to $2f$, and its size increases from 0 to the same size as the object.

If the object is moved still closer, to within f units in front of the lens, $1/f = 1/f + 1/i$, $i = \infty$, and image size is $\infty/o = \infty$. Similarly it can be shown that object distances less than f produce images of finite magnification but with negative sign; i.e., the image is virtual (in front of the lens).

In summary, as the object distance moves from infinity to f, the image distance moves from f to infinity and its size increases from zero to infinity. The change in image distance is of special significance. The photographer focuses images by appropriately varying the distance between the lens and film. Some fishes similarly focus near objects by moving the lenses of their eyes. The human eye focuses near objects by increasing the power of the lens to shorten the focal distance.

THE REFRACTIVE MECHANISM OF THE EYE

Figure 15–7 shows a horizontal section through a human eyeball. Light rays from the outside successively pass through the cornea, the aqueous humor, the lens, and the vitreous humor before falling on the retina. Consequently, light rays undergo a complex series of bendings and unbendings, depending on the curvature and the indices of refraction of the interposed structures. The major refraction occurs at the air-corneal interface, where the greatest change of index of refraction (air = 1.000, cornea = 1.376) occurs; this amounts to about + 45 diopters. In the aqueous humor the index of refraction is 1.336, so the power is slightly negative (-5.9 diopters). The refraction by the lens is again positive but is complicated both because its two surfaces have different curvatures and because its index of refraction is graded from surface to center: in the absence of accommodation, the two surfaces provide about +17 diopters, a rather small contribution relative to that of the air-corneal junction. Nevertheless, the lens is highly important, not so much for its refractive power per se, but because its power (and hence its focal length) can be varied to focus images of near objects. The mechanism for increasing the refractive power of the lens, called *accommodation*, is discussed later.

Tracing light rays through the various refractive structures of the eye is tedious and can be avoided by the use of a model,

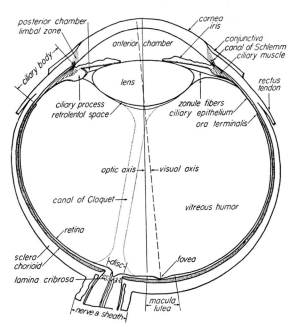

Figure 15–7. A horizontal section through the equator of the right eye. (From Ruch and Patton, eds., *Physiology and biophysics*, Philadelphia, W. B. Saunders Co., 1965.)

called the *reduced eye*, in which the several refractive surfaces are replaced by a single imaginary lens with a principal focus equal to that of the normal unaccommodated eye for parallel rays of light. The starting point in designing such a simplified model is to know the distance from cornea to retina in a normal eye, because by definition a normal eye focuses parallel rays on the retina; this distance averages 24.4 mm. A single lens with an index of refraction of water placed 1.5 mm behind the cornea and with a radius of curvature of 5.7 mm focuses parallel rays at 24.4 mm. The optical center of this system is 7.2 mm behind the cornea and 17.2 mm anterior to the retina. The reduced eye of course describes only the unaccommodated eye, but it greatly simplifies diagrams of abnormal eyes.

ACCOMMODATION

In the relaxed eye light rays from a distant object are focused upon the retina. As the light source moves closer to the lens, the focal point moves behind the retina. Then the retinal image is no longer the sharp apex of the cone of the refracted light rays but rather a ring or circle ("blur circle") that becomes increasingly larger, the nearer the object. Vision becomes blurred or indistinct, just as does a projected image when the screen is too near

the projector. A sharp image of near objects can be achieved if: (1) the distance between the retina and refracting surface increases, or if (2) the amount of refraction increases. The latter can be effected by (a) increase of the index of refraction of one or more of the media or by (b) increase of the radius of curvature of one or more refracting surfaces.

The human eye focuses near objects by increasing the convexity of the lens (mainly its anterior surface). The lens is held in place behind the iris by the thin zonal strands of the suspensory ligament, which bridge between the elastic capsule of the lens and the ciliary body (Fig. 15–8). In the relaxed eye the zonula is taut, holding the lens in a semiflattened shape. The tension of the zonula, however, is decreased by contraction of the smooth muscle of the ciliary body. One set of ciliary fibers is circular; their contraction reduces the diameter of the ciliary body and thus slackens the zonula. Another set of muscle fibers is longitudinally arranged; their contraction pulls the attachments of the zonula closer to the base of the iris and reduces zonular tension. Contraction of both circular and longitudinal fibers thus relaxes the zonula and allows the elastic lens to bulge passively into a more nearly spherical shape; the magnitude of the change is a function of the strength of ciliary contraction. The resulting rounding, or fattening, of the lens increases its

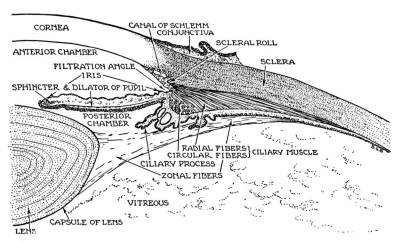

Figure 15–8. The ciliary body, lens, and iris. (From Ruch and Patton, eds., *Physiology and biophysics,* Philadelphia, W. B. Saunders Co., 1965.)

power, shortens the focal length, and brings the image of near objects into focus on the retina.

The efficiency of accommodation depends on the elasticity of the lens, which varies with age. The lens, like the spirit, loses some of its resiliency with age, and the accommodative dividends of ciliary effort wane with senility, a condition known as *presbyopia*. The effect of age on magnitude of accommodation can be readily gauged by measurement of the *near point, i.e.*, the minimum distance from the cornea at which a clear image can be formed by maximum accommodative effort. In a normal 15-year-old subject the near point is about 8 cm; in a septuagenarian, about 1 m. Translated into powers: the youth can by accommodation increase the power of his eye from about 60 diopters to 72 diopters; the aged, from 60 to 61 diopters. From youth to senility our lenses deteriorate at a rate of about a quarter of a diopter a year. Presbyopia, the farsightedness of age, is readily corrected with convex converging lenses, which compensate for the lack of power in the inelastic ocular lens.

The ciliary muscle is innervated by parasympathetic postganglionic neurons located in the ciliary ganglion. The preganglionic neurons are in the Edinger-Westphal nucleus; their axons reach the ganglion via cranial nerve III. Like other parasympathetic postganglionic neurons, those supplying the ciliary muscle are cholinergic, and the acetylcholine (ACh) receptors of the ciliary muscle can be readily blocked with atropine eyedrops. Accommodative adjustments of ocular refraction to focus near objects are then paralyzed, and objects nearer than about 20 ft are indistinctly seen. Ophthalmologists sometimes paralyze accommodation to determine the optical properties of the completely relaxed eye.

Ciliary contraction is one of the three adjustments that are collectively termed the accommodation reflex; the other two adjustments are *ocular convergence* and *pupillary constriction.*

Convergence refers to the inward rotation of the two eyes as the object of gaze moves from a distant to a near object, an adjustment that keeps the image in the two eyes focused on the foveae. A failure of accurate convergence leads to double vision, or *diplopia*, for reasons that will be discussed in Chapters 17 and 22. Convergence requires contraction of the medial rectus muscles and relaxation of the lateral recti. These two sets of muscles are innervated by somatic components of cranial nerves III and VI, respectively; their coordinated action during convergence is thus an example of reciprocal innervation with excitation of oculomotor neurons and inhibition of abducens motoneurons.

The third component of accommodation is analogous to the use of the diaphragm of the camera—pupillary constriction, or *miosis*. The iris has two sets of smooth muscles: a circular or sphincter muscle, which acts to constrict the pupillary aperture, and a radial component, contraction of which dilates the pupil. Pupillary size is determined by the balanced action of these two sets of muscles. The sphincter muscle is innervated by postganglionic parasympathetic neurons in the ciliary ganglion, the axons of which reach the iris through the short ciliary nerves in company with those destined for the ciliary muscles. The preganglionic neurons are located in the Edinger-Westphal portion of the oculomotor nucleus and reach the ganglion via cranial nerve III. The radial muscle of the iris is innervated by sympathetic postganglionic neurons in the superior cervical ganglion; their axons reach the eye via the carotid plexus and the ophthalmic branch of cranial nerve V. The sympathetic preganglionic cell bodies are in the intermediolateral cell column of the upper thoracic cord and reach the superior cervical ganglion via upper thoracic white rami and the cervical sympathetic chain.

Pupillary constriction, the so-called *near reflex* of the iris, aids in forming clear images of near objects in two ways. First, by obstructing marginal light rays it serves, as already mentioned, to diminish chromatic and spherical aberration, both of which tend to become more troublesome as the lens becomes more rounded and hence stronger. Secondly, the diaphragm action of the iris increases the depth of focus of the eye. A pencil of rays entering the eye is bent into a cone of rays that

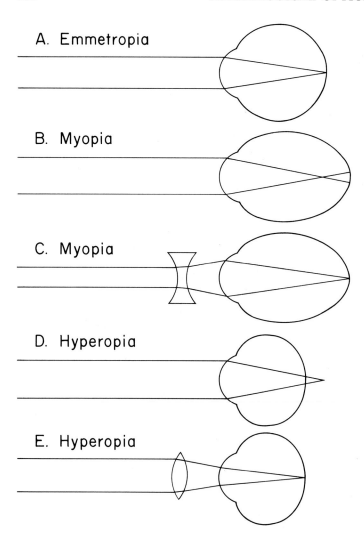

A. Emmetropia

B. Myopia

C. Myopia

D. Hyperopia

E. Hyperopia

Figure 15–9. Normal vision (*A*) and optical defects uncorrected (*B* and *D*) and corrected by appropriate lenses (*C* and *E*).

ideally has its apex on the retina. When the apex is behind the retina, blur circles are formed (Fig. 15–9*D*). If the circles are small, they are not perceived as different from a point. The size of a blur circle is diminished if the marginal rays are obstructed so that the base of the cone (and hence the size of the blur circle) is reduced. In this way the iris diminishes the perceptual blurring of objects nearer or farther than the point of ideal focus. For example, when the eye is focused on an object 1 m away, objects within the range from 5 m to 56 cm are seen with relative clarity if the pupil size is 1 mm. For the same conditions with a pupil size of 4 mm, the depth of focus is only over the range of 1.4 m to 78 cm.

The three components of the accommodation reflex (ciliary contraction, convergence, and pupillary constriction) are all mediated by cranial nerve III, employing both its somatic and autonomic components. The input to the oculomotor nucleus that brings about the integrated discharge resulting in accommodation is not clear but presumably involves the occipital cortex and corticofugal paths to the pretectal area.

OTHER PUPILLARY REFLEXES

The near reflex is only one reflex response of the iris; two others are the *light reflex* and the *pupillodilator reflex*. The former is a reflex response to change of illumination of the eye; the pupil constricts as light intensity increases and dilates as it dims. If light enters only one eye, the other being shaded, both pupils constrict; the response of the illuminated eye is called the *direct light reflex* and that of the contralateral eye, the *consensual light reflex*. The receptors for the light reflex are the photoreceptors of the retina; both rods and cones are involved. The further course is as follows: the receptors connect with bipolar cells, and the latter impinge on ganglion cells (see Chapter 16). The axons of the ganglion cells traverse the optic nerve and optic tract in company with the visual fibers, but prior to reaching the lateral geniculate body they part from the optic tract to form synaptic connections with cells in the pretectal area ventral and rostral to the superior colliculus. Pretectal neurons connect with cells in the Edinger-Westphal nuclei of both sides. The remainder of the pathway is through cranial nerve III, the ciliary ganglion, and the short ciliary nerves. The light reflex may be lost from a lesion of either the afferent or efferent limb of the reflex arc; the lesions are readily distinguished, since the former abolishes both direct and consensual responses to stimuli on the affected side, whereas the latter leaves the consensual response intact.

The mechanism of accommodative miosis is not identical with that of the light reflex, since the two responses can be differentially and independently impaired. An example is the *Argyll-Robertson pupil* that occurs in syphilis. The pupil is constricted and fails to respond to light but responds normally in accommodation. The converse of the Argyll-Robertson pupil occurs in diphtheritic neuritis; that is, accommodative miosis fails, and the light reflex remains intact. The sites of the lesions underlying these dissociations are controversial, but they clearly indicate that the accommodative response of the pupil is not simply a result of the increased illumination resulting from bringing the luminous object closer to the eye.

The pupillodilator reflex is elicited by noxious stimulation. It also occurs in emotional states of fright or alarm. The change in pupil size is governed by re-

ciprocal inhibition of the parasympathetic (oculomotor) supply and excitation of the sympathetic supply.

The parasympathetic fibers innervating the pupillary sphincter are cholinergic and are readily blocked by atropine eyedrops, which not only paralyze accommodation but widely dilate the pupil. In fact, the atropine-containing extract of the belladonna (literally, "beautiful woman") plant was used cosmetically by Italian belles to dilate their pupils, a practice that rendered their eyes romantically lustrous but exceedingly farsighted. A more legitimate usage of atropine eyedrops is to permit ophthalmoscopic examination of the fundus without obstruction from a constricted iris.

REFRACTIVE ERRORS AND THEIR CORRECTION

In a normal eye, relaxed from all accommodative effort, parallel light rays are focused on the retina 24.4 mm behind the cornea. Closer objects are focused by an increase in the power of the lens and a shortening of the focal distance to correspond to the corneoretinal distance. Faulty vision occurs if the image falls either behind or in front of the retina, and this may result from a refractive power inappropriate for a normal corneoretinal distance or conversely from normal refraction combined with an eyeball that is either abnormally long or abnormally short. We have already described presbyopia, in which the refractile power of the lens is at fault. Two common optical defects mainly or exclusively due to variance of eyeball length are myopia and hyperopia.

In *myopia*, the eyeball is too long, and distant objects are focused in front of the retina (Fig. 15–9). Beyond the focal point the rays, of course, diverge, and the image on the retina is a blur circle rather than a point. As the object moves closer, the focal point moves back and eventually falls on the retina, but beyond this abnormally short far-point of vision, everything is blurred. For this reason myopic patients are said to be nearsighted. The condition is readily corrected with a concave diverging lens, which in combination with the convergent action of the eye produces a focal point farther than normal behind the cornea on the abnormally distant retina.

In *hyperopia* the eyeball is abnormally short (Fig. 15–9), so that in the relaxed eye distant objects are focused behind the retina. By accommodative effort the hyperope can see distant objects, but as the object moves closer, he exhausts his accommodative capacity, and images of close objects are blurred; *i.e.*, he has an abnormally distant near-point of vision. Presbyopes and hyperopes have a similar problem for different reasons; the former lacks adequate accommodative reserve because his lens is inelastic, the latter because he is compelled to use up his accommodative effort in focusing distant objects normally seen without effort. In either case the defect is readily corrected with convex (converging) lenses to increase the refractive power of the eye.

A common optical defect due to a defect in the refractive mechanisms is *astigmatism*, in which the curvature of the refracting surface (*e.g.*, the cornea) departs from that of a true sphere and more nearly resembles that of a segment cut from the surface of an egg. Such a surface has two different major radii of curvature at right angles to each other—a long radius in the vertical axis of the egg and a short radius in the horizontal plane. Accordingly, parallel rays in the horizontal plane focus in front of those striking the eye along the vertical plane. What is needed to correct the defect is a lens that increases convergence in the less curved plane. Such a lens can be made by a section through the long axis of a cylinder; it is known as a *cylindrical lens.* Such a lens placed with its curved surface in the plane of the less curved surface of the cornea compensates for the refractive discrepancy and permits sharp focus of all rays striking the cornea, regardless of plane of incidence.

ADDITIONAL READING

Campbell, C. J., Koester, C. J., Rittler, M. C., and Tackaberry, R. B. *Physiological optics.* New York, Harper & Row, 1974.

Davson, H. The eye as an optical instrument. Chap. 57 in *Starling's human physiology*, Davson, H., and Eggleton, M. G., eds., Philadelphia, Lea & Febiger, 1968.

Davson, H. *Physiology of the eye.* London, Churchill, 1963.

Weymouth, F. W. The eye as an optical instrument. Chap. 19 in *Physiology and biophysics*, Ruch, T. C., and Patton, H. D., eds., Philadelphia, W. B. Saunders Co., 1965.

APPENDIX:
The Lens Equation

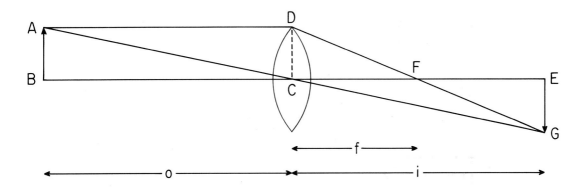

Triangles ABC and GEC are similar; hence,

$$\frac{AB}{GE} = \frac{BC}{EC} = \frac{o}{i} \tag{1}$$

Triangles CDF and EGF are similar; hence,

$$\frac{DC}{EG} = \frac{CF}{FE} = \frac{f}{i-f} \tag{2}$$

$DC = AB$, so

$$\frac{DC}{EG} = \frac{AB}{EG} = \frac{CF}{FE} = \frac{f}{i-f} \tag{3}$$

Substituting (1) into (3),

$$\frac{o}{i} = \frac{f}{i-f} \quad \text{or} \quad \frac{i}{o} = \frac{i-f}{f} \tag{4}$$

Dividing (4) by i,

$$\frac{1}{o} = \frac{1-\frac{f}{i}}{f} \tag{5}$$

Adding $\frac{1}{i}$ to both sides of (5),

$$\frac{1}{o} + \frac{1}{i} = \frac{1-\frac{f}{i}}{f} + \frac{1}{i} = \frac{1}{f}$$

Therefore,

$$\frac{1}{f} = \frac{1}{o} + \frac{1}{i}$$

CHAPTER 16

RETINAL PROCESSES IN VISUAL FUNCTION

HARRY D. PATTON

THE DUPLICITY THEORY

STRUCTURE OF THE RETINA

VISUAL THRESHOLDS

DARK ADAPTATION

THE ROD PIGMENT, RHODOPSIN

CONE PIGMENTS

ELECTRICAL RESPONSES OF RETINAL ELEMENTS

GANGLION CELLS

THE RETINA AND VISUAL ACUITY

In the preceding chapter the eye was likened to a camera, the retina, as a first approximation, corresponding to the photographic film. In fact, the analogy begins to break down seriously at the retinal level, for many subtle features of retinal function have no clear counterparts in the camera.

The retina contains not only photosensitive receptors, the rods and cones, but also the secondary and tertiary neurons of the visual pathway, the bipolar cells and ganglion cells; three out of five of the cells of the visual pathway are located in the retina. In addition to the receptors and the relay cells, the retina contains cells (horizontal cells) that establish lateral connections between receptors and others (amacrine cells) that in turn establish lateral connections between ganglion cells. These interneurons permit interaction between elements located in different parts of the retina and add to the visual process a complexity and refinement unparalleled in photography.

THE DUPLICITY THEORY

The retina contains two kinds of receptors—rods and cones—that are not only morphologically distinctive but also endowed with quite different functional properties. In essence the retina is a double sense organ, a concept that is known as the *duplicity theory* of retinal function. Because the duality of rod and cone function underlies so many of the peculiar properties of the visual system, salient features of the duplicity theory are summarized here and will be further developed in the remainder of this chapter.

The cones have relatively high thresholds and function mainly in conditions of daylight, or *photopic*, illumination. Cones are found throughout the retina but are concentrated in the fovea, where they are smallest and most closely packed together. Many foveal cones have "private pathways" to the central nervous system; *i.e.*, there is little or no convergence of different foveal cones on a common bipolar cell nor of different bipolar cells on common ganglion cells. Privacy of foveal pathways, once thought to be absolute, is now known to be relative; *i.e.*, foveal bipolar and ganglion cells receive input from fewer receptors than do their counterparts in extrafoveal sites. Perhaps "semiprivate" is a better description. Cones are responsible for high-acuity form and detail vision and for color vision.

Rods, on the other hand, have exquisitely low thresholds and function under conditions of twilight or *scotopic* illumination. Indeed, rods have achieved near maximum sensitivity, some being responsive to a single quantum of energy. Rods are lacking in the fovea and none has a private (or even semiprivate) pathway to the brain. In the peripheral retina many receptors (both rods and cones) may converge on a single bipolar cell, and many bipolar cells may converge on a single ganglion cell. Scotopic rod vision is poor in detail and achromatic.

In essence, then, the eye contains two systems, one underlying color and detail vision but requiring relatively high illumination, the other underlying twilight vision, which is poor in detail and lacks color but is exquisitely sensitive (Table 16–1).

STRUCTURE OF THE RETINA

The retina lines the interior surface of the optic globe as far forward as the ciliary body (see Figure 15–7), where it terminates in a wavy or serrate border, called the ora serrata. The retina is perforated at the optic nerve head, where the accumulated axons of the retinal ganglion cells penetrate the retina, choroid, and sclera on their way into the brain; the receptor-free nerve head is responsible for the functional blind spot of the visual field.

In histological section the retina is prominently laminated (Fig. 16–1). It is a confusing perversity of anatomical nomenclature that the terms *outer* and *inner* are used to designate distances of layers from the center of the eyeball. That is, the outer layers are those that lie deep in the retina close to the choroid, and the outermost is the pigment cell layer, a single layer of epithelial cells, with pigment-laden, finger-like processes that penetrate between the outer segments of the receptor cells (Fig. 16–2). The dark pigment presumably minimizes reflection of light. The pigment layer (considered by some to be a part of the choroid rather than of the retina) is loosely bound to the other retinal layers and is a common site of pathological detachment of the retina.

Internal to the pigment layer is the receptor layer, containing the rods and cones. Both rods and cones have elongated *outer* and *inner segments* connected by an eccentric constricted region, which in cross section has the characteristics of a cilium (Figs. 16–3 and 16–4) in electron micrographs. The outer segment of the rod is narrow and uniform in diameter; that of the cone is flask-shaped, being wide at the base and tapering to a blunt tip. Electron micrographs reveal that the outer segments of both rods and cones contain a thickly packed series of discs resembling a pile of stacked coins (Figs. 16–3 and 16–4). High-power micrographs show that each disc is composed of two continuous membranes separated by a small space—like a collapsed membranous sac, with the cen-

TABLE 16–1. Comparison of Rods and Cones

	Cones	Rods
Threshold	Relatively high.	Exquisitely low.
Distribution	Ubiquitous, concentrated at fovea.	Nonfoveal, peripheral retina only.
Convergence	Limited in fovea.	Extensive.
Illumination	Photopic (daylight).	Scotopic (twilight).
Function	Central vision. Color vision. Detail vision.	Peripheral vision. Achromatic vision. Poor detail vision.

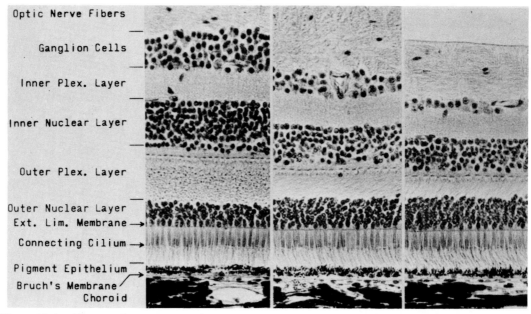

Optic Nerve Fibers

Ganglion Cells

Inner Plex. Layer

Inner Nuclear Layer

Outer Plex. Layer

Outer Nuclear Layer
Ext. Lim. Membrane →

Connecting Cilium →

Pigment Epithelium
Bruch's Membrane
Choroid

Figure 16–1. Microscopic appearance of monkey retina. The section at the *left* is near the fovea; that at the *right,* near the optic disc. The *middle section* is from a site intermediate between the other two. The bottom of the figure faces the sclera; the top faces the vitreous humor. Although all layers are present in each section, their thicknesses vary with position. In the periphery *(right)* the ganglionic and inner nuclear layers become thinner and the outer nuclear layer becomes thicker because of a higher rod–cone ratio in the peripheral retina and a consequent higher density of peripheral receptors. (From Brown *et al., Cold Spr. Harb. Symp. quant. Biol.,* 1965, *30, 457–482.*)

tral space almost obliterated. The outer segments are the photosensitive portion of the receptors and contain the light-sensitive visual pigments attached to the disc membranes. The rod pigment is rhodopsin (see later). Although, as we shall see, there is physiological evidence for three cone pigments with different spectral sensitivities, there is no morphological basis for distinction between cones.

In both rods and cones the discs are formed by infoldings of the outer segment surface membrane. In rods the invaginated folds separate from the outer membrane and seal, so that, except for the most basal discs, their flattened cavities have no connection with the extracellular space (Fig. 16–3). In cones discs maintain their external connections and do not become free-floating.

In rods the discs undergo continuous and surprisingly active turnover; new folds constantly form at the base of the outer segment. Newly formed discs become free-floating and are gradually pushed distally toward the tip, where they

are sloughed and ingested by the pigment cells. The process is strikingly displayed in radioautographs of rods from animals receiving injections of labeled amino acids, which are rapidly incorporated into the protein moiety of visual pigment. The labeled molecules first appear in the inner segment where protein synthesis is thought to occur. They then migrate through the connecting cilium and show up as discrete transverse bands corresponding to new discs. The discs thus labeled can be clearly followed at ensuing intervals as they progress toward the tip and subsequently in fragments within the pigment cells. Turnover is brisk. In tree shrew retina the outer segment turns out a new disc every 20 min. Each newborn disc has a longevity of about a week, being importunately nudged from below each day about 1.6 μm closer to inevitable exile and extinction at the tip.

Cone discs do not display such readily traceable behavior. Labeled amino acids are incorporated diffusely into cone discs, a finding which prompted the postulate that cone discs, once formed, are immortal.

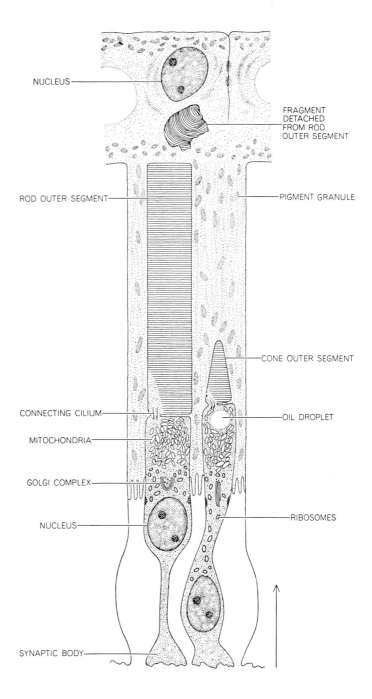

NUCLEUS

FRAGMENT
DETACHED
FROM ROD
OUTER SEGMENT

ROD OUTER SEGMENT

PIGMENT GRANULE

CONE OUTER SEGMENT

CONNECTING CILIUM

OIL DROPLET

MITOCHONDRIA

GOLGI COMPLEX

NUCLEUS

RIBOSOMES

SYNAPTIC BODY

Figure 16–2. The relation between rods, cones, and pigment epithelium in frog retina. (From *Visual Cells,* by Richard W. Young. Copyright © 1970 by Scientific American, Inc. All rights reserved.)

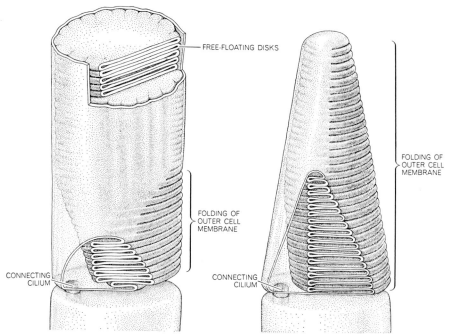

Figure 16–3.   Outer segments of rod *(left)* and cone *(right)*. In both receptors discs are formed by infolding of plasma membrane. In rods the folds pinch off so that discs become free-floating within the outer segment. Cone discs persist as folds; the disc space communicates with extracellular space. (From Visual Cells, by Richard W. Young. Copyright © 1970 by Scientific American, Inc. All rights reserved.)

However, careful studies indicate that cones, too, either slough their tips or have them nipped off by the pigment cells. How the discarded cone discs are replaced is not clear.

There is reason to suspect that retinitis pigmentosa, a blinding retinal degenerative disease, characterized by accumulation of pigment and cellular debris with accompanying receptor degeneration, may reflect a failure of epithelial phagocytosis to keep pace with the extrusion of senescent discs. Retinal degeneration probably results from starvation, for the accumulation of pigment and debris in the outer retina widens the diffusion distance over which nutrients must migrate from capillaries in the choroid layer to reach the outer segments.

The inner segments of the receptors contain numerous mitochondria. The inner segment of the rod has a narrow neck that expands to enclose a nucleus; the receptor nuclei form the thick band of rounded profiles described in light micrographs as the *outer nuclear layer*. The cone nuclei are larger than those of the rods

and are arranged in a single row at the outer edge of the outer nuclear layer. Beyond the nuclear layer the inner segments extend into a fibrous region, the *outer plexiform layer*, and terminate in expansions (the *rod spherule* and the *cone pedicle*), which form synaptic contact with the dendrites of the bipolar cells. The expansions are cup-shaped, with the bipolar dendrite invaginated into the cup. Spherules and pedicles contain many vesicles.

The bipolar cell bodies make up the inner nuclear layer. Diffuse bipolar cells in the peripheral retina receive input from several receptors. Midget bipolar cells are found in the foveal region; each receives input from a single foveal cone. The axons of bipolar cells form synapses with the dendrites of ganglion cells in the inner plexiform layer. The ganglion cells form the innermost cell layer next to the vitreous layer; those in the peripheral retina receive input from several diffuse bipolar cells, but those in the foveal region form synapses with only one midget bipolar cell. The axons of the ganglion cells sweep

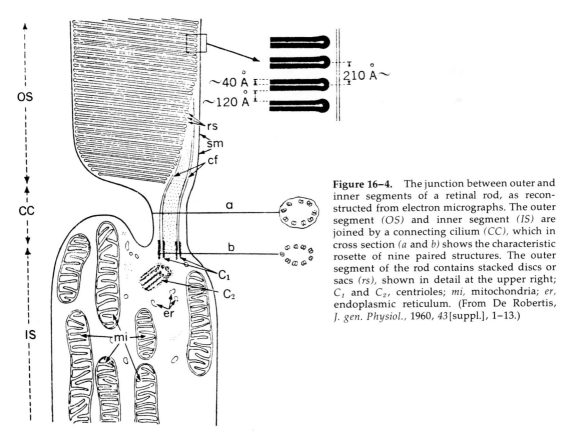

Figure 16–4. The junction between outer and inner segments of a retinal rod, as reconstructed from electron micrographs. The outer segment *(OS)* and inner segment *(IS)* are joined by a connecting cilium *(CC)*, which in cross section (*a* and *b*) shows the characteristic rosette of nine paired structures. The outer segment of the rod contains stacked discs or sacs *(rs)*, shown in detail at the upper right; C_1 and C_2, centrioles; *mi*, mitochondria; *er*, endoplasmic reticulum. (From De Robertis, *J. gen. Physiol.*, 1960, 43[suppl.], 1–13.)

across the surface of the retina to enter the optic nerve head, which is situated about 2.5 mm to the nasal side of the fovea. The nerve head is also the site of entrance and exit of the central retinal artery and vein, the branches of which course over the surface of the retina to penetrate the center of the optic nerve head and run with the nerve through the outer coats of the eye, emerging once again within the orbit near the optic foramen. In this course these vessels supply a rich capillary network to the nerve fibers. The optic nerve is invested with extensions of the dura and arachnoid membranes, so that the vessels, in parting from the nerve, run through the subarachnoid space. Increased intracranial pressure due to the impeding of venous outflow often causes edema of the nerve, which is manifested by swelling and blurring of the margins of the optic nerve head. This condition is called *papilledema* (or a "choked disc"); it can be observed and measured with the ophthalmoscope.

In addition to the receptors and bipolar cells and ganglion cells, the retina contains, as already mentioned, interareal association cells. The horizontal cells lie in the upper part of the inner nuclear layer and via dendrites, which course laterally, make connections with rod spherules and cone pedicles; the amacrine cells in the inner nuclear layer make similar lateral connections between the dendrites of ganglion cells. Finally the retina is held together by large glial cells (the cells of Müller), whose processes extend from the inner surface of the retina between the retinal elements to form tight connections around the base of the inner segments of the receptors. These latter connections, once erroneously thought to be a continuous membrane, form in light micrographs a visible horizontal streak between the inner segments and the outer nuclear layer, called the *outer limiting membrane*.

In summary, the retinal portion of the visual path includes from outer to inner layers: the receptors, the bipolar cells, and the ganglion cells, with horizontal and amacrine cells providing lateral linkages between receptors and ganglion cells, respectively (Fig. 16–5).

A surprising feature of retinal structure is that the photosensitive outer segments

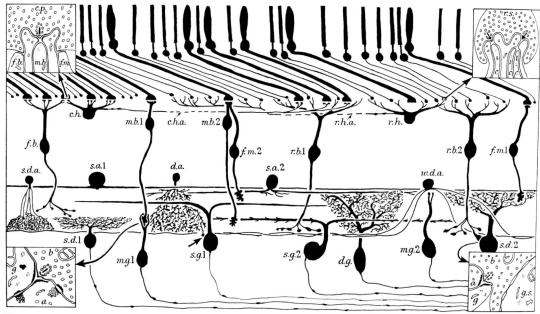

Figure 16–5. Diagram of neuronal connections in the nonfoveal vertebrate retina. Rod and cone inner segments are at the top (outer segments are not shown); their oblique course reflects the lateral displacement of inner elements at the fovea, which lies beyond the right margin of the diagram. Cells labeled with the letter *b* represent various kinds of bipolar cells; *m.b.* is a midget bipolar cell that receives input from only one cone, as do also the flat midget bipolar cells *(f.m.1* and *f.m.2)*. Note that *c.h.* and *r.h.* are horizontal cells connected to cones and rods, respectively. Cells labeled with *a* are varieties of amacrine cells, and those with *g* are ganglion cells.

Insets: Above left, Synapse between cone pedicle *(c.p.)* and bipolar cells *(f.b., m.b., f.m.). Above right,* Synapse between rod spherules *(r.s.)* and postsynaptic cells *(c). Lower left,* Axodendritic synapse between bipolar cell *(b),* ganglion cell *(g)* and amacrine cell *(a). Lower right,* Axosomatic synapse between bipolar cell *(b)* and ganglion cell *(g.s.)* in addition to axodendritic contacts. (From Boycott and Dowling, *Phil. Trans. [Lond.],* 1969, Ser. B, *255,* 109–184.)

lie deepest in the retina, so that incoming light must penetrate the tangled mass of fibers, cell bodies, and blood vessels to reach the photosensitive pigments attached to the discs. This seeming architectural blunder is partially amended in the fovea. The fovea is the part of the retina we use when we are looking at an object, because the convergent action of the extraocular muscles normally positions the eyes so that light from the object of visual attention falls on both foveae (see Chapter 17). At this site the ganglion cells and bipolar cells intervening between receptors and incoming light are pulled obliquely aside, causing a cup-shaped thinning of the retina, which exposes the foveal receptors (Fig. 16–6). Blood vessels and ganglion cell axons also skirt the rim of the fovea and hence avoid casting shadows on the receptors.

The fovea is the portion of the retina with highest visual acuity; *i.e.,* foveal images provide maximum clarity of detail and discrimination of contours. The excentration of superficial layers between receptors and incoming light, the densely packed population of pure cones of minimal size, and the existence of foveal "private paths" are all anatomical specializations favoring high acuity in the most used part of the retina.

An incidental consequence of foveal structure is that it establishes in the optic nerve a separation of the axons derived from the upper and lower halves of the retina. Fibers above the equator swing in whirligigs over the top of the fovea to reach the nerve head and those from the lower half swing underneath (see Figure 17–5). The axons of the ganglion cells receiving input from the fovea, one for

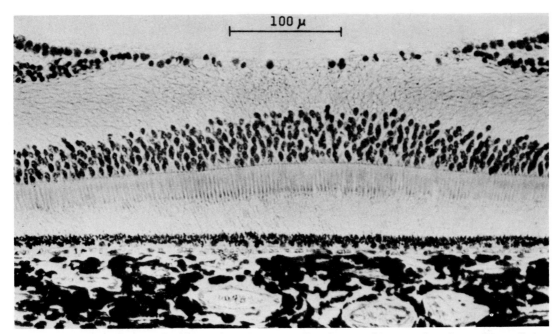

Figure 16–6. Photomicrograph of fovea of monkey retina. Ganglionic and inner nuclear elements are pulled to the side, and the length of the inner segments is increased. (From Brown *et al., Cold Spr. Harb. Symp. quant. Biol.,* 1965, *30,* 457–482.)

each of the 50,000 minute and densely packed foveal cones, run (nasally) directly along the equator to the nerve head and thus become interposed between the axons from the upper and lower hemispheres. As we shall see in the next chapter, this topographical organization established at the retinal level persists in modified form throughout the central visual pathways.

VISUAL THRESHOLDS

To describe the sensitivity of the eye, it is necessary to specify the wavelength of the test light; monochromatic sensitivity varies continuously throughout the visible spectrum, which extends from about 400 to 700 mμ. Thresholds are therefore expressed as curves, called *visibility curves,* relating sensitivity to wavelength. In addition the rod and cone systems have different spectral sensitivities, and since they function optimally under different conditions of illumination, it is not surprising that the visibility curve varies, depending on the previous history of the eye. If the eye is dark-adapted—*i.e.,* has been exposed to total darkness for 30 or more minutes—

and if the spectral tests are conducted with brief dim test lights, a curve known as the *scotopic visibility curve* is obtained, and this covers the range from about 400 to 625 mμ, with maximum sensitivity at 507 mμ (blue-green). The same eye when light-adapted (*i.e.,* exposed to normal daylight illumination) has a *photopic* visibility curve shifted to the right of the scotopic curve, with a range from about 425 to 700 mμ and a maximal sensitivity at 555 mμ (yellow-green). The two curves are shown in Figure 16–7. It should be noted that the ordinate values are normalized; *i.e.,* for both curves the maximal sensitivity is given a value of 1.0; if the sensitivities were expressed in absolute values, the scotopic curve would have a much higher peak because of the enormous relative hypersensitivity of the dark-adapted eye.

The shift in spectral sensitivity when the dark-adapted eye is exposed to higher levels of illumination is known as the Purkinje shift, after Johannes Purkinje, who first described it a century and a half ago. The Purkinje shift is a cornerstone for the duplicity theory. The scotopic curve represents rod vision, and photopic visibility represents cone vision.

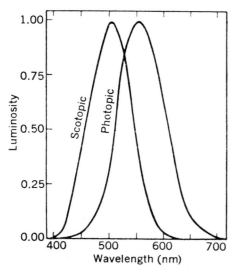

Figure 16–7. Spectral visibility curves of the human eye. The ordinate scale is relative; 1.0 represents maximal sensitivity for each condition of testing. Data are standards adopted by the International Commission on Illumination. (From Optical Society of America, *The science of color,* New York, Thos. Y. Crowell, 1953.)

As will shortly be shown, the visibility curves are also valuable quantitative indices in identifying visual photosensitive pigments. This is because the initiation of the visual process is by photic breakdown of visual pigment in the disc membranes of the receptor outer segments, a process in which light is absorbed. Isolated photosensitive pigments extracted from retina can be characterized by determination of their spectral absorption curves, which describe the amount of light absorption as a function of wavelength. Close correspondence of the absorption curve of an extracted substance with one or the other visibility curve thus constitutes strong presumptive evidence that the extracted pigment is identical with a functional photopigment of the eye. By a refinement of technique (called *microspectrophotometry*) the absorption spectrum of single rod or cone outer segments can be determined. Absorption by materials other than the photosensitive pigment can be estimated (and eliminated) by difference spectrometry, *i.e.,* by comparison of absorption before and after prolonged exposure to monochromatic light, which bleaches the pigment. Microspectrophotometry is especially valuable in identification of cone

pigments because the primate retina has three kinds of cones with different pigments; extracts contain mixtures of pigments.

DARK ADAPTATION

The Purkinje shift suggests that different receptors operate in scotopic and photopic conditions. Further evidence can be obtained by measurement of the progressive decrease in visual threshold that occurs in darkness, a process known as *dark adaptation.* That sensitivity changes is a commonplace observation; when, on a sunny day, we enter a dimly lighted theater, vision is so poor that an usher is required to get us to a seat. In a few minutes vision so improves that we can quite easily spot and move to a better seat if we wish.

The reverse of dark adaptation is light adaptation — a decreased visual sensitivity following exposure to bright light. Again it is common experience that when we emerge from the dark into bright light, we are for a time bedazzled, until the light-adaptive process desensitizes the retina.

Dark adaptation is measured by the drop in threshold to a brief test light stimulus as a function of time spent in a completely dark environment. Characteristically the dark-adaptation curve has two components (Fig. 16–8, *upper graph*): a rapid drop in threshold of 2 to 3 log units (100 to 1000 times) that stabilizes in about 5 min and a second abrupt drop of another 3 log units, beginning at about 8 min and reaching a relatively stable base by 30 min. Note that the fully dark-adapted eye is at least 100,000 times more sensitive than the light-adapted eye.

Some features of the dark-adaptation curve are readily accounted for by the duplicity theory. The early component appears to be due to changes in the cones, the later component to adaptation of rods. Three lines of evidence are offered. First, if the test light is colored, the visual sensations are chromatic throughout the early component but abruptly become achromatic when the second limb appears (Fig. 16–8, *filled* and *open circles*). Second, if the test object is a red light (to which rods are insensitive), and if it is focused exclusively

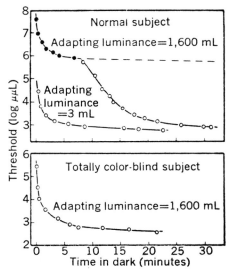

Figure 16–8. Dark adaptation of normal *(upper graph)* and cone-free *(lower graph)* retinae. *Upper graph,* Curve above is from normal subject exposed to equivalent of sunlight on a bright day prior to dark exposure. *Filled circles,* chromatic vision; *open circles,* achromatic vision. *Dashed line* shows how curve plateaus when test light is red spot focused on the fovea. Curve below is from normal subject exposed, before testing, to light dim enough to make reading difficult.

Lower graph, Curve is from color-blind subject fully light-adapted before test. (From Hecht *et al.,* J. gen. Physiol., 1948, *31,* 459–472.)

the rod and cone neural pathways to the brain. Recent experiments in which generator potentials to equivalent light flashes were recorded in individual rods and cones indicate that the rod is indeed a more efficient transducer than the cone is, producing a generator potential of 280 μV per quantum absorbed, as compared with 45 μV per quantum for the cone.

The duplicity theory satisfactorily explains many of the features of the adaptation curve. However, it is still unclear exactly what determines the abrupt shift from cone dominance to rod dominance. For example, comparison of the curves for the normal and the cone-free retina (Fig. 16–8) indicates that in the latter, rod thresholds have dropped far below those of cones at 5 min, although in the normal retina cone vision continues to dominate. It has been established that the photosensitive pigment of cones regenerates more rapidly than does that of rods (rhodopsin) and that the shift from cone dominance to rod dominance does not occur until rhodopsin accumulation is about 90 per cent complete. Since bright light bleaches both rhodopsin and cone pigments, the relatively slow rate of rhodopsin regeneration plays some role in the lag of rod dominance. Beyond this, however, some other factor must hold rod function in abeyance in the normal retina, for otherwise the rapid rod adaptation seen in the cone-free retina should be manifest in the normal retina. Somehow cones appear to suppress rod function — perhaps through the horizontal cells.

Dark adaptation is often immensely important in human performance. For example, the increased visual sensitivity is vital to such functions as night flying and motor vehicle operation. A simple physiological way to maintain the benefits of adaptation is to cover essential instrument panels with red glass, for the rods are insensitive to red light. Similarly, a darkroom worker who must alternate between dark and lighted rooms can avoid intermittent light adaptation by wearing red goggles in the lighted room.

THE ROD PIGMENT, RHODOPSIN

It is well established that the breakdown of a photosensitive pigment concentrated

on the rod-free fovea, the second component fails to occur (Fig. 16–8, *dashed line*). Finally, in rare individuals completely lacking retinal cones, a smooth, unbroken adaptation curve is obtained that plateaus at the low threshold level of the second component (Fig. 16–8, *lower graph*). One can conclude that in photopic conditions the cone system dominates, providing detail and color; but in the twilight realm of scotopic illumination the rod system begins to function and, because of its low threshold and extreme efficiency in detecting light, dominates vision. In plentiful light we can prodigally afford to enjoy the color and detail of cone vision; in darkness we economically sacrifice color and detail to avail ourselves of the exquisite, though colorless and blurred, sensitivity of the rods.

A basic question is whether the relatively greater sensitivity of the rod system is due to greater efficiency of the receptor itself or to some difference in the efficiency of in the receptor outer segments is the initial event in the production of the generator potential. It has long been known that a freshly removed dark-adapted retina has a purplish color, and that upon exposure to light it bleaches to become colorless. The fact that the retina is colored indicates that something in it, a pigment, is differentially absorbing light and reflecting the wavelengths characteristic of its color. The fact that extended light exposure bleaches the pigment suggests that light absorption produces a chemical change in the pigment, breaking it down into nonabsorptive products that reflect light at all wavelengths. Recently developed methods depending on measurement of reflected light permit measurement of the pigment content of the human retina *in situ*. Not only can it be shown that pigment content varies with the extent of dark adaptation but spectral analysis of absorption (calculated from reflectances) yields a curve that agrees well with the scotopic visibility curve, with maximal absorption and maximal sensitivity at 507 mμ.

The purple color of the dark-adapted retina is due to reflection from the rod pigment. Microspectral absorption analysis of single rods reveals further that the pigment is concentrated in the outer segments of the rods. The rod pigment can be differentially extracted from a dark-adapted retina by chemical means and subjected to spectral absorption analysis *in vitro*. Figure 16–9 shows the nearly perfect correspondence of the absorption spectrum of extracted pigment with the scotopic visibility curve. Such experiments, coupled with the finding that destruction of the layer of the outer segments abolishes the photic responses of all retinal elements, leave little doubt that photochemical bleaching of receptor pigment in the outer segments constitutes the essential first step in generating visual messages.

The rod pigment is called visual purple, or *rhodopsin*; it is a protein, similar to carotene compounds, and has attached a pigment group that gives it both its color and its light-absorptive properties. The chemical steps in the photic breakdown of rhodopsin and its regeneration in the dark have been extensively studied. The details should be sought in a textbook of biochemistry, but in skeleton outline: the absorption of light by rhodopsin through a series of steps breaks rhodopsin down to a colorless pigment, retinene, and a protein component, opsin. Retinene is then reduced by alcohol dehydrogenase and diphosphopyridine nucleotide (DPN) to vitamin A, which is stored in the cells of the pigment epithelium. In the dark,

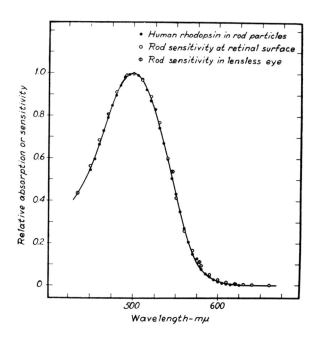

Figure 16–9. Comparison of the absorption spectrum of human rhodopsin *in vitro (filled circles)* with the scotopic visibility curve *(open circles)*. The visibility curve was corrected for light absorption in ocular media to represent light striking the retina rather than that entering the eye, hence the difference from the scotopic curve in Figure 16–7. Data were also obtained from a lensless eye for elimination of absorption by the yellow lens. (From Wald and Brown, *Science*, 1958, *127*, 222–226.)

vitamin A, both from the pigment cells and from the circulation, is reconverted, again through a number of steps, into retinene, which then combines with opsin to reconstitute rhodopsin, which is then available for another photoexcitatory cycle. The photic sensitivity of the system thus depends on relative rates of breakdown and reconstitution of rhodopsin. Only under scotopic conditions is there sufficient pigment for the rods to function.

Although it is clearly established that pigment breakdown is the initial step in the visual process, just how the chemical event leads to the electrical response of the rod is still not entirely clear, especially since, as will be discussed below, the generator responses of retinal receptors have

some surprising properties not found in any other known receptors.

CONE PIGMENTS

Chemical isolation and characterization of the photosensitive cone pigments has progressed more slowly than that of rhodopsin. A pigment called *iodopsin* has been isolated from chicken retina, which contains only cones. The pigment has a maximal absorption that agrees well with the peak of the photopic visibility curve.

A more fruitful technique for studying cone pigments is difference microspectrophotometry. So studied, cones from monkey and human retina fall into three

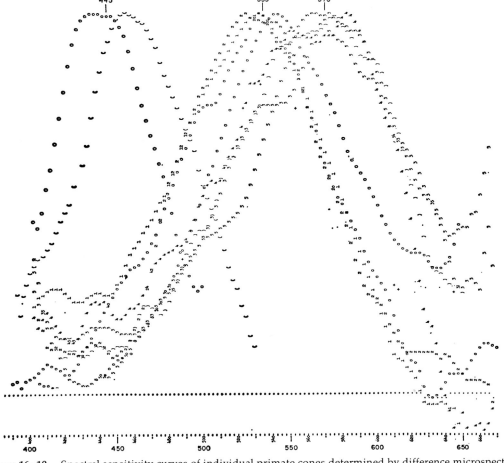

Figure 16–10.   Spectral sensitivity curves of individual primate cones determined by difference microspectrophotometry. Maximum absorption of all cones normalized to the same value on the ordinate. (From Marks *et al., Science*, 1964, *143*, 1181–1182. Copyright 1964 by the American Association for the Advancement of Science.)

groups, with spectral curves peaking at 440, 535, and 570 mμ. *i.e.,* in the blue, green, and red portions of the spectrum (Fig. 16–10). This means that there are really three cone pigments and that the photopic visibility curve is compounded from three different but overlapping systems.

Special interest attaches to the discovery of three cone pigments, because a red-green-blue theory of color vision was proposed almost a century ago by Young and by Helmholtz. Impressed by the fact that all of the visible hues can be produced by appropriate mixtures of two or more of the three primary colors red, green, and blue, Young and, subsequently, Helmholtz suggested that the retina possesses three cone types sensitive to these hues and that the sensory experience of other hues results from appropriately mixed excitation of populations of "color-coded" cones. Physiological data now seem to support a theory based wholly on psychophysical data.

The existence of the three-pigment system provides a ready explanation for color blindness that is due to a lack or deficiency of one or more color-specific pigments.

ELECTRICAL RESPONSES OF RETINAL ELEMENTS

Despite the exquisitely small size of retinal elements, their electrical responses to light can be measured with intracellular micropipettes. After obtaining a record, the experimenter can eject a dye from the pipette to mark the cell from which the record was obtained. In some instances when the recording conditions are sufficiently stable, the spectral sensitivity of impaled cells can be tested.

A surprising finding in such studies is that receptors, bipolar cells, and horizontal cells are incapable of generating action potentials. The response of these elements to photic stimulation is a graded non-propagated potential change, and all-or-nothing propagated responses are not encountered in the retinal chain until the amacrine cells and ganglion cells are tapped (Fig. 16–11). It is, however, clear that the graded responses in bipolar and horizontal cells are synaptically trans-mitted, since neither responds to light when the receptors are destroyed.

A second surprise is that the generator potentials of receptors and the graded synaptically transmitted responses of the horizontal cells are *hyperpolarizing*, rather than depolarizing, responses (Fig. 16–11). The photic responses of bipolar cells depend on the spatial pattern of the light stimulus (Fig. 16–11). Moreover, unlike the responses of all other studied receptors to stimulation, the hyperpolarizing generator potential of rods and cones is accompanied by an increase rather than a decrease in membrane resistance. Apparently the absorption of light in the outer segment somehow blocks membrane channels that are open in the dark.

These perverse and unorthodox features of retinal behavior have been clarified by an indirect approach-study of extracellular current distribution, a procedure which is somewhat simplified by the orderly geometric configuration of the receptor array. Penn and Hagins found that in retinae kept in total darkness a sizeable extracellular current flows from the region of inner segments to outer segments. This *dark current* is Na^+-borne and is extinguished in Na^+-free media. Its presumed intracellular course is inward through the outer segments, which have an unusually high permeability to Na^+ (in the dark), and outward through the more proximal parts of the receptors (inner segments and rod spherules). Such a regional influx of Na^+ through the outer segments tallies with the observation that resting potentials of rods in the dark are low. In essence, the high Na^+ permeability of the outer segment is comparable to a persistent excitatory postsynaptic potential (EPSP), a consideration which leads to the surprising deduction that the darkened receptor constantly releases depolarizing transmitter onto bipolar and horizontal cells.

Although such a mechanism whereby transmitter is released when we are seeing nothing seems outrageously extravagant and contrary to the spirit of fuel conservation, experimental evidence supports it. Secondary elements (bipolar cells and horizontal cells) have low resting potentials in

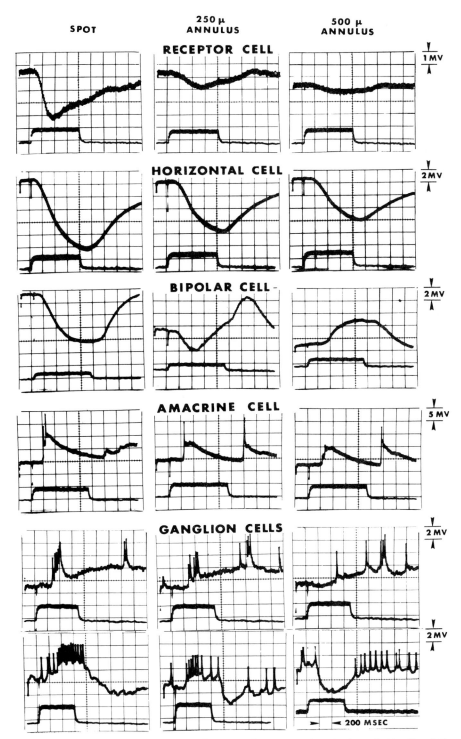

Figure 16–11. Intracellular recordings from cells in mud-puppy retina during photic stimulation. *Bottom trace* of each pair signals light flash. In *upper trace,* downward deflection indicates increase in membrane potential (hyperpolarization). Depolarizing spikes in amacrine and ganglion cells are action potentials. (From Werblin and Dowling, *J. Neurophysiol.,* 1969, *32,* 339–355.)

the dark, and procedures that block transmitter release (*e.g.,* immersion of the retina in a low-Ca^{++}, high-Mg^{++} medium) significantly polarize them. A further deduction is that dark-adapted bipolar cells may also be releasing transmitter onto ganglion cells and amacrine cells. Since the response of these latter cells to light is (at last) conventionally depolarizing, the bipolar cell transmitter is presumed to be a hyperpolarizing agent.

The influence of light is to reduce the dark current by diminishing the permeability of the outer segments to Na^+; the result is relative hyperpolarization of the receptor and increased electrical resistance of the cell. Secondarily, depolarizing transmitter release diminishes so that the secondary cells establish higher membrane potentials (hyperpolarize). Finally, relative hyperpolarization of bipolar cells curtails release of hyperpolarizing transmitter

onto ganglion cells with resultant depolarization, which may lead to spike generation. The peculiarity of the retina is that it responds to its adequate stimulus not by affirmative action but by a series of restraints and prohibitions on secretory mechanisms that run free in the dark.

Hagins has proposed an ingenious mechanism to explain the diminution of Na^+ current across the dark-adapted outer segment when it is exposed to light (Fig. 16–12). He proposes that the high permeability to Na^+ in outer segments requires a low cytoplasmic Ca^{++} concentration, a suggestion in accord with the observation that in many epithelial tissues low-resistance gap junctions (between cells) are effectively sealed when cytoplasmic Ca^{++} concentration rises. He postulates that in the dark-adapted rod Ca^{++} is sequestered in the discs by an active pumping mechanism, keeping the cytoplasmic concen-

(a) DARK

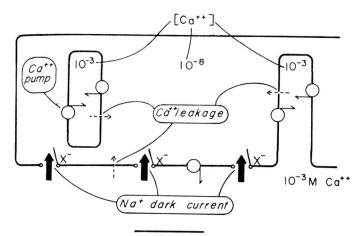

(b) LIGHT

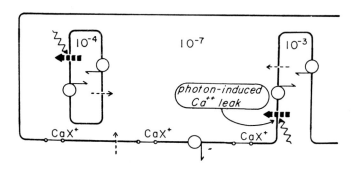

Figure 16–12. A proposed mechanism for excitation in rods and cones. For generality, the model incorporates both the infolded disc characteristic of cones *(right)* and the closed free-floating disc typical of rods *(left)*. In either case photo pigment is a constituent of the disc membrane. Numbers give estimated Ca^{++} concentrations.

In the dark *(above)*, Ca^{++} is concentrated in the disc space by a Ca^{++} pump, and Na^+ inflow through open Na^+ gates *(X^-)* occurs, giving rise to dark current. In the light *(below)*, pigment breakdown permits leak of Ca^{++} across disc membrane, and elevated intracellular Ca^{++} closes Na^+ gates, turning off dark current. (From Hagins, *Ann. Rev. Biophys. Bioeng.,* 1972, *1,* 131–154.)

tration low. The function of the disc is thus comparable to that of the sarcoplasmic reticulum in muscle. Light, by inducing conformational change of rhodopsin (which is a constituent of the disc membrane), permits sequestered Ca^{++} to leak into the cytoplasm and to close the Na^+ gates. In cones the disc spaces communicate with the extracellular fluid, and the pump-sequestered Ca^{++} is extracellular Ca^{++}; otherwise, the mechanism is the same as that in the rod.

The amplitude of the generator potential in receptors varies with the intensity and wavelength of light. Curves relating magnitude of rod hyperpolarization to wavelength satisfyingly resemble the scotopic visibility curve. Spectral analysis of the generator responses of cones reveals three types, with maximal sensitivity in the blue, green, and red portions of the spectrum (Fig. 16–13). Thus there is again heartwarming agreement between psychological theory (Young-Helmholtz) based on color mixing, the absorption spectrum of cones, and their spectral sensitivity as measured by potential change to light.

Intracellular study of the spectral sensitivity of horizontal cells in light-adapted retinae reveals a third surprise. In some of these elements not only the amplitude but the polarity of the light-evoked response varies with wavelength. Figure 16–14 shows two examples; in one, the maximal depolarizing response is to the red part of the spectrum and the maximal hyperpolarizing response to the green—a red-green cell. The other cell is a yellow-blue cell. Such behavior suggests the interesting possibility of another mechanism for color signaling in addition to the band-sensitive cones. Although, as pointed out by Young and Helmholtz, all the visible hues can be produced by appropriate mixtures of red, green, and blue, it is also true that the pairs red-green and blue-yellow are complementary colors; i.e., mixtures of the members of each pair are colorless. Appropriate mixtures of red and green would be expected to turn off the red-green horizontal cell, for red depolarizes it and green hyperpolarizes it. The blue-yellow cells are even more interesting, for they could provide the explanation why yellow is subjectively as distinctive as

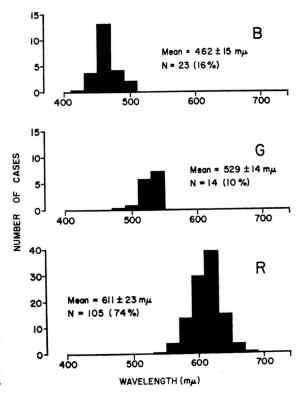

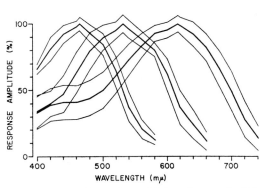

Figure 16–13. Spectral sensitivity of cones in fish retina, as measured by amplitude of the generator potential. *Upper graphs,* Frequency histograms of wavelengths giving maximal response.

B, blue; *G,* green; *R,* red. *Lower graph,* Mean generator amplitude plotted against wavelength for three classes of cones. *Heavy line* is mean per cent of maximal; *thin lines* represent standard deviations. (From Tomita *et al., Vision Res.,* 1967, 7, 519–531.)

red, green, and blue: a yellow experience is signaled by a depolarizing response in the yellow-blue units. Interestingly, just such a four-color theory was proposed by E. Hering in the last century. Hering's

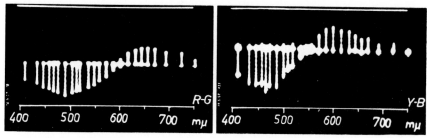

Figure 16–14. Postsynaptic responses of horizontal cells in fish retina to monochromatic light flashes. The sweep speed of the oscilloscope was very slow, so that the potentials appear as vertical bars; downward deflection indicates hyperpolarization; upward, depolarization. The "turnover" point for the cell in the first record is between red and green (R-G); for the second cell, between yellow and blue (Y-B) parts of the spectrum. (From Svaetichin and MacNichol, *Ann. N.Y. Acad. Sci.,* 1958, *74,* 385–404.)

theory, because it suggested that complementary colors induce opposing effects in retinal cells, is often referred to as the *opponent-process theory.*

GANGLION CELLS

Amacrine and ganglion cells behave in a more conventional fashion than do other retinal elements; their synaptic potentials are depolarizing and trigger threshold spikes that are all-or-nothing and propagated. Ganglion cell responses to diffuse illumination of the retina are of three types: on responses, off responses, and on-off responses. Discharge of on cells accelerates during illumination, off cells give a burst of spikes at the termination of stimulation, and on-off cells discharge at the beginning and end of photic stimulation.

Stimulation of the retina with punctate light sources indicates that the response of each ganglion cell depends on the stimulus site. A common pattern is a contiguous retinal area, excitation of which produces on responses surrounded by a fringe area for off responses. An intermediate area yields on-off responses (Fig. 16–15). Stimuli applied simultaneously to the center and surround counteract each other. The total retinal area in which light spots influence discharge is called the *receptive field* of the ganglion cell, and the unit just described is said to have an "on-center, off-surround" receptive field. Equally numerous in the primate retina are ganglion cells that have the reverse arrangement of receptive field, *i.e.,* "off-center, on-surround."

The competitive interaction between central and peripheral parts of the receptive fields is another example of lateral inhibition, described earlier in cutaneous somatosensory pathways. In the retina the interareal association neurons (horizontal and amacrine cells) probably subserve

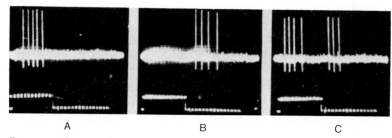

A   B   C

Figure 16–15. Response of a retinal ganglion cell to spot illumination of different parts of its receptive field. *Upper beam* indicates extracellular record of ganglion cell activity; *lower beam* signals intensity and duration of light flash and time (20 msec). In *A,* flash focused on retina beneath electrode gives "on response." In *B,* same flash delivered 0.5 mm away gives "off response." In *C,* intermediate region is stimulated, yielding "on-off response." Cell is of the "on-center, off-surround" type. (From Kuffler, *J. Neurophysiol.,* 1953, *16,* 37–68.)

lateral inhibition. It is further postulated that lateral inhibition enhances contrast in messages generated by visual images. For example, a luminous bar on the retina not only generates discharge of units whose on-fields it strikes but inhibits adjoining units, so that the contrast between illuminated and shaded areas is preserved and emphasized in the neural messages.

THE RETINA AND VISUAL ACUITY

In general terms, *visual acuity* measures the ability of the visual system to detect boundaries and contours. Operationally, visual acuity is a measure of the minimum separation between two luminous lines on the retina that can be detected as two (the *minimum separable*); it is analogous to the two-point threshold for cutaneous tactile stimuli. Because the separation between retinal images formed by two luminous points diminishes as their distance from the eye increases, acuity is often expressed in terms of the angle subtended by points at the optical center of the eye (the *minimum angle of resolution*). Another measure of acuity is the *minimum visible*, the thickness of a luminous line or shadow (expressed in terms of subtended angle) that can be detected. Under optimal circumstances the minimum angle of resolution may be as low as 3 sec and the minimum visible 0.5 sec.

In practice, acuity is gauged on a relative scale by means of the Snellen test, well known to all who have applied for a driver's license. The Snellen chart consists of a series of letters of graded size. Beside each row is a number that indicates the distance at which a somewhat arbitrarily designated normal eye can recognize the letters. At that distance the distinctive lines of the letters and their spacing subtend a visual angle of 1 min. For example, the *E* subtends a total of 5 min, 1 min each for the horizontal bars and 1 min for each of the two intervening spaces. The subject reads as far down the graded lines as he can, and his acuity is expressed as the ratio between the distance of the chart from the eye (usually 20 ft or 6 m) and the designated distance, to give a 1-min angle. Thus

a subject who can read at 20 ft only what a normal subject can read at 40 ft is said to have 20/40 vision.

The factors that determine visual acuity can be divided into those that are purely optical and those that are physiological or anatomical. Among the first category are spherical and chromatic aberration, optical defects (myopia, hyperopia, astigmatism), and pupil size, all of which were discussed in the preceding chapter.

A major factor in the second category is what is often referred to as *retinal grain* (comparable to grain of a photographic film), which is a function of receptor size and packing. In coarse-grained film precise contours are blurred because the silver particles are too large to reveal fine regional differences of exposure. Similarly, if the retinal images of two bright lines separated by a shadow fall on the same or adjacent layers of cones, a message is generated that is identical with that set up by a single luminous image three times

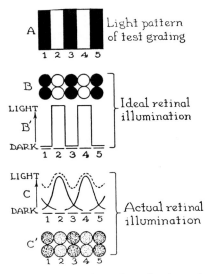

Figure 16–16. Hypothetical mechanism of visual acuity. *A* shows test pattern consisting of alternate dark and light bands separated by the width of one foveal cone. *B* shows effect of pattern on retina when light scatter and eye movements are ignored, and *B'* illustrates hypothetical illumination of rows of cones. *C'* shows the pattern of cone illumination and shading under actual conditions, and *C* illustrates the resulting activity; the dotted line is an algebraic summation of the two curves. (From Ruch and Patton, eds., *Physiology and biophysics*, Philadelphia, W. B. Saunders Co., 1965.)

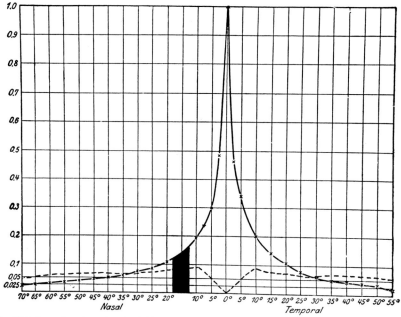

Figure 16–17. Relative visual acuity in different parts of the retina. *Solid line,* cone (photopic) vision; *dashed line,* rod (scotopic) vision. Black bar represents the blind spot. (From Wertheim, Z. *Psychol.,* 1894, 7, 172–187.)

wider and two-thirds the luminance of the individual lines. When the lines are separated by a shadow equal to the width of a receptor, as in Figure 16–16B and B', the ambiguity is resolved and in fact the retinal separation at the minimum angle of resolution corresponds satisfactorily to the measured diameter of foveal cones (1 to 2 μm). Actually, involuntary movements of the eyes, which amount to 5 to 17 per min even during voluntary fixation, smear the borders so that the pattern is one of relative rather than absolute lighting and shading, as shown in Figure 16–16C

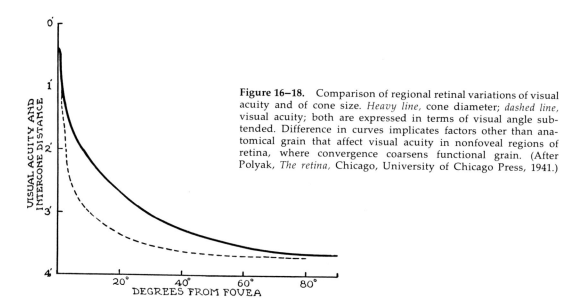

Figure 16–18. Comparison of regional retinal variations of visual acuity and of cone size. *Heavy line,* cone diameter; *dashed line,* visual acuity; both are expressed in terms of visual angle subtended. Difference in curves implicates factors other than anatomical grain that affect visual acuity in nonfoveal regions of retina, where convergence coarsens functional grain. (After Polyak, *The retina,* Chicago, University of Chicago Press, 1941.)

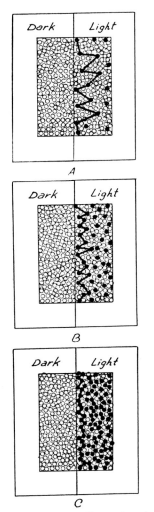

Figure 16–19. Diagrams illustrating the influence of the level of illumination of the functional grain of the retina and perception of contour. Intensity of illumination increases from above downward, resulting in increased numbers of activated retinal units *(filled circles)*. At low illumination, the pattern of discharge caused by the dim light bar is indistinguishable from that produced by the irregular contour joining recruited units. With recruitment of greater numbers of units at higher illumination, definition of contour becomes sharper. (From Ruch and Patton, eds., *Physiology and biophysics,* Philadelphia, W. B. Saunders Co., 1965.)

and C'. Interestingly, these movements improve rather than blur vision, for when, by optical tricks, the retinal image is stabilized, perception fades. This phenomenon is correlated with the finding, described in the next chapter, that visual cortical cells respond only to images moving across the retina.

The importance of retinal grain is indicated by the variation of acuity as a function of retinal region (Fig. 16–17). In the center of the fovea cones are of minimum dimensions (about 1 μm) and are undiluted by rods; here photopic visual acuity is maximum. Acuity drops precipitously in the parafoveal and peripheral retina. Scotopic acuity is low throughout compared with cone-mediated photopic acuity but is maximal in the parafoveal retina about 10 degrees from the center of the fovea (which is itself blind in twilight vision). For this reason night work is best performed with the eyes fixed slightly off target.

In the peripheral retina not only cone size but the increasing amount of convergence limits visual acuity, for it increases the retinal area feeding individual ganglion cells. Figure 16–18 shows that with increasing distance from the fovea, relative visual acuity drops more rapidly than does the distance between cones because convergence makes the ultimate grain coarser than the anatomical grain.

Another factor that alters the functional grain of the retina, and hence visual acuity, is illumination. As illumination increases, acuity mounts because greater numbers of receptors are excited (Fig. 16–19). Low levels of illumination probably activate mainly large receptor-bipolar-ganglion cell units because excitatory effects of convergent receptors may sum at the bipolar and ganglion cell levels. With higher levels of illumination, elements driven by cones with semiprivate pathways are recruited, and the full benefits of maximally fine retinal grain accrue.

ADDITIONAL READING

Brown, K. T.   Physiology of the retina. Chap. 67 in *Medical physiology,* Mountcastle, V. B., ed., St. Louis, The C. V. Mosby Co., 1968.
Davson, H.   The visual process. Chap. 58 in *Starling's human physiology,* Davson, H., and Eggelton, M. G., eds., Philadelphia, Lea & Febiger, 1968.
Ruch, T. C.   Vision. Chap. 20 in *Physiology and biophysics,* Ruch, T. C., and Patton, H. D., eds., Philadelphia, W. B. Saunders Co., 1965.

CHAPTER 17

VISUAL FIELDS AND CENTRAL VISUAL PATHWAYS

HARRY D. PATTON

VISUAL FIELDS AND THEIR MEASUREMENT	LESIONS OF THE OPTIC PATHWAYS	SPECTRAL SENSITIVITY OF CENTRAL VISUAL NEURONS
BINOCULAR VISION; HOMONYMOUS RETINAL POINTS	RECEPTIVE FIELDS OF GENICULATE AND STRIATE NEURONS	Ganglion Cells Lateral Geniculate Neurons Neurons in Striate Cortex
CENTRAL VISUAL RELAYS AND RECEPTIVE AREAS	DEVELOPMENTAL INFLUENCES ON VISUAL CORTICAL ORGANIZATION	PRESTRIATE CORTICAL AREAS

The messages generated in retinal ganglion cells are conducted centrally in their axons, which reach the lateral geniculate body by way of the optic nerve and optic tract. In the nerve and tract (and especially the latter) the axons bearing messages from different portions of the retina are clustered together in a definite topographical pattern. We have already noted (Chap. 16) that fibers from the fovea become interposed between those serving the upper and lower halves of the retina. Beyond the optic chiasm an even more prominent topographical pattern appears, for fibers from hemiretinae divided along the vertical meridian become separated. Those from the nasal half of each retina decussate in the optic chiasm to reach the optic tract and lateral geniculate body of the opposite side, whereas those from the temporal hemiretinae pursue a strictly ipsilateral

course. Consequently, a unilateral lesion of the central pathway caudal to the chiasm blinds the ipsilateral temporal and the contralateral nasal hemiretinae. That is, complete interruption of the left optic tract produces partial blindness in each eye, temporally on the left and nasally on the right. *It is accepted practice, however, to describe such defects not in terms of regional retinal blindness but in terms of gaps in the visual field*, which will now be defined.

VISUAL FIELDS AND THEIR MEASUREMENT

The *monocular visual field* is defined as the total extent of the external world perceived by one eye without movement of the head or change of ocular fixation. The basic reference point of the visual field is

232

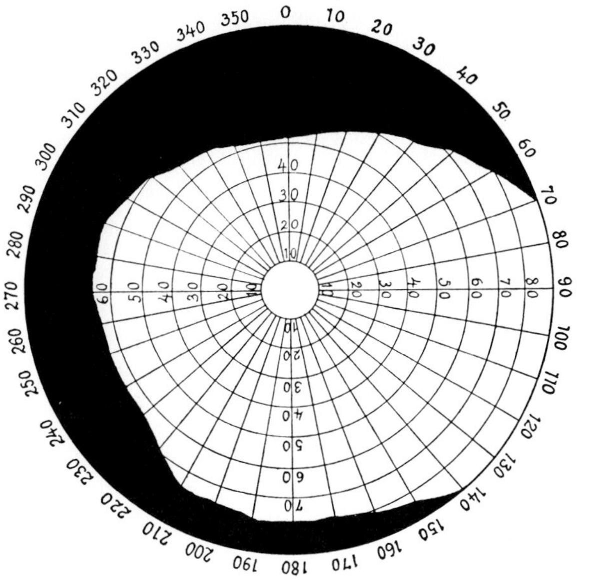

Figure 17–1. Perimetric chart, showing the normal visual field of the *right* eye. The temporal field is to the right; the nasal, to the left of chart. Numbers along the horizontal and vertical meridians are degrees of visual angle from the center of the fovea. (From Ruch and Patton, eds., *Physiology and biophysics,* Philadelphia, W. B. Saunders Co., 1965.)

the visual axis, an imaginary line passing perpendicular to the cornea to the center of the fovea (see Figure 15–7).

One method of measuring the visual field employs the *tangent screen,* a concentrically circular wall hanging with the pattern shown in Figure 17–1. The subject is seated in a well-lighted room with his head fixed by a chin rest to align the tested eye at the level of, and 1 m in front of, the center of the pattern. He is instructed to focus on the central point with that eye, the other being covered. In these circumstances the concentric circles delineate equiangular displacements from the visual axis in 10-degree steps, and the radii depict deviations from the vertical meridian. A small target (contrasting in color to the screen) is moved in from the periphery of the screen along each of the radii, and the subject is asked to report when it comes into his fixed field of vision. The examiner checks the report by moving the target outward until it disappears. The limits of vision measured on the screen along each of the radii are transcribed as points to a small replica suitable for inclusion in the patient's record, and the measured points are connected to outline the boundaries of the visual field. Each eye is tested separately.

A somewhat more portable device for measuring visual fields is the *perimeter,*

which has a chin rest and a semicircular framework supporting a metal strip marked in degrees. The semicircle can be rotated around its center to change the radial deviation. Otherwise, the testing procedure is the same as with the tangent screen. Mapping of visual fields, whether done with screen or perimeter, is called *perimetry.*

In a rough, but often useful, bedside test the examiner and patient face one another at a distance of about 1 ft and focus on each other's eyes. With the examiner's right eye and the patient's left eye shut, the examiner moves his finger in along various radii and checks the patient's reports against his own (presumably normal) field. The procedure is repeated for the other eye.

If our eyes projected on stalks like those of the crayfish, the visual field would be circular; because, however, they are recessed in the orbit, portions of the peripheral field are obliterated by the nose and by the supraorbital and infraorbital ridges. Only the temporal field is unobstructed, permitting vision through a full 90 degrees. Figure 17–1 shows a normal field for the right eye. Not shown (although easily mapped) is the blind spot that lies centered on the equator and 15 degrees to the temporal side of the center of the field. Fine mapping sometimes picks up spidery irregularities along the margins of the blind spot due to shadows cast by the larger vessels entering and leaving the nerve head.

The nerve head lies 15 degrees to the *nasal* side of the fovea (see Figure 15–7), but the blind spot is 15 degrees to the *temporal* side of the field. This relationship emphasizes a vitally important rule: *temporal field points are seen by the nasal retina and the nasal field is seen by the temporal half of the retina. Similarly, objects in the upper field project onto the lower hemiretina and those in the lower field are seen by the upper retinal half.* Partial retinal blindness thus causes a defect in the opposite part of the visual field. By convention visual defects are designated according to the field defect, not the retinal defect.

BINOCULAR VISION; HOMONYMOUS RETINAL POINTS

Although visual fields are determined separately for each eye, we of course view the world through two eyes. In binocular vision a considerable part of the external world is viewed by both eyes; *i.e.,* the monocular visual fields overlap extensively. Figure 17–2 shows the binocular visual field, the hatched area indicating the over-

lap. The crescent-shaped unhatched areas on the two sides are seen only by the nasal half of the ipsilateral retina because the nose shades the temporal half of the contralateral retina. You can confirm this by holding an object in the temporal part of your binocular field and then shutting the ipsilateral eye when the object disappears.

For clear visualization of an object in the central binocular field, where overlap of monocular fields prevails, the images must fall on what are called *corresponding* or *homonymous* parts of the retina. Otherwise, double vision, or *diplopia*, occurs. There is a simple way to identify homonymous retinal points, simultaneous excitation of which produces a single visual image. Obviously the two foveae are homonymous points, for objects focused on them are seen as one. Imagine each retina split in half along the vertical meridian; if the nasal half of each bisected retina is superimposed upon the temporal half of the retina of the contralateral eye, homonymous points are superimposed; *i.e.,* the nasal hemiretina of one eye and the temporal hemiretina of the opposite eye are homonymous. Similarly, if the retinae are divided along the horizontal equator, the upper halves are homonymous, and so are the lower halves.

As we shall see presently, visual messages generated by simultaneous excitation of homonymous points eventually converge

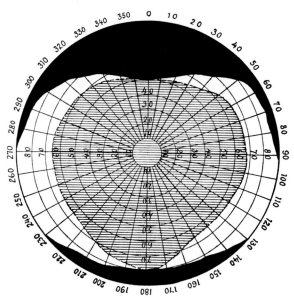

Figure 17–2. Perimetric chart to show the extent of the normal binocular visual field. The *crosshatched area* is the portion of the visual field seen by both eyes; *clear areas* at the sides are the temporal monocular crescents seen only by the nasal portions of each retina. (From Ruch and Patton, eds., *Physiology and biophysics,* Philadelphia, W. B. Saunders Co., 1965.)

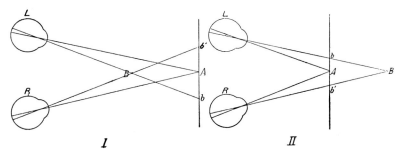

Figure 17–3. Diagram illustrating that objects located either short of (*I*) or beyond (*II*) the plane of ocular fixation cast images on noncorresponding retinal points, causing diplopia. In *I*, the eyes are focused on point *A* and light from *B* falls on noncorresponding temporal parts of the retina; double images of *B* are seen at *b* and *b'*. In *II*, ocular fixation is on *A*, so that retinal images of *B* fall on noncorresponding nasal points of the retina; double images are seen at *b* and *b'*. (From Ruch and Patton, eds., *Physiology and biophysics,* Philadelphia, W. B. Saunders Co., 1965.)

on common cortical cells, and this appears to be the prerequisite for normal single-image vision. It is for this reason that accuracy of the convergence mechanism discussed in Chapter 15 is critical for clear vision. The extraocular muscles reflexly adjust eye position so that light from an object of visual attention falls on the two homonymous foveae. You can convince yourself of the importance of accurate convergence by pushing on one eyeball to displace it from its alignment — the result is diplopia.

Clinically, failure of the eyes to position so that the image falls on corresponding retinal points is called *strabismus*, or *squint.* Strabismus may be either paralytic or nonparalytic. Paralytic strabismus may be due to lesions of the neural elements supplying the extraocular muscles (cranial nerves III, IV, and VI) or to neuromuscular failure in myasthenia gravis. Nonparalytic strabismus (extraocular muscle imbalance, or heterophoria) is usually of unknown cause. Curiously, patients with congenital strabismus do not experience diplopia even when the ocular misalignment clearly results in noncorresponding retinal images, because information from only one eye is used, that from the other being mysteriously suppressed. Sometimes one eye is consistently favored; if so, vision in the unfavored eye may become permanently impaired to the point of uselessness (*amblyopia*), a possibility that makes early correction of congenital strabismus of more than cosmetic importance. Alter-

natively, the favored eye is randomly alternated; if so, usefulness of each eye is retained. The mechanism of suppression is mysterious; later in this chapter we will describe the effect that experimental strabismus induced in newborn kittens has on the development of visual pathways.

In a somewhat less obvious way suppression of visual images, which might be expected to cause diplopia, occurs in normal subjects. If two objects (*e.g.,* forefingers) are held about 6 inches apart and 1 ft from the eyes, focusing on one results in a double image of the other. Figure 17–3 shows that light from objects short of, or beyond, the plane of focus falls on noncorresponding points. Normally we suppress the resulting double images and are aware of diplopia only when, as in this experiment, we attend to objects outside the range of optical focus.

CENTRAL VISUAL RELAYS AND RECEPTIVE AREAS

The axons of retinal ganglion cells reach the lateral geniculate body by way of the optic tract, which, as we have already noted, carries fibers from the temporal half of the ipsilateral eye and the nasal half of the contralateral retina. As mentioned previously (Chap. 15), the axons forming the afferent limb of the pupillary reflex are exceptions; they depart from the tract to relay in the pretectal nucleus rather than in the geniculate body. The lateral geniculate nucleus of primates is readily recognized from its conical shape and its distinctive laminar structure. It consists of six discrete layers of cell bodies (numbered from base to apex) separated by strata of fibers (Fig. 17–4). Lateral geniculate neurons are unique in that they degenerate

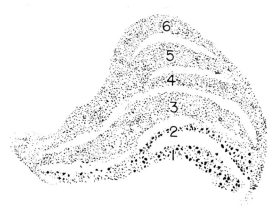

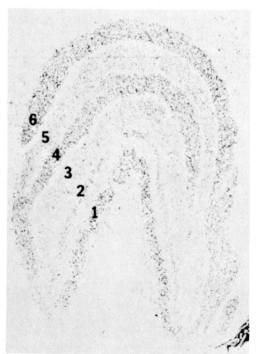

Figure 17–4. The primate lateral geniculate nucleus, intact and degenerate after removal of one eye. *Upper,* Drawing from cell-stained normal nucleus in man. The right side is medial. *Lower,* Cell-stained section of lateral geniculate nucleus of a monkey 6 days after removal of the ipsilateral eye. Layers 2, 3, and 5 show severe antegrade degeneration. (*Upper,* From Truex and Carpenter, *Human neuroanatomy.* © 1969, The Williams & Wilkins Co., Baltimore. *Lower,* Mathews *et al., J. Anat.,* 1960, *94,* 145–169.)

irreversibly when the presynaptic axons (ganglion cells) supplying them are destroyed (*transynaptic,* or *antegrade, degeneration*). The reason for this peculiar reaction is obscure, but it provides a fruitful neuroanatomical method for tracing the projections of different parts of the retina onto the nucleus.

For example, when one eye is removed and time is allowed for degeneration, layers 2, 3, and 5 of the *ipsilateral* geniculate (Fig. 17–4) and layers 1, 4, and 6 of the *contralateral* geniculate show a conspicuous lack of cells. This finding indicates that, at the geniculate body, visual information from the two retinae is still segregated, a conclusion that is confirmed by single-cell recording from geniculate neurons during focal stimulation of the retinae. As will be developed presently, visual impulses derived from homonymous binocular retinal points do not converge onto common neurons until the visual cortex is reached.

By making discrete punctate retinal lesions and searching the geniculate nuclei for foci of transneuronal atrophy, anatomists can map precisely the topographical projection of the retina onto the geniculate body. Such studies indicate that the separation of upper and lower retinal representations by foveal projections is established at the retinal level and persists throughout the nerve, the tract, and its termination in the lateral geniculate nucleus. That is, the terminations of lower retinal projections are lateral, those of upper projections are medial, and the foveal terminations are wedged between and dorsal to the two peripheral halves (Fig. 17–5). The separation of upper and lower retinal projections in nerve, tract, and geniculate is not sufficiently pronounced that one set of fibers is likely to be damaged selectively, but it provides the beginning of a topographical segregation that is significantly exaggerated, as described below, in the geniculocortical projection system.

The axons of geniculate neurons project to the striate cortex surrounding the lips of the calcarine fissure on the mesial surface of the occipital lobe. Collectively the fibers are called the *geniculocalcarine tract,* or *optic radiation;* they hook around and over the temporal horns of the lateral ventricles and then course posteriorly as a dorsoven-

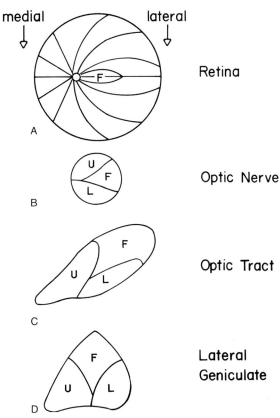

medial ↓   lateral ↓

Retina

A

Optic Nerve

B

Optic Tract

C

Lateral
Geniculate

D

Figure 17–5. Topographical organization of retina (A), optic nerve (B), optic tract (C), and lateral geniculate nucleus (D). A, Course of retinal ganglion cell axons swinging around the fovea (F). Foveal fibers become wedged between fibers from upper (U) and lower (L) retinal halves, and this general arrangement persists in the optic tract and lateral geniculate nucleus.

body, where the spatial separation of upper and lower retinal representations is less prominent.

The primary visual cortex flanking the calcarine fissure is often referred to as *striate* cortex because in vertical sections the cortical gray matter shows in its center a prominent white band of fibers visible even to the naked eye (the *line of Gennari*). The band is composed of the terminal ends of the radiation fibers. The projection onto the striate area is strictly organized; the fibers from the upper retina terminate in the superior lip of the fissure and those from the lower retina terminate in the inferior lip. The fibers from the central retina (fovea and parafovea, collectively called the *macular representation*) terminate caudally in the occipital pole, with upper and lower portions being distributed to superior and inferior lips (Fig. 17–7). The area of cortex devoted to representation of different parts of the retina is graded; the macular representation is largest, paralleling the relatively high visual acuity of the central retina (see Figure 16–14).

LESIONS OF THE OPTIC PATHWAYS

Because of the changing topographical organization of the visual pathways at different levels, a discrete lesion often produces in the visual field a distinctive defect that provides the neurologist with a valuable localizing clue. A punctate lesion in the retina near the nerve head (*e.g.*, a small hemorrhage or a tubercle) produces a blind area or *scotoma* that has a pinwheel or wedge shape in accordance with the "drainage" pattern of ganglion cell axons into the nerve head (Fig. 17–5). If the lesion is below the horizontal meridian, the defect is in the upper field and *vice versa*.

Complete severance of the optic nerve results in simple blindness of the ipsilateral eye, but interruption of the optic tract causes blindness in half of each monocular visual field because of the redistribution of fibers in the optic chiasm. Thus, division of the left tract causes blindness in the left nasal and right temporal fields (Fig. 17–8), a defect called a *right homonymous hemianopsia* because it involves homonymous parts

trally flattened sheet of fibers in the white matter of the temporal lobe to reach the occipital lobe (Fig. 17–6). In the radiation, the fibers carrying information from the upper half of retina are superior, those from the lower half are inferior, and the foveal fibers are in between. Because the radiation is flattened into a dorsoventrally oriented ribbon and because the numerous foveal fibers occupy a significant amount of this extent, the fibers from the upper and lower retinal halves are spatially separated, and one or the other may be selectively damaged by appropriately situated temporal lobe lesions. The result is a visual field defect, to be described below, that is distinctively different from those produced by lesions of the tract or of the geniculate

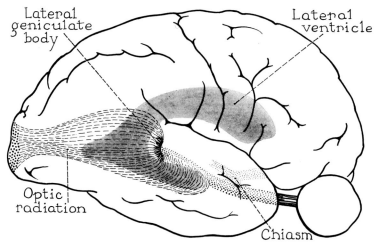

Figure 17–6. The course of the optic radiation (geniculocalcarine tract) in man. Fibers running in temporal subcortical white matter to occipital cortex are shown in surface projection as if the brain were transparent. The upper retinal representation is superior, the lower is inferior, and the foveal is sandwiched between. (From Sandford and Bair, *Arch. Neurol., Psychiat.* [*Chic.*], 1939, *42,* 21–43.)

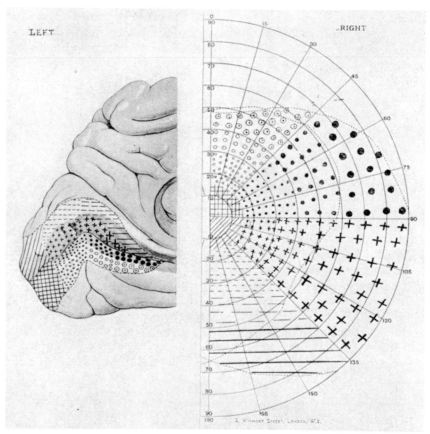

Figure 17–7. Cortical representation of the contralateral half of the binocular visual field in man. Figure on *left* shows calcarine fissure on mesial surface of left occipital lobe. Symbols indicate representation of parts of the field marked with corresponding symbols. (From Duke-Elder, *A textbook of ophthalmology,* Vol. 1, St. Louis, The C. V. Mosby Co., 1939.)

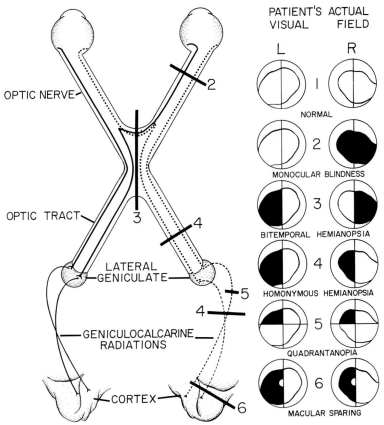

Figure 17-8. Optic pathways and the visual field defects resulting from lesions at different sites. (From Curtis *et al., An introduction to the neurosciences,* Philadelphia, W. B. Saunders Co., 1972.)

of the retina. A lesion of the crossing fibers of the chiasm causes a hemianopsia which is not homonymous; vision is lost in both temporal fields—a *bitemporal hemianopsia* (Fig. 17-8). Bitemporal hemianopsia often accompanies expanding tumors of the pituitary gland that compress the adjacent chiasm.

Lesions of the radiation or of the cortex may cause homonymous quadrantic field defects because the separation of fibers from upper and lower retinal halves allows selective injury. For example, interruption of radiation fibers in the right inferior radiation or destruction of the lower lip of the right calcarine fissure causes a *left upper quadrantanopia* (Fig. 17-8). Complete interruption of the tract of course yields a hemianopsia indistinguishable from that following a tract lesion, but a quadrantic defect is a clear sign of a lesion caudal to the geniculate body.

Lesions of both upper and lower calcarine cortex sometimes produce a hemianopsia that appears to spare central vision—a so-called *hemianopsia with macular sparing* (Fig. 17-8). The reason is a mystery; perhaps macular splitting is an artifact due to inadequate fixation of the eye during testing.

In man, complete removal of the occipital lobes causes complete irreversible blindness; vision is the only sensory modality that is totally dependent on cerebral cortex. In the monkey occipital lobectomy is followed by loss of all form and detail discrimination and of color discrimination, but the animal can still discriminate between light and dark panels. The residual function apparently permits the animal to differentiate (like a photocell) the total amount of light entering the eye because he cannot distinguish between two lighted panels of different brightness but of sufficiently different area that the total luminous flux is the same. The limited visual capacity of the destriate monkey presumably depends on subcortical visual connections (colliculus or reticular formation).

RECEPTIVE FIELDS OF GENICULATE AND STRIATE NEURONS

Recordings from single geniculate neurons during punctate exploration of the retina with white light reveals no surprises, for the receptive fields of geniculate neurons are remarkably similar to those of ganglion cells. That is, geniculate receptive fields consist of an excitatory center with an inhibitory surround or the reverse; they are, however, somewhat larger than those of ganglion cells, probably because of convergence at the geniculate level. The fields of geniculate neurons are monocular, with no evidence of convergence of crossed and uncrossed fibers on the same cell. In es-

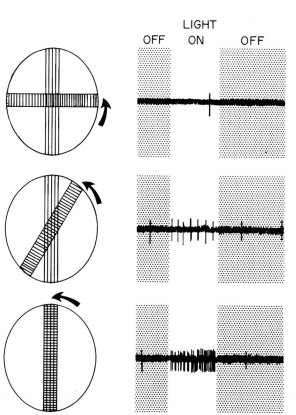

Figure 17–10. Behavior of striate neuron when stimulus orientation relative to field axis is varied. Field is oriented vertically, as indicated by long vertical lines. Response is maximal when stimulus bar *(crosshatched)* is aligned parallel with field axis. (After Hubel, *Sci. Amer.*, 1963, *209*, 54–62.)

sence, geniculate neurons appear to be simple relays, adding little to the complexity already established at the retinal level.

The receptive fields of visual cortical neurons are different. Usually cortical cells fire poorly or not at all to diffuse illumination of the retina, a finding that suggests that inhibitory portions of the field dominate. Exploration with punctate spots of light reveals that cortical cell fields, unlike those of ganglion and geniculate neurons, are not circular but rather are linearly arranged as adjacent barlike excitatory and inhibitory areas. Typical arrangements are shown in Figure 17–9. A consequence of the elongated configuration is that cortical cells are optimally discharged by *straight-line* contours, such as a dark bar on a bright background or a boundary between light and darkness.

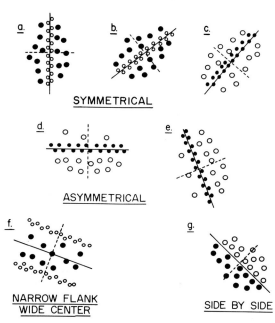

Figure 17–9. "Simple" receptive fields of striate cortical neurons. *Open circles* indicate excitatory points; *filled circles,* inhibitory points. The solid line is the axis of the field and represents the orientation of a line or border that causes optimal firing. (After Hubel and Wiesel, *J. Physiol.*, 1959, *148*, 574–591.)

Moreover, the cell is sensitive to the *orientation* of the stimulus; responses are maximal when the linear stimulus is parallel to the field orientation and are minimal or absent when it perpendicularly intersects both inhibitory and excitatory parts of the field (Fig. 17–10). When the optimal orientations are determined for each sequential cell encountered in an electrode penetration perpendicularly through the striate cortex, they are found to be either identical or similar; the cortex is composed of a mosaic of vertical cellular columns, each column containing cells more or less selectively sensitive to lines of light of a given orientation (Fig. 17–11). Perhaps

this organization is the basis of contour perception, for any visual contour could theoretically be constructed from a large number of straight line segments of appropriate orientations.

A second characteristic of cortical cells is that they often respond only — or, at least, optimally — to moving lines, and frequently they are sensitive to the *direction* as well as to the *orientation* of the movement. An example is shown in Figure 17–12. Sensitivity to movement is probably due to facilitation that results when the stimulus moves progressively across the excitatory field, and directional sensitivity may be due to asymmetrical fields, such

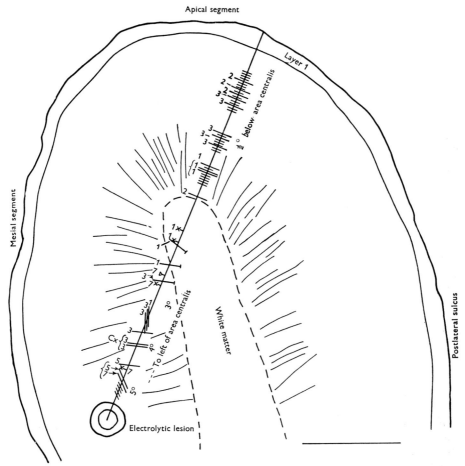

Figure 17–11. Reconstruction of a recording electrode tract through the visual cortex of a cat. Lines intersecting the tract represent sites at which striate cells were isolated and indicate the axes of their receptive fields. The tract begins approximately parallel to the entering geniculocalcarine fibers, shown as radial lines near white matter. Through this course, the field orientation of all isolated units is the same. In the lower part, the tract penetrates white matter and then reenters the gray matter at an angle oblique to the deep fiber bundles. Field orientations vary as the electrode samples units from different cell columns arranged parallel to fiber bundles. (From Hubel and Wiesel, *J. Physiol.*, 1962, *160*, 106–154.)

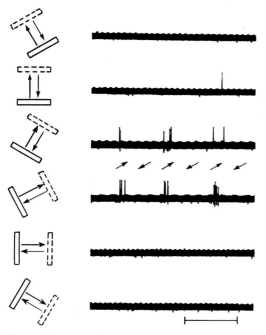

Figure 17–12. Records from a directionally sensitive cell in the cat's visual cortex. Figurines on the left represent the stimulus triangle, which was moved back and forth over the receptive field, as indicated by arrows. Optimal orientation was approached in the third row and reached in the fourth row from the top. The cell responded only to movement upward and to the right and ignored movement in the opposite direction. (From Hubel and Wiesel, *J. Physiol.*, 1959, *148*, 574–591.)

as shown in Figure 17–9*g*; oblique movement from above and downward would affect excitatory and inhibitory areas sequentially, whereas the reverse movement would activate the inhibitory areas first and suppress the subsequent action on the excitatory strip.

Not all cortical cells have simple receptive fields such as those shown in Figure 17–9. Complex fields cannot be divided by punctate exploration into segregated excitatory and inhibitory regions; rather, the entire field is a homogeneous mixture of excitatory and inhibitory points. Units with complex fields are exquisite line detectors, often responding differentially to the position of the line in the field, *e.g.*, on responses when the line is in one half of the field and off responses when it is in the other half. Hubel and Wiesel suggest that cells with simple fields receive their inputs directly from the

geniculate nucleus and that those with complex fields are cells receiving inputs secondarily from a number of simple-field neurons.

Another feature of the receptive fields of cortical cells is that many are binocular; at the cortical level fibers bearing information from both eyes finally converge on common neurons. In cat cortex the two fields of binocularly driven cells are situated in *corresponding portions* of the two retinae. Moreover, the optimal orientation and direction of the stimulus is the same for each of the two fields; that is, if a cell responds best to a bar of light moved downward in the two o'clock direction in the left retina, it will respond best to a downward two o'clock movement in the homonymous region of the right retina. Such precise similarities leave little doubt that convergence of information engendered by binocular retinal images onto common cortical cells is the basis for single-image vision and that the chiasm makes such fusion possible.

In animals with eyes laterally displaced so that there is no overlap of visual fields, no such fusion can occur; Melville, in *Moby Dick*, devotes an intriguing chapter to speculation about the visual experience of the whale, which, because of the lateral location of the eyes, perforce sees two unfused external worlds, one for each eye. Melville would be pleased to know that although the whale has an optic chiasm, the crossing of fibers is unrelated to retinal origin—all the fibers cross so that the whale's visual worlds split asunder at the eye remain disparate, though crossed, in the brain. Perhaps the whale, like the child with strabismus, alternately suppresses one or the other of his two non-overlapping visual images and thus avoids diplopia. Cells with binocular fields are not always equally well driven from the two eyes; many are dominated by inputs from either the ipsilateral or contralateral eye (see below). The extremes of dominance are represented by those cells with strictly monocular fields; among these, cells with contralateral and ipsilateral monocular fields are about equally represented.

The site of fusion of information from the two eyes varies with species. In the cat 84 per cent of visual cortical cells have

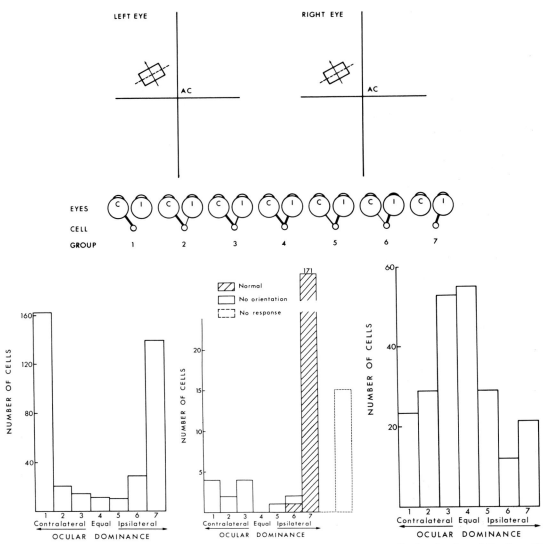

Figure 17–13. Ocular preferences of visual cortical neurons in normal, visually deprived, and "walleyed" cats. *Upper diagram* shows the method of classifying cells according to ocular dominance, ranging from strictly contralateral *(1)* through mainly contralateral *(2 and 3)*, equal *(4)*, and mainly ipsilateral *(5 and 6)*, to strictly ipsilateral *(7)*. *Below left,* distribution of ocular dominance of 223 cells from striate cortex of normal adult cats. *Below middle,* ocular dominance of 199 cells in striate cortex of kittens visually deprived by suturing of the contralateral eyelids for the first 8 to 14 weeks of postnatal life. *Below right,* ocular dominance of 384 striate neurons in kittens with experimentally induced neonatal divergent strabismus. (From Hubel, *Physiologist,* 1967, *10,* 197–45.)

binocular fields, although many show a preference for inputs from one or the other eye (Fig. 17–13). In the striate cortex of monkeys, the numbers of cells with binocular fields is less and varies with depth in the cortex. Cells in layer IV, upon which the incoming geniculostriate fibers terminate, have monocular fields like those of geniculate cells. The fields of neurons superficial and deep to layer IV are usually binocular but with a distinct preference for one eye or the other, the preference corresponding to the selective preference of the layer IV cells sandwiched between them. The resultant organization is a vertical column of cells each having a like ocular preference. Moreover, when viewed face-on, these columns are confluent and form stripes or slabs of cortex with regularly alternating preference for the right or left eye. In the monkey, the striate cortex is not the "end of the line," for it in turn projects onto the adjacent peristriate areas (described later). Peristriate cells have mainly binocular fields more nearly like those of striate cortex in the cat. A simple (or grossly oversimple) view is that in the primate, which has a more elaborate cortex, binocular confluence is delayed and established farther downstream than in the cat.

DEVELOPMENTAL INFLUENCES ON VISUAL CORTICAL ORGANIZATION

Clinical experience suggests that visual function is significantly influenced by early postnatal environmental factors. For example, a congenital cataract left untreated through early childhood leads to visual loss that lingers persistently, and sometimes ineradicably, when the cataract is removed. By contrast, removal of a blinding cataract developed in adulthood promptly restores unimpaired vision. The contrasting visual effects of congenital and acquired strabismus have already been mentioned. Taken together, such observations indicate that early postnatal development plays a vital role in visual function, which can be explored further by electrophysiological studies in experimental animals. For this purpose, the newborn kitten is chosen because the cat is born with closed eyelids that normally open between the 8th and 10th postnatal day, an event that can be unilaterally delayed by suturing of the lids. The ocular dominance of striate neuronal receptive fields can then be compared with those of kittens in which both eyes are allowed to open normally.

Normal field dominances of cortical cells can easily be divided into seven classes, as shown in Figure 17–13. Surgical closure of one eye on the day of eye opening and maintained until the day of testing 8 to 14 weeks later produces the striking alteration of field dominances shown in Figure

17–13. Of 199 cells, only 13 responded at all to stimuli presented to the previously occluded eye. Of these, 12 responses were abnormal in that the fields failed to display the normal sensitivity to the orientation of the stimulus. By contrast 171 cells responded only to inputs from the ipsilateral eye, which had been allowed to open normally. In the same animals exploration of the lateral geniculate body revealed a normal number of cells responding to stimuli to the previously occluded eye. Despite the normal behavior of geniculate neurons, histological inspection revealed a striking atrophy of cells in the layers receiving input from the occluded eye. Behavioral tests also indicated that the deprived eye was either blind or seriously defective; when the normal eye was blindfolded so that the kitten was obliged to depend on the deprived eye, it bumped into objects, fell off tables, and failed to follow moving objects.

Other experiments establish the following further details about the effects of visual deprivation. (1) The defect is due to loss of a function present at birth rather than failure of postnatal maturation, for the receptive fields of visual cells in a newborn, visually naïve kitten are indistinguishable from those of a normal adult. (2) The period of vulnerability is confined to the first few postnatal months; an adult cat survives as much as 3 months of lid closure without defect, and a kitten deprived for less than 6 weeks is similarly normal. (3) The critical deprivation is lack of experience with form vision, not lack of light; occlusion of one eye with a translucent but opaque contact lens, which prevents formed images but reduces incident light only slightly, produces a disturbance as severe as that following lid closure. Indeed, not only ocular dominance but also the preferred orientation of the stimulus is determined by early experience. Newborn kittens were raised for several months in total darkness save for an 8-hour daily exposure to a face mask that projected horizontal lines onto one eye and vertical lines onto the other. Their striate cells had monocular receptive fields that responded only to vertically or horizontally oriented stimuli, the rectilinear preference being identical with that to which the eye had been exposed in the mask.

Equally striking (and no less mysterious) are the effects of neonatal strabismus experimentally induced by section of both internal rectus muscles in newborn kittens. When tested after several months of divergent squint, the animals displayed a striking increase of cells with monocular fields (79 per cent compared to 20 per cent for a normal animal) (Fig. 17–13). A similar abnormality is induced if the eyes are prevented from working together by daily alternating occlusion of one eye or the other. Apparently, cells with binocular fields but with a preference for one or the other eye become the sole property of the dominant eye when concurrent binocular function is chronically prevented.

SPECTRAL SENSITIVITY OF CENTRAL VISUAL NEURONS

In the experiments on which the foregoing discussion are based white light was employed as the visual stimulus. Moreover, the experimental animal was frequently the cat, which is color-blind or, at best, "color-stupid," since in behavioral tests it learns painfully slowly and imperfectly to make color discriminations. Monkeys, which have a three-cone retina and a spectral sensitivity (as measured behaviorally) that duplicates that of man with satisfactory precision, are thus the experimental animals of choice. In Chapter 16 we pointed out that the existence of three cone types having photopigments with maximal sensitivity in the long (red), medium (green), and short (blue) wavelengths lends support to the Young-Helmholtz theory, which postulates that the perception of color depends on the population of cones excited by a given spectral band. Implicit in the theory is the assumption that the message generated in at least some of the color-coded cones reaches the cortex intact without ambiguous mixing because of convergence of distinctive messages on common elements in the geniculate body and cortex.

In Chapter 16 we also noted that some secondary retinal elements display another kind of selective spectral response in which

certain wavelengths produce hyperpolarization and others, depolarization, the turnover point varying in different cells (see Figure 16–11). Such cells are called *opponent-response* units, and they are reminiscent of Hering's theory, which postulated just such an opponent mechanism (although he guessed wrongly that it might occur in receptors). Thus both Hering and Young-Helmholtz theories have elements of truth, the opponent mechanism of Hering being added centrally onto the trichromatic receptor system of Young and Helmholtz. The opponent response of horizontal and bipolar cells suggests that two kinds of cones converge on opponent cells but that the cones liberate different transmitters. However, to implicate opponent responses in color coding, it is necessary to show that the polarity of the graded responses of bipolar cells has a counterpart in the conducted messages of ganglion cells and of geniculate and striate neurons. In short, spectral analysis of unit responses in monkeys demonstrates that central neuron action potentials do indeed show opponent responses. In fact, such analysis in monkeys provides the experimenter with more detail and complexity than he really wants, or, in any case, more than he can persuasively interpret at present (Fig. 17–14). The following is a brief summary of the findings.

Ganglion Cells

Ganglion cells may be opponent or nonopponent in type. Nonopponent cells respond indiscriminately to all wavelengths in both center and surround. Opponent ganglion cells are of two types, one that receives from green-and-red-sensitive cone systems, and another that responds to either green, blue, or red selectively in its center and is inhibited by a different cone system from its periphery. The first type gives only a poorly sustained phasic burst of impulses to sustained stimulation; the latter responds tonically. Because opponent cells have slower conduction velocities than do nonopponent cells, it is postulated that they derive from smaller

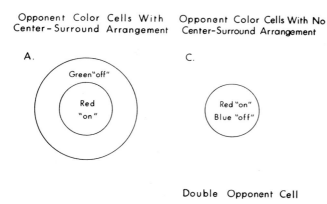

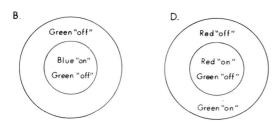

Figure 17–14.   Types of receptive fields of opponent color-coded cells in the primate visual system. (From Daw, *Physiol. Rev.*, 1973, 3, 571–611.)

cells, possibly from the midget ganglion cells found mainly in the fovea.

Lateral Geniculate Neurons

About 70 per cent of lateral geniculate neurons are opponent cells, some having a center-surround field arrangement. Most of the latter are red-green cells and are spatially as well as spectrally opponent with the following combinations: red on-center, green off-surround; or red off-center, green on-surround; or green on-center, red off-surround; or green off-center, red on-surround.

Neurons in Striate Cortex

About half of the striate neurons show opponent responses. Many are similar to geniculate cells, with circular fields excited by one wavelength and inhibited by another. Some may receive input from all three cone systems; *e.g.*, red and blue may excite and green may inhibit. Some opponent cells are line detectors and are sensitive to orientation as well as to color. Finally, some show so-called "double-opponent" behavior; *e.g.*, the center may

be "on" to red and "off" to green, with the reverse arrangement in the surround.

While it is not yet possible to weave these complex relations into a clear, workable theory of color perception, the data clearly indicate that cortical cells receive a plethora of color information.

PRESTRIATE CORTICAL AREAS

In addition to the striate cortex (area 17 of Brodmann) two other adjacent cortical areas are related to vision in less direct and well defined ways. A band of cortex bordering the calcarine striate cortex on the mesial surface and extending onto the lateral surface as a band covering all but the caudal tip of the posterior occipital lobe is called 18. Another strip, area 19, is a more rostrally situated lateral band that invades posterior parietal and temporal cortex. Both areas contain cells that are like the orientation-sensitive edge-detectors of striate cortex; they are all of the complex type. Many have what Hubel and Wiesel call "hypercomplex" fields, which means that the cells are sensitive not only to orientation of the line but to its length; extension of the line inhibits a discharge that a shorter line sets up.

Some of the crude visually oriented

behavior remaining in the destriate monkey appears to depend on prestriate cortex. Although the destriate animal fails to recognize stationary objects, it still responds with eye and head movements to moving objects; these vestigial responses disappear after additional extirpation of prestriate cortex.

Area 18 is the portion of the visual system that is linked to the opposite hemisphere by the corpus callosum. The role of the interhemispheric callosal connections in transfer of monocular learned behavior was first demonstrated by Meyers and Sperry in a classic experiment. They found that a monkey trained to perform a visual discrimination with one eye covered can subsequently perform perfectly when the stimulus is presented to the previously covered eye. That is, cues presented to one eye can elicit behavior learned through the opposite eye. Moreover, interocular transfer is unimpaired by section of the chiasm, so that only the ipsilateral hemisphere receives direct input during the training period. However, if both the chiasm and the posterior corpus callosum are divided prior to training, the animal is completely incapable of discriminating with the untrained eye.

ADDITIONAL READING

Daw, N. W. Neurophysiology of color vision. *Physiol. Rev.*, 1973, *53*, 571–611.

DeValois, R. L. Analysis and coding of color vision in the primate visual system. *Cold Spr. Harb. Symp. quant. Biol.*, 1965, *30*, 567–579.

Hubel, D. Effects of distortion of sensory input on the visual system of kittens. *Physiologist*, 1967, *10*, 17–45.

Poggio, G. F. Central neural mechanisms in vision. Chap. 68 in *Medical physiology*, Mountcastle, V. B., ed., St. Louis, The C. V. Mosby Co., 1968.

Ruch, T. C. Binocular vision and central visual pathways. Chap. 21 in *Physiology and biophysics*, Ruch, T. C., and Patton, H. D., eds., Philadelphia, W. B. Saunders Co., 1965.

CHAPTER 18

AUDITION AND ITS DISTURBANCES

HARRY D. PATTON

COMPARISON OF HEARING AND VISION

Just as the visual system detects electromagnetic waves (light), the auditory system is designed to detect mechanical waves (sound) in the medium surrounding the ear. Unlike light waves, sound waves will not travel in a vaccum but require either a gas, solid, or liquid medium; the ear employs all three routes. Sound is produced by vibrating objects. The vibrations alternately compress and rarefy the surrounding medium, and these compressions and rarefactions spread as pressure waves, just as ripples spread in water when a pebble is dropped into it. Pressure waves mechanically vibrate the auditory receptors, causing them to discharge impulses that give rise to hearing. The ear is thus a highly specialized mechanoreceptor.

In the eye light waves pass through, and are altered by, ocular structures (cornea, ocular fluids, and lens) interposed between the outer world and the retinal receptors; similarly, in the ear auditory vibrations traverse, and are modified by, a complex conduction system (external auditory canal, tympanic membrane, the ossicular system, and the cochlear perilymph and endolymph) before reaching the auditory receptors, the hair cells. The sensitivity of the eye varies with the stimulus wavelength; so does that of the ear, although auditory sensitivity is usually expressed as a function of frequency (which is inversely proportional to wavelength). As we shall see later, the variation of auditory sensitivity with frequency is largely due to properties of the conduction system, which transmits some frequencies more efficiently than others. Whether hair cells in dif-

248

ferent parts of the cochlea have different thresholds to displacement, comparable to the different photic sensitivities of rods and cones, is an unanswered question. The psychological correlate of photic wavelength is color; of sound frequency, pitch. Like photoreceptors, cochlear hair cells have exquisitely low thresholds; in the range of maximal sensitivity (1000 to 2000 Hz), vibratory displacements of the hair cells in the basilar membrane of 10^{-10} cm are audible. For comparison, the diameter of a Na^+ ion is approximately 100 times as much!

SOUND WAVES

Any vibrating body generates sound waves that travel in air (20°C) at 344 m/sec. The pattern of vibration (and hence of the pressure waves) has several variables, each having significant perceptual correlates. The simplest pattern is a sinusoidal vibration such as that produced by a tuning fork or by an electronic oscillator; such sounds are called *pure tones*. A pure tone has two variables: frequency and magnitude. As already mentioned, the subjective correlate of frequency is *pitch*. The higher the frequency, the higher the pitch; doubling the frequency of a tone raises its pitch by one octave. Magnitude of vibration is related to, but is not the sole determinant of, subjective *loudness*. For a fixed frequency, the greater the magnitude, the greater the loudness. But when one compares the relative loudness of two pure tones of different frequency, the simple relationship between magnitude and loudness breaks down because, as already mentioned, auditory sensitivity is a function of frequency. When tones of different pitch are compared, both magnitude and frequency are determinants of relative loudness.

Most musical sounds are not of simple sinusoidal pattern (pure tones) but rather have a more complex (although periodically repeating) wave form: such sounds are called *complex tones*. Vibrating strings, horns, organ pipes, and the human voice all produce complex tones. All complex musical tones can be analyzed into a funda-

mental sinusoidal frequency superimposed on which are harmonics, *i.e.*, sinusoidal frequencies that are multiples of the fundamental frequency. For example, a plucked guitar string may vibrate not only between the fret and the bridge, producing the fundamental frequency, but also in segments that are integral fractions (one half, one third, and so forth) of the length. The vibratory frequency of these subsegments increases as the length of the segment decreases, producing the harmonics that are superimposed on the fundamental frequency. The magnitude of the harmonic vibrations (and hence their prominence in the resultant complex tone) depends on the physical properties of the vibrating object and on the way it is set into motion. Complex tones thus vary not only in frequency and magnitude but also in *wave form*, depending on their harmonic content. The subjective correlate of wave form is *timbre*, or *quality*. Timbre permits us to distinguish notes of the same fundamental frequency (and hence the same pitch) when played on different instruments, for example, on a violin and an oboe.

Finally, sounds in which the wave form is complex but nonperiodic are called *noises*; the hissing sound of escaping steam, the crackling of a burning log, and the sound of crashing glass are examples.

Frequency and Intensity of Sound Waves

To describe a pure tone physically, we need to specify its frequency and intensity. *Frequency* is simply expressed as the number of vibrations per second. By international agreement adopted in 1960, a cycle per second is called a hertz (Hz), in honor of the German physicist Heinrich Hertz—an unfortunate substitution of an eponym for a self-explanatory designation.

Specification of *intensity* (not to be confused with its psychological correlate, loudness) is more involved. The intensity of a sound wave depends on its energy content, or ability to do work. Power is the unit used to describe the comparable parameter in electrical (watts, W) and mechanical (horsepower) systems. Absolute acoustic power is an awkward designation both because the range of values pertinent to hearing is surpassingly broad and because the absolute values are infinitesimally small. For example, for a 1000-Hz tone the range from the minimum audible sound to the maximum tolerable is from about 0.000,000,000,000,000,1 to 0.01 W/cm²—an unwieldy span of 10^{14}-fold, from nearly nothing to barely a smidgeon. For these reasons a logarithmic scale that merely designates the ratios between sound intensities in powers of ten is used; the unit is the bel (B), named in honor of Alexander Graham Bell. Thus 1 B means a 10-fold change; 2 B, 100-fold; 3 B, 1000-fold; and so forth. More commonly the decibel (dB), one tenth of a bel, is employed: 10 dB connotes a 10-fold change; 20 dB, a 100-fold change; and so on. When, as is usual, pressure, rather than power, is measured, the number of decibels is doubled because power (the base of the decibel) is proportional to the square of the pressure, and the log of P^2 is $2 \log P$. Thus a 10-fold change in pressure is 20 dB.

Since the decibel system of notation describes ratios, it is useful for relative comparison of two intensities or pressures; but some reference level is needed to describe a single intensity or pressure. The standard reference level is the threshold for a 1000-Hz tone, 10^{-16} W/cm², or (in pressures) 0.0002 dyn/cm². Because of its relative ease of measurement, the pressure standard is more frequently used and is designated SPL (for sound pressure level).

An example may help. The components of ordinary conversational speech at a distance of 1 m range from about 40 to 60 dB (SPL), or 4 to 6 B (SPL). Since the reference is pressure, the log of the intensity ranges from 40/20 to 60/20, or from 2 to 3. The intensity range is thus from 100 to 1000 times that of the threshold for a 1000-Hz tone.

Appreciation of the decibel system, like that of a new spouse, requires time, patience, and experience. To help you on your honeymoon, Figure 18–1 locates some familiar sounds on the decibel scale.

AUDITORY THRESHOLDS, AUDIOMETRY

We have already mentioned that auditory sensitivity varies with frequency of the sound wave mainly because the conduction system transmits some frequencies more efficiently than others. The clinical procedure whereby the acuity of hearing is tested through the range of frequencies normally audible is called *audiometry*, and the graphic result of such a test is called an *audiogram*.

Precise audiometry is difficult because the exquisite sensitivity of the ear requires measurements of infinitesimally small energy steps. Also, the results are highly dependent upon the conditions under which the test is conducted and the degree to which extraneous background sound can be controlled. As Figure 18–2 shows, thresholds obtained under the conditions prevailing in most audiometry tests are 15 to 20 dB greater than those obtained under ideal conditions. Also illustrated in Figure 18–2 is a feature of sound recognition that becomes important in severe hearing loss, *viz.*, that even a totally deaf subject can detect an intense sound by "feeling" the movements of the tympanic membrane without actually hearing the sound. The threshold of feeling (sometimes called the *pain threshold* because the "feeling" of intense sound is unpleasant) is, of course, very much higher than that

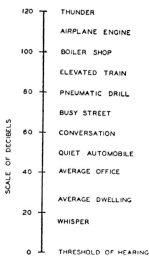

Figure 18–1. Decibel equivalents of familiar sounds. (From Stevens and Davis, *Hearing, its psychology and physiology*, New York, John Wiley & Sons, 1938.)

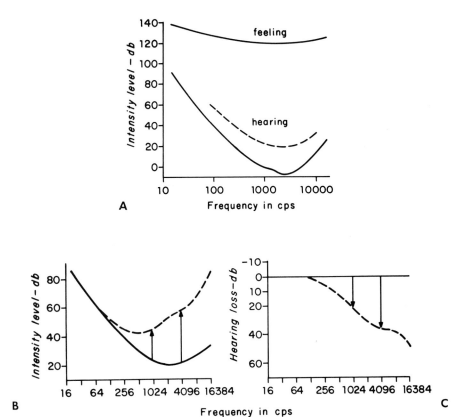

Figure 18–2. Auditory sensitivity in man. *A,* The heavy lines show the thresholds of feeling ("pain") and of hearing, as determined under ideal testing conditions; the dashed line shows the hearing threshold determined under usual testing conditions.

B and *C,* How the audibility curve (*B*) is converted to the hearing loss curve (*C*). The heavy line shows data from a normal subject; in the hearing loss graph it is converted to zero on the ordinate. Dashed line shows data from a subject with high-tone hearing loss; arrows on the right figure show the magnitude of loss. (*A,* After Licklider, in *Handbook of experimental psychology,* Stevens, ed. New York, John Wiley & Sons, 1951. *B* and *C,* From Ruch and Patton, eds., *Physiology and biophysics,* Philadelphia, W. B. Saunders Co., 1965.)

of hearing and is also much less sensitive to frequency since it is less subject to frequency-sensitive conductive losses.

The clinician is usually less interested in absolute hearing acuity than in his patient's hearing relative to that of a normal subject in the same circumstance. Consequently, it is common to plot hearing either in terms of per cent of normal or in terms of "hearing loss" in decibels below the average normal. A series of frequencies (usually at octave intervals) is generated by an electronic oscillator and presented through earphones to the subject. The examiner varies the intensity, and the subject is asked to flash a light when he hears a sound. The intensity dial is calibrated in decibels above or below the normal threshold for that frequency. Figure 18–2 shows (in *B*) the result of an audiometry test in terms of thresholds and (in *C*) an audiogram in which the same results are expressed as hearing loss. The subject providing the interrupted curve had a higher-than-normal threshold to high frequencies (greater than 128 Hz), as shown in *B*. In *C* the same data are expressed as hearing loss.

Auditory acuity is profoundly affected by age. Characteristically, advancing age is accompanied by decreased sensitivity to high tones, as shown by the dotted curves in Figure 18–2*B* and *C*. Although the high-tone deafness of the elderly is "normal" in the sense that it is expected, it is nevertheless a pathological consequence of the aging process, in which the cochlear receptive cells in basal turns (where, as discussed later, high frequencies are received) degenerate. In contrast, hearing loss due to impairment of conduction through the ear usually results in a relatively flat audiogram, *i.e.*, the deficit is approximately the same at all frequencies.

ANATOMY OF THE PERIPHERAL AUDITORY APPARATUS

The peripheral auditory apparatus comprises the outer ear, middle ear, and inner ear (Fig. 18–3). The outer ear consists of the *pinna* (or auricle) and the external *auditory canal*, which ends blindly at the *tympanic membrane*, or *eardrum*, covering the external auditory meatus. The tympanum is oval and funnel-shaped, with its apex (*umbo*) directed upward and inward because of the attachment of the foot (*manubrium*) of the malleus to its inner superior surface.

The middle ear (Fig. 18–4) is an air-filled bony cavity in the temporal bone, closed save for a communication with the nasopharynx through the Eustachian (auditory) tube. The tube is normally closed at the pharyngeal end but opens during swallowing and yawning. It serves the purpose of keeping middle ear pressure at atmospheric levels. The noteworthy contents of the middle ear are the auditory ossicles (*malleus*, *incus*, and *stapes*) and two muscles, one attached to the malleus (*tensor tympani muscle*), and the other to the stapes (*stapedius muscle*). The malleus, incus, and stapes are linked together by hingelike attachments to bridge the gap across the middle ear from the tympanum to the oval window in the vestibule of the inner ear. Vibrations induced in the drum by sound waves entering the canal are transmitted by the ossicular chain to the membrane covering the oval window of the cochlea and thence to the fluid (perilymph) filling the cochlear channels. The tensor tympani muscle is innervated by a branch of the cranial nerve V and arises in a bony canal in the medial wall of the middle ear dorsal to the Eustachian tube; its tendon turns at a right angle to bridge the cavity and attach to the malleolar manubrium (Fig. 18–4). Contraction of the muscle pulls the drum dorsomedially and tenses it. The stapedius muscle is innervated by a branch of cranial nerve VII and extends from the posterior wall of the middle ear to the head of the stapes.

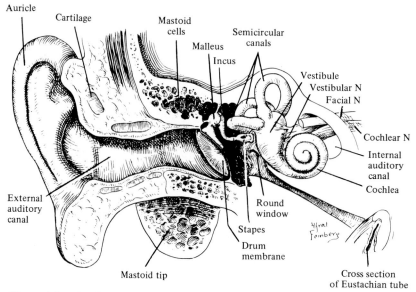

Figure 18–3. The peripheral auditory apparatus. The cochlea is turned slightly to show its coils. The Eustachian tube runs forward as well as downward and inward. (From Davis and Silverman, *Hearing and deafness,* New York, Holt, Rinehart, and Winston, 1970.)

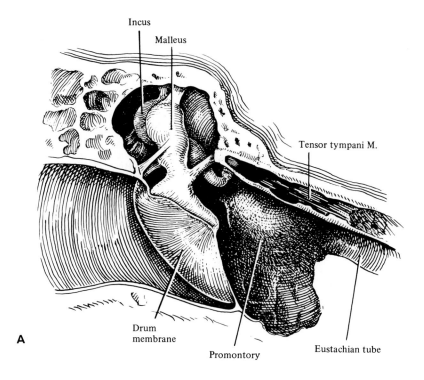

Incus

Malleus

Tensor tympani M.

Drum
membrane

A

Promontory

Eustachian tube

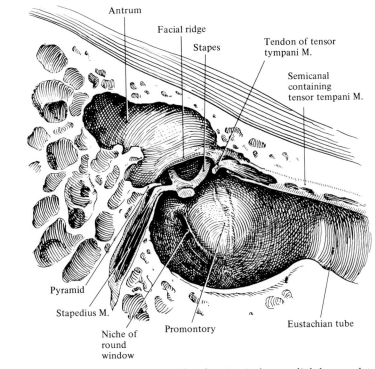

Antrum

Facial ridge

Stapes

Tendon of tensor
tympani M.

Semicanal
containing
tensor tempani M.

Pyramid

Stapedius M.

Niche of
round
window

Promontory

Eustachian tube

B

Figure 18–4. The middle ear and its contents. *A*, This drawing is from a slightly more lateral angle than that of Figure 18–3. Note the connection of the tensor tympani muscle. *B*, This figure depicts a view from the external canal with the drum and the malleus and incus removed. Note the attachment of the stapedius muscle to the stapes. (From Davis and Silverman, *Hearing and deafness*, New York, Holt, Rinehart, and Winston, 1970.)

Its contraction rocks the stapes out of the oval window (Fig. 18–4). The actions of the two muscles tend to stiffen the ossicular chain and to reduce energy transmission, particularly of low frequencies. They are reflexly activated by intense sounds (70 dB and greater) and presumably serve a protective function by reducing the impact of devastating intensities on the delicate inner ear.

The inner ear is a structure of minute proportions and intricate architecture, so that it is both hard to see and virtually impossible to describe intelligibly. But every textbook writer tries—and so shall we. The bony cavity in the temporal bone housing the inner ear structures is called the *osseous labyrinth* (Fig. 18–5). It contains a fluid, called perilymph. Floating in the perilymph is a membranous bag, the *membranous labyrinth*, which is in turn filled with *endolymph*. The bony labyrinth com-

prises three parts: the three *semicircular canals*, the *vestibule*, and the *cochlea*. The corresponding encased membranous structures are the three *semicircular ducts* (in the canals), the *utricle* and *saccule* (in the vestibule), and the *cochlear duct* (or *scala media*), which extends into the spiral cochlea as a blind tube. The semicircular ducts, the utricle, and the saccule contain receptors innervated by the vestibular portion of cranial nerve VIII. These receptors, concerned with equilibrium and unrelated to hearing, are dealt with elsewhere; presently attention is focused on the cochlea, which houses the auditory receptors.

The cochlea (Fig. 18–6) spirals like a snail or conch shell for two and a half turns around its central pillar, or *modiolus*; the cochlear duct extends blindly, like a glove finger, to the apex of the spiral channel. A vertical section from apex to base through

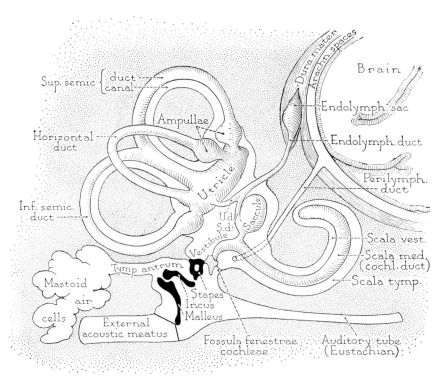

Figure 18–5. The relationship of the osseous and membranous labyrinths. The former is filled with peri-lymph and at the vestibule communicates with the subarachnoid space via the perilymphatic duct. The membranous labyrinth floats in the perilymph and contains endolymph. Only part of the coiled cochlea is shown. Note that the cochlear duct (scala media) is part of the membranous system. It ends blindly at the cochlear apex and contains endolymph. The perilymph-filled scala vestibula communicates with the vestibule and, through the helicotrema, with the scala tympani, which ends at the round window. (From Bast and Anson, *The temporal bone and the ear*, Springfield, Ill., Charles C Thomas, 1949.)

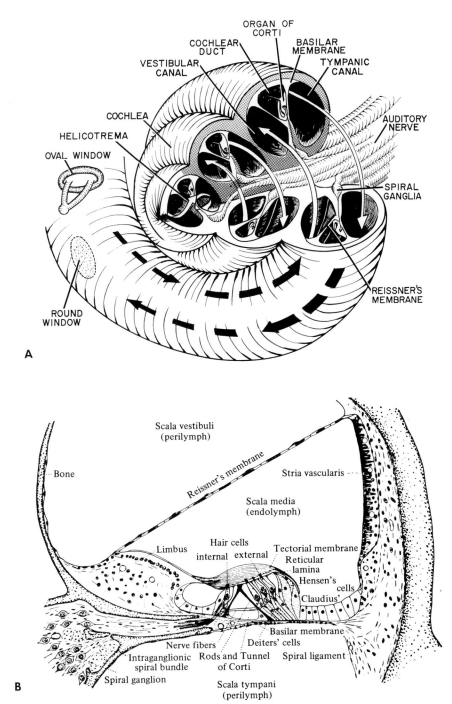

Figure 18–6. The cochlea and the organ of Corti. *A*, Diagram of cochlea cut through to show the partition of the cavity by the basilar membrane and cochlear duct (scala media). Arrows show the pathway of transmission of pressure waves originating at the oval window. *B*, The cochlear partition and the organ of Corti. (*A*, From Curtis, Jacobson, and Markus, *An introduction to the neurosciences,* Philadelphia, W. B. Saunders Co., 1972. *B*, From Davis and Silverman, *Hearing and deafness,* New York, Holt, Rinehart, and Winston, 1970.)

the central modiolus opens the spiraling tunnel in a cross section; one such section is shown in Figure 18–6. A bony shelf projects from the modiolus into the channel and forms the central attachment of a delicate membrane, the *basilar membrane,* which stretches horizontally across the opening and attaches to the lateral wall by the *spiral ligament.* The basilar membrane divides the opening approximately in half: the lower half is called the *scala tympani* and is filled with *perilymph;* the upper half accommodates the *cochlear duct,* which is filled with *endolymph.* The superior wall of the cochlear duct, the delicate *Reissner's membrane,* further subdivides the upper half and separates its endolymph from the perilymph of the *scala vestibuli,* which is continuous with that of the vestibule. The lateral wall of the cochlear duct is lined by columnar cells, collectively called the *stria vascularis;* their metabolic activity maintains the composition and electrical potential of the endolymph. At the apex of the cochlea, the scala vestibuli and scala tympani communicate through a tiny opening, the *helicotrema;* at the base the scala tympani ends blindly at the round window, being partitioned from the middle ear by a membranous covering.

The perilymph of the scala vestibuli is compressed when the stapes moves inward at the oval window. Although Reissner's membrane is an effective chemical barrier separating endolymph and perilymph, it is acoustically nothing, and simplified diagrams of the ear often pretend that it does not exist; compression in the scala vestibuli is transmitted undiminished across the cochlear duct to the basilar membrane and causes it to bulge into the scala tympani. In turn the membranous covering of the round window bulges into the middle ear. Decompression produces the opposite displacement of basilar membrane and round window. Because of the small size of the helicotrema and the reluctance of the viscous perilymph to move through it (particularly at high frequencies), displacement is almost entirely *across* the basilar membrane, the ultimate point of "give" being the compliant membrane of the round window.

The sensory structure of the cochlea, the *organ of Corti* (Fig. 18–6), is attached to the dorsal surface of the basilar membrane and is derived from the floor of the cochlear duct, just as the similar sensory structures of the noncochlear part of the inner ear are derived from the utricular, saccular, and semicircular portions of the membranous labyrinth. In the middle of the membrane are the *rods, or pillars, of Corti,* cells stiffened with intracellular filaments and joined at the top to form a triangular arch around a central space, the *tunnel of Corti.* Flanking the pillars are columns composed of elongated cells of two types, the supporting *phalangeal cells* and the *hair cells.* Lateral to the tunnel the phalangeal cells (*Deiters' cells*) form cuplike lateral shelves on which the *outer hair cells* rest; they also send upward between the hair cells thin, stiff projections with platelike terminations. These join the platelike terminations of the rods of Corti to form the stiff upper surface of the organ of Corti, *the reticular lamina,* or *cuticular plate.* The outer hair cells are arranged in three to five rows; the *inner hair cells* are aligned medial to the tunnel in one row.

Overlying the organ of Corti is the *tectorial membrane,* a stiff, gelatinous, and fibrous flap hinged medially to the limbus atop the bony modiolar ridge. Despite earlier contentions to the contrary (prompted by fixation artifacts), the hairs, or stereocilia, of the hair cells (see later) are embedded in, or attached to, the undersurface of the tectorial membrane, so that they are bent by to-and-fro lateral movement of the hair cells relative to the tectorial membrane as the basilar membrane vibrates up and down. The basilar membrane medial and lateral to the hair cells is paved with soft, compliant columnar cells (*Hensen's cells and Claudius' cells*).

The hair cells are the auditory mechanoreceptors. The superior surface of each cell is adorned with up to 80 hairs, or *stereocilia,* each about 1 μm in diameter, arranged in the pattern of a U or W, with the angular points directed laterally (Fig. 18–12). Their distal ends attach to the tectorial membrane, and their roots project into the distal end of the hair cells. It is believed that the to-and-fro movement of the stereocilia is the critical event in generating auditory messages, as it is in the

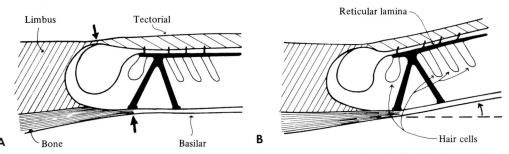

Figure 18–7. Movements of the cochlear partition and bending of stereocilia. *A,* Partition is at rest; arrows indicate the hinge points of tectorial and basilar membranes. *B,* Upward movement of partition (decompression in scala vestibuli) bends hairs laterally. Lateral shear is thought to initiate discharge; medial shear, silence. (From Davis and Silverman, *Hearing and deafness,* New York, Holt, Rinehart, and Winston, 1970.)

similar receptor organs of the utricle, saccule, and semicircular canals, but the details of the transducer mechanism are, as we shall see, still uncertain. The base of the hair cells receives two kinds of nerve endings derived from fibers reaching the organ from the central modiolus, which houses the *spiral ganglion* containing the somata of the primary auditory neurons. One type of ending is relatively large and laden with vesicles; the other endings are small and are free of vesicles. The larger, granular terminals are *efferent* endings of axons arising from cells in the superior olivary nucleus, whereas the smaller, clear terminals are afferent endings of the cells in the spiral ganglion. The olivocochlear efferent projection, as we shall see later, depresses the excitability of the hair cells.

In summary, the intricate pathway followed by sound vibrations giving rise to hearing is as follows. The airborne pressure waves set up by a vibrating object traverse the external auditory canal and set the tympanic membrane in vibration. The oscillations are transmitted by the ossicles across the middle ear to the oval window, where they induce pressure waves in the perilymph of the scala vestibuli. Acting through Reissner's membrane, the pressure waves impinge on the basilar membrane. Displacement of the basilar membrane alters the pressure in the perilymph of the scala tympani, a change which is accommodated by bulging of the elastic membrane of the round window in and out of the middle ear. Because of the attachment of the hairs to the tectorial membrane and because of the different

hinge points of basilar and tectorial membranes, the movement of the basilar membrane causes a shearing displacement of the hairs, the adequate stimulus for the hair cells (Fig. 18–7). When the stapes rocks outward, the organ of Corti moves upward, the hairs bend laterally, and nerve impulses are discharged. The opposite movement turns the discharge off.

CONDUCTION THROUGH THE EXTERNAL AND MIDDLE EARS

Since the sound wave must successively traverse air, the ossicles, and fluid (perilymph) to deflect the basilar membrane, it is not surprising that it undergoes some transformations in conduction. Apart from the influence of head position (shading and diffraction) on the incident wave, the first significant alteration occurs in the external auditory canal, which, being a tube closed distally by the tympanum, acts approximately like a miniature organ pipe. A blind organ pipe resonates at a frequency that depends on the pipe length; *i.e.,* it accentuates the fundamental frequency of the pipe. This is because waves striking the dead end are reflected and can reinforce or diminish incoming waves, depending on the phase relations of incident and reflected waves. The fundamental resonant frequency of the pipe has a wavelength four times the length of the tube (certain of the harmonics may also be accentuated).

For the auditory canal, which is 2.7 cm long, the calculated fundamental resonant frequency is 3185 Hz. In fact, the auditory canal is not a perfect resonator because, unlike a rigid closed pipe, the tympanum is elastic and displaceable. This factor lowers the resonant frequency to about 3000 Hz. The result is that a 3000-Hz tone produces a pressure which is considerably greater at the drum than at the entrance to the canal. The resonant tuning of the ear canal is not sharp, the amplification dropping off rather gradually on either side of the resonant frequency; from 2000 to 5500 Hz the amplification amounts to 5 to 12 dB, an advantage gained simply by the introduction of a resonant tube between the drum and the incident waves. The resonant properties of the external canal, which thus preferentially amplify the pressures of a band of frequencies, are partly responsible for the shape of the audibility curve.

The oscillations of the drum are transmitted across the middle ear to the oval window by the ossicular chain (Fig. 18–8). The malleus and incus vibrate as a unit around an axis passing through their ligaments and impart a rocking, piston-like motion to the stapes, which swings like a door with its hinge at the posterior border of the oval window. Since the manubrium is longer than the arm of the incus, displacement at the oval window is

less than at the drum, but the force is amplified about 1.3 times. Also, the effective area of the drum is 16 times that of the oval window, so that the overall pressure amplification of the ossicular system is about 21 times—a gain of about 25 dB.

The ossicular system nicely solves the problem of transmitting pressure waves from a gaseous medium (air) to a liquid medium (perilymph), a transfer which would otherwise be hampered by reflection of most of the energy. Even so, some energy is lost in reflection and friction, especially at the high and low frequencies, but transmission losses are minimal in the range of 1000 to 2000 Hz. Taken together, the resonance of the external canal and the mechanical properties of the ossicular chain keep sensitivity acute to the middle range of frequencies that predominate in human speech (about 400 to 3000 Hz).

Alternate Routes of Conduction

Although the ossicular chain is the dominant pathway across the middle ear, air conduction also occurs. Because the stapes shields the oval window, airborne pressure waves act mainly at the round window of the scala tympani and in the normal ear oppose the waves set up in the perilymph of the scala vestibuli by the ossicular route. In fact, shielding the round window from airborne waves improves hearing. The perilymph can also be set into vibration by oscillations conducted through the bony structure of the skull, a fact that is exploited in the design of some hearing aids. The retention of bone conduction (as tested by placement of a tuning fork against the skull) enables the physician to distinguish between *conduction deafness* and *sensorineural deafness*, due to damage to cochlear structures or to cranial nerve VIII.

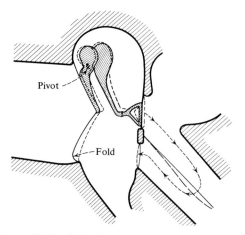

Figure 18–8. Ossicular transmission across the middle ear. For simplicity the cochlea is represented uncoiled and the acoustically ineffectual Reissner's membrane is omitted. (From Silverman and Davis, *Hearing and deafness*, New York, Holt, Rinehart, and Winston, 1970.)

Conduction Deafness

Conduction deafness may result from obstruction of the canal with wax or a foreign object or from middle ear disease; in either case, bone conduction bypasses the obstruction. The most common middle ear disease is infection (*otitis media*), which, if chronic, may cause adhesions and scarring and may permanently reduce mobility of the drum or the ossicles. *Aero-otitis* results from rapid changes of altitude when the Eustachian tube is closed. Because the static pressure in the middle ear does not match that of the atmosphere, the drum either bulges outward or funnels inward. Descent from high altitude is especially troublesome, for a relative vacuum develops in the middle ear and the subject may have difficulty opening the Eustachian tube to adjust the pressure; the funneling of the drum inward causes pain and impairs hearing.

Another middle ear disease causing conduction deafness is *otosclerosis*, a condition in which abnormal bone growth immobilizes the stapes in the oval window. Hearing is impaired, but less than might be expected because air conduction to the round window continues to function. Air conduction is, however, less than maximally efficient, because with the stapes stoppering the oval window and with the round window serving as the entry port, the perilymphatic system has no point of "give," a condition necessary for displacement of the basilar membrane. Surgically providing a "give" point was the purpose of the original "fenestration" operation, in which a hole was drilled in some part of the perilymphatic channel (usually one of the semicircular canals, which can conveniently be approached through the mastoid bone) and covered with periosteum to form a compliant window. Hearing was promptly and dramatically improved, but the benefits were disappointingly short-lived because the artificial covering tended soon to scar and to lose its elasticity. A better procedure is to use the round window as the give point and to create a new entry port into the horizontal canal by making a window covered with skin from the auditory canal.

COCHLEAR MECHANISMS

Wave Propagation in the Basilar Membrane; the Place Theory of Pitch Discrimination

The final step in the sequence of events leading to the generation of auditory messages is a shearing displacement of the stereocilia of the hair cells as the basilar membrane moves up and down. One clearly established fact indicates that the transduction process must differ radically from that underlying generation and transmission of telephone messages. In the telephone the electrical signals duplicate the frequencies imposed on the microphone diaphragm, and these frequencies are reconverted to sound waves by movements of the diaphragm of the receiver. The telephone thus transmits electrical analogs of the *frequency pattern* of sound. But auditory nerve fibers supplying the hair cells are limited by the refractory period to an upper frequency limit of approximately 1000 impulses per second, far short of the upper range of auditory perception and discrimination (about 20,000 Hz).

It was Helmholtz who first resolved this problem by suggesting that different parts of the basilar membrane are differentially displaced by different frequencies and that the discrimination of pitch depends not primarily on frequency analysis but rather on spatial discrimination of what portion of the basilar membrane is maximally displaced, the locus varying for different frequencies. This is known as the *place theory* of pitch perception. Looked at in this way, discrimination of two pitches is comparable to two-point tactile discrimination in skin and to the minimum separable in vision.

Helmholtz based his theory mainly on the structure of the basilar membrane. In the basal turns the fibers of the membrane are relatively short (from medial to lateral) and seem to be tightly stretched.* Toward the apex the membrane appears broader, slacker, and more heavily laden with cellular elements that might be expected to damp the oscillations as do the windings on the bass strings of the piano. Helmholtz, who played a major role in the design of pianos, suggested that the basilar membrane is differentially tuned through its extent: the short, taut, unloaded fibers

---

*This was an erroneous deduction. The membrane is not under tension at either base or apex. It is, however, stiffer and less compliant at the base than at the apex.

of the basal turns, to high frequencies, and the longer, laxer, loaded fibers at the apex, to low frequencies. He suggested that a sound wave of given frequency causes the appropriately tuned portion of the membrane to vibrate sympathetically, or to resonate, much as a sound wave of frequency corresponding to the fundamental of an individual piano string can make it vibrate. Resonant behavior of the kind proposed by Helmholtz can occur only if the resonators, like the strings of a musical instrument, are independent of each other, a condition not encountered in the basilar membrane, in which the fibers are longitudinally bound together as a continuous membrane.

It was George von Békésy who elucidated the mechanism by which the cochlear partition (basilar membrane and organ of Corti) vibrates differentially in response to sound waves of different frequencies, an achievement that won him the Nobel Prize in 1961. His studies were carried out on cochleae removed from cadavers, placed in a bath and drilled to permit direct microscopic measurement of movements of the basilar membrane at various points from base to apex. A mechanical oscillator placed in the vestibule provided vibrations of known frequency. Békésy's analysis established firmly that pressure waves induced in the perilymph by oscillation of the oval window initiate in the basilar membrane traveling waves which proceed from the base toward the apex (Fig.

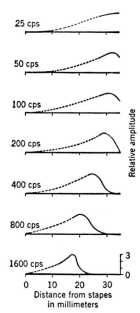

Figure 18–10. Magnitudes of envelopes of traveling waves elicited in basilar membrane by pressure oscillations of different frequencies. (From Von Békésy, *Experiments in hearing,* Wever, tr. and ed., New York, McGraw Hill Book Co., 1960.)

18–9). His measurements proved that the amplitude of the wave at different sites along the membrane from base to apex varies with the frequency of the sound wave. With high frequencies the wave reaches maximal amplitude (causes maximal displacement) in the basal turns and dies out before reaching the apical turns. Conversely, with low frequencies the wave displaces the basal turns minimally and reaches maximal amplitude toward the apex. Systematic investigation shows that each frequency through the audible range has a "place" of maximal displacement on the membrane. Figure 18–10 shows the spatial distribution of displacement induced in the membrane through a range of frequencies from 25 to 1600 Hz. Presumably, higher and lower frequencies also have appropriate "places" on the membrane, although these are technically difficult to measure with accuracy.

Békésy's experiments established clearly that the basilar membrane responds differentially to different frequencies and that the place theory is a reasonable basis for pitch discrimination. According to this

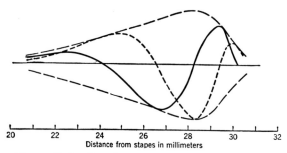

Figure 18–9. Traveling wave in basilar membrane. Solid and short dashed lines represent the same wave at two successive instants of time. The long dashed line outlines the envelope and indicates that displacement is maximal at about 28.5 mm from the stapes. (After Von Békésy, *J. acoust. Soc. Amer.,* 1947, *19,* 452–460.)

theory we recognize pitches by sensing the point of maximal displacement. Like other sensory systems, the auditory system employs the rate of action potential discharge to signal magnitude of displacement. Thus the trick of recognizing a pitch is to detect which hair cells along the membrane are initiating maximal rates of action potential discharge in their corresponding auditory nerve fibers. The theory is further substantiated, as we shall later describe, by studies of acoustic responses of single auditory nerve fibers, each of which shows maximal discharge rate to a given frequency, which varies with the site of fiber termination along the membrane.

Electrical Responses of the Cochlea

In 1930 Weaver and Bray, while recording electrical potentials from the auditory nerve of the cat, made the astonishing discovery that pure tones applied to the ear produced potential oscillations that were remarkably accurate analogs of the sound wave. Indeed, when the electrodes were connected through an amplifier to a loudspeaker, the cat's ear served as a passable microphone, and speech or music entering the ear emerged as understandable broadcasts from the speaker. Weaver and Bray's experiment created a storm. Since they believed they were recording action potentials from the auditory nerve, their experiment seemed to contradict the place theory and to support a "telephone" theory in which sound wave frequencies are supposed to evoke identical frequencies of action potential discharge, just as the oscillations of a telephone receiver induce oscillations of current in the line. We have already mentioned that a major stumbling block to telephone theories is the inability of nerve fibers to follow the high frequencies of audible sounds. (Auditory nerve fibers can of course follow low frequencies, and there is evidence that cadence of firing may indeed be useful for encoding low-frequency sounds.) The contradiction was in due time resolved when it was shown that the potentials underlying the Weaver and Bray phenomenon are not action potentials at all but rather are nonpropagated potentials of hair cells generated by the movements of the organ of Corti. They can be recorded optimally by electrodes tapping between the round window and ground. Such potentials are known as *cochlear microphonics.*

The voltage oscillations of the cochlear microphonic are often superimposed on a base line that shifts slowly in either a positive or a negative direction, depending on recording sites. The slow base line shifts, called positive and negative summating potentials, like the cochlear microphonics, derive from the hair cells rather than from nerve fibers. Their underlying mechanisms and significance are not clear.

The mechanism and significance of the cochlear microphonic are similarly controversial. What seems clear is that the cochlear microphonic depends on the integrity of the hair cells, for it is lacking from portions of the cochlear apparatus in which the hair cells have been selectively damaged by intense sound or by ototoxic drugs (see later). It is also lacking in deaf "waltzing mice," which genetically lack an organ of Corti. Through a considerable range of intensities the cochlear microphonic amplitude clearly reflects the intensity of sound, and when focally recorded from different sites on the basilar membrane, it can be used to map the tonotopic organization from base to apex (Fig. 18–11). It is thus a sensitive index of physical displacement of the hair cells.

A second pertinent point is that the endolymph bathing the superior surface of the scala media is some 80 mV positive to the perilymph. This positive endocochlear potential appears to be generated by the cells of the stria vascularis, although how is not clear. It clearly exists in waltzing mice and in drug-deafened animals, despite the lack of hair cells and of cochlear microphonics. An electrode placed in the organ of Corti below the cuticular plate registers some 60 to 80 mV negativity relative to the perilymph. If we assume that this negativity represents intracellular recordings of the hair-cell membrane potential (a moot point), a driving voltage of 140 to 160 mV would exist across the ciliated surface of the hair cell. It is at this ciliated surface that the cochlear

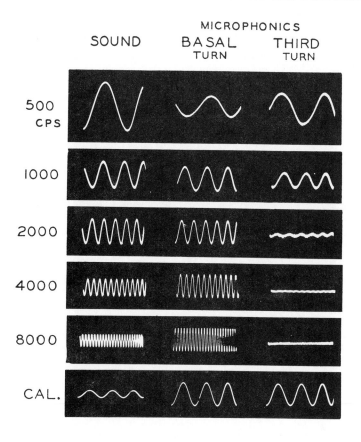

Figure 18–11. Microphonic responses of the guinea pig cochlea recorded at different sites during stimulation of the ear with different frequencies of sound waves. (From Tasaki, *J. Neurophysiol.*, 1954, *17*, 97–122.)

microphonic is generated because the recordings made just above and just below the reticular plate are mirror images.

Davis has incorporated these various observations into a hypothetical model of the cochlear transducer mechanism. He proposes that the voltages generated by the stria vascularis (endocochlear potential) and by the hair cell (membrane potential) in series provide the driving force for a current passing from the scala media through the cuticular surface of the hair cell and out somewhere near the base of the hair cell. Outward current at the base depolarizes the membrane and liberates a transmitter onto the afferent endings. The magnitude of the current (and hence the amount of transmitter liberated) is assumed to vary with the resistance of the cuticular surface membrane, which in turn depends on the position of the hair. Upward movement of the membrane (outward movement of the stapes) moves the hair laterally, decreases resistance, and increases the leakage current; the opposite movement increases resistance and decreases the leakage current. It is proposed that these fluctuations in leakage current underlie the cochlear microphonic, which is viewed as the receptor potential of the ear.

It should be noted that in Davis' theory the hair cell behaves not as an excitable cell, for like rods and cones it cannot support action potentials. Rather it serves as a variable resistor regulating flow of current driven by other sources just as a carbon microphone varies current flow by varying the resistance to current flow driven by stable direct current (DC) batteries. Viewed in this way, the role of the hair cell resembles that of the retinal photoreceptors in modulating the dark current. The hair cells are variable resistors sensitive to mechanical distortion of the hairs; the resistance of the rods and cones varies with illumination.

Damage to the Organ of Corti

The delicate hair cells are subject to injury by a number of agents and conditions. Often the damage is restricted to portions of the organ and can be mapped clearly in scanning electron micrographs of the dorsal surface of the cochlear partition as areas in which hair cell cilia are lacking.

When hair cell damage is localized, the audiogram is characterized by "tonal gaps," *i.e.*, by hearing loss confined to the frequencies mediated by the damaged portion of the organ. It has already been mentioned that elderly subjects suffer high-tone loss because of degeneration of hair cells in the basal part of the cochlea.

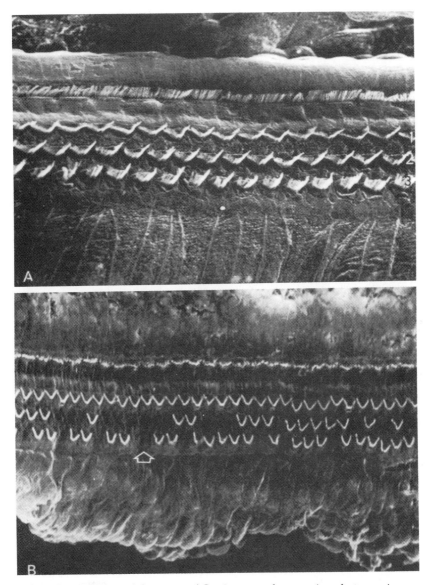

Figure 18–12. The dorsal surface of the organ of Corti, as seen by scanning electron microscopy. *A*, Normal organ. The modiolus is toward the top. The stereocilia of the single row of hair cells appear at top; then below the space occupied by the pillars the cilia of three rows of outer hair cells are seen arranged in the typical *U* or *W* configuration. *B*, Similar view from animal exposed to the noise of a starting pistol. Hairs are missing from some cells (*arrow*) in second and third rows. (From Angelborg and Engström, in *Basic mechanisms in hearing*, Møller, ed., New York, Academic Press, 1973.)

Geriatric high-tone deafness is presumably due to vascular inadequacy of the basal cochlea. On the other hand, subjects exposed to loud noises in industrial plants and performers in rock bands lose hair cells in the middle parts of the cochlea and suffer hearing losses to midfrequencies, around 4000 Hz. Figure 18–12A shows a normal guinea pig cochlea with one row of inner hair cells and three rows of outer hair cells. Figure 18–12B shows loss of cilia from outer hair cells in a guinea pig exposed to the sound of a starting pistol. Selectivity of noise damage is presumably due to physical damage accruing to those portions of the membrane responding to the damaging frequencies, which are amplified by the resonant and mechanical properties of the outer and middle ear.

Finally, the hair cells are destroyed in a predictable order by chronic treatment with some antibiotics derived from actinomycetes (such as streptomycin, dihydrostreptomycin, neomycin, and kanamycin). The -mycin drugs are known to interfere with protein synthesis, but the reason for their ototoxicity is not clear. Outer hair cells are destroyed before inner cells; the row nearest the tunnel of Corti is damaged the earliest. The progression is then to the middle and lateral outer hair cell layers and finally to the inner hair cells. Along the length of the membrane the basal region sustains damage first, so that tonal gaps occur in the higher registers. Continued poisoning leads to progressive damage toward the apex, and the frequency cutoff moves to include the lower frequencies. For this reason, the use of -mycin antibiotics should be accompanied by close monitoring of auditory acuity. Other drugs that are ototoxic, although much less so than the -mycin drugs, are quinine and aspirin. There is reason to believe that drug and physical effects can be additive, so that even nontoxic doses of quinine or aspirin in a rock band artist may increase the damage.

Action Potentials of Auditory Nerve Fibers

The afferent endings on the base of the hair cells derive from bipolar cells in the spiral ganglion in the cochlear modiolus.

Their central processes emerge from the base of the cochlea as the cochlear nerve. Their distal processes travel through tunnels in the spiral lamina and emerge through fine perforations on its dorsal aspect just medial to the inner pillar of the tunnel of Corti, at which point they lose their myelin coats. About 95 per cent of these fibers directly innervate the local inner hair cells, 20 fibers to a cell (Fig. 18–13). The remaining 5 per cent cross under the tunnel to the outer part of the organ, turn at right angles, and pursue a spiral course along it. A single fiber may thus traverse a path as long as 0.6 to 0.7 mm; in its last 200 μm it gives off repeated branches to innervate about 10 outer hair cells. This surprising disproportion of innervation focuses attention on the richly innervated inner cells as opposed to the more numerous, but diffusely and sparsely innervated, outer cells. Both inner and outer hair cells also receive efferent terminals; these are discussed later.

By inserting microelectrodes into the cochlear nerve, one can record the activity of single afferent fibers and measure their responses to graded auditory stimuli of different frequencies. A surprising finding is that most auditory primary afferent fibers display a random "spontaneous" resting discharge (up to 100 spikes per second) even in a soundproof room and in the absence of any intentional auditory stimulation. This "idling" discharge is reminiscent of the prodigal spontaneous discharge of retinal elements in complete darkness. In both systems biologically significant messages appear to be superimposed on a background of random noise. Perhaps the leakage current postulated by Davis accounts for the "spontaneous" discharge.

When single fibers innervating limited portions of the organ of Corti are driven by different pure tones applied to the ear, each is found to respond to a band of frequencies, but the thresholds for discharge vary drastically within the band, with one frequency having the lowest threshold. That is, each unit has a preference for one "best frequency," and the best frequencies (as well as the breadth of the effective band) vary from unit to unit. The "tuning curves" of sixteen units are shown in Figure 18–14. Each curve is a V,

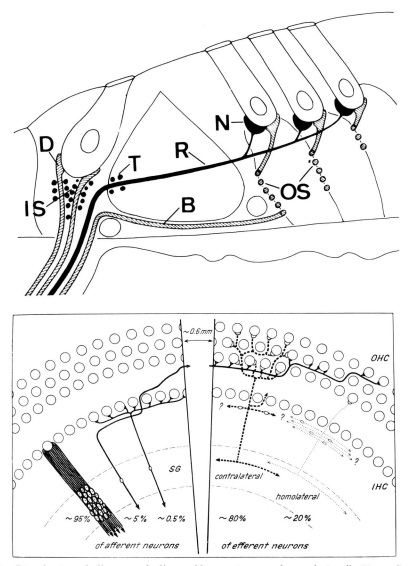

Figure 18–13. Distribution of afferent and efferent fibers to inner and outer hair cells. *Upper diagram,* Afferent fibers are crosshatched; efferent fibers, solid. *D,* direct afferent fibers to inner hair cells; *IS,* inner spiral efferent fibers; *I,* tunnel spiral efferent fibers; *R,* upper tunnel efferent fibers to outer hair cells (*N*); *B,* basal fibers (afferent); *OS,* outer spiral afferent fibers.

    Lower diagram, Quantitative distribution of afferent (*left*) and efferent (*right*) fibers to inner and outer hair cells. (*Upper diagram,* From Spoendlin, in *Basic mechanisms in hearing,* Møller, ed., New York, Academic Press, 1973. *Lower diagram,* From Spoendlin, Arch. klin. exp. Ohr-Nas-Kehlkopfheilkunde, 1971, *200,* 275–291.)

with the nadir representing the best frequency. It is reasonable to suppose that the different curves are from fibers supplying hair cells located at different sites along the basilar membrane. Parenthetically, it should be noted that the envelope connecting the best frequencies is a reasonable approximation of the normal audibility curve, an approximation that might be

expected to improve with the addition of more units.

Inhibition of Hair Cell Discharge; the Olivocochlear System

We have already mentioned that nerve endings at the base of hair cells are of two morphological types: small nonvesicular

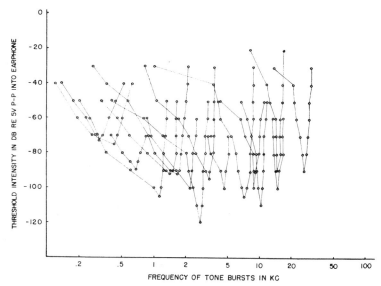

Figure 18–14. Tuning curves of 16 auditory nerve fibers from the cat. All tones within the triangle increased the firing of the unit, but the intensity required to alter unit firing varied sharply with frequency. The nadirs represent "best frequencies" of the units. (From Kiang *et al., Ann. Otol.* [St. Louis], 1962, *71*, 1009–1062.)

endings adjacent to accumulations of vesicles on the hair cell side and large endings containing vesicles. The location of the vesicles suggests that the former are afferent fibers and that the latter are efferent fibers ending on the receptors. Experimental analysis supports this conclusion.

Rasmussen first demonstrated the existence of efferent fibers in the cochlear nerve. They originate mainly from the cell bodies in the contralateral superior olive, cross the midline in the floor of the fourth ventricle at the level of the nucleus of cranial nerve VII to join the acoustic nerve, and run with it uninterruptedly through the spiral ganglion to the cochlea. Those distributed to the inner hair cells terminate on the bases of the receptors alongside the afferent terminals, whereas those destined for the outer hair cells bridge the tunnel of Corti and terminate *on the afferent fibers* near their point of contact with hair cells (Fig. 18–13). In addition to the crossed fibers, others arise from the ipsilateral olive; these constitute 20 to 25 per cent of the total and appear to be mainly distributed to inner hair cells. Both ipsilateral and contralateral fibers diverge extensively by branching to pro-

vide many terminal knobs; for the outer hair cells, which receive the more abundant efferent supply, some 40,000 knobs derive from about 500 crossed fibers in the olivocochlear bundle. Olivocochlear fibers respond to auditory stimuli applied to either ear, the threshold usually being 40 dB (SPL) or greater. Like afferent fibers they display tuned behavior and have a best frequency corresponding to that of the portion of the cochlea supplied.

Electrical stimulation of the efferent fibers where they cross in the medulla either blocks or reduces the neural response to auditory stimuli without depressing the microphonic. (In fact, the microphonic is somewhat increased in amplitude.) During stimulation of the bundle the threshold of individual primary elements is elevated from 1 to 25 dB, the depression being most striking in elements having best frequencies in the range of 6 to 10 kHz. Neural responses to auditory stimuli exceeding intensities of 70 dB are little influenced. For this reason it has been postulated that the efferent system plays a role in diminishing the masking effect of background noise, *i.e.*, it improves the signal-to-noise ratio when the signal is intense and the noise is low.

CENTRAL AUDITORY PATHWAYS

The primary auditory nerve fibers, upon entering the brainstem, promptly form synaptic connection with secondary neurons in the cochlear nuclei—the beginning of a remarkably complex and confusing network diffusing auditory input to a surprising number of central structures.

The cochlear nuclear complex occupies the dorsolateral portion of the medulla just caudal to the inferior cerebellar peduncle and comprises three nuclear groups: a dorsal nucleus and two ventral nuclei, the anteroventral and the posteroventral. Each receives input from the cochlea, and in each the projection is tonotopically organized, with the high frequencies represented dorsally and the low frequencies ventrally. That is, the tuning curves of dorsally located cells have higher best frequencies than do those of ventrally situated cells. The basilar membrane is thus faithfully projected onto the cochlear complex, not once, but three times, an extravagance of as yet unknown significance.

Beyond the cochlear nuclei the central auditory pathways become almost unbearably complex and puzzling, as summarized in the diagram in Figure 18–15. Basically, two sets of ascending projections arise from the secondary neurons of the cochlear neurons, a crossed and an uncrossed. The crossed path (the main one) arises from both ventral and dorsal nuclei and, crossing the midline in the trapezoid body, either enters the contralateral lateral lemniscus directly or relays in the nucleus of the trapezoid body or in the superior olive before projecting into the lateral lemniscus. The uncrossed pathway either projects directly into the ipsilateral lateral lemniscus or, like the contralateral path, relays in the superior olivary complex. The lateral lemniscus of each side thus contains crossed and uncrossed axons of second- and third-order neurons.

Lateral lemniscal fibers project either directly or indirectly (via relays in dorsal or ventral nuclei of the lateral lemniscus) onto the inferior colliculus, which is an obligatory relay site for all auditory fibers.

The cells of the inferior colliculus mainly project onto the medial geniculate body of the same side, but some cross in

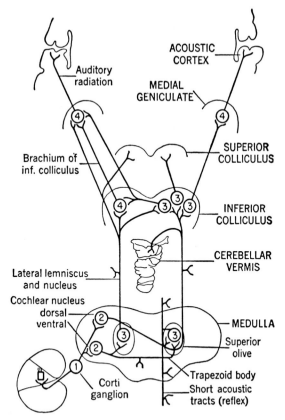

Figure 18–15. Central auditory pathways. Numbers label first-, second-, third-, and fourth-order neurons. (From Davis, in *Handbook of experimental psychology*, Stevens, ed., New York, John Wiley & Sons, 1951.)

the commissure of the inferior colliculus to reach the contralateral medial geniculate. The medial geniculate is another obligatory relay site; *i.e.*, all auditory fibers funnel through it. The medial geniculate cells send axons to the auditory cortex, located on the superior lip of the temporal lobe.

The functional properties of cells in each of the principal nuclei above the cochlear nucleus have been explored and at each site the cochlea is tonotopically represented at least twice. For example, two tonotopic organizations have been mapped in the superior olive, in the nuclei of the lateral lemniscus, in the inferior colliculus, and in the medial geniculate nucleus. Topping off this prodigal multiple representation of the cochlea is the projection to the auditory cortex; in the cat five separate tonotopically organized areas have been defined!

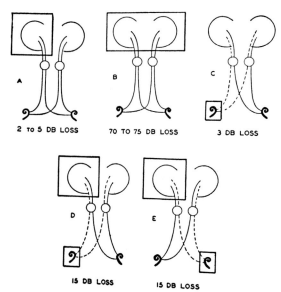

2 TO 5 DB LOSS   70 TO 75 DB LOSS   3 DB LOSS

15 DB LOSS   15 DB LOSS

Figure 18–16. Summary diagram of experiments in which hearing loss was measured after various lesions of the auditory cortex and the cochleae. The results indicate the extent to which bilateral representation "protects" hearing function from impairment by unilateral lesions. (After Stevens and Davis, *Hearing, its psychology and physiology*, New York, John Wiley & Sons, 1938.)

In summary, three principles of organization characterize the auditory system at each level of its course from cochlea to cortex: (1) tonotopic organization, (2) multiplicity of tonotopic representation, each level comprising from two to five separate maps of the cochlea, and (3) extensive bilateral representation as a result of crossing and recrossing of fibers.

The significance of these remarkable features is unknown, but they provide fertile ground for speculation. First, the redundancy provided by multiple representation and bilaterality unquestionably provides security of transmission of auditory information. Where, for example, could a discrete lesion be placed in the brainstem that would alter sensitivity to

high-frequency tones? The answer is nowhere (Fig. 18–16). Because of multiple and bilateral representation of the cochlea, a lesion large enough to interrupt all high-frequency information from the cochlea would be so devastating that the hearing defect would be a relatively minor neurological consideration.

Simple hearing functions such as threshold sensitivity, recognition of pure tones, frequency discrimination, and intensity discrimination are not severely impaired by rather large experimental lesions of central auditory structures (Fig. 18–16). However, some complex discriminations are not completely protected by the redundancy of representation. For example, cortical lesions (albeit large ones) do disrupt discriminations of patterned sequences of tonal stimuli. In man, speech perception is sensitive to central lesions. Finally, discriminations requiring interpretation of binaural stimuli are disturbed by central neural lesions. Of the simpler behaviors in this category, sound localization has been studied most extensively, mainly because it is relatively easy to investigate in laboratory animals.

Sounds are localized by two cues: difference in arrival time (or phase) of sounds at the two ears and difference in intensity on the two sides. In the cat a discrete lesion of the trapezoid body impairs the animal's ability to use difference in arrival time as a cue for localization. A unilateral lesion of the lateral lemniscus disrupts the animal's ability to localize sounds from differential intensity cues. Finally, either a lesion transecting the projection from the inferior colliculus or a unilateral lesion of auditory cortex deprives the animal of the capacity to "appreciate the directionality of a sound source." In this respect it is interesting to recall that the major effect of a postcentral cortical lesion on somatosensory function in man is a disturbance of spatial discrimination and localization.

ADDITIONAL READING

Davis, H., and Silverman, S. R. *Hearing and deafness.* 3rd edition, New York, Holt, Rinehart, and Winston, 1970.

Goldstein, M. H., Jr. The auditory periphery, in *Medical physiology*, Mountcastle, V. B., ed., St. Louis, The C. V. Mosby Co., 1974.

Møller, A. R. *Basic mechanisms in hearing.* New York, Academic Press, 1973.

Towe, A. L. Audition and the auditory pathway, in *Physiology and biophysics*, Ruch, T. C., and Patton, H. D., eds., Philadelphia, W. B. Saunders Co., 1965.

CHAPTER 19

SUPRASEGMENTAL CONTROL OF MOVEMENT

WAYNE E. CRILL

INTRODUCTION TO THE MOTOR SYSTEMS

The segmental and peripheral apparatus underlying movement are discussed in Chapters 6, 9, and 10. In this and in the next two chapters we will look at the control of movement by higher neurostructures.

In man, the motor units and segmental reflex pathways necessary for coordinated voluntary movement and maintenance of posture are largely under the control of suprasegmental structures. This increasing importance of suprasegmental structures in higher animals is called *encephalization* of the nervous system. The term *motor systems* is usually reserved for the descending pathways of the cerebral cortex and brainstem, along with the basal ganglia and cerebellum. These are the structures that will be discussed in this portion of the text. Nevertheless, it should be appreciated that both at the segmental and at higher levels, major afferent pathways project to these motor structures and are necessary for normal motor function. Some inputs, such as the I_a afferent fibers, are part of the negative feedback control system, in this instance, to keep muscle length constant. The afferent inputs to higher motor structures subserve more complex functions, which we are just beginning to understand. It is clear that normal motor behavior requires continuous information about the status of the motor apparatus (muscle length and so forth), body position, and its relationship to the outside world.

Figure 19–1 shows a highly schematic but useful first view of the motor systems. The descending suprasegmental pathways originate in either the cerebral cortex or the brainstem. Most of the brainstem pathways projecting to the spinal cord also receive input from the cerebral cortex. The basal ganglia (Chap. 20) and the cere-

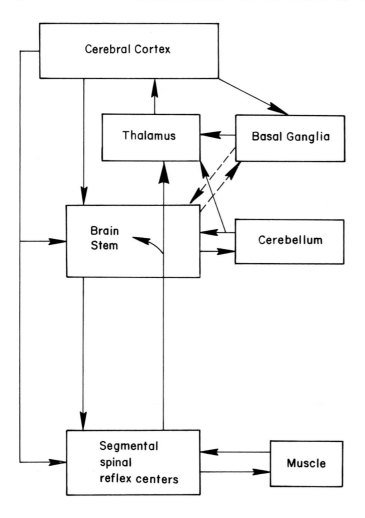

Figure 19–1. A highly schematic flow diagram of the motor systems. The arrows should not be taken to represent direct monosynaptic connections.

bellum (Chap. 21) are two large supra-segmental structures that do not directly project to the segmental motor apparatus. These two large portions of the motor systems process information from other parts of the nervous system and project back to the sites of origin of the descending suprasegmental pathways in the cerebral cortex and brainstem. The importance of the basal ganglia and the cerebellum in motor behavior is illustrated by the spectacular deficits in motor control that occur when these structures are damaged either experimentally or by disease.

DESCENDING SUPRASEGMENTAL PATHWAYS

As we can see in Figure 19–1, the cerebral cortex can influence motoneurons and

segmental structures by several pathways: directly by the corticospinal and corticobulbar pathways, and indirectly through descending tracts originating in the brainstem, *i.e.,* the rubrospinal, the vestibulospinal, and the reticulospinal tracts.

The Corticospinal and Corticobulbar Tracts

The corticospinal and corticobulbar tracts are the only direct pathways projecting from the cerebral cortex to segmental interneuron and motoneuron pools in the brainstem and spinal cord. The fibers have their cell bodies in the cerebral cortex; the axons pass through the corona radiata and are somatotopically organized in the internal capsule (Fig. 19–2). The cortico-

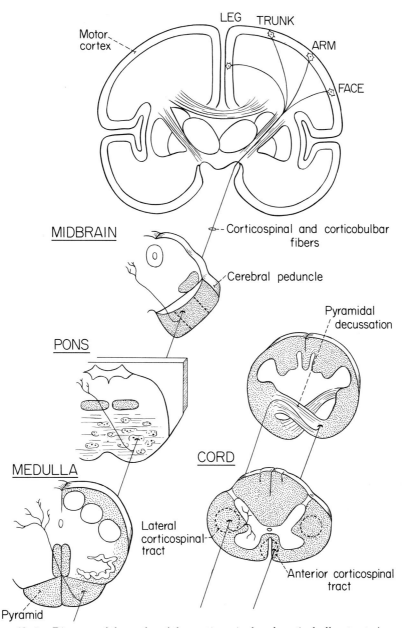

Figure 19–2. Diagram of the paths of the corticospinal and corticobulbar tracts in man.

bulbar fibers are near the knee of the capsule, and the corticospinal fibers pass nearby through the posterior limb of the capsule. The corticospinal fibers pass successively through the middle two thirds of the ipsilateral cerebral peduncle, the basis pontis, and the medullary pyramid. At the caudal end of the pyramid, the majority of the fibers cross the midline and enter the lateral column of the spinal cord to form the lateral corticospinal tract. The other fibers do not cross in the pyramidal decussation but descend in the ventral column of the spinal cord as a ventral, or anterior, corticospinal tract. These fibers ultimately cross the midplane at spinal segmental levels and terminate in the gray matter of spinal cord segments. Very few fibers in the anterior corticospinal tract descend below the level of the thoracic spinal cord.

In the brainstem, the corticobulbar fibers swing dorsally and cross the midline near the level of the motor nuclei of the cranial nerves that they innervate. A general pattern emerges. The corticobulbar and corticospinal fibers that originate in the contralateral cerebral cortex supply input to all spinal and most cranial nerve motoneuron pools. On the basis of anatomical, physiological, and clinical evidence there is no difference between the cortical input to brainstem motoneuron nuclei and that to spinal motoneuron pools. Thus, these two pathways are often collectively referred to as the *pyramidal tract*, although strictly speaking the term should refer only to those fibers passing through the medullary pyramids.

In addition the corticobulbar fibers originating from both ipsilateral and contralateral cortex supply input to many brainstem motoneurons, notably the motoneurons of the nucleus ambiguous (which innervates the pharyngeal muscles) and the motoneurons of the facial nucleus that innervate the muscles of the upper face. This is presumed to be the reason that a unilateral corticobulbar lesion causes weakness of the lower face and tongue but not of the frontalis and pharyngeal muscles.

In humans, the pyramidal tract contains approximately one million fibers. Sixty per cent of the fibers originate anterior to the central sulcus (Brodmann areas 8, 6, and 4); the rest are from the parietal lobe (Brodmann areas 3, 1, 2, 5, and 7). Although most (94 per cent of) pyramidal tract fibers are myelinated, only 10 per cent are larger than 4 μm in diameter, and only 2 per cent originate from Betz cells and therefore have axons larger than 10 μm in diameter (Fig. 19–3). Thus, most of the pyramidal tract fibers are relatively small, myelinated fibers coming from broad areas of frontal and parietal cortex around the central sulcus.

In primates, fibers from the parietal lobe (classic sensory areas) terminate more dorsally in the spinal gray matter than do fibers from the frontal lobe (motor areas). Only the largest pyramidal tract fibers, probably those from Betz cells of the frontal lobe, make direct monosynaptic connections with the motoneurons. In the

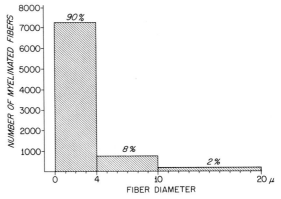

Figure 19–3. Histogram of the spectrum of myelinated fibers in the pyramidal tract. (After Lassek, *J. comp. Neurol.*, 1942, *76*, 217–225.)

cat few, if any, pyramidal tract axons project directly to alpha motoneurons. Moreover, the monosynaptic connections of corticospinal fibers are primarily · with alpha motoneurons that innervate muscles in the distal portions of the extremity, that is, those muscles that are used in the most precise and fine types of movements. These connections are excitatory.

The pyramidal tract also influences more widely distributed muscles in the extremities, acting through segmental internuncial neurons. Those muscles that are used to resist the effects of gravity (the physiologic extensors) are inhibited, and the physiologic flexors are excited by pyramidal tract stimulation. Thus, through segmental connections those portions of the pyramidal tract that are concerned with voluntary movement can overcome segmental postural mechanisms and at the same time exert some excitatory influence on the muscles used for fine motor behavior. Like other descending suprasegmental pathways, the pyramidal tract also has an effect upon fusimotor neurons. Although there are minor exceptions, the general rule for both the pyramidal tract and other descending pathways is that descending pathways influence both the alpha motor and fusimotor neurons going to a given muscle in a similar fashion.

It should be evident from this discussion that the corticospinal tract is not a homogeneous tract with one physiological function. It is composed of several populations of fibers differing in both size and site of origin in the cerebral cortex. Different groups of fibers project to functionally different neuron pools at the segmental levels. In addition, collateral fibers from pyramidal tract axons project to many brainstem nuclei, such as the red nucleus, the pontine nuclei, and the inferior olivary nucleus, all of which are part of the cerebellar systems. Some pyramidal tract fibers modulate afferent input transmitted through relays, such as the dorsal column nuclei and neurons in the dorsal horn. To assume that the pyramidal tract is the sole pathway serving voluntary movement is as unrealistic as the opposite opinion that the corticospinal tract is not concerned with voluntary movement at all. The largest fibers, which directly connect with motoneurons, are probably concerned with fine, agile finger movements. It is interesting that monosynaptic connections with alpha motoneurons by pyramidal tract axons occurs only in primates and in lower mammals that have a fair amount of digital dexterity, such as the raccoon and kinkajou.

One of the best ways to examine the role of the pyramidal tract in motor behavior is to cut it selectively. In experimental animals this is relatively easily accomplished at the medullary level, where the tract is isolated. In man the commonest lesions are due to vascular accidents, which rarely destroy the tract selectively. Bucy approximated the pyramidotomized state in humans by cutting the fibers in the middle third of the cerebral peduncle to relieve hemiballismus. The results from these neurosurgical procedures are similar to those following transection of the pyramidal tract at the level of the medullary pyramid in normal chimpanzees. Immediately after the transection there is a profound contralateral hemiparesis. However, after about 10 days and continuing often for several months, there is progressive recovery, to the point at which the patient has difficulty only in moving individual fingers, with little other detectible impairment of motor activity. In humans and chimpanzees there is a slight increase in muscle tone. This is not of the magnitude frequently seen in patients with larger, more poorly defined lesions of the

descending pathways. The superficial abdominal reflex (contraction of the abdominal muscles following cutaneous stimulation of the abdomen) is absent; so is the cremasteric reflex (contraction of the cremaster muscle evoked by stroking of the inside of the thigh). The *Babinski sign* is present, that is, dorsal flexion of the great toe evoked by a noxious stimulus applied to the lateral aspect of the sole of the foot. The normal response is plantar flexion of all the toes. The Babinski sign is one of the most important physical signs in neurology and specifically indicates dysfunction of the pyramidal tract. Because the pyramidal tract does not complete its myelination until about one year of age, the Babinski sign is normally present during the first year of life. The above findings are all contralateral to the side of the sectioned pyramid or peduncle.

The role of the pyramidal tract can also be evaluated by stimulation experiments. For example, Woolsey and his colleagues sectioned one pyramidal tract in monkeys and then studied the effects of electrical stimulation of the precentral (motor) cortex in these animals. For the cortex ipsilateral to the sectioned pyramidal tract, the threshold for stimulus evoked movement was increased. Also no distal movements could be evoked from the cortex with no pyramidal connections to spinal segments.

For a variety of reasons, none of which is supported by experimental evidence, clinicians have assumed that the bulk if not all of the descending suprasegmental fibers concerned with voluntary movement are located in the pyramidal tract. An infarction in the internal capsule that disrupts most of the descending suprasegmental pathways from the cerebral cortex causes an intense hemiparesis, usually associated with severe spasticity. This symptom complex is often referred to in the clinic as the *pyramidal syndrome*. It is true that *part* of this syndrome—the Babinski sign and the loss of the abdominal reflex, the cremasteric reflex, and fine voluntary movements—can be correctly attributed to a lesion involving the pyramidal tract fibers. The rest of the syndrome, the severe paralysis and the marked spasticity, must be attributed to lesions in other descending pathways, which we will discuss later. This misuse of the term *pyramidal syndrome* has led to the use of another imprecise term in the clinic — the *extrapyramidal syndrome,* or *extrapyramidal signs.* The clinician often uses this term to refer to abnormal motor movements and changes in motor tone primarily associated with lesions of the basal ganglia (discussed in the next chapter). Specifically the extrapyramidal system comprises all of the motor systems except the pyramidal tract; thus, it includes the descending pathways originating in the brainstem, the basal ganglia, and the cerebellum. Since very different signs and symptoms are associated with disease processes localized in each one of these structures, there can be no single extrapyramidal syndrome. It is best not to use this term at all but to refer to the areas of the brain that we know cause specific signs and symptoms on the basis of good clinical pathological correlations and experimental procedures in animals.

The Rubrospinal Tract

The red nucleus is located in the tegmentum of the midbrain dorsomedial to the cerebral peduncles and the substantia nigra. Its name comes from its fleshy red color in the freshly cut brain. The axons of large neurons in this nucleus cross the midline of the neuroaxis at the level of the red nucleus and pass down the lateral brainstem into the lateral column of the spinal cord, forming the rubrospinal tract. The rubrospinal fibers are extensively intermingled with the corticospinal fibers in the lateral column of the spinal cord. They do not make direct connections with motoneurons but end on interneurons closely associated with motoneurons in the lateral portion of the ventral gray matter of the anterior horn. Excitation of the rubrospinal tract facilitates both alpha and gamma motoneurons projecting primarily to flexor muscles mostly in the distal portions of the extremity.

Lawrence and Kuypers showed in monkeys (that had sustained but recovered from pyramidotomy) that cutting the rubrospinal tract leads to almost complete paralysis of the distal musculature but has little effect upon strength of the axial muscles.

Neurons in the red nucleus receive input from the cerebellar nuclei, particularly the interpositus nucleus, and from the cerebral cortex, largely via collaterals of the pyramidal tract axons. Thus, this is one indirect pathway that has a significant influence upon activity at the segmental spinal level that receives major input from the cerebral cortex and from structures that control movement, such as the cerebellum. The distribution of the terminals of the rubrospinal tract axons and their effect upon motoneurons innervating different types of muscles are remarkably similar to those of the corticospinal tract. For example, both systems facilitate motoneurons (both alpha and gamma) innervating flexor muscles and inhibit motoneurons projecting to extensor, or antigravity, muscles.

There is no well-defined clinical syndrome related to selective destruction of the rubrospinal tract. The severe hemiparesis resulting from lesions of the internal capsule is undoubtedly partly due to disruption of corticorubral pathways. The severe ipsilateral paralysis below the level of lesions in the lateral columns of the spinal cord also is partially due to interruption of the descending rubrospinal pathways.

The Vestibulospinal Tracts

Two subdivisions of the vestibular nuclei send projections from the brainstem to the spinal cord. The major pathway originates from the *lateral vestibular nucleus* (Deiter's nucleus) and passes caudally in the ventromedial brainstem to the anterior column of the spinal cord. This pathway does not cross the midline. The *lateral vestibulospinal tract* makes synaptic connections with ipsilateral interneurons and alpha and gamma motoneurons on the ipsilateral side of the anterior horn. These are the motoneurons that innervate axial muscles. Stimulation of the lateral vestibulospinal tract excites motoneurons innervating extensor muscles and inhibits those projecting to flexor muscles. There is no significant input from the cerebral cortex to the lateral vestibular nucleus. The major inputs to this nucleus come from the cerebellum and vestibular system. It is the only nucleus outside the cerebellum that receives direct input from Purkinje cells of the cerebellar cortex. In addition, the midline cerebellar nuclei also project to the lateral vestibular nucleus (see Chapter 21).

The descending fibers from the *medial vestibular nucleus* are often referred to as the *medial vestibulospinal tract*. Fibers from this nucleus can only be followed as far as the midthoracic area. They pass bilaterally down the most medial portion of the anterior columns of the spinal cord. It appears that their major function is to influence the neck and spinal muscles.

The Reticulospinal Tracts

Two well-defined areas of the lower brainstem, one in the pons and the other in the medulla, are the origin of descending reticulospinal pathways. The *pontine reticulospinal pathway* projects to spinal segments ipsilaterally in the ventral portion of the spinal cord. These fibers excite alpha and gamma motoneurons of extensor muscles. The *medullary reticulospinal pathway* projects bilaterally in the lateral spinal columns.

THE CEREBRAL CORTEX

The cortical control of movement in man and other higher animals has received particular attention in the clinic and the research laboratory for over a hundred years. In 1870 Fritsch and Hitzig first demonstrated in the dog that electrical stimulation of the cerebral cortex evokes movements. These studies were rapidly extended to subhuman primates by the famous British physiologist David Ferrier, working at the West Riding Lunatic Asylum. In this century the general pattern of responses was confirmed in humans by Penfield.

Those areas of cortex in some way related to movement are often called *motor cortex*. This term is often used without definition. A precise definition requires

many qualifications. The area from which movement can be evoked by electrical stimulation depends upon the stimulus parameters and the level of anesthesia. These regions do not necessarily correlate with the findings after lesions. It is true, however, that the precentral cortex has the lowest threshold to electrical stimulation.

Throughout the last hundred years, beginning with the incisive reasoning of the famous English neurologist Hughlings Jackson, the concept has evolved of a cerebral cortical area that is the major final output for voluntary movement from the cerebral hemisphere, projecting to brainstem motor centers (*e.g.*, red nucleus, reticular nuclei) and brainstem and spinal cord segmental structures. On the basis of clinical-pathological correlations and stimulation studies, this area is in the precentral regions of the frontal lobe. The motor cortex is not necessary for all types of movements: both simple and complex types of reflex motor behavior are possible when this area has been destroyed, but in humans voluntary movement requires it. It is not the area where the neurocircuitry for complex coordinated movements is located (if such an area exists at all), nor the area where the initial neural impulses leading to movement originate. The motor cortex is not just a simple neural relay to other descending systems of the segmental motor apparatus.

The objective of the neuroscientist interested in the motor cortex has been to understand the exact nature of the relationship of this part of the brain to movement. To do so, we must know the spatial and synaptic organization of the motor cortex, the interconnections it has with other parts of the brain and lower motor centers, and the behavior of the neurons in these regions during various types of movement. The following is a synthesis of the evidence available that is related to these questions.

Somatotopic Organization

Both lesion and stimulation studies indicate that the motor cortex is somatotopically organized; that is, different cortical regions ultimately project (often through many relays) to motoneurons innervating muscles in a spatially restricted part of the body. Moreover, the general spatial relationship among these cortical areas is similar to the spatial relationship among the muscles.

The most lateral parts of the precentral cortical regions influence facial muscles, and the medial parts of the hemispheres are concerned with leg movement. Between the face and leg regions are the areas related to voluntary movement of trunk and upper extremity. Moreover, the parts of the body with the most precise motor movement—tongue, mouth, hands, and feet—are represented in the motor cortex more posteriorly (in and near the central sulcus) than is the trunk. Finally, the areas responsible for evoking tongue, mouth, thumb, and hand movements are larger than those responsible for movements of the proximal extremities and trunk. The pattern of organization is illustrated in Figure 19–4. Experimentally produced lesions in similar areas cause deficits in the appropriate structures.

It must be emphasized, however, that the superimposed homunculus represents an oversimplification of the motor organization of the precentral cortex. For example, it was recognized by Hughlings Jackson that destructive lesions cause a loss of the most "voluntary functions"; that is, a lesion in the arm area is always associated with profound weakness in the thumb and hand. The amount of distal weakness and the extent of involvement of more proximal structures in the extremity reflect the size of a cortical lesion. A lesion under the shoulder area of the homunculus illustrated in Figure 19–4 *does not* cause selective weakness of the shoulder muscles. Similarly, seizure activity beginning in the upper arm area of the motor cortex does not lead to convulsive movements of shoulder muscles first but rather to convulsive movements involving the thumb and hand. This illustrates the complex nature and detailed fine organization of the motor cortex and must be kept in mind when data from physiological stimulation experiments are presented.

As expected from this discussion, experimental studies on high subhuman primates have shown wide fields of repre-

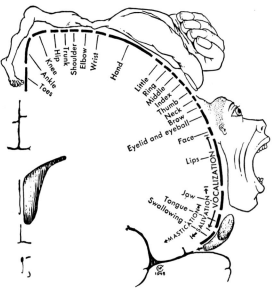

Figure 19–4. The locations and relative sizes of parts of the human motor cortex from which movements of different parts of the body can be elicited by electrical stimulation. (From Penfield and Rasmussen, *The cerebral cortex of man*, New York, The Macmillan Co., 1950.)

sentation for movements of the thumbs, index fingers, feet, and face. It has been concluded that the low-threshold projections from the motor cortex preferentially excite motoneurons causing these movements. It should also be noted that in most animals the major movements evoked by cortical stimulation are flexion type movements of the distal extremity.

For a more detailed insight into the organization of pathways projecting from the motor cortex, investigators have studied the effects of electrical stimulation of the descending suprasegmental pathways upon individual motoneurons. Phillips and Porter formulated the concept of colonies of corticomotoneuronal units on the basis of their examination of monosynaptic EPSP's produced in motoneurons by cortical stimulation. These effects must be carried only by the relatively few large fibers in the pyramidal tract that make direct connections to motoneurons, that is, by a very small percentage of the total descending suprasegmental motor fibers. They found that cortical colonies projecting to distal motoneurons of the forearm and hand muscles evoked much larger

EPSP's in the motoneurons supplying forearm and hand muscles than in other motoneurons. In some instances no direct effect from cortical stimulation could be found in motoneurons projecting to proximal muscles of the extremity. In addition, corticomotoneuronal colonies projecting to the motoneurons of distal muscles tended to occupy smaller cortical territories than did those projecting to the motoneurons of proximal muscles. During neurosurgical procedures under local anesthesia it is possible to stimulate the cerebral cortex in conscious man and observe the response and also to obtain introspective reports from the subject. Cortical stimulation in man evokes discrete movements that are usually not associated with a subjective desire to move.

Our understanding of the physiological nature of cells in the motor cortex has been expanded by the recent development of techniques that allow extracellular recording from single cortical neurons in fully conscious, behaving animals. Evarts pioneered the use of these techniques in investigations of the pyramidal tract neurons in animals. He found that large pyramidal tract neurons identified by antidromic stimulation tended to fire phasically with active movement of the animal's contralateral arm, whereas the smaller, more slowly conducting pyramidal tract neurons tended to fire tonically. By using techniques that enabled him to dissociate the position of the wrist during simple flexion extension movements from the force exerted by flexor and extensor muscles, he was able to show a high correlation between the frequency of discharge of pyramidal tract neurons and the force exerted by a particular muscle. Records from single neurons in the motor cortex from a number of laboratories indicate that, in general, activity in neurons of the precentral cortex begins from 60 to 80 msec earlier than the movement.

SPINAL TRANSECTION

The importance of suprasegmental descending pathways upon segmental circuits may be observed clinically and experimentally when they are disconnected by a complete spinal cord transection. Immediately after spinal cord transection in man, all voluntary motor activity in the parts of the body innervated by the segments below the section is lost. All sensation from the isolated segments is abolished. In addition, the reflexes served by the segments below the transection disappear for a variable period of time. Stretching muscles passively and tapping tendons no longer cause reflex contraction of muscles. Noxious stimuli applied to the skin do not evoke flexion responses. This condition of areflexia is called *spinal shock.*

The duration of spinal shock is a function of cerebral dominance, which is closely related to an animal's position on the phylogenetic scale. For example, if the spinal cord is cut in amphibians, reflex depression is barely detectable, whereas in carnivores spinal shock may last an hour or so. In humans the reflexes are depressed for several weeks.

The excitability of central neurons is determined by the summed effect of tonic activities in hundreds or thousands of synaptic terminals, some excitatory and others inhibitory. The existence of areflexia after spinal transection illustrates that the *net effect* of disconnecting descending pathways is to remove excitation at the motoneuron level. Even synchronous activity of excitatory I_a fibers from muscle spindles evoked by sudden stretching of a muscle no longer can excite motoneurons.

With time the depression of segmental reflexes disappears. Usually, the first reflexes to return after a period of spinal shock are the flexion reflexes mediated by polysynaptic pathways. One of the earliest reflexes to appear is the Babinski sign. With time the flexion reflexes evoked by cutaneous stimulation become more prominent. In many cases relatively mild cutaneous stimulation below the level of the transection evokes massive flexion of the legs and emptying of the bowel and bladder (mass reflex). There is some evidence that mass reflexes are less of a problem in patients receiving meticulous nursing care and therefore not suffering from either skin pressure ulcers or urinary tract infections.

Along with the appearance of the flexion reflexes, stretch reflexes become moderately brisk and are often associated with other signs of spasticity: the clasp-knife response, clonus, and brisk tendon jerks. In spinal lesions the excitability of stretch reflexes, although clearly exaggerated, never reaches the magnitude seen with some higher lesions (decerebrate). In man, long after the disappearance of spinal shock there is a greater increase in flexion reflexes than in stretch reflexes.

In addition to the extensive effects on somatic motor and sensory function by spinal transection, widespread alterations occur in visceral functions. After transection, the bladder wall becomes atonic. This is associated with increased sphincter tone. The continued production of urine leads to extensive dilatation of the bladder, until intravesicular pressure overcomes sphincter resistance. Progressive increase in bladder wall tone is associated temporally with the return of somatic reflexes. At this stage reflex bladder contraction overcomes sphincter tone, and emptying of the bladder may be evoked by cutaneous stimulation.

The control of vasomotor reflexes by segments below the transection is also lost during the period of spinal shock. With time tonic automatic activity returns and postural hypotension is less of a problem.

Spinal transection also eliminates the effective use of the portions of the body innervated by segments below the level of the transection for temperature control.

BRAINSTEM LESIONS

The functional relationship between the descending suprasegmental pathways from cerebral structures and various levels of the brainstem is illustrated by lesions in the brainstem. Complete transection at the lower medullary level causes changes in spinal segmental functions similar to those produced by complete spinal cord transection. This lesion also interrupts areas of the brain controlling respiration and is usually not compatible with survival unless ventilatory support is available.

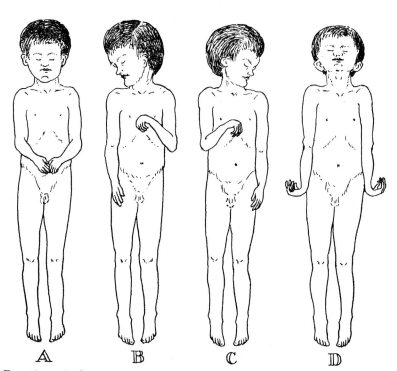

Figure 19–5. Decorticate rigidity in man: *A,* decorticate posturing; *B* and *C,* tonic neck reflexes; *D,* decerebrate posturing. (From Fulton, ed., *A textbook of physiology,* Philadelphia, W. B. Saunders Co., 1955.)

Section of the brainstem at the inter-collicular level, the classic decerebrate lesion of Sherrington, produces almost immediate extensor rigidity in animals. The animal can stand but shows no dynamic response to forces that tend to disturb posture. A slight push will easily topple the animal. Humans with similar lesions also show the syndrome of decere-brate rigidity. The legs, arms, and neck are hyperextended, and the arms are also hyperpronated (Fig. 19–5). It can be shown that decerebrate rigidity requires afferent input at the segmental level. Sec-tion of the dorsal roots in the decerebrate animal causes flaccidity. More detailed in-vestigation of this segmental input reveals that the afferent input must come from the muscle, not the cutaneous structures. To produce these changes, the decerebrate lesion must either remove tonic inhibition or cause increased excitation of segmental stretch reflexes involving extensor alpha motoneurons, or both. Pathways responsi-ble for this change in excitatory—inhibitory balance must be located between the mid-brain and the lower medulla. Serial hemi-sections of the brainstem at progressively lower levels reveals that, once either the lower pons or the upper medulla is hemi-sected, decerebrate rigidity disappears. This occurs on the same side as the lesion. Available evidence indicates that the hemisection lesion disconnects the lateral vestibulospinal and pontine reticulospinal pathways for the segmental level. Recall that both pathways are excitatory to pools of motoneurons innervating extensor muscles and project ipsilaterally to the segmental level. Thus, the midbrain inter-collicular lesion removes tonic inhibition of those brainstem pathways having a net excitatory effect on extensor motoneuron pools.

Decerebrate animals also show postural reflexes (the *tonic neck reflexes*). Rotation of the head on the body increases extension of the arm and leg on the side to which the chin is turned and decreases extensor rigidity of the extremities of the other side (Fig. 19–5). Extension of the neck in-creases extension of the forelimbs and causes relative relaxation of the hind limbs. The reverse occurs with ventro-flexion of the neck. Similar responses are often seen in patients with severe bilateral cerebral lesions.

In addition to classic spasticity, both decerebrate humans and animals display paroxysms of hyperextension of the ex-tremities when both extensor and flexor muscles become rigid. These waves of decerebrate rigidity are often called *decerebrate fits*, or sometimes *cerebellar fits*. There is no evidence that they are epileptic in nature. They can easily be precipitated by noxious stimuli, such as supraorbital pressure or occlusion of the airway. A possible explanation is that noxious stimuli may bilaterally activate the tonic neck re-flexes.

Higher lesions in humans, at the level of the internal capsule or following de-struction of the cerebral cortex, cause postural changes that are often referred to as *decorticate posturing*. When the lesion is in the internal capsule the signs are con-tralateral to the lesion, whereas with diffuse laminar necrosis of the cerebral cortex the signs are bilateral. The de-corticate posture in humans is character-ized by flexion of the elbow and wrist and metacarpophalangeal drawings, but usu-ally extension of the interphalangeal joints. These patients also show marked spasticity.

CLINICAL–PATHOLOGICAL CORRELATIONS

Most diseases that affect the nervous system can interrupt the descending suprasegmental motor pathways. The major signs of lesions in these pathways are weakness or paresis of voluntary motor behavior. In addition, the physician ex-amines the tone of the muscle at rest and in response to passive stretch; he tests the muscle response to phasic stretch evoked by tapping of the tendon with a reflex hammer; and he looks for changes in motor reflexes evoked by cutaneous stimu-lation.

Lesions at various levels of the neuroaxis cause different patterns of abnormalities. For example, early in the course of their illnesses, patients with low brainstem or spinal lesions often may complain of spontaneous or evoked flexion responses in the legs. Decerebrate posturing indicates dysfunction at the upper brainstem level, and decorticate posturing suggests a higher lesion.

Lesions of the descending suprasegmental pathways cause most weakness in the distal muscles of the extremity, those used for the most voluntary functions, to paraphrase Hughlings Jackson. Since these lesions are likely to interrupt the corticospinal tract, the Babinski sign and loss of abdominal and cremasteric reflexes are often present.

Major conclusions about the site of the lesion can also be made on the basis of the distribution of the motor involvement. Brainstem and spinal cord lesions often cause bilateral motor impairment, since the descending pathways going to each side of the body are relatively close together below the pons. For example, motor involvement of both legs should prompt suspicion of a lesion somewhere in the thoracic spinal cord. (However, such a deficit can be caused also by a midline cortical lesion affecting the medial aspects of the motor cortex in both cerebral hemispheres.) Obviously, the presence of suprasegmental motor deficits in the facial muscles means that the lesion must be above the level of the pons. Lesions at the level of the cerebral peduncles and higher often cause weakness only on the contralateral side of the body, producing a hemiparesis (weakness) or hemiplegia (paralysis).

Although the postural changes and distribution of the motor deficit are extremely valuable in localizing the site of the lesion, the most valuable signs are those indicating direct involvement of segmental structures. These signs result from the direct involvement of cranial nerve nuclei or fibers, or spinal segmental structures. For example, a patient with a lesion in one cerebral peduncle will show a contralateral hemiparesis involving face, arm, and leg. The same lesion often interrupts the fibers of the third cranial nerve, which leaves the brainstem at this level. Thus, the presence of the hemiparesis in addition to a contralateral third-nerve palsy allows the physician to locate the lesion precisely in the midbrain. Spinal cord lesions frequently cause suprasegmental signs below the lesion and segmental signs (muscular atrophy or loss of stretch reflexes) at the level of the lesion.

ADDITIONAL READING

Lawrence, D. G., and Kuypers, H. G.   The functional organization of the motor system in the monkey. I. The effects of bilateral pyramidal lesions. *Brain,* 1968, *91,* 1–36.

Phillips, C. G.   The Ferrier lecture: Motor apparatus of the baboon's head. *Proc. roy. Soc. (Lond.),* 1969, Ser. B, *173,* 141–174.

Porter, R.   Functions of the mammalian cerebral cortex in movement. *Prog. Neurobiol.,* 1973, *1,* 1–51.

Wiesendanger, M.   The pyramidal tract. Recent investigations on its morphology and function. *Ergebn. Physiol.,* 1969, *61,* 72–135.

THE BASAL GANGLIA

WAYNE E. CRILL

ANATOMY

Over the years the term *basal ganglia* has been applied to many different subcortical nuclei in the cerebral hemisphere, even the thalamus. Now the term is reserved for specific gray masses both deep in the cerebral hemispheres and in the upper brainstem. The basal ganglia include the caudate nucleus, putamen, globus pallidus (pallidum), claustrum, subthalamic nucleus, and substantia nigra (Fig. 20–1). The caudate, putamen, pallidum, and claustrum have a streaked appearance in myelin-stained sections and are therefore called the *striate body*, or *corpus striatum*. Together the putamen and globus pallidus often are referred to as the *lentiform nuclei* because

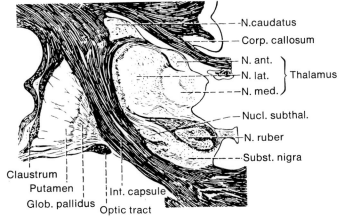

Figure 20–1. Coronal section through the basal ganglia, thalamus, internal capsule, and upper brainstem. Stained for myelin. (From Brodal, *Neurological anatomy in relation to clinical medicine*, New York, Oxford University Press, 1969.)

N.caudatus
Corp. callosum
N. ant.
N. lat. } Thalamus
N. med.
Nucl. subthal.
N. ruber
Subst. nigra

Claustrum
Putamen
Glob. pallidus
Int. capsule
Optic tract

281

of their lenslike shape. However, a more meaningful grouping is based on the histology and phylogenetic development of the basal ganglia. The caudate nucleus and putamen have a similar pale gross appearance and histological structure. Both of these nuclei have appeared relatively recently in terms of the phylogenetic development of the brain, and they are both derived from the telencephalon. The caudate nucleus and putamen are called the *neostriatum*, or sometimes just *striatum*, whereas the phylogenetically earlier-appearing pallidum develops from the basal plate of the neural tube and is referred to as the *paleostriatum*.

The internal capsule separates the medially placed caudate nucleus and the laterally placed putamen, except at their anterior-inferior extremes. The claustrum is just medial to the insular cortex and separated from the putamen by a thin band of white matter, called the *external capsule*. The subthalamic nucleus is medial to the internal capsule and ventral to the thalamus. The substantia nigra is darkly pigmented in the freshly cut brain and located dorsomedial to the cerebral peduncle. Its dark color is due to melanin pigment in large neurons.

Our knowledge of the connections between elements of the basal ganglia is in many aspects incomplete. Where the anatomical data are reliable, great complexity is indicated. The fine details need not plague us here, but there is a general pattern of connections that is important. It was once thought that the basal ganglia are major relays in the multisynaptic descending suprasegmental pathways leading from cortex to spinal cord and brainstem segments. The concept is not supported by recent anatomical studies.

The major connections through the basal ganglia are from cerebral cortex to caudate and putamen, to globus pallidus, to thalamus, and back to motor and premotor cerebral cortex. All parts of the cerebral cortex project to the caudate and putamen in a topographic manner. The frontal cortex sends efferent fibers to the head of the caudate and anterior putamen. The posterior portions of the cortex project to the caudal portion of the neostriatum. There are major connections

from the neostriatum to the medial pallidum. Large fiber bundles lead from the pallidum to the *nucleus ventralis anterior* (VA) and the *nucleus ventralis lateralis* (VL) of the thalamus. These specific thalamic nuclei in turn project to the motor areas of the frontal cortex. The pallidum is interconnected with the subthalamic nucleus and substantia nigra. A pathway that has received attention recently and will be discussed below is the nigral-striatal tract from the substantia nigra to the caudate and putamen. From the pattern of these connections alone, it is clear that the basal ganglia do not directly affect motoneuron pools but rather influence motor cortex via thalamic relays. Since the nucleus ventralis lateralis is a major relay for cerebellar output (Chapter 21) destined to reach motor cortex, integration of basal ganglia and cerebellar output probably occurs at this level.

CLINICAL SYNDROMES

At present the data available from physiological studies of the basal ganglia and its connections do not make a coherent story. Therefore, we must rely upon extensive clinical–pathological correlations for some understanding of this part of the motor system.

Hughlings Jackson first grasped the concept that higher levels of the central nervous system frequently have a suppressing influence on the lower levels. A lesion in one area may allow other levels to function in an unrestrained manner. Diseases of the basal ganglia present many examples of release from higher control. These will be called *positive signs*. In addition to causing release phenomena, central lesions also directly destroy and impair the function of specific nuclei or tracts. These deficits will be called *negative signs*. The best example of this type of effect is the weakness caused by dysfunction of the descending suprasegmental pathways. Nearly all clinical syndromes due to disease of the basal ganglia include positive and negative signs. The diseases of the basal ganglia cause marked abnormalities in motor function but generally do not cause major alterations in muscle strength. The motor dysfunction in this group of diseases is characterized by involuntary movement disorders (positive signs) that occur either at rest or with muscle activation and that usually disappear during sleep. There are also changes in muscle tone and altered postural reflexes (negative signs). For most of the disorders only clinical descriptions are available; however, we are finally beginning to understand the physiological and chemical abnormalities in Parkinson's syndrome. Both kinds of data are presented here.

Chorea

Chorea is an involuntary movement disorder (dyskinesia) characterized by rapid semipurposeful movements largely restricted to muscles of the distal extremity and face, although trunk and proximal muscles of the extremity may sometimes be affected. The movements are often incorporated into normal actions and may not be recognized by the inexperienced observer. Muscle tone measured by passive movement is usually decreased in this condition.

Sydenham's Chorea. Sydenham's chorea is a reversible choreiform disorder that usually runs its course in a few months but occasionally persists for 1 or 2 years. It occurs as a complication of acute rheumatic fever and consequently is now a rare disorder. There are only a few pathological studies of this condition because of the high probability of survival. These cases have shown some vasculitis, perivascular infiltrates, and neuronal degeneration in the caudate nucleus, putamen, thalamus, substantia nigra, and subthalamic nucleus. The correlations between clinical findings and pathological lesions restricted to a particular nucleus of the basal ganglia are poor.

Huntington's Disease. Huntington's disease is a devastating illness characterized by progressive chorea and dementia (loss of intellectual function). The disease is inherited in an autosomal dominant pattern. Unfortunately, the symptoms frequently do not appear until after the affected individuals have had their children. During precolonial times in New England many of the patients with

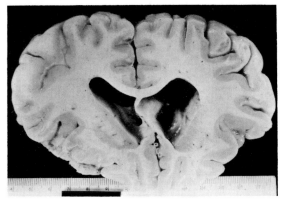

Figure 20–2. Coronal section through the brain of a patient with Huntington's disease. Note the marked atrophy of the caudate nucleus. (From Curtis, Jacobson, and Marcus, *An introduction to the neurosciences*, Philadelphia, W. B. Saunders Co., 1972; courtesy of Dr. E. R. Ross, Loyola University, Chicago.)

Huntington's disease were burned as witches.

The brains of these patients show loss of neurons and gliosis in the cerebral cortex and striatum, particularly the caudate nucleus (Fig. 20–2). Recent studies have shown a decrease in the enzyme glutamic acid decarboxylase in the brains of patients with Huntington's chorea. This enzyme is responsible for the conversion of L-glutamic acid to γ-aminobutyric acid, a putative central nervous system transmitter. The decrease may reflect a specific enzyme defect or may be just a nonspecific finding due to loss of neurons containing this enzyme.

Ballism

Ballism is an involuntary movement disorder that is usually unilateral (hemiballismus), involving the proximal muscles, and is characterized by violent flailing and flinging of the extremities. The movements can be difficult to distinguish from those in chorea. Some neurologists, particularly those from England, call this condition *hemichorea*. The frequent sudden onset of hemiballismus suggests a vascular etiology. Pathological examination of the brains of patients that die with hemiballismus often reveals small infarctions in and around the subthalamic nucleus on the side contralateral to the movement disorder.

Athetosis

Athetosis is characterized by slow, twisting movements of the extremities, hands, and feet. The attitude of hyperextension is often present. Many patients with chorea have some athetosis, hence the term *choreoathetosis*. A common cause of this movement disorder is anoxia occurring before, or associated with, birth. Sometimes it is caused by a marked neonatal rise in bilirubin because of hemolysis of red blood cells due to Rh or some other blood incompatibility between mother and fetus. The neurological complications of this condition are called *kernicterus*. Pathological examination of the brains of patients suffering from presumed neonatal anoxia reveals atrophy and gliosis of the putamen. With myelin stains the putamen and less commonly the caudate and thalamus have a marbled appearance (*état marbré*, status marmoratus).

Dystonia

Dystonia describes tonically rigid posture. This motor abnormality occurs as a sign in many neurological conditions. *Dystonia musculorum deformans* is a disease that is inherited in an autosomal dominant pattern, with a penetrance of 0.5 to 0.7. It first appears in childhood or in the teenage years. The patients often have a severe kyphoscoliosis. The disease may lead to severe deformation of the body or in some cases may stabilize with only minimal signs, *e.g., writer's cramp*.

Parkinson's Disease

Parkinsonism is the most common syndrome due to disease of the basal ganglia. There are many known causes, each resulting in a similar clinical syndrome. The patients show positive signs, such as rigidity and tremor, and negative signs, such as impaired postural reflexes and bradykinesia.

The muscles in Parkinson's disease, in contrast to spasticity, show increased tone throughout the range of passive movement. In the patient with spasticity, the increased tone to passive stretch of a muscle requires activation of the muscle spindle mechanism. Because at rest length the spindles may not be excited, the muscle often feels flaccid to direct palpation and is electrically silent. Moreover, because the spindles have a significant velocity-sensitive component, stretching the muscle slowly in the spastic patient evokes asynchronous afferent input from the spindle that is not sufficient to activate motoneurons. Therefore, the examiner does not feel increased tone with slow passive movements. In the patient with Parkinsonism there is continual activation of the motoneurons. Electrical activity is present in the resting muscle and resistance to stretch is present throughout the range of passive movement, regardless of speed. This type of increased tone is often called *lead pipe*, or *plastic, rigidity*. It should not be concluded that patients with Parkinsonism have no segmental reflex component contributing to increased tone. It has been shown that blocking the gamma efferent fibers decreases the rigidity or increased tone present in Parkinson's disease. However, it is also clear that the increased tone in Parkinson's disease is not solely explained by activation of the stretch reflex mechanism, as occurs in classic spasticity.

The tremor in Parkinson's disease may involve the face but is usually primarily restricted to the distal extremities. In the hand it is characterized by the extension of the interphalangeal joints and flexion of the metacarpophalangeal joints with the fingers beating against an extended thumb. The frequency of this tremor is about 5 cycles per second. When the extremity is passively moved, the rigidity varies with time. This rhythmic interruption of tone is called *cogwheel rigidity*. Some investigators believe that the cogwheeling is caused by superimposition of the tremor upon the rigidity; others believe that they are independent phenomena. The tremor in Parkinson's disease is most prominent during specific static postures. It often disappears during active movement; it is therefore called a *rest tremor*.

The negative signs in Parkinson's disease are more incapacitating than the more immediately obvious and spectacular positive signs just discussed. Akinesia or bradykinesia (absence or slowness of movement) is usually present in patients with Parkinson's disease. The patients have a lack of facial expression and blinking and have difficulty in initiating voluntary movement. Early observers of Parkinsonism considered that the slowness of movement was caused by the rigidity; however, there is no predictable relationship between rigidity and bradykinesia. Although the bradykinesia is evident in the patient's response to commands for voluntary movement, the motor responses to unexpected stimuli such as a startle may be quite rapid.

Patients with Parkinson's disease also show significant abnormalities in postural fixation and maintenance of equilibrium. *Postural fixation* refers to the fixation of a portion of the body on adjoining segments. For example, in normal posture the head and trunk are held in an upright position. Parkinsonian patients frequently show a general flexed attitude, particularly involving the trunk and neck. They can, upon command, assume an erect posture, but if left alone for a few minutes, they slowly drift into a general flexed attitude. Richter demonstrated this same flexed position in monkeys suffering from a severe bilateral degeneration of the globus pallidus.

The erect posture of humans is stable because the center of gravity is kept in line with the vertical projection of the basal stance. When disturbing external forces tend to displace our center of gravity, we adjust our stance by complex reflex responses involving the basal ganglia and other suprasegmental structures. These postural reflexes, which can be evoked in a normal erect person by a small shove, are frequently absent or impaired in patients with Parkinson's disease. The loss of postural reflexes can also be demonstrated on a tilt table. Even when the table is slowly tilted, the kneeling patient does not make corrective postural responses necessary to keep him from falling.

The gait in Parkinson's disease is also abnormal. The patients cannot make the dynamic changes in postural reflexes necessary during walking and easily lose their balance. They also have difficulty in initiating walking. Once they begin, they take small shuffling steps and do not display the normal associated movements, such as swinging the arms. Martin has suggested that part of the gait abnormality is due to the loss of associated movements, such as lateral rocking of the body, which is a part of normal locomotion.

Righting reflexes are also impaired in patients with Parkinson's disease. Normal attempts to roll from the supine into a prone position involve first a turning of the head, followed closely by torsion of the trunk. Many patients with Parkinson's disease show significant impairment of this reflex behavior. Similar reflexes are used in normal turning in the erect position. Parkinsonian patients often find themselves trapped in the corner of a room because they are unable to turn around.

Only rarely can a specific cause for Parkinson's disease be identified. Many victims of the great encephalitis epidemic from 1917 to 1924 developed the disease, the signs of which appeared either soon after the acute illness or with a latency of as long as 10 years. Parkinsonism also occurs as part of the symptom complex caused by manganese or carbon monoxide poisoning. A reversible form of the disease occurs in many patients receiving phenothiazine drugs for psychiatric disorders. However, no cause can be found in the bulk of the patients; they are said to have *idiopathic Parkinson's disease*. Forno and Alvord have suggested that there are two distinct types of idiopathic Parkinson's disease, based on the neuropathological findings in the substantia nigra. One group has cytoplasmic inclusion bodies with a clear halo (called Lewy bodies), and the other has intraneuronal Alzheimer neurofibrillary tangles. A consistent major pathological finding in Parkinson's syndrome is depigmentation of the substantia nigra.

Neurochemistry of Parkinson's Syndrome. Clinical pharmacological observations and more recent neurochemical studies have shown that many of the abnormalities of Parkinson's syndrome and other disorders of the basal ganglia may be related to alterations in putative neurotransmitters, such as acetylcholine and catecholamines.

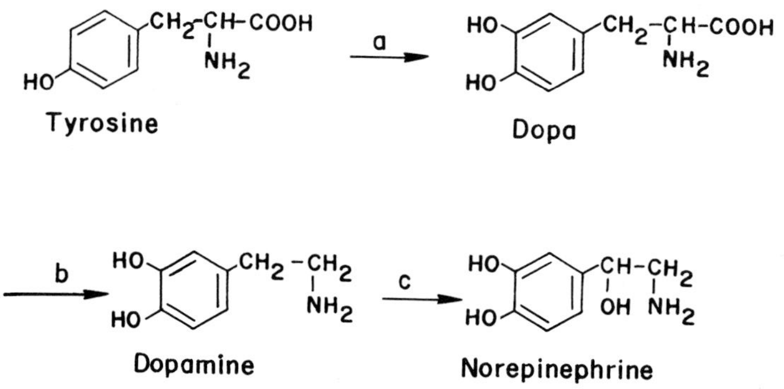

Figure 20–3. Metabolic pathway for synthesis of catecholamines. Enzymes for each step are: *a*, tyrosine hydroxylase; *b*, dopa decarboxylase; and *c*, dopamine β-oxidase. (From Sourkes, Parkinson's disease and other disorders of the basal ganglia, in *Basic neurochemistry*, Albers *et al.*, eds., Little, Brown & Co., 1972.)

The concentration of acetylcholine, choline, and the enzymes required for the synthesis and breakdown of acetylcholine are high in the neostriatum, particularly in nerve terminals. Clinicians have known for a number of years that parasympathomimetic drugs exacerbate Parkinsonism and that anticholinergic drugs provide some relief. Charcot, a 19th century French neurologist, found that Parkinsonian patients improved with atropine treatment. In the laboratory the iontophoretic application of acetylcholine to neurons in the caudate nucleus causes increased firing of these cells. Microinjection of acetylcholine into the caudate of animals produces tremor of the head and extremities.

Dopamine is a naturally occurring monoamine. It now appears that in addition to being a precursor for norepinephrine (Fig. 20–3), it also has its own physiologic functions. About 80 per cent of the dopamine in the brain is located in the basal ganglia. The highest concentration of dopamine is in the caudate nucleus and putamen; somewhat less dopamine is present in the substantia nigra and globus pallidus (Table 20–1). The concentrations of synthetic enzymes for dopamine are also high in the caudate and the substantia nigra. Fluorescent histochemical techniques have localized the dopamine in nerve terminals of the neostriatum and in cell bodies of the substantia nigra.

This evidence is the basis for postulation of a dopaminergic nigral-striatal pathway. Experimental lesions of the ventral medial tegmentum of the midbrain cause a decrease in striatal dopamine closely correlated to the amount of nerve cell degeneration present in the substantia nigra.

In animals, the iontophoretic application of dopamine inhibits both spontaneously active cells in the caudate and neurons stimulated to fire by the local application of acetylcholine.

It was a logical step during the course of these experimental studies to measure the concentration of dopamine in the basal ganglia of Parkinsonian patients (see Table 20–1). Dopamine concentration in the neostriatum and substantia nigra was very low, particularly in patients with postencephalitic Parkinsonism.

This kind of indirect evidence is the basis for the hypothesis that there is a balance between cholinergic and dopaminergic effects in the basal ganglia. Any shift in this balance of activity, either an increase in the effects of acetylcholine or a deficiency in the dopaminergic mechanism, is postulated to lead to Parkinsonian symptomatology. Thus, one would expect drugs that have anticholinergic effects or which potentiate dopaminergic actions to help patients with Parkinson's disease. As noted already, it has been known for many years

TABLE 20–1. Concentrations of Dopamine in Parts of the Brain in Normal Man and Parkinsonian Patients*

Brain Region	Normal†	Parkinsonian†
Caudate nucleus	3.50	0.32
Putamen	3.57	0.23
Globus pallidus	0.30	0.14
Substantia nigra	0.46	0.07
Dentate nucleus	0.02	
Medulla oblongata	0.17	

*From Sourkes, in *Basic neurochemistry*, Albers, Siegel, Katzman, and Agranoff, eds., Boston, Little, Brown & Co., 1972.

†In micrograms per gram fresh weight of tissue.

that anticholinergic drugs give some relief to Parkinsonian patients.

If indeed many symptoms of Parkinson's disease are due to decreased dopamine, the obvious next step is to replace this putative transmitter. Unfortunately, dopamine does not cross the blood-brain barrier. Therefore, the immediate precursor L-dopa (levo-3,4-dihydroxyphenylalanine) has been administered to patients with Parkinson's disease. The therapeutic effect of this treatment is many times better than has previously been obtained with any other drug. Much of the ingested L-dopa is converted to dopamine by systemic dopa decarboxylase (Fig. 20–3); therefore, the maximum therapeutic effect often requires a very high dosage (average 4 g per day) and is associated with systemic side effects, such as nausea and vomiting. Identical therapeutic effects can be obtained by administering a systemic (not CNS) dopa decarboxylase inhibitor (carbidopa) along with L-dopa. The required dosage of L-dopa is reduced by 75 per cent, and many of the systemic side effects are avoided. Patients who were previously unable to walk, dress, or feed themselves have been significantly improved by L-dopa therapy. However, observations over periods of 5 to 6 years indicate that L-dopa does not prevent the steady, slow progression of the disease process. Drug therapy is only a relatively effective form of symptomatic therapy.

The interrelationship of the movement disorders associated with diseases of basal ganglia is illustrated by the signs and symptoms that appear in patients who are receiving too much L-dopa. These patients develop reversible dyskinesias characterized by perioral movements and choreiform movements of the extremities. A slight reduction in the dosage usually reduces these side effects. Most patients prefer to have the movements from overdosage rather than the bradykinesia from undertreatment.

Drug-Induced Parkinsonism. Reserpine-induced Parkinsonism has been known for a number of years and has many of the characteristics of Parkinson's disease, such as akinesia, rigidity, and tremor. Reserpine depletes the brain of catecholamines; therefore, there is a marked decrease in striatal dopamine in animals and people treated with this drug. It is interesting that the injection of L-dopa into reserpine-treated animals transiently restores striatal dopamine and reverses the symptoms.

Phenothiazines (*e.g.*, chlorpromazine) and butyrophenones (*e.g.*, haloperidol) induce Parkinsonism in man. These drugs, which are commonly used in psychiatric practice, do not reduce brain dopamine significantly, except in high dosage. These antipsychotic drugs block dopamine receptors; therefore, they cause a functional impairment of the dopaminergic pathways. Parkinsonian symptoms are usually relieved when the drug is withdrawn, but there is now evidence that in some patients the movement disorders may, unfortunately, persist long after antipsychotic therapy is discontinued (tardive dyskinesia).

On much less firm scientific ground is the general concept that abnormal movements such as those that occur in Huntington's and Sydenham's chorea may be due to overactivity of dopaminergic pathways. It is true that some patients with chorea show modest improvement during treatment with reserpine, phenothiazines, or butyrophenones.

Hepatolenticular Degeneration (Wilson's Disease)

This is a familial disorder that is inherited in an autosomal recessive pattern. Wilson's disease is associated with both central nervous system and liver dysfunction due to copper accumulation. These patients have low circulating levels of ceruloplasm, a circulating copper-binding globulin, and increased levels of nonceruloplasm copper in their sera. Copper is deposited in the brain, liver, and kidney. Liver involvement produces common signs of hepatocellular disease and ultimately of cirrhosis. Brain deposition of copper is primarily in the basal ganglia. Symptoms vary from rigidity to tremor and athetosis. The tremor often has an excessive excursion and is therefore described as *wing beating*. Deposition of copper in the cornea at the scleral junction produces a greenish brown pigmentation called the *Kayser-Fleisher ring*, which is one of the few pathognomonic physical findings in medicine. It is important to recognize this dis-ease, because further neurological and liver deterioration can be prevented by treatment of the patients with penicillamine, a chelator of copper.

ADDITIONAL READING

Calne, D. B. *Parkinsonism; physiology, pharmacology and treatment.* London, Edward Arnold, Ltd., 1970.

McDowell, F. H., and Markham, C. H., eds. Recent advances in Parkinson's disease. *Contemp. Neurol. Ser.*, 1971, *8*, 1–245.

McDowell, F. H., ed. Symposium on levodopa in Parkinson's disease. *Neurology*, 1972, *22*(5), Part 2.

Martin, J. P. *The basal ganglia and posture.* Philadelphia, J. B. Lippincott Co., 1967.

CHAPTER 21

THE CEREBELLUM

WAYNE E. CRILL

CEREBELLAR MORPHOLOGY

CEREBELLAR CIRCUITRY

FUNCTIONAL
ORGANIZATION

EFFECTS OF CEREBELLAR
DYSFUNCTION

The cerebellum is a prominent supra-segmental structure that is present in all vertebrates. Its size relative to the rest of the brain is greatest in the electric fishes and higher primates. In mammals the cerebellum lies in the posterior fossa covered by the tentorium cerebelli and is dorsal to the hindbrain. Based on studies of patients and animals with cerebellar lesions, it is generally accepted that in mammals the cerebellum controls motor behavior. After cerebellectomy, there is no loss of either sensory perception or in-tellectual function, but the most prominent abnormality is a loss of the smoothness and precision of movements.

Extensive afferent input comes to the cerebellum from spinal, brainstem, and cerebral centers. After neural processing has occurred in the cerebellar cortex and nuclei, the output is transmitted largely to the sites of origin for the descending suprasegmental pathways, e.g., the cortico-spinal, vestibulospinal, and reticulospinal pathways. Some physiologists have sug-gested that the cerebellum compares afferent information from the periphery with the motor output from the cerebral hemispheres and brainstem and is con-tinually updating and correcting neural

output so that the movement has precision both in time and space. Although this theory of cerebellar function is not proven, the characteristics of cerebellar deficiency are most logically explained by such a theory.

CEREBELLAR MORPHOLOGY

The cerebellum consists of two lateral hemispheres on either side of a narrow midline ridge called the *vermis* (Fig. 21–1). On the superior surface, the vermis is elevated and is continuous with the hem-ispheres. The inferior surface is deeply grooved, forming the *vallecula*. The cere-bellar surface is composed of many ridges, or folia, separated by deep fissures gen-erally running in a transverse direction. The cerebellum can be likened to an accordian folded in the anterior-posterior direction with the cephalad and caudal ends bent underneath until they nearly meet above the fourth ventricle (Fig. 21–2). One can best understand the anatomical relationship of the cerebellar divisions by imagining an unfolded cerebellum pro-jected upon a flat surface (Fig. 21–3). If the cerebellum could be unfolded in this man-

289

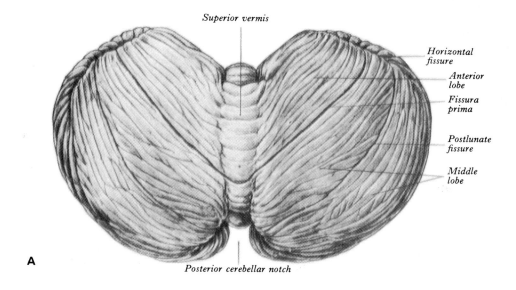

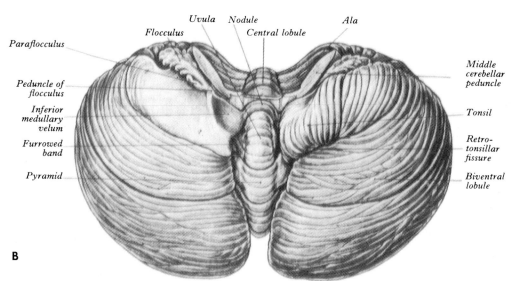

Figure 21–1. *A,* Dorsal view of the human cerebellum. *B,* Ventral view of the cerebellum. Note that on the ventral surface the posterior end (nodule) and anterior end of the vermis nearly meet each other. (From Warwick and Williams, *Gray's anatomy,* 35th ed., Philadelphia, W. B. Saunders Co., 1973.)

ner, in humans, it would be 120 cm long and 17 cm wide.

The cerebellum is divided into the corpus cerebelli and flocculonodular lobes (Fig. 21–3). The flocculonodular lobe is phylogenetically the oldest portion of the cerebellum and is separated from the corpus cerebelli by the posterior lateral fissure. In the intact cerebellum the midline nodule is deep under the cerebellum, and the two flocculi extend laterally ad-

jacent to the foramina of Lushka. The corpus cerebelli is divided into an anterior lobe and a posterior lobe by the primary fissure. Although the majority of fissures run in a horizontal direction, we shall see that much of the functional organization is in an anterior-posterior direction.

The cerebellum is attached to the brainstem by three large fiber bundles on each side of the midline, called *brachia,* or *peduncles.* The superior, middle, and in-

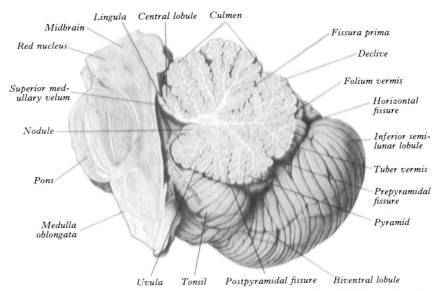

Figure 21-2. Sagittal section of cerebellum and brainstem. (From Warwick and Williams, *Gray's anatomy*, 35th ed., Philadelphia, W. B. Saunders Co., 1973.)

ferior cerebellar peduncles connect the cerebellum to the midbrain, pons, and medulla oblongata, respectively. All afferent fibers projecting to and efferent fibers leaving from the cerebellum are contained in the cerebellar peduncles.

When a sagittal section is made of the cerebellum, the cut surfaces show an outer

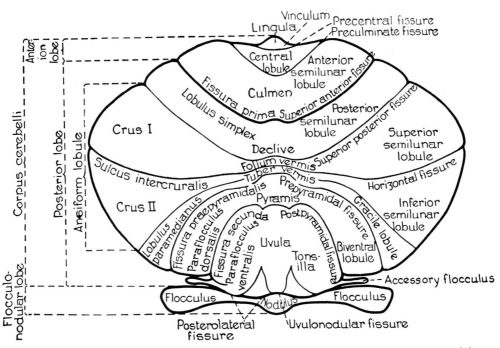

Figure 21-3. Unfolded cerebellum, showing major lobes and divisions. (From Larsell, *Anatomy of the nervous system*, 2nd ed., New York, Appleton-Century-Crofts, 1951.)

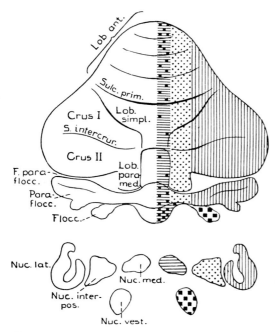

Figure 21-4. The unfolded cerebellum (*above*) with the cerebellar nuclei (*below*) receiving Purkinje cell projections. Note the sagittal organization of the Purkinje cell projections. (From Janson and Brodal, *Avh. norske Vidensk. Akad.*, 1942, Kl,I [3].)

layer of gray matter, the cerebellar cortex, most of which is concealed by the deep fissures. Located deep in the white matter of the cerebellum, just above the fourth ventricle, are nuclear masses collectively called the *deep cerebellar nuclei*. In mammals (Fig. 21-4), there are three distinct cerebellar nuclear masses on either side of the midline: a lateral nucleus (dentate nucleus), an intermediate nucleus (interpositus nucleus), and a medial nucleus (fastigial nucleus). In humans, the intermediate group can be divided into two collections of cells called the *nucleus embolliformis* and the *globosus nucleus*.

CEREBELLAR CIRCUITRY

The basic neural circuit of the cerebellum is relatively easy to understand and with only minor modifications is consistent throughout all vertebrates (Fig. 21-5). Afferent fibers enter the cerebellum through the inferior and middle cerebellar peduncles and project to the cerebellar

cortex. After one or two synaptic relays in the cortex, incoming information converges upon Purkinje cells, the sole output of the cortex. The axons of Purkinje cells project to neurons in the proximate deep cerebellar nuclei; that is, the output of the lateral hemisphere projects to the dentate nucleus, the vermis to the fastigial nucleus, and the intermediate regions to the interpositus nucleus. With this medial-to-lateral projection of the cortex to deep nuclei, we have the first suggestion of the sagittal organization of the cerebellum (Fig. 21-4).

With few exceptions all the axons leaving the cerebellum arise from neurons in the cerebellar nuclei. These efferent fibers are located either in the superior or inferior cerebellar peduncle. Neurons of the cerebellar nuclei also receive inputs from collaterals of cerebellar cortical afferent fibers. One minor exception to this basic

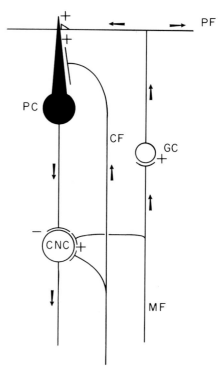

Figure 21-5. Basic neuronal circuit of the cerebellum. *PC,* Purkinje cell; *PF,* parallel fiber; *GC,* granule cell; *MF,* Mossy fibers; *CF,* climbing fibers; *CNC,* cerebellar nuclear cell. Cortical interneurons are omitted. Plus sign (+) indicates excitatory synapses and minus sign (−) inhibitory synapses.

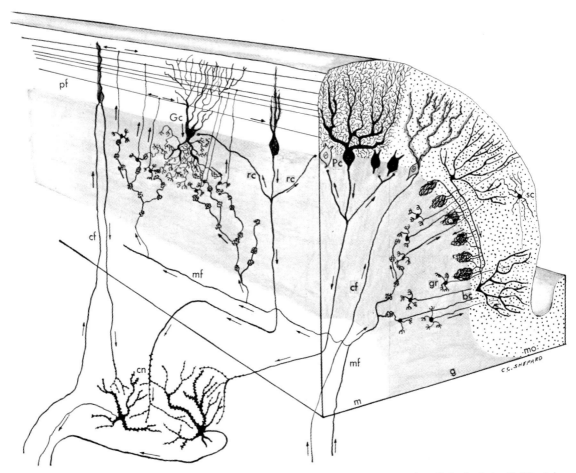

Figure 21–6. A portion of a single cerebellar folium. *Pc,* Purkinje cell; *gr,* granule cell; *bc,* basket cell; *SD,* stellate cell; *Gc,* Golgi cell; *mf,* mossy fiber; *cf,* climbing fiber; *pf,* parallel fiber; *rc,* recurrent collateral fiber; *mo,* molecular layer; *g,* granular layer; *m,* medullary layer (white matter); *cn,* cerebellar nuclear cell. (From Fox, The structures of the cerebellar cortex, in Crosby, Humphrey, and Lauer, eds., *Correlative anatomy of the nervous system,* New York, The Macmillan Co., 1962.)

circuit is illustrated in Figure 21–4. Some Purkinje cells in the vermal region of the corpus cerebelli and in the flocculonodular lobe bypass the cerebellar nuclei and synapse with neurons in the vestibular nuclei of the brainstem. Analogous to the basic pattern, the vestibular neurons receiving direct projections from Purkinje cells also receive collateral input from cerebellar afferent fibers.

The cerebellar cortex is composed of three layers: the largely acellular outer molecular layer, the inner, densely packed granule cell layer, and the interposed sheet of large Purkinje cells (Fig. 21–6). The detailed circuitry of cerebellar cortex is identical in all areas of the cerebellum.

The only axons leaving the cerebellar cortex arise from the large Purkinje cells. These axons make *inhibitory connections* with neurons in the deep cerebellar nuclei and the vestibular nuclei. The pear-shaped Purkinje cells have massive dendritic trees. They are one of the most complex types of neurons in the nervous system. They branch extensively in a plane perpendicular to the direction of the folia.

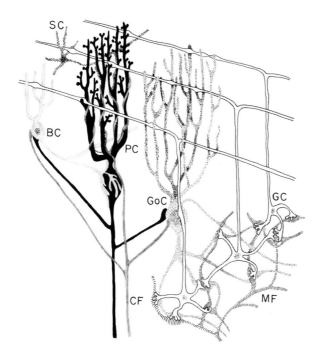

Figure 21-7. The interconnections of the five different neuronal types in the cerebellar cortex. *PC*, Purkinje cell; *SC*, stellate cell; *BC*, basket cell; *GC*, granule cell; *GoC*, Golgi cell. (After Llinas, *Sci. Amer.*, 1975, *232*, 58.)

The output Purkinje cells are influenced by inputs of two anatomically and physiologically distinct types, the mossy fibers and climbing fibers (Figs. 21-5 to 21-7). As we shall see later, the complex structure is matched by unusual physiological properties. Purkinje cells can signal to the cerebellar nuclei which input is active.

Mossy fibers are the axon terminals of all cerebellar cortical afferent fibers except those from the inferior olive nucleus. Mossy fibers branch extensively in the cerebellar white matter, so that a single axon projects to several folia. Mossy fibers make excitatory synaptic connections with short dendrites of the small granule cells in the granule cell layer. Axons of the granule cells project superficially through the Purkinje cell layer into the molecular layer and bifurcate like a T, extending 1 to 2 mm in each direction, always running parallel to the direction of the folia; hence, these axons of the granule cells are termed *parallel fibers*. They pass through and make excitatory connections with successive Purkinje cells like the telephone wires (parallel fibers) between successive telephone poles (Purkinje cells). Each Purkinje cell receives contact from 80,000 to 100,000 different parallel fibers. There are more granule cells in the cerebellar cortex than

previously thought to be present in the entire nervous system. The finely graded excitatory input mediated by the mossy-fiber–parallel-fiber system evokes repetitive firing with conventional type action potentials in Purkinje cells (Fig. 21-8).

The cerebellar cortex also contains inhibitory interneurons of three different types (Fig. 21-7). Stellate and basket cells have similar structures. Their cell bodies are located in the molecular layer, with the dendritic trees extending superficially and the axons projecting transverse to the direction of the folia (in the same plane as the Purkinje cell dendritic branches). These interneurons make inhibitory synaptic connections with Purkinje cells. They are oriented so as to inhibit Purkinje cells on either side of an active band of parallel fibers. Golgi cells have somas that are located in the superficial portion of the granule cell layer. Their dendrites extend into the molecular layer and receive excitatory contacts from parallel fibers. Golgi cell axons make inhibitory synaptic connections with the dendrites of granule cells. The dendrites and axon branches of Golgi cells extend in a radially symmetrical pattern, in contrast to the planar pattern of the other inhibitory interneurons and Purkinje cells.

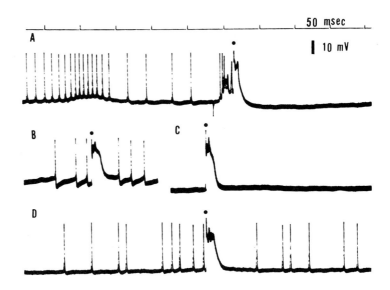

Figure 21–8. Tracings of intracellular potentials recorded from cerebellar Purkinje cells. Dots mark responses evoked by climbing-fiber connections. The shorter action potentials are evoked by Purkinje cell input arriving via the mossy fiber–granule cell pathway. The response at the end of tracing *A* is evoked by stimulation of ipsilateral cerebral cortex. All other responses occurred spontaneously. (From Martinez, Crill, and Kennedy, *J. Neurophysiol.*, 1971, *34*, 348–356.)

The climbing-fiber input arises from neurons in the contralateral inferior olive nucleus and is in every way a contrast to the mossy-fiber system. All olivary axons enter the cerebellum through the inferior cerebellar peduncle. A single olivary axon branches to make excitatory connections with only about 10 Purkinje cells, but each Purkinje cell receives only one climbing-fiber input. The climbing fiber entirely entwines the dendritic trees of a Purkinje cell, making 150 to 200 different synaptic excitatory contacts. As might be expected, this is an extremely powerful synaptic connection.

The excitatory postsynaptic potential (EPSP) evoked by a single climbing fiber impulse has an amplitude greater than 25 mV, well above the Purkinje cell's threshold. Therefore, a single impulse in a climbing fiber axon always evokes an action potential in the 10 or so innervated Purkinje cells. It is an obligatory synapse. The response of the Purkinje cell is a complex spike like that shown in Figure 21–8. The complex spikes evoked by climbing fibers and simple spikes evoked by parallel fibers allow the experimentalist to identify

readily the responses generated by the Purkinje cells. Unfortunately, the physiological significance of these two distinct cerebellar input systems is not understood. Some investigators have suggested that the climbing-fiber system is a means of testing the summed excitatory and inhibitory synaptic activity present at any instant in time. Others have proposed that the climbing-fiber system is concerned with rapid, ballistic movements, whereas the mossy-fiber system regulates slow, tonic movements.

FUNCTIONAL ORGANIZATION

According to phylogenetic development and the characteristics of the mossy-fiber system, the cerebellum can be divided into three major divisions: the archicerebellum, or the vestibulocerebellum; the paleocerebellum, or spinocerebellum; and the neocerebellum, or pontocerebellum.

The archicerebellum is the flocculonodular lobe, and an adjacent portion of the vermis called the *uvula* (Fig. 21–3). It is interconnected with the vestibular system and is phylogenetically the oldest portion of the cerebellum. It receives input both from the vestibular nuclei and from primary vestibular afferent fibers. Purkinje cell axons project to the fastigial nucleus, whose neurons in turn leave the cerebellum and make connections with the vestibular nuclei. Some Purkinje cells of the flocculonodular lobe bypass the fastigial nucleus and make direct contacts with neurons in the vestibular nuclei. All incoming and outgoing connections of the archicerebellum travel in the inferior cerebellar peduncle.

This portion of the cerebellum regulates eye movements and controls neck and axial muscles. Although it is unusual for a lesion to destroy this portion of the cerebellum selectively, animals that have had the flocculonodular lobe removed do not develop sickness induced by motion. They also show dysequilibrium without abnormalities in fine movements of the extremities. When the head is placed in some positions, persistent nystagmus appears (positional nystagmus). The clinical disorder that most selectively impairs this portion of the cerebellum is the medulloblastoma, a tumor that commonly occurs in children and arises in the roof of the fourth ventricle. As would be expected, the earliest signs of medulloblastoma are dysequilibrium, positional nystagmus, and the obstruction of the flow of spinal fluid through the fourth ventricle.

The next oldest portion of the cerebellum is the paleocerebellum, or spinocerebellum. It receives input from the spinal cord and projects back to it. This portion of the cerebellum includes the vermis and adjacent intermediate regions of the corpus cerebelli, particularly in the anterior lobe (Fig. 21-9). Mossy fibers that project into the spinocerebellum are terminals of the dorsal spinocerebellar tract, the cuneocerebellar tract, the ventrospinocerebellar tract, and the rostral spinocerebellar tract.

The dorsal spinocerebellar tract (DSCT) originates from neurons in Clarke's column (T1 to L2 in man). These neurons receive inputs from Group Ia and Group II afferents from muscle spindles and Group Ib fibers from Golgi tendon organs in the lower extremity and trunk. The axons from neurons in Clarke's column project up the ipsilateral dorsal spinocerebellar tract, enter the cerebellum through the inferior cerebellar peduncle, and project to the ipsilateral cerebellar cortex in the anterior lobe. Many dorsal spinocerebellar tract fibers carry exclusive information from Group Ia afferents of a single muscle and its synergists. The homologous pathway transmitting information from the upper limb, neck, and trunk is the cuneocerebellar tract, arising in the lateral cuneate nucleus. The cuneocerebellar tract also enters the ipsilateral inferior cerebellar peduncle and projects to ipsilateral vermal and intermediate portions of the anterior lobe just posterior to the termination of the dorsal spinocerebellar tract.

The other major spinal tract projecting to the cerebellum is the ventrospinocerebellar tract (VSCT). It arises from neurons in the intermediate gray matter of the cord. Axons ascend in the cord ipsilateral and some contralateral to their cell of origin. The ventrospinocerebellar tract does not enter through the inferior cerebellar peduncle but rather passes through the medulla and enters the cerebellum through the superior cerebellar peduncle projecting to the vermal and intermediate regions of the anterior lobe. The equivalent of the ventrospinocerebellar tract for the arm is the rostral spinocerebellar tract. It has only been identified physiologically. Many fibers in the ventrospinocerebellar tract are activated by Group Ib afferents, usually coming from many muscles in the same extremity. Also, exteroceptive information from the skin is transmitted by this pathway to the cerebellum.

Purkinje cells in the paleocerebellum project to the fastigial nucleus and in some instances directly to the dorsal portion of the lateral vestibular nucleus. In all instances they are inhibitory. Neurons in the fastigial nucleus project to either other cells in the lateral vestibular nucleus (the origin of the lateral vestibulospinal tract) or reticular neurons (the origin of the reticulospinal pathways). Thus the paleocerebellum is reciprocally connected with the spinal cord.

Selective lesions of the cortex of the anterior lobe of the cerebellum remove inhibition of the midline deep cerebellar

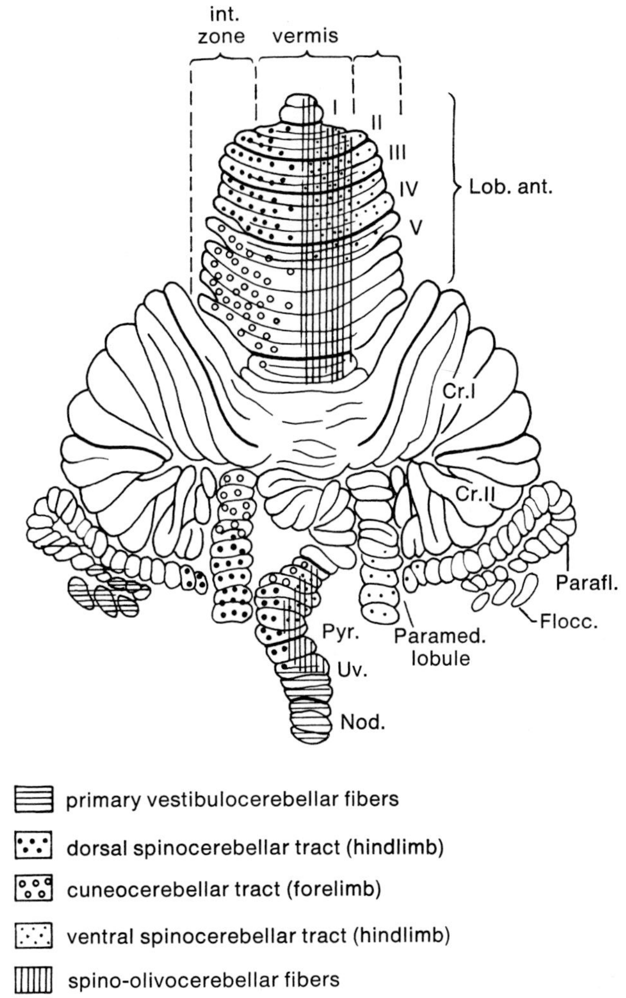

Figure 21–9. The unfolded cat cerebellum, showing the projections of spinocerebellar, vestibulocerebellar, cuneocerebellar, and spino-olivocerebellar pathways. *Cr. I,* Crus I; *Cr. II,* Crus II; *Parafl.,* Paraflocculus; *Flocc.,* Flocculus; *Pyr.,* Pyramis; *Uv.,* Uvula; *Nod.,* Nodulus. (From Brodal, *Neurological anatomy,* 2nd ed., New York, Oxford University Press, 1969.)

nuclei and the lateral vestibular nucleus. This lesion markedly increases decerebrate rigidity in carnivores, switching it from a gamma to an alpha type of rigidity. Gamma rigidity (facilitation of gamma motoneurons) disappears after section of the dorsal roots, whereas alpha rigidity (facilitation of alpha motoneurons) does not. Recall that the vestibulospinal and the reticulospinal tracts are primarily excitatory to motoneuron pools in the spinal cord that project to extensor muscles.

In man, the disease process that most selectively causes dysfunction of this portion of the cerebellum is seen in alcoholic cerebellar degeneration (Fig. 21–10). This syndrome, caused by chronic and excessive alcohol intake, presents largely as an abnormality in coordination of the legs. The gait is ataxic and wide-based.

The neocerebellum includes both cerebellar hemispheres and is reciprocally connected to the cerebrum. Collaterals of the pyramidal tract and cortical bulbar fibers synapse with neurons in the pontine nuclei. The afferent pontocerebellar fibers (mossy fibers) originate in the contralateral pons. The axons of the pontine neurons cross the midline in the basis pontis and enter the cerebellum through the middle cerebellar peduncle. Purkinje cells in the intermediate and lateral portions of the cerebellar hemispheres project to the interpositus and lateral nucleus of the cerebellum, respectively. Axons from neurons in these two cerebellar nuclei leave the cerebellum through the superior cerebellar peduncle, crossing the midline in the decussation of the superior peduncle in the midbrain. Collaterals from axons of inter-

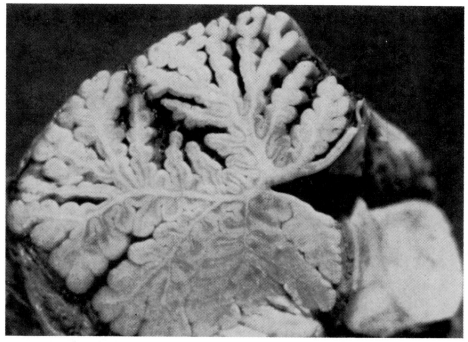

Figure 21–10.   Median sagittal section of a human cerebellum, showing atrophy of the anterior lobe. Note the increased space between folia in the anterior portion compared with that in the posterior portion at the bottom of the photograph. (From Victor, Adams, and Mancall, *Arch. Neurol.*, 1959, *1*, 579, 599, 600.)

positus neurons also project to the red nucleus. The terminals of axons from the lateral and interpositus nuclei continue and end in the ventrolateral (VL) nucleus of the thalamus. Recall that the ventrolateral nucleus projects to the precentral or motor cortex. Thus, the cerebral-neocerebellar interconnections are characterized by two midline crossings: (1) the pontocerebellar fibers and (2) the nuclear fibers in the superior peduncle. A cerebellar hemisphere is thus interconnected with the cerebral hemisphere (primarily motor portions) on the contralateral side. From these interconnections it should be clear that lesions of the neocerebellum will cause abnormalities on the ipsilateral side of the body.

All Purkinje cells of the cerebellum receive climbing-fiber input from the inferior olive nucleus. Those portions of the inferior olive nucleus that project to the cerebellar hemispheres receive the major portion of their input from descending pathways. The paleocerebellum, or spinocerebellum, receives its climbing-fiber input from olivary nuclei receiving afferent connections from spino-olivary tracts.

EFFECTS OF CEREBELLAR DYSFUNCTION

Patients with either cerebellar degeneration or lesions in cerebellar peduncles show abnormalities in motor control. They have some weakness and decrease in muscular tone, but the most spectacular abnormality is loss of the fine control of muscular activity. Many terms are used to describe abnormalities of cerebellar function. The most commonly used terms are listed below. Several of these deficits may be present in the same patient.

Cerebellar ataxia is a general term used to describe the disturbances in the coordination of volitional movement. Although this term correctly describes the abnormality in muscle groups in all portions of the body, it is often used clinically to refer to the abnormality in gait seen in patients with cerebellar dysfunction. Patients with cerebellar disease show a wide-based gait characterized by staggering and reeling. It should be noted that an ataxic gait may be caused by lesions in other parts of the nervous system, such as sensory systems (sensory ataxia) and frontal lobes (frontal ataxia). The absence of sensory signs and other evidence of cerebral dysfunction in the presence of other cerebellar signs helps the clinician identify a problem with gait as being caused by cerebellar dysfunction.

Hypotonia, asthenia, decomposition of movement, dysergia, and *dysmetria* are terms used to describe abnormalities of specific parameters in motor function. In contrast to lower mammals, which usually show an increase in muscle tone after lesions of the cerebellum, humans frequently have *hypotonia,* or a decrease in muscle tone. This is measured by the passive movement of a joint. It may be manifested by *pendular knee jerks,* in which the to-and-fro excursion of the lower leg following tapping of the patellar tendon continues beyond the one or two swings present in normal individuals Fig. 21–11.

Asthenia (Fig. 21–12) refers to the moderate amount of weakness present in patients with cerebellar dysfunction. A delay in the initiation and termination of the force exerted by a single group of muscles can usually be demonstrated. Patients with cerebellar disease frequently show *decomposition of movement,* that is, an impaired cooperation of all the muscle groups involved in a single complex motor act. The act is broken into a series of elemental movements that are usually performed sequentially. For example, when

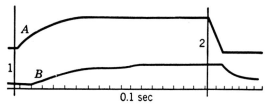

Figure 21–12. Myograms showing the temporal course of initiation and termination of grip in a patient with a unilateral cerebellar lesion. Vertical lines *1* and *2* mark signals to start and stop gripping. *A* is the tracing taken contralateral to the cerebellar lesion. Note the slower onset and relaxation in addition to a smaller maximum force in *B,* which was taken from the hand ipsilateral to the cerebellar lesion. (From Ruch, Chap. 5 in *Handbook of experimental psychology,* Stevens, ed., New York, John Wiley & Sons, 1951.)

the patient comes to a step, he may first raise his leg to an appropriate height before he moves the foot forward to place it upon the step, and only then does he extend his lower leg.

Dysergia is an abnormality similar to decomposition of movement but is usually used to describe lack of cooperation between closely related muscle groups. The abnormality is particularly prominent when the supine patient attempts to raise one leg, place the heel on the opposite knee, and slide it down the shin. *Dysmetria* describes abnormality in the range of movement. The patient either undershoots or overshoots a spatial target. One of the best tests for this abnormality is the alternate touching of the examiner's finger and the patient's nose with the index finger of one hand.

Another group of abnormalities that are often seen in patients with cerebellar disease include problems restricted to one type of motor behavior, such as speech or rapid movements. *Dysdiadochokinesia* refers to an abnormality in rapid alternating movements (Fig. 21–13). It is tested for by having the patient alternately slap his thigh with his palm and the dorsal surface of his hand. The slow starting and stopping of muscle tension, dysmetria, and dysergia all combine to cause dysdiadochokinesia. *Scanning speech* is present in patients with cerebellar disease, is characterized by an irregular volume and rhythm of speech,

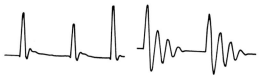

Figure 21–11. Tracing of lower leg excursion caused by tapping the patellar tendon in a normal person (*left*). The two traces on the *right* are from a patient with a cerebellar lesion, illustrating the much slower dampening of the lower leg excursion. (From Holmes, *Lancet,* 1922, *202,* 1177–1182.)

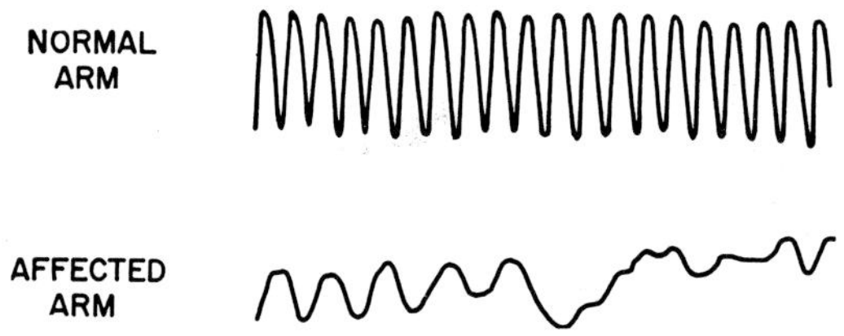

Figure 21–13. Dysdiadochokinesia. Tracings showing movements of the forearm during attempted rapid alternating pronation and supination. (From Holmes, *Lancet*, 1922, *203*, 59–65.)

and is due to dyscoordination in the control of the flow of air past the vocal cords. An *intention tremor* is often seen in patients with cerebellar disease and is only evident when the patient is doing volitional movements. Similar results from a combination of dysergia and dysmetria are best seen in the finger-to-nose test. This abnormality is prominent in patients with lesions in the dentate nucleus or in the superior cerebellar peduncle. *Titubation* refers to an abnormality in maintaining a sitting or an erect posture. The trunk is not stationary but frequently jerking forward and backward, and the patient has to make continual corrections in order to keep an erect position. The *rebound phenomenon of Holmes* is demonstrated by having the patient apply a constant force against resistance. When the resistance is suddenly removed or the examiner releases his hold, the patient lacks the ability to make a rapid check, and the arm will go an excessive distance in the direction in which the patient is applying force. This results from the delay in stopping the movement.

In contrast to the movement disorders observed in patients with basal ganglia disease, the abnormalities in motor control characteristic of cerebellar lesions are present only when muscles are being used.

The patient rests quietly in bed, and ataxia appears only when he tries to maintain posture or perform skilled movements.

Although we have a good understanding of the cerebellar circuitry with respect to its anatomical and physiological properties, we do not understand the functional significance of the rectangular lattice formed by the mossy-fiber and parallel-fiber inputs to Purkinje cells or the role of the spacially restricted climbing-fiber input to single Purkinje cells. The concept that the cerebellum regulates motor behavior comes from lesion experiments and clinical[1] pathological correlations of deficits, such as those previously described.

A potentially rewarding technique is the extracellular recording from single neuronal units in awake animals (monkeys) performing specific behavioral tasks. In these studies it is clear that the Purkinje cells and cerebellar nuclear cells alter their activity in relation to somatic movement. Some cells increase their firing rates, whereas others decrease their activity. The precise relationship between the alteration of firing pattern and movement is variable. Because even the most simple movement is composed of elemental motor actions, it is impossible to ascribe a specific function to a Purkinje cell that alters its firing rate during a movement.

One set of experiments, however, carried out by Lisberger and Fuchs, has shown a specific action of Purkinje cells in the control of movement. Unitary responses from the flocculus are only timed with activity in the vestibular nerve when the animal is suppressing the vestibulo-ocular reflex in the light (see Chapter 22). It is possible that one can solve the cerebellar puzzle by first deciphering its relationship to the control of ocular motor activity.

ADDITIONAL READING

Brodal, A. *Neurological anatomy in relation to clinical medicine.* 2nd edition, New York, Oxford University Press, 1969, Chap. 5.

Eccles, J. C., Ito, M., and Szentágothai, J. *The cerebellum as a neuronal machine.* New York, Springer-Verlag, 1969.

Llinas, R. R. The cortex of the cerebellum. *Sci. Amer.* 1975, *232*(1), 56–71.

CHAPTER 22

THE OCULOMOTOR AND VESTIBULAR SYSTEMS

WAYNE E. CRILL

THE OCULOMOTOR SYSTEM

The neural systems that are responsible for the fine and precise movements of the eyes must include mechanisms to move both eyes as a unit and also must contain interconnections so that the visual image falls on identical regions of each retina. The oculomotor system is interesting because its fundamental mechanisms are better understood than other aspects of the motor system and also because abnormalities in oculomotor control are extremely useful in neurological diagnosis.

The ocular muscles are innervated by three cranial nerves: III (oculomotor nerve), IV (trochlear nerve), and VI (abducens nerve). The nucleus of the abducens nerve (Fig. 22–1C) is just below the floor of the fourth ventricle. The facial nerve loops around the nucleus of cranial nerve VI. The fibers of VI leave the brainstem at the pontomedullary junction, pierce the dura, and travel through the lateral portion of the cavernous sinus. They enter the orbit through the superior orbital fissure and innervate the lateral rectus muscle.

The nucleus of the trochlear nerve is in the mesencephalon at the level of the inferior colliculus and emerges on the dorsal aspect of the brainstem, crosses the midline, travels around the midbrain, and pierces the dura (Fig. 22–1B). It also passes through the lateral portion of the cavernous sinus and enters the orbit through the superior orbital fissure, innervating a superior oblique muscle.

The nucleus of the oculomotor nerve is in the midbrain at the level of the superior colliculus just ventral to the aqueduct (Fig. 22–1A). The nerve fibers from cranial nerve III traverse the red nucleus and leave the midbrain at the lateral portions of the interpeduncular fossa. The fibers pierce the dura and also travel in the lateral portion of the cavernous sinus, passing through the superior orbital fissure to innervate the superior rectus muscle, the levator palpebrae superioris, the inferior rectus muscle, the inferior oblique muscle, and the medial rectus muscle. The third

301

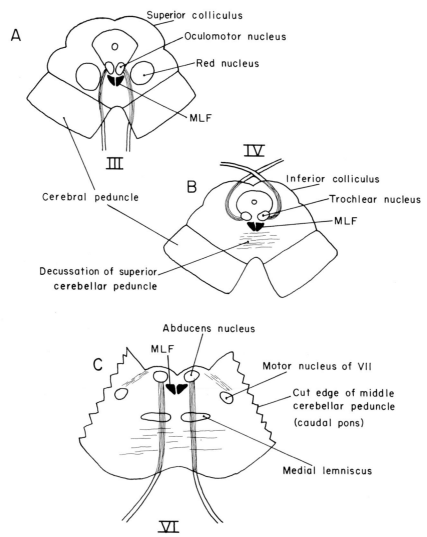

Figure 22–1. Diagrammatic cross sections at the levels of the nuclei for the (A) oculomotor nerve (III), (B) trochlear nerve (IV), and (C) abducens nerve (VI). *MLF* locates the medial longitudinal fasciculus.

nerve also contains parasympathetic fibers innervating the pupillary sphincter and ciliary muscles.

The superior and inferior recti extend in a direction parallel to the axis of the orbit. This direction of pull (the orbital axis) is about 23 degrees lateral to the ocular axis. Since the superior and inferior recti insert on the anterior half of the globe, they act as pure elevators and depressors, respectively, when the eye is abducted 23 degrees (ocular axis parallel to orbital axis). As the ocular axis deviates more and more medially, the superior and inferior recti cause more and more intorsion.

The oblique muscles are attached to the anterior medial aspect of the orbit and insert on the *posterior lateral* portion of the globe (Fig. 22–2*A*). The oblique muscles tend to become relatively pure elevators and depressors as the eye is adducted. However, since each oblique muscle inserts on the posterior half of the globe, the superior oblique muscle depresses the eye and the inferior oblique one elevates the eye when it is adducted. The oblique muscles cause ocular rotation when the eye

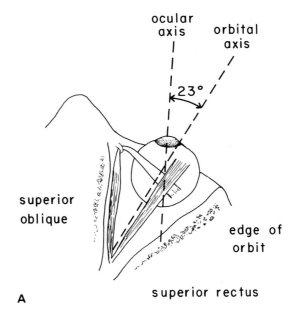

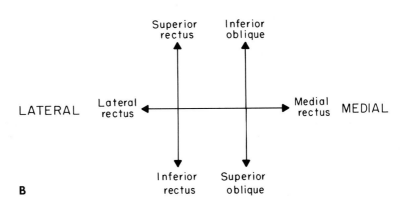

Figure 22–2. *A,* Dorsal view of the orbit, globe, superior rectus muscle, and superior oblique muscle. Note the relationship of the ocular axis to the orbital axis with regard to insertion of each muscle. *B,* Primary direction of pull by each of the six extraocular muscles.

is abducted. As shown in Figure 22–2*B*, each muscle is best tested with the ocular axis parallel to the muscle's primary direction of pull.

Eye movements may be divided into two major categories. Conjugate, or version, eye movements are characterized by the visual axes remaining parallel to each other. Disconjugate, or vergence, eye movements cause the visual axes to intersect. For example, convergence from a distant to a near point involves about 8-degree adduction of each eye.

There are two types of version eye movements. The eyes may move from one fixed position to another either by rapid jumps between successive fixations (sac-

cades) or by smoothly tracking a moving object (smooth-pursuit movements).

Saccadic eye movements are extremely fast; the eyes move 40 degrees in only 100 msec. Saccades are the only version eye movements that can be made voluntarily in the absence of a moving target. It is with saccades that we read or view a stationary scene. During a saccade, visual acuity is depressed so that extraneous information is eliminated while the eyes are moving. You can demonstrate the effect of rapid eye movements without visual suppression by tapping your eyeball and causing passive movement. The decreased acuity occurs before the onset of the saccade. On the basis of these observations,

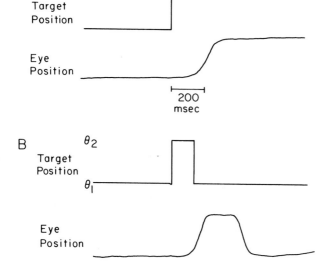

Figure 22–3. Tracings of visual target position and eye position.

it has been assumed that the motor system that is responsible for saccadic movements sends a corollary discharge to the visual system and decreases visual acuity. Presumably, vision is suppressed at the level of the lateral geniculate body.

After the target has changed position, the latency of the saccadic eye movement is 200 to 500 msec (Fig. 22–3A). The latency determines the minimum separation of successive saccades and therefore has implications in improving one's reading speed. For example, if you make three saccades per second and only read one word per fixation, the upper limit for reading speed is 180 words per minute. Reading clinics improve speed by having their clients practice including as many words as possible in a single fixation.

The neural systems subserving saccadic eye movements acquire information about target position by a sampled data system. If, as shown in Figure 22–3B, the target moves first to position θ_2 and then back to θ_1 within the 200-msec latency period, the eyes still move to fix on position θ_2, even though the target has returned to position θ_1. The nervous system must then resample target position, and another 200-msec latency occurs before the eyes move back to position θ_1.

Saccadic eye movements are ballistic, and the velocity cannot be affected by voluntary effort. Saccades are relatively resistant to drugs but are altered in some diseases; for example, many patients with Huntington's chorea lose their saccadic eye movements. Progressive supranuclear ophthalmoplegia is a less common disease in which one of the primary clinical signs is loss of saccadic eye movements.

The other type of version movements is called a *smooth-pursuit movement* and is used to track moving targets. Smooth-pursuit movements are slower than saccades; the maximum velocity is about 50 degrees per second. In contrast to the visual acuity during saccadic movement, that during a pursuit movement is good. Smooth-pursuit movements cannot be made without the stimulus of a moving target. The nervous system is continually sampling target position during smooth-pursuit movements. The latency between displacement of the moving target and the pursuit movement by the eyes is 130 msec. Whereas sedative drugs, such as barbiturates, have little effect upon saccadic movements, they severely depress smooth-pursuit movements and divide the following motion into a series of saccades.

Physiological studies of the unitary activity of motoneurons in the oculomotor, trochlear, and abducens nuclei reveal the same types of responses relative to the individual muscles innervated by each group of neurons. An intense burst of 400 to 600 spikes per second precedes the onset and lasts the duration of each saccade. The duration of the burst is proportional to the size of the saccade. Steady firing is at a slower rate during fixation, and the frequency is proportional to the angular displacement of the globe in the direction of the muscle innervated.

Because the eyes must move in precision with each other and there is little margin for error, the motor nuclei to the ocular muscles are yoked together by fibers in the medial longitudinal fasciculus (MLF). The anatomical and physiological characteristics of these interconnections are now well understood; the details can be found in more extensive texts. The bulk of the fibers in the medial longitudinal fasciculus originate in the tectal areas of the midbrain and the vestibular nuclei. Suprasegmental neural signals leading to eye movements must feed into the medial longitudinal fasciculus, either at its cephalad or caudal extreme.

The major inputs to the medial longitudinal fasciculus and hence the nuclei of the ocular muscles arise from the cerebral structures, superior colliculus, brainstem reticular formation, vestibular structures, and cerebellum.

Classical neurological teaching ascribes the supranuclear control of voluntary conjugate eye movements (saccades) in the horizontal direction to the frontal eye fields located in Brodman's area 8. Patients with destructive lesions in this area have transient difficulty making voluntary horizontal version movements to the side contralateral to the lesion. Moreover, stimulation in one frontal eye field causes contralateral conjugate saccades with a latency of about 25 msec. The poorly defined pathway can be followed anatomically by stimulation to the level of the pons. At the level of the midbrain the direction of the evoked eye movement reverses, so that the stimulation in the pons causes the eyes to deviate conjugately to the side of the stimulus. Lesions in the reticular formation cause a paralysis of horizontal conjugate gaze to the side of the lesion. These observations have led to the postulate that a frontal mesencephalic pathway that controls horizontal conjugate gaze feeds into

the medial longitudinal fasciculus at the level of the abducens nucleus. This concept is of practical value at the bedside, but unfortunately it must be an oversimplification.

Recordings from neurons in the frontal eye field reveal that less than 10 per cent of the unitary firing is related to eye movements; moreover, the neurons show bursts of activity that do not precede saccadic eye movements.

Recent work indicates that the superior colliculus is an important structure that probably has a major role in the conversion of visual input into oculomotor commands. The dorsal position of the colliculus receives direct retinal and cortical projections. (In the lower vertebrates all optic tract fibers project to the superior colliculus.) The neurons in the dorsal colliculus respond best to movement in their receptive fields. In the deeper output layers of the colliculus, the units respond with a burst of spikes during saccades in a specific direction.

The neural systems that control conjugate gaze in the vertical plane are less well understood. However, lesion experiments in monkeys and clinical pathological correlations in humans indicate that the lesions around the posterior commissure are highly correlated with paralysis of vertical gaze.

In addition to the saccadic and smooth-pursuit movements, two other subsystems control eye movements. The vergence system is used to track approaching objects, and each eye moves in the opposite direction. The eye movements in this system are slow (about 20 degrees per second). The anatomical basis for this system is poorly defined but probably involves the parieto-occipital cortex.

The vestibular system (see later) is a nonoptic reflex system that compensates for head motion. It keeps the eyes fixed on a visual target. With destruction of a single labyrinth or the vestibular nerve, patients complain of jumbled vision when the head is moving.

Nystagmus refers to oscillating eye movements that are usually conjugate. The nystagmoid movements are evoked in normal patients by either visual or vestibular stimuli and consist of slow movements in one direction followed by a rapid jerk in the opposite direction. Optokinetic nystagmus is produced by looking at moving stripes in a revolving drum. Occipital parietal lesions impair the slow phase of optokinetic nystagmus, and frontal lesions impair the fast phase. Stimulation of the semicircular canals evokes nystagmus with a short latency. The slow phases of vestibular and optokinetic nystagmus appear similar, but higher velocities can be obtained by vestibular stimulation. Moreover, the vestibular system is a more precise system. Compare tracking a rapidly oscillating target with viewing a fixed target while oscillating your head (vestibular).

The cerebellum has a major influence in the control of eye movements. The primary signs of cerebellar deficiency are overshooting and undershooting of the saccadic movements and decomposition of the smooth-pursuit movements into a series of saccades.

In summary, lesions outside the nuclei innervating the extraocular movements and their interconnections through the medial longitudinal fasciculus are referred to as *supranuclear*. These deficits are characterized by abnormalities and conjugate gaze. Destructive cerebral lesions impair version movements to the contralateral side, whereas supranuclear brainstem lesions are associated with paralysis of conjugate gaze to the side of the lesion.

Lesions of the medial longitudinal fasciculus that do not involve the nuclei of the abducens, trochlear, and oculomotor nerves are called *internuclear* (Fig. 22–4). The pathways subserving lateral conjugate gaze feed into the medial longitudinal fasciculus at the level of the abducens nucleus and cross the midline ascending in the medial longitudinal fasciculus to the portion of the oculomotor nerve innervating the medial rectus muscle. Lesions of the medial longitudinal fasciculus on one side between the abducens and the oculomotor nuclei are characterized by disconjugate gaze when the patients attempt to look to the contralateral side. The nucleus of contralateral cranial nerve VI receives normal supranuclear input so that the contralateral eye abducts; however, input to the nucleus of ipsilateral cranial

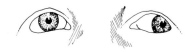

ATTEMPTING TO GAZE TO THE LEFT

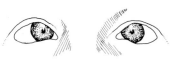

INTACT CONVERGENCE

Figure 22–4. Internuclear ophthalmoplegia. Lesion is in the patient's right medial longitudinal fasciculus.

nerve III is blocked by the lesions in the medial longitudinal fasciculus so that the ipsilateral eye does not cross the midline. In these patients, it can be shown that the lesion does not directly involve neurons innervating the medial rectus muscles because they can still converge. Bilateral internuclear ophthalmoplegias are often found in patients with multiple sclerosis.

THE VESTIBULAR SYSTEM

The vestibular portion of cranial nerve VIII transmits messages from receptors in the vestibular labyrinth to the central nervous system. This information about the spatial orientation of the body, along with visual and proprioceptive input, is used to adjust muscle tension and resist the effect of gravitational forces.

It is important for the clinician to understand the vestibular system because many patients complain of dizziness and because the physician can make deductions about the anatomical location of neurological lesions on the basis of physical signs related to specific influences of the vestibular system on oculomotor control and segmental reflex activity. *Vertigo*, one of the many symptoms collectively included in the complaint of dizziness, is the extremely disturbing abnormal perception of the body's orientation in space relative to the external environment.

The sensory receptors of the vestibular system are in the labyrinth of the inner ear

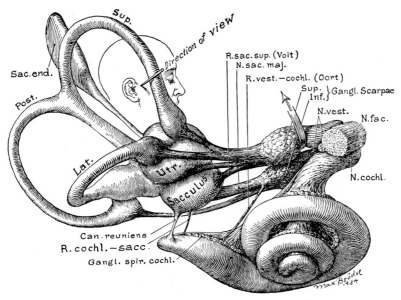

Figure 22-5. The right human labyrinth. (From Hardy, *Anat. Rec.*, 1935, *59*, 403–418.)

(Fig. 22–5). Each vestibular labyrinth embedded in the petrous bone includes the three semicircular canals and the saclike utricle and saccule. Each of these structures has a sensory epithelium containing the receptor hair cells and supporting cells. The vertical anterior and posterior semicircular canals are perpendicular to each other and to the horizontal canal.

The *ampulla* is a dilatation located at one end of each semicircular canal and contains the receptor organ, or *crista ampullaris.* A gelatinous mass, called the *cupula,* covers the hair cells of each crista ampullaris. The ciliated hair cells have numerous short stereocilia and a single longer kinocilium (Fig. 22–6) that is always located on one side of the hair cell. In a single crista ampullaris, the eccentricity of the kinocilium of each of the adjacent hair cells is in the same direction; thus, the end organ is said to be polarized. Movement of the endolymph fluid in the thin-walled membranous labyrinth bends the cupula either toward the utricle or away from the utricle toward the canal. Deflection of the cupula then bends the cilia toward the side of the kinocilium and increases electrical activity in the vestibular nerve fibers innervating the hair cell receptor. Deflection of the cilia in the opposite direction decreases activity in the vestibular nerve fibers.

Impulse frequency in the vestibular fibers is linearly related to the angular de-

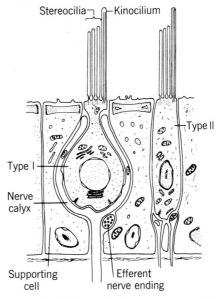

Figure 22–6. Schematic drawing of vestibular epithelium (from electron micrographs), showing two types of hair cells. (From Brodal, *Neurological anatomy in relation to clinical medicine,* New York, Oxford University Press, 1969.)

flection of the cupula. Although the adequate stimulus for the semicircular canal is angular acceleration of the head, the viscous effect of the small canal diameter dissipates so much energy that cupula deflection is more closely related to head velocity. In other words, for the normal range and speed of head movements, the semicircular canals functionally transform angular acceleration into a velocity term so that cupula deflection and, therefore, firing frequency of vestibular nerve fibers are linearly related to head velocity.

Direct recording from single vestibular nerve fibers in monkeys reveals a high spontaneous firing rate (Fig. 22–7). The experiments clearly demonstrate that the appropriate stimulus, angular acceleration, is linearly related to firing frequency. However, this can be demonstrated only with angular accelerations of longer duration and greater magnitude than occur in physiological situations.

The hair cells in the ampulla of the horizontal canal are polarized with the kinocilium toward the utricle; therefore, excitation of vestibular fibers from the horizontal canal occurs when the endolymph in this canal moves toward the ampulla. Excitation of fibers from the vertical canals is caused by movement of endolymph fluid away from the ampulla toward the canal.

The effect of angular rotation of the head on movement of the endolymph fluid is illustrated in Figure 22–8. For example, when the head is rapidly rotated or accelerated to the left, the movements of the endolymph fluid and cupula lag behind skull rotation because of inertia.

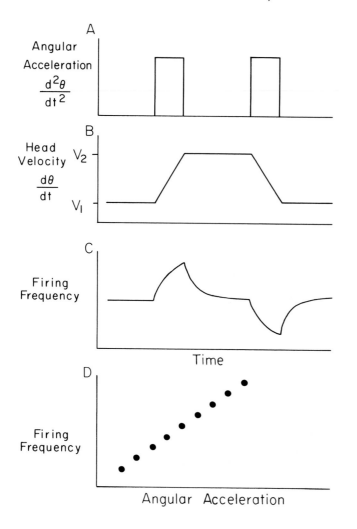

Figure 22–7. Responses of a single nerve fiber in the vestibular nerve of a squirrel monkey in a rotating chair. *A*, Angular acceleration of the chair; *B*, angular velocity of the chair; *C*, instantaneous firing frequency of a single nerve fiber; and *D*, steady-state firing frequency of a single vestibular fiber, plotted against angular acceleration. (After Goldberg and Fernandes, *J. Neurophysiol.*, 1971, 34, 635–660.)

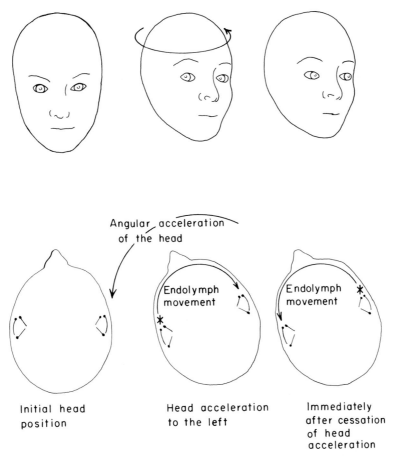

Figure 22–8. Acceleration of the head to the left in relation to movement of endolymph. The bottom row of figures is viewed from above. Because of the inertial torque of the endolymph fluid, it lags behind the movement of the canal. The asterisk (*) indicates the excited horizontal canal.

Thus, there is a net movement of the endolymph fluid (with respect to the canal) away from the ampulla in the right horizontal canal and toward the ampulla in the left horizontal canal. Therefore, nerve fibers in the crista ampullaris on the left side are excited during acceleration to the left. When head rotation decelerates, or slows, the endolymph fluid continues to move toward the left, and the right crista ampullaris is transiently excited.

The sensory epithelium in the utricle and the saccule is called the *macula*. It contains hair cells similar to those of the crista ampullaris. In addition, otoliths, crystals of calcium carbonate, are embedded in the gelatinous material covering the macular hair cells. The utricular macula is oriented mainly in the horizontal plane;

thus, movement with the head in the upright position causes very little deflection of the cilia of utricular and saccular hair cells. However, when the head is tilted; the effect of gravity on the otolith deflects the cilia of hair cells in the utricle. Assuming minimal adaptation of the receptor, one would expect a change in tonic firing frequency of vestibular fibers from the utricle as long as gravitational action on the otolith of the hair cells causes deflection of stereocilia and kinocilia. For this reason, the utricular and saccular end organs often are called *static vestibular receptors*. The exact head position, or movement, that maximally stimulates the saccule is not known.

The parent cell bodies of the fibers in the vestibular nerve projecting to the central nervous system are located in Scarpa's ganglion in the internal auditory canal. Axons in the vestibular nerve project to the vestibular nuclear complex in the lateral pons and medulla. A few axons also pass through the vestibular nuclei directly to the flocculonodular lobe of the cerebellum. The vestibular nuclei compose four main nuclear groups: medial, lateral (Deiters'), superior, and inferior. The vestibular nuclei are interconnected with the spinal cord by the medial and lateral vestibular spinal tracts, with the nuclei of cranial nerves III, IV, and VI and motoneuron pools in the neck by the medial longitudinal fasciculus, and with the cerebellum by the "inner" cerebellar peduncle, the juxtarestiform body. Although the details of these connections are fairly well understood, they will not be considered here and may be obtained from any standard textbook in neuroanatomy.

However, the net effect of these connections is relevant. If the vestibular fibers from the left horizontal semicircular canal are selectively stimulated, motoneurons in the contralateral abducens nucleus and in the portion of the ipsilateral oculomotor nucleus innervating the medial rectus are excited; that is, the eyes deviate conjugately to the right side. The effects are mediated through the medial longitudinal fasciculus.

This observation, when related to the properties of the horizontal canal illustrated in Figure 22–8, provides an explanation for the vestibulo-ocular reflex. Angular acceleration of the head to the left increases the firing frequency of vestibular nerve fibers from the left horizontal canal. These vestibular nerve afferents ultimately excite the motoneurons in the right abducens nucleus and the motoneurons innervating the left medial rectus. Thus, the response of the eyes when the head is accelerated to the left is to remain fixed on an object. It is interesting that the firing frequency of motoneurons innervating the eye muscles is directly related to eye position. Clearly, the integrative function of the nervous system is illustrated by this example, since the vestibular system and other brainstem structures must operationally integrate (in the mathematical sense) angular acceleration twice to produce an output that is a function of position. As discussed above, the actual output of the vestibular afferents is directly related to velocity of the head because of the physical characteristics of the semicircular canal. Thus, the first integration occurs at the end organ itself (velocity is the time integral of acceleration). The synaptic mechanism and site where angular velocity is integrated into a position term are not known.

The vestibulo-ocular reflex is the basis of a valuable clinical test used to evaluate the function of the vestibular labyrinth and its connections with the oculomotor muscles. If the head is alternately rotated approximately 60 degrees to the right and left, the eyes will conjugately oscillate 90 degrees out of phase with the head. This is called the *doll's eye maneuver* and is illustrated in Figure 22–8. Cortical influences upon oculomotor movements can suppress the doll's eye response in the awake patient; however, this problem can be eliminated by closure of the eyelids, and the movement of the eyes can be felt through the closed eyelids. The reflex is extremely brisk in patients who are unconscious from bilateral cerebral dysfunction but who still have the vestibulo-ocular reflex pathway intact.

The awake person can suppress the vestibulo-ocular reflex by visual fixation. The flocculus of the cerebellum is involved in inhibiting this reflex. Flocculectomy abolishes the ability to suppress the reflex. Purkinje cells in the flocculus only modulate their firing frequency with cranial nerve VIII during fixation when the vestibulo-ocular reflex is suppressed.

The physiological function of the vestibular system is to inform the nervous system about static and changing gravitational forces so that the motor system can maintain equilibrium. These adjustments via the complex reflex pathways just discussed are continually occurring and usually do not reach conscious awareness. At least, since we have learned that the output of this system is appropriate, sudden movement does not cause untoward sensations. However, if the output of the vestibular system is excessive, such as occurs during and immediately after rapid rotation or in an imbalance of input from the two sides caused by pathological processes, the illusion of movement occurs, producing the symptom of *vertigo*. The effect of this input may be so strong that the patient is thrown violently to the ground. Vertiginous sensations are familiar to those readers who have, for one reason or another, not appropriately monitored an evening's alcohol intake. The extremely disturbing symptoms of the flying-bed syndrome usually curb alcohol intake in the future. This syndrome also illustrates the importance of spatial cues from other sensory systems. Vertigo does not usually appear until the inebriated subject lies down in a dark room or closes his eyes, decreasing visual input. The experienced bed pilot soon learns that the alcohol-induced vertigo may be diminished by keeping the lights on and his eyes open. Even in the normal person, the sudden loss of visual and proprioceptive information about the body's position in space may transiently cause vertigo.

Vertigo is often associated with nausea and sometimes vomiting. The systematic association of vertiginous sensations with head movement or body position and the consistency of the illusion of motion are signs suggesting vestibular involvement. Vertigo should be differentiated from the less specific complaints of dizziness, giddiness, or lightheadedness.

The effect of the vestibular system upon oculomotor control is a valuable clinical sign, since abnormalities may be detected by simple bedside tests and frequently implicate neural dysfunction in a spatially restricted region of the central nervous system. The input to the central nervous system from excitation of the horizontal canal will tonically excite motoneurons innervating the ipsilateral medial rectus and contralateral lateral rectus muscles, and the eyes will tonically deviate away from the side of the increased vestibular input. In the awake person and animal, cerebral cortical mechanisms serving rapid saccadic conjugate eye movements will overcome the tonic vestibular input so that the eyes will rapidly move back to the center of gaze. Thus, tonic vestibular input on one side will cause oscillatory conjugate eye movements or nystagmus consisting of a slow movement away from the side of the increased vestibular input and a fast saccadic return (jerk nystagmus). Clearly, the slow phase of vestibularly induced nystagmus is the active movement caused by the increased vestibular activity. This must be remembered if you wish to understand the mechanism or deduce from clinical observation the site of lesions. Regrettably, clinical terminology does not help the student, since *the direction of nystagmus is denoted by the direction of the fast component;* that is, nystagmus that is clinically labeled right-sided should imply a relative hyperactivity of the right vestibular input.

Jerk nystagmus has distinct fast and slow components and usually indicates damage to either the labyrinth, vestibular nerve, or vestibular nuclei. In labyrinthine disease, the direction of nystagmus is usually independent of the direction of gaze. With more central lesions, nystagmus is in the direction of gaze. Vertical nystagmus is a sign of disease of the central nervous system. When both phases of nystagmus have nearly the same velocity, it is called *pendular.* Congenital ocular disease may disturb fixation mechanisms and cause pendular nystagmus with forward gaze.

THE CALORIC TEST

The semicircular canals may be selectively stimulated for evaluation of the intactness of the pathways between the vestibular end organ and the extraocular muscles. The head is tilted 60 degrees from the vertical plane with the face up, so that the horizontal semicircular canals are vertical. The external auditory canal is irrigated with warm water, and convection currents are induced in the endolymph fluid by the warm fluid. The warm endolymph rises in the vertically positioned horizontal canal, moving *toward* the ampulla. Thus, the firing frequency of vestibular fibers innervating the horizontal crista ampullaris increases. This maneuver evokes nystagmus with a slow phase toward the contralateral side. Conversely, irrigation of the external auditory canal with cold water when the head is in the same position causes nystagmus in the opposite direction. When cerebral cortical function is depressed and the connections between the vestibular receptor and the extraocular muscles are intact, the fast phase of this nystagmus is absent. In this situation, the eyes tonically deviate to one side or the other, depending on the temperature of water used.

ADDITIONAL READING

Bach-y-Rita, P., and Collins, C., eds. *The control of eye movements.* New York, Academic Press, 1971.

Cogan, D. G. *Neurology of the ocular muscles.* 2nd edition, Springfield, Ill., Charles C Thomas, 1956.

Young, L. R. Role of the vestibular system in posture and movement, in *Medical physiology*, Mountcastle, V. B., ed., St. Louis, The C. V. Mosby Co., 1974.

CHAPTER 23

THE CEREBRAL CORTEX, CONSCIOUSNESS, AND SLEEP

WAYNE E. CRILL

THE CEREBRAL CORTEX

The *cerebral cortex*, or *pallium*, is the gray mantle covering the telencephalon. Three major divisions of the pallium are phylogenetically first discernible in amphibians. The *archicortex*, the anlage of the hippocampus, is located medially, and the *paleocortex*, or *piriform cortex*, is located laterally in lower vertebrates. Between these two divisions in the dorsal area is the anlage of the *neocortex*. The precise definition of the *rhinencephalon* (see Chapter 27) varies with different authors but generally includes the archicortex and paleocortex.

The new, six-layered neocortex is primarily a mammalian development and is most prominent in primates (90 per cent of the cortex in humans). Because of its dominance, it displaces the phyloge-netically older regions of cortex medially. Man's neocortex has a surface area of 2000 cm² and varies in thickness from 2 to 4.5 mm. *Isocortex* and *homogenetic cortex* are synonyms for *neocortex*. With the extensive increase in cortical volume, infolding occurs; consequently, much of the cortex is located in deep fissures, or sulci.

The discovery of regional differences in neocortical anatomy started with the 1776 observation by Gennari of grossly visible striae running parallel to the cortical surface in the occipital lobe. With the development of better microscopes in the past century, structural investigations of the nature of the neocortex flourished. These early cytoarchitectural studies were based on the histological techniques of Nissl, Golgi, and Weigert and demonstrated that the neocortex has six layers and neurons

313

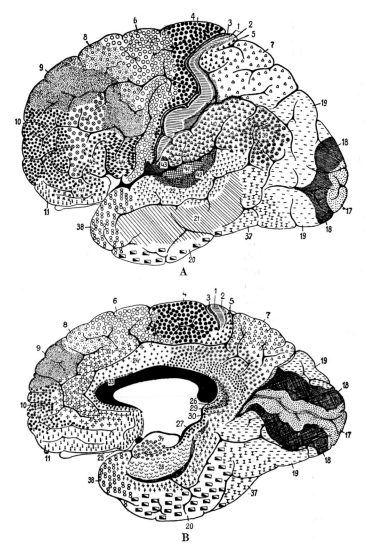

Figure 23–1. Cerebral cortical cytoarchitectural map of Brodmann. (From Ranson and Clark, *The anatomy of the nervous system; its development and function,* Philadelphia, W. B. Saunders Co., 1959.)

of four different types. Cytoarchitectural maps of the neocortex have been developed by many neuroanatomists, but the most popular system is Brodmann's division of the cortex into no less than 52 areas (Fig. 23–1). Only a few of these divisions have identified physiological significance, but the system remains the most popular.

Cortical Neurons

On the basis of size, shape, location, and form of dendritic trees, four types of cortical neurons have been identified (Fig. 23–2). *Pyramidal cells* have a triangular soma with the apex directed toward the cortical surface. The soma varies in diameter from 15 to 100 μm. The largest pyramidal cells are located in the motor cortex and are called *Betz cells.* The dendritic tree is characterized by a long dendrite, originating from the apex of the soma and directed toward the cortical surface, and a basal dendritic arborization. The axons of pyramidal cells have recurrent collateral fibers that project back to the cortex. Only a small fraction of the cortical pyramidal cells have axons in the pyramidal tract. The axons of pyramidal cells leave the cortex and project either to other areas of cortex or to more distant

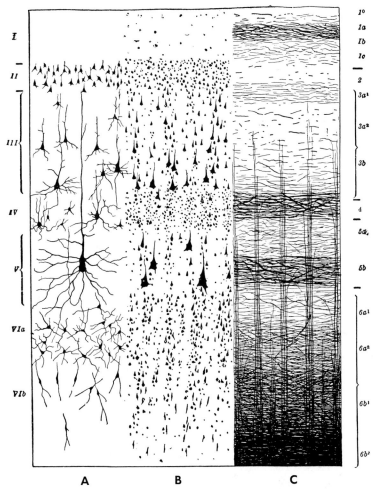

Figure 23–2. Schematic diagram showing the structure of the cerebral cortex obtained by (*A*) Golgi stain, (*B*) Nissl stain, and (*C*) myelin stain. (From Ranson and Clark, *The anatomy of the nervous system; its development and function*, Philadelphia, W. B. Saunders Co., 1959.)

parts of the nervous system. A relatively few pyramidal cells (*Martinotti's cells*) have axons that do not leave the cortex.

Stellate, or *granule*, cells have a star-shaped dendritic tree and axons that remain in the cerebral cortex. Most of the cortex neurons are either pyramidal or stellate cells.

The *fusiform cells* are cigar-shaped, with small dendritic branches arising from each pole. They are oriented perpendicular to the cortical surface and are in the deepest cortical layer.

The *horizontal cells of Cajal* are similarly shaped but are oriented parallel to the surface and are located in the most super-

ficial cortical layer. Their axons also run parallel to the cerebral surface.

Cortical Layers

Using the appearance of soma stains, anatomists have divided the neocortex into six layers (listed here from the outside surface inward).

The molecular layer (I) is composed mostly of fibers and contains dendritic terminals from cells in deeper layers and a few cortical afferent fibers. The sparse horizontal cells of Cajal are located in this layer.

The outer granular layer (II) contains many small pyramidal cells and granule cells.

The pyramidal cell layer (III) contains medium-sized pyramidal cells. Axons of some neurons in this layer leave the cerebral cortex.

The inner granular layer (IV) consists of densely packed stellate cells. Most of their axons project to the dendrites passing through this layer from cell bodies in layers V and VI. This layer is most highly developed in the primary sensory receiving areas of cortex and is nearly absent in motor cortex.

The ganglionic layer (V) contains pyramidal cells and a few stellate cells and Martinotti's cells. This layer also contains the giant Betz cells. Axons from pyramidal cells in this layer leave the cortex as either projection, commissural, or association fibers.

The fusiform cell layer (VI) contains cells of various shapes but consists mostly of fusiform cells.

When the cortex is stained for myelin there are two prominent tangential bands, the outer and inner lines of Baillarger, located in layer IV and the deep portions of layer V. In the visual cortex, the outer line of Baillarger is so thick that it can be seen with the naked eye. In this region it is called the *line of Gennari*. It is because of the prominent line of Gennari that visual cortex is frequently called *striate cortex.*

On the basis of the cytoarchitecture of the cerebral cortex, several generalizations can be made about its structure and function. Most of the cortex contains six clearly identifiable areas of homotypical cortex. In other areas the recognized specialization is associated with six less discernible layers (heterotypical). For example, the cortex in the posterior frontal lobe (motor cortex) has a distinct lack of granular layers II and IV (agranular cortex). The larger cortical efferent systems originate in agranular cortex. On the other hand, the specialized sensory receiving areas are characterized by poorly developed pyramidal and ganglionic layers (III and V) and a richness in granule cells (layers II and IV). This type of heterotypical cortex is called *granular cortex*, or *koniocortex*. It is best exemplified by the visual striate cortex.

Four major types of axons are found in the cerebral cortex. *Corticofugal fibers* project out of the cerebral cortex (*e.g.,* the cortical spinal tract). *Corticopetal fibers* come to the cortex from the thalamus. *Association fibers* connect different cortical regions of the same hemisphere. *Commissural fibers* connect homologous portions of the two cerebral hemispheres.

Nearly all the subcortical cerebral brainstem and spinal cord gray masses receive projection fibers from the cerebral cortex (the vestibular nuclei and pallidum are exceptions). One of the most prominent projection systems in man is the pyramidal tract, but there are also cortical projections to the thalamic nuclei, caudate nucleus and putamen, red nucleus, reticular formation, pontine nuclei, cranial nerve nuclei, inferior olive nuclei, colliculi, and dorsal column nuclei. The projection fibers arise mainly from layers III and V. Most of the corticopetal fibers arise from the thalamus and terminate mainly in layers III and IV. The less specific thalamic afferents project to many layers.

Cortical association fibers may be very short, remaining in the cortex. Longer fibers traverse the white matter to connect one gyrus to its neighbor (U-fibers). Still longer association fibers connect distantly separated areas of cortex, such as those linking the temporal cortex to the frontal lobes and those between the peristriate regions and the temporal cortex.

The largest fiber bundle of the nervous system, the corpus callosum, contains commissural connections between the two cerebral hemispheres. The specific somatosensory cortex and striate cortex do not receive commissural fibers. The distribution of commissural fibers in the monkey is shown in Figure 23–3. Association and commissural fibers project primarily to layers II and III, although terminals may be given to other layers.

It has been postulated that the cells of the cerebral cortex are organized into functional units, called *columns*. This concept is based on the anatomical orientation of the cortex. The major cells of the cerebral cortex, the pyramidal cells, are radially symmetrical with respect to their basal dendrites and apical dendrite. The bulk of the interconnecting interneurons

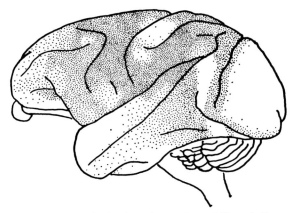

Figure 23–3. Projection of commissural fibers to the cortex of the left hemisphere of the monkey. (From Myers, in *Functions of the corpus callosum*, Ettlinger, ed., Study Group No. 20, London, The CIBA Foundation, 1965.)

have axons that project in a vertical direction. Similarly, the major cortical afferents project vertically through the cortex, giving collaterals to cells at various levels in a column. This concept is supported by physiological experiments, particularly in the visual cortex, where cells oriented vertically to each other have receptive fields of similar types. However, whether or not other cortical areas have a basic columnar organization is a controversial question.

CEREBRAL CORTICAL POTENTIALS

Intracellular recordings of potentials from neurons in the cerebral cortex show resting potentials of about 60 mV, inside negative. The action potentials overshoot the zero potential and, on the basis of available evidence, have underlying ionic mechanisms similar to those in better-studied preparations (Chap. 5). The all-or-nothing response to a threshold stimulus is presumably due to the regenerative properties of the Hodgkin's cycle. Graded depolarizing, or excitatory, postsynaptic potentials (EPSP's) and hyperpolarizing, or inhibitory, postsynaptic potentials (IPSP's) also can be recorded from cortical neurons. When the postsynaptic potentials of cortical cells are compared with those of the more thoroughly studied spinal

motoneurons, some differences are noted. In cortical neurons the inhibitory postsynaptic potentials are larger and have longer durations. Intracellular recording from cortical neurons reveals marked fluctuations in the resting potential, presumably due to the continuous bombardment by somewhat synchronized synaptic activity.

Technically easier to record but less well understood is the electrical activity registered between a larger electrode placed directly on the cortical surface and a distant indifferent electrode placed on inactive tissue such as bone or skin. Such a system responds to currents caused by synchronous potential changes in populations of neuronal elements underlying the active electrode. *Evoked potentials* are the electrical responses thus recorded following direct stimulation of either sense organs or afferent fibers that project to the area of cortex being studied. The *electrocorticogram* is ongoing (spontaneous) electrical activity not evoked by stimulation.

The most-studied and best-understood evoked cortical response is the primary evoked potential (Fig. 23–4). It is a positive-negative wave recorded on the cortical surface after stimulation of a major sensory pathway or of a specific thalamic relay nucleus. Although the volley of impulses in the afferent fibers may contribute somewhat to the primary evoked response, the neuronal currents mainly responsible for this response are synaptic currents generated in cortical cells. Experimental evidence indicates that the initial positive wave of the primary evoked potential is a surface reflection of excitatory postsynaptic potentials occurring deep in the cerebral cortex. The later negative wave is caused by currents flowing from delayed hyperpolarizing, inhibitory postsynaptic potentials in the depths and excitatory postsynaptic potentials occurring near the cortical surface. Because action currents in single cortical cells are of short duration relative to synaptic potentials and because there is some variation in the orientation of cortical cells, it is unlikely that they cause significant currents to flow on the cortical surface. Cortical neuronal spikes therefore contribute little to the evoked cortical response. By using electronic

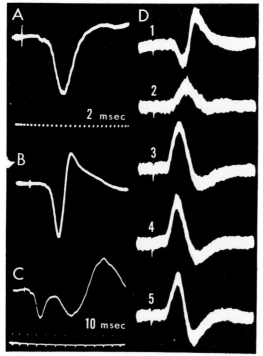

Figure 23–4. Cortical primary evoked responses recorded from the cat: *A*, response recorded from somatosensory area I; *B*, primary evoked response from somatosensory area II; *C*, primary evoked response and secondary discharge from area I; *D*, superimposed tracings of microelectrode recording in 480-μm steps from the surface down to a depth of 1920 μm (*1* to *5*). The primary discharge reverses sign with depth. The site of reversal indicates that the current source for the primary response occurs near the cortical surface. (From Ruch and Patton, eds., *Physiology and biophysics,* Philadelphia, W. B. Saunders Co., 1965.)

averaging devices to separate small synchronized signals from noise, one can record evoked potentials from the scalp without exposing the cortex.

THE ELECTROENCEPHALOGRAM

In addition to the responses evoked by stimulation of afferent pathways, ongoing spontaneous activity can be recorded from the cortical surface. These recorded potential oscillations are termed *electrocorticograms* when they are recorded directly from the cortex and *electroencephalograms* (EEG's) when they are recorded from the surface of the scalp. In the early

1930's Hans Berger first demonstrated that the cerebral potentials could be recorded from the scalp (Fig. 23–5).

EEG potentials vary in frequency and amplitude with the placement of the electrode, with the behavioral state of the subject, and with the biochemical and structural status of the underlying cortex. For example, to determine whether or not the cortex is electrically silent, indicating cerebral death, one doubles the normal bipolar electrode separation of 5 to 6 cm to increase the size of any recorded signal. Most unconscious patients have a generalized slowing of the EEG, and destructive cerebral lesions cause focal slowing of the EEG.

The frequency of the EEG oscillations varies from 1 to 35 Hz, and the amplitude of scalp voltages ranges from 50 to 100 mV. The rhythms are classified on the basis of their frequency. The *alpha rhythm* range is 8 to 13 Hz. It waxes and wanes in amplitude and is spatially distributed over the posterior regions of the cerebral hemisphere. The alpha rhythm is most prominent during relaxed wakefulness with the eyes closed. Rhythms faster than 13 Hz are called *beta rhythms.* They occur over wide regions of cortex and are prominent in individuals taking sedative drugs. When a subject in a state of relaxed wakefulness either opens his eyes or concentrates on specific mental problems the alpha activity is replaced by low-voltage beta rhythms. This change in EEG rhythms is called *activation,* or *desynchronization,* of the EEG, or *alpha blocking.*

Other rhythms slower than the alpha range (*theta,* 3 to 7 Hz, and *delta,* 0.5 to 3 Hz) are only rarely present in normal, awake, adult subjects. Slower rhythms normally predominate in sleep. When slow rhythms are present in awake adults, they are indicative of either metabolic or structural abnormalities.

As in the case of the evoked potentials, the currents responsible for the EEG are primarily generated by synaptic activity. It should be appreciated that all the currents recorded from the surface originate in the cortex in close proximity to the recording electrodes. However, these rhythms may be significantly influenced by activity in remote structures projecting

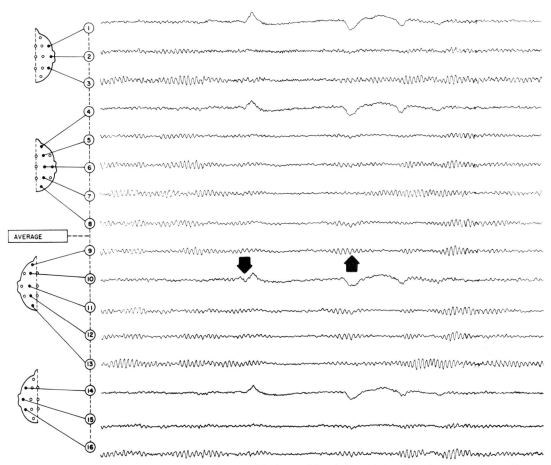

Figure 23–5. EEG from a normal patient showing blocking of the alpha activity when the eyes are open (*downward arrow*) and reappearance of the alpha activity when the eyes are closed (*upward arrow*).

to the cerebral cortex. The fact that potential oscillations are so prominent suggests a synchronization of cortical electrical activity.

CONSCIOUSNESS

Although we frequently use the term *consciousness*, it is difficult to define satisfactorily. It is clearly a neural phenomenon characterized by an awareness of self and environment. Animals other than man show conscious behavior; however, where in the phylogenetic line it first appears is uncertain. It is a measure of an organism's capacity to choose selectively one course of action in favor of another.

Two aspects of consciousness are arousal and the content of consciousness. *Arousal*, or the closely related term *wakefulness*, is a variable quantity. Terms such as *clouding of consciousness*, *stupor*, and *coma* refer to different levels of consciousness. The presence of consciousness can be tested only by measurement of the content of consciousness. Perception of one's environment and memory are examples of the content of consciousness. There is a fairly good correlation between the EEG rhythms and the degree of arousal, but there are exceptions, as we shall see later.

The neural substrate of arousal includes the cortex, the thalamocortical system, and the reticular formation of the brainstem. The content of consciousness is a cortical function. The thalamocortical system includes the cerebral cortex and the nonspecific thalamic nuclei. These are a collection of thalamic nuclei that do not project solely to specific sensory receiving areas; they include the intralaminar nuclei, the midline nuclei, and the reticular thalamic nucleus. Whereas stimulation of the specific nuclei gives rise to the localized primary evoked response, stimulation of the nonspecific nuclei evokes in cortex a widely distributed, long-latency, recruiting response. This is a surface, negative response that becomes progressively larger but also waxes and wanes with successive stimuli (Fig. 23–6). Because the recruiting response can be evoked only by stimuli in the frequency range of 6 to 12 Hz (close to the alpha rhythm) and because higher-frequency stimulation in the nonspecific nuclei causes desynchronization of the EEG, it has been postulated that these regions of the thalamus may act as pacesetters of the cortex. Other experiments suggest that the thalamocortical system is activated by an ascending system of neurons located in the reticular formation of the upper brainstem.

In the core of the brainstem are complexly structured regions of the nervous system called the *reticular formation*. The area contains a diffuse cellular network comprising cells of various shapes and sizes and with axons traveling in many different directions. Although obvious architectonic differences exist between relatively small areas, the general pattern of this region of the nervous system is reticulated. Specific regions of the reticular formation project to different structures, such as the thalamus, spinal cord,

and cerebellum. Some cells of the reticular formation have axons that project in both the ascending and descending directions. Much of the reticular formation receives collaterals from many ascending afferent pathways and in turn projects to wide areas of the cerebral cortex via the nonspecific thalamic nuclei.

Morruzzi and Magoun showed that stimulation of the bulbar reticular formation at frequencies exceeding 12 Hz activated the EEG. Moreover, such stimulation in sleeping animals led to behavioral awakening in addition to desynchronization of the EEG. Destructive lesions of the same areas (Fig. 23–7) produced unresponsive animals. Such experiments, combined with the abundant clinical evidence that destructive lesions in the tegmentum of the upper pons and midbrain produce coma, are the basis for the concept of an *ascending reticular activating system* that in some way drives the thalamocortical system and maintains consciousness.

It should be appreciated that this vitally important portion of the nervous system is in an extremely vulnerable location, the notch of the tentorium, where herniation may cause damage.

Clinical Correlations

Plum and Posner have divided disease processes that cause coma into three major categories: supratentorial lesions, lesions of the posterior fossa, and metabolic disorders. Structural damage to the cerebral hemispheres above the tentorium causing

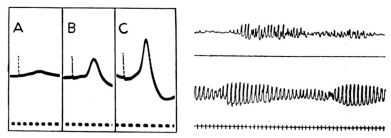

Figure 23–6.   *Left,* Cortical recruiting response evoked by successive shocks applied to the intralaminar thalamic region. Negativity is upward. *Right,* A spontaneously occurring response (*upper trace*) and a continuously occurring waxing and waning response (*lower trace*) evoked by repetitive shocks applied to the intralaminar thalamic region. Frequency of stimulation is shown on the bottom trace. (From Morison and Dempsey, *Amer. J. Physiol.,* 1942, *135,* 281–292.)

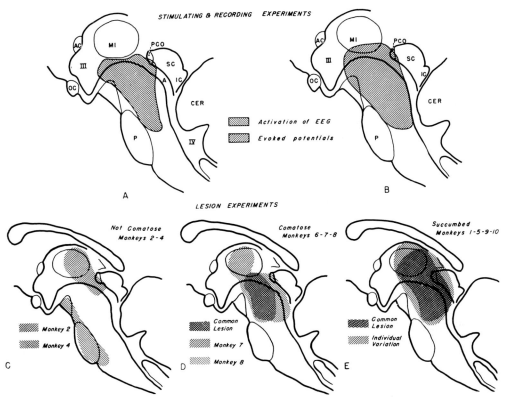

Figure 23–7. Summary diagrams showing brainstem regions related to several aspects of sleep and consciousness. *A*, Regions in which high-frequency stimulation caused EEG activation and arousal of sleeping animals. *B*, Areas from which evoked potentials were recorded after various peripheral stimuli. *C*, Site of lesions that did not produce coma. *D*, Site of lesions causing coma. *E*, Sites of lethal lesions. (From French and Magoun, *Arch. Neurol. Psychiat.* [*Chic.*], 1952, *68,* 591–604. Copyright 1952, American Medical Association.)

altered states of consciousness must either directly involve the thalamocortical system bilaterally at the level of the thalamus or indirectly involve it through the shifting of brain structures caused by mass effects. It is unusual for structural damage to the cerebral cortex itself or its underlying white matter to be extensive enough to cause coma. Patients in coma from widespread cortical disease, as occurs in some degenerative disorders of the nervous system and in metabolic abnormalities such as anoxia, are clinically similar to patients in coma due to primary metabolic abnormalities.

Supratentorial Lesions. McNealy and Plum have presented an orderly description of the sequential changes found in patients who have become comatose because of mass cerebral lesions.

The initial symptoms and signs reflect

the parenchymal destruction of the brain. For example, a large destructive process in the middle portion of the left hemisphere is likely to cause language dysfunction, right hemiparesis, sensory abnormalities on the right side, and possibly right homonomous hemianopsia. Cerebral edema associated with either infarction, abscess, or tumor often causes a shift of intracranial contents. The left hemisphere can herniate under the falx cerebri, causing pressure effects in the right hemisphere; the medial temporal lobe can be displaced into the notch of the tentorium; or the upper midbrain can be displaced caudally through the tentorial notch. Any or all of these changes may compromise the functioning of vital bilateral structures that are responsible for the maintenance of consciousness.

As herniation continues over minutes

to days, the following sequence of clinical signs occurs. Early there are, in addition to the signs and symptoms of the primary lesion, clouding of consciousness and other signs of bilateral brain dysfunction, such as a release of primitive reflexes (sucking and snouting). Bilateral deep cerebral dysfunction is often associated with cyclic changes in the respiratory pattern, varying from apnea to hyperventilation (Cheyne-Stokes respiration). At this stage the vestibulo-ocular reflex (Chap. 22) is prominent because of loss of cortical suppression. Marked agitation may be an early sign of impending herniation due to a cerebral mass. Isolated herniation of the temporal lobe may cause relative early compression of the third cranial nerve as it passes through the incisura of the tentorium, producing unilateral pupillary dilation.

As midbrain function is lost, these clinical signs appear: loss of pupillary light reflexes and bilateral signs of involvement of descending motor pathways (Babinski's sign, decerebrate or decorticate posturing). At this stage, the patient may show sustained hyperventilation. Dysfunction of the nerves innervating the extraocular muscles and their interconnections through the medial longitudinal fasciculus are often associated with dysconjugate gaze. The vestibulo-ocular reflex and caloric response are lost. More compression of the caudal brainstem may be associated with irregular depth and rate of breathing and finally apnea. When the level of dysfunction reaches the pontomedullary junction, decerebrate rigidity gives way to flaccidity (disruption of the lateral vestibulospinal and pontoreticulospinal tracts).

Extra-axial cerebral lesions, such as subdural hematoma and subdural empyema, can cause a similar sequence of changes; but, because these lesions are outside the parenchyma of the brain, unilateral focal cerebral signs early in the course of the illness are usually relatively mild.

Lesions of the Posterior Fossa.
Lesions (such as infarction, hematoma, tumor, and abscess) occurring in the posterior fossa are also associated with unconsciousness. These lesions may either directly involve the ascending reticular activating system of the brainstem or cause its dysfunction by pressure effects. Occasionally, small lesions of the posterior fossa clinically simulate supratentorial lesions by obstruction of the outflow of cerebral spinal fluid in the fourth ventricle, causing acute hydrocephalus. The hallmark of lesions of the posterior fossa is the occurrence of early signs referable to dysfunction of structures in the brainstem or cerebellum. For example, isolated single or multiple cranial nerve abnormalities, cerebellar signs, bilateral motor signs, sensory loss characteristic of brainstem lesions (loss of pain and temperature sensation on one side of the face and the other side of the body), or vestibular signs and symptoms are characteristic of lesions in the posterior fossa. The orderly sequence of signs occurring in rostral caudal deterioration from supratentorial masses is absent.

Metabolic Coma.
The signs and symptoms of coma due to metabolic brain dysfunction are varied. The list of causes is extensive and ranges from exogenous compounds such as sedative drugs and poisons to endogenous metabolic abnormalities associated with failure of various bodily functions (renal, hepatic, etc.). Although there are many exceptions, patients with altered states of consciousness due to metabolic abnormalities usually do not show signs of focal involvement of either motor, sensory, or cranial nerve pathways early in the course of their illness. The neurological signs that occur are symmetrical, and frequently the offending agent can be identified by history or by laboratory tests. Moreover, the sequence of signs often selectively involves specific functions of the central nervous system in a nonanatomical pattern. For example, if a patient takes an overdose of barbiturates, he is first drowsy and confused; his gait is ataxic (uncoordinated), and he has nystagmus. With time, as consciousness is lost, the pupillary light reflexes persist; but, because of the selective depression of vestibulo-ocular function by barbiturates, the caloric response is difficult to evoke and the vestibulo-ocular reflex is usually absent.

Although it would be incorrect to say that clinical experience with unconscious patients is not of great value, it is true that when the clinician is faced with difficult diagnostic problems involving consciousness, consideration of sound pathophysiologic principles will often lead him to the correct diagnosis. He must be able to recognize whether altered consciousness is due to direct involvement of the brainstem structures or caused by compression by an expanding remote lesion. The astute, early detection of the latter cause can lead to corrective neurosurgical intervention. For a detailed, lucid, and practical approach to this problem, the reader is referred to the book by Plum and Posner.

SLEEP

After the discovery of the ascending reticular activating system, it was assumed that changes in the activity of this system could explain the special normal behavioral changes related to consciousness, specifically sleep. It was therefore suggested that sleep results from a decrease in tonic activity of the ascending reticular activating system. This passive theory of sleep implies that sleep and coma are basically the same. It should be clear even to the casual observer that they are not.

The EEG recording taken during sleep may be divided into four stages of progressively slower electrical activity associated with the increasing depth of sleep (Fig. 23–8). These stages are now generally referred to as the *four stages of slow-wave sleep*. When these stages were the only ones known, it was relatively easy to explain the phenomena as decreases in the activity of the ascending reticular activating system.

However, more recent data indicate that sleep, like consciousness, is an active process. When the brainstem is transected at the midpontine level just rostral to the trigeminal input, the animal has insomnia and an activated or desynchronized EEG. Transection at the cervical medullary junction, however, leaves the animal with relatively normal sleep-wakefulness patterns. These observations suggest that sleep is controlled by the lower brainstem.

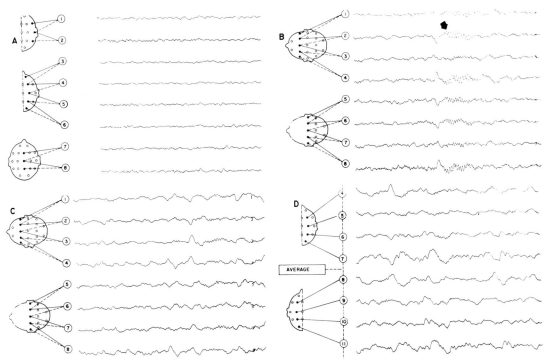

Figure 23–8. Sequential EEG records showing (A) Stage I, (B) Stage II, (C) Stage III, and (D) Stage IV of slow-wave sleep. The arrow in B illustrates sleep spindles.

Another observation indicating that slowing of the EEG during sleep is not due to removal of the activating effect of the ascending reticular system is the discovery of another type of sleep, characterized by a desynchronized EEG.

This stage is called rapid-eye-movement (*REM*) sleep because it is accompanied by episodic, rapid, saccadic eye movements. It is also called *paradoxical* sleep because the EEG suggests that the patient is in a relatively light sleep, whereas actually REM sleep is deeper than stage IV slow-wave sleep, as measured by arousal threshold. REM sleep usually appears within an hour after the onset of sleep and lasts from 5 to 30 min. REM sleep recurs about every 90 min throughout the night, and the duration of REM bouts increases as the night progresses. Patients awakened during REM sleep often say that they have been dreaming. Blood pressure, heart, and respiratory rates slowly decrease during slow-wave sleep. During REM sleep there are marked fluctuations in these vital signs. It has been suggested that nocturnal myocardial infarction and cerebral hemorrhage are more likely to occur during REM sleep. Spinal reflexes are markedly inhibited during REM sleep. There seems to be a biological need for REM sleep; if subjects are repeatedly awakened just as they enter REM sleep, they enter the REM stage sooner after falling asleep again.

Recent research strongly suggests that biogenic amines are involved in the biochemistry of sleep. Neurons of the median raphe nuclei of the brainstem contain large amounts of 5-hydroxytryptamine (5-HT). Lesions of these nuclei of animals cause insomnia that is relieved by administration of a precursor to 5-HT. Moreover, the drug *p*-chlorphenylalanine, which blocks the synthesis of 5-HT, causes a marked decrease in both slow-wave sleep and REM sleep. Thus, it is assumed that the raphe system and 5-HT are intimately involved in the mechanisms of slow-wave sleep.

Neurons of the locus coeruleus contain high concentrations of norepinephrine (NE). Bilateral destruction of the locus coeruleus in cats causes selective suppression of REM sleep without apparent effect on slow-wave sleep. Moreover, the drug reserpine, which depletes the brain of both 5-HT and NE, produces insomnia. If a precursor of 5-HT is given after reserpine, slow-wave sleep returns but REM sleep does not. The interrelationships of the various stages of sleep are illustrated in Figure 23–9.

The Narcolepsy Syndrome

This is a relatively benign but disturbing clinical condition involving abnormalities of sleep patterns. Patients with narcolepsy fall asleep easily at inappropriate times no matter how hard they attempt to stay awake. The syndrome also includes the symptoms of cataplexy, sleep paralysis, and hypnogogic hallucinations. *Cataplexy* is sudden weakness and loss of postural control, usually associated with emotional excitement. It is not unusual for it to occur in response to hearing a good joke. A baseball player treated by the author frequently falls flat on his face after hitting the ball. *Sleep paralysis* is a sensation of being unable to move upon awakening. Stimuli, such as being touched, usually

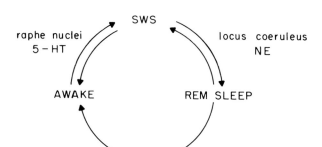

Figure 23–9. The interrelationship of the various stages of sleep. Note that a normal individual may enter into slow-wave sleep (*SWS*) and intermittently enter rapid-eye-movement (*REM*) sleep, but he does not go directly from the awake state to the REM sleep. (*5-HT*, 5-hydroxytryptamine; *NE*, norepinephrine; see text.)

cause the feeling of paralysis to disappear. *Hypnogogic hallucinations* are extremely vivid dreams occurring in the twilight setting just as a patient enters sleep. The EEG of patients with the narcolepsy syndrome usually, but not invariably, shows early entry into REM sleep just as they fall asleep. Drugs such as amphetamines are helpful to patients with a narcolepsy syndrome, but unfortunately, in many instances it is difficult to distinguish the true narcoleptic from the drug abuser.

ADDITIONAL READING

Brodal, A. *Neurological anatomy in relation to clinical medicine.* 2nd edition, New York, Oxford University Press, 1969.

Mountcastle, V. B., ed. *Medical physiology.* St. Louis, The C. V. Mosby Co., 1974.

Plum, F., and Posner, J. B. *The diagnosis of stupor and coma.* 2nd edition, Philadelphia, F. A. Davis Co., 1972.

Shepherd, G. M. *The synaptic organization of the brain: An introduction.* New York, Oxford University Press, 1974.

Warwick, R., and Williams, P. L. *Gray's anatomy.* 35th British edition, Philadelphia, W. B. Saunders Co., 1973.

CHAPTER 24

EPILEPSY AND SEIZURE STATES

WAYNE E. CRILL

Patients with destructive lesions of the nervous system may have "negative" signs (*e.g.*, paralysis or loss of sensation) secondary to interruption of specific excitatory neuropathways, or they may have "positive" signs (*e.g.*, spasticity or chorea) due to destruction of inhibitory pathways. Another class of symptoms and signs occurs in patients with neurological disease and is related to the excitable properties of neurons. A variety of pathological states increase the excitability of neurons and lead to their spontaneous discharge. If the spontaneous discharge of large populations of cortical neurons becomes synchronized, an epileptic seizure occurs.

DEFINITIONS

Before the classification and pathophysiology of epileptic disorders can be discussed, several terms must be defined.
Seizure is commonly used by nonmedical personnel to refer to a sudden attack of variable cause, including myocardial infarction, syncope, stroke, or convulsions. Most medically oriented individuals use the term *seizure* for the transient dysfunction of the central nervous system that is

associated with the abnormal increased firing of neurons. A more precise term would be *epileptic seizure. Ictus* is a synonym for *seizure. Convulsion* refers to the most dramatic type of epileptic seizure, characterized by tonic and clonic contraction of most skeletal muscles. In most convulsions there is loss of consciousness.
Epilepsy is a condition in which individuals are predisposed to recurring seizures. The potential for seizures is an inherent property of the human brain, and convulsions will occur in normal individuals when they are subjected to severe physical and chemical stresses. Convulsions precipitated by chemical abnormalities such as hypoglycemia or hyponatremia are indistinguishable from those occurring in patients with epilepsy. Excessive electrical stimulation of the brain, used in electroconvulsive therapy, also evokes convulsions. These types of seizures are not usually classified as epilepsy.

CLASSIFICATION

Clinicians have used numerous systems for the classification of epilepsies. Most of these methods have been exceedingly complex and cumbersome. The classification that follows is relatively simple and based on the current International Classification of Epileptic Seizures.* This scheme is based on clinical signs and symptoms in the patient and abnormalities in his electroencephalogram (EEG); it is the most useful classification for managing patients and understanding the underlying pathophysiology.

With rare exceptions epileptic seizures can be divided into two major groups. Seizures that began locally in the cortex are called *partial seizures*, or focal epilepsy; seizures that began bilaterally, without local onset, are called *generalized seizures*. To understand better the distinction between these two major classes of epilepsies, let us look at the sequence of clinical and electrical events that occur in the typical patient.

Patients with partial epilepsy show no

---

*Gastaut, H. Classification of the epilepsies. Proposal for an international classification. *Epilepsia*, 1969, *10*:14–21.

neurological signs between spells (the interictal period), unless the seizures are caused by a large, destructive lesion. In these cases the patients have "negative" symptoms appropriate for the size and location of the lesion. However, the EEG often shows transient spikes larger than the background voltage and lasting 15 to 180 msec (Fig. 24–1). These spikes can be localized to an anatomically restricted area of cortex and reflect the synchronized discharge of a small group of neurons. There are no subjective or objective signs associated with the spikes, presumably because the discharge is brief and only a small collection of individual neurons is involved. It is the occurrence of these spikes during the interictal period that makes the EEG so valuable in the diagnosis of focal epileptic disorders.

Occasionally, for largely unknown reasons, the spikes are associated with afterdischarges and can be recorded from larger areas of cortex. With this more extensive involvement of cortex, the patient often experiences symptoms. The signs depend on the location of the discharge.

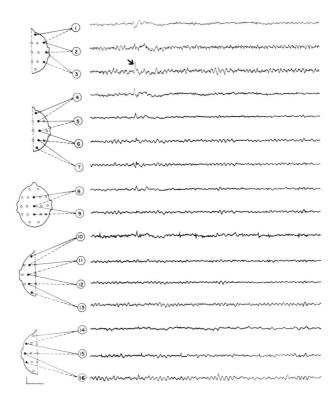

Figure 24–1. Electroencephalogram showing single epileptiform spike in the right frontotemporal region (*arrow*). This tracing is from a 42-year-old man who had periodic lapses of memory associated with stereotyped behavior (lip smacking and attempts to disrobe). Calibration: 50 μV and 500 msec.

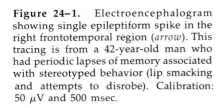

For example, if the increased spiking is in the visual cortex, the patient may see flashing lights. If the discharge is in the sensory or motor cortex, abnormal sensations or movements occur. If the seizure activity is confined to the temporal lobe, the patient often experiences recurring bizarre thoughts or displays complex types of behavior. The objective manifestations or subjective experiences during the initial portion of the seizure give the clinician valuable clues about the location of the seizure focus. The localized discharge can stop, producing only a partial seizure, or progressively involve larger areas of cortex, producing the expected increase in symptoms. When the epileptic activity involves both hemispheres, a generalized motor convulsion occurs. In this case, the symptoms and signs occurring before the focal seizure becomes generalized are called the *aura*. During the generalized

convulsion, the EEG shows high-voltage and high-frequency transients. After the seizure has terminated, the patient is often confused or obtunded, and background EEG rhythms are slowed. Postictal neurological deficits are frequently present and may last from several hours to a few days. These postictal abnormalities also have some localizing value.

In contrast to patients with focal epilepsy, those with *generalized seizure disorders* have no symptoms nor signs that herald the sudden occurrence of bilaterally synchronous high-voltage polyspike or spike and wave activity on the EEG (Fig. 24–2). The generalized seizure can be convulsive; the patient has a sudden loss of consciousness, a generalized contraction of skeletal muscle, transient apnea, an increase in heart rate and blood pressure, excessive salivation, and often loss of bowel and bladder control. The generalized convul-

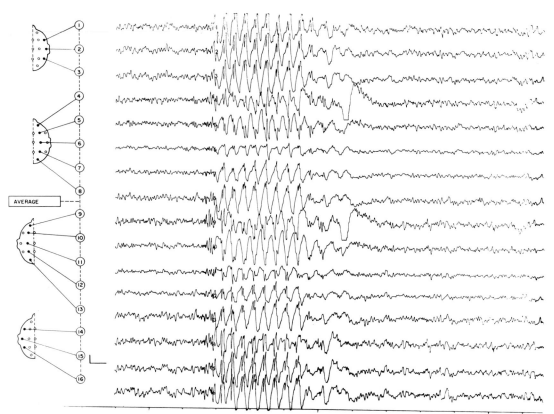

Figure 24–2. Electroencephalogram showing bilaterally synchronous onset of polyspike and spike and wave activity in a 38-year-old man with absence spells, generalized convulsions, and myoclonic jerks since childhood. Calibration: 50 μV and 500 msec.

sion lasts from a few seconds to a few minutes. It clinically differs in no way from the generalized convulsion occurring as the end result of a focal process. Patients with generalized epilepsy also show interictal changes in EEG. Intermittently, transient, bilaterally synchronous polyspikes or spikes and waves are recorded on the EEG. If this generalized burst lasts less than 1 to 2 sec, the patient experiences no symptoms.

In some patients, mostly children, generalized seizures may be nonconvulsive and take the form of absence attacks. The EEG abruptly changes from normal activity to bilaterally synchronous, 3-Hz, high-voltage spikes and waves that last from 5 to 30 sec (Fig. 24–2). During the abnormal discharge the patient is unaware of his environment and stares blankly into space. He does not lose postural control but may show muscle jerks or eye blinks at a frequency of 3 Hz. This specific syndrome is termed *petit mal*. Interestingly, this type of seizure is easily precipitated by metabolic changes, such as the hypocarbia induced by hyperventilation. Petit mal responds to a specific group of anticonvulsants and appears to be an inherited trait characterized by a dominant pattern with poor penetrance. Patients with generalized epilepsy may also have either myoclonic jerks or akinetic seizures. Myoclonic jerks are characterized by sudden synchronous jerks of the extremities and sometimes the trunk. In akinetic seizures the patient has a sudden loss of postural tone and falls to the ground.

PATHOPHYSIOLOGY

Many different animal models have been used in studies of the pathophysiology of epileptic disorders. The epilepsy of most animal models more closely resembles partial, or focal, epilepsy than generalized epilepsy. Since the neuroglial scars following trauma and the gliosis found around brain tumors and arteriovenous malformations are often associated with foci of epileptic activity, it is not surprising that researchers have attempted to produce epileptic animals by inducing focal cortical gliosis. The subpial injection of alumina cream induces seizures that most faithfully mimic the natural history of focal epilepsy in humans. Because it takes weeks for this lesion to develop into an active seizure focus, extensive work has been devoted to more rapidly developing epileptic foci induced by local freezing or the application of drugs such as strychnine or penicillin. In these latter models focal EEG spiking appears within minutes after the application of the drug.

Regardless of the experimental method used to induce focal epilepsy, the cellular events recorded with microelectrodes are relatively similar in each of the models. The interictal spikes recorded with surface electrodes are associated with paroxysmal depolarization shifts (PDS's) in single cells of the focus (Fig. 24–3). Superimposed upon this depolarization is a high-frequency burst of action potentials. The periodic depolarization shift is followed by a long hyperpolarization. In cells surrounding the active focus, the entire interictal event is associated only with a long hyperpolarization. Possibly this surround inhibition is a factor preventing the spatial spread of the seizure. In the case of the penicillin focus, which has been most extensively studied at the cellular level, the transition to a seizure is characterized by progressive loss of the hyperpolarization following the paroxysmal depolarization shift. Finally, individual neurons show a long-lasting depolarization of 20 to 30 mV that inactivates the sodium mechanism of the Hodgkin cycle. This is associated with the tonic phase of the seizure. During the clonic phase of the seizure the membrane potential intermittently returns to resting potential for progressively longer periods of time until the seizure ceases. A similar sequence of events occurs in cortical cells during the seizure induced by repeated electrical stimulation.

A single shock applied directly to the cerebral cortex evokes an action potential followed by a long afterhyperpolarization. With repetitive stimulation the afterhyperpolarization becomes a depolarization. Double and triplet firing occurs with each stimulus. A sustained membrane polarization appears, and the neurons fire at extremely high rates. Finally, depolarization block ensues.

A

EEG

B

INTRACELLULAR

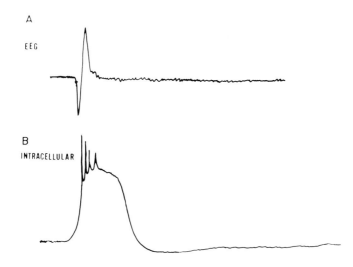

Figure 24-3. Experimental epileptogenic focus. The *top trace* is the electrocorticogram and the *bottom trace* is the intracellular recording from an adjacent cortical neuron. This figure illustrates the temporal association of the interictal cortical spike with a paroxysmal depolarization shift recorded from a single cortical neuron. Traces are drawn from records.

A major question facing epilepsy researchers is the nature of the interictal and ictal slow depolarizations. Several possible membrane and synaptic processes could explain the periodic slow depolarizations. For example, altered synaptic input could cause the depolarization. Either increased postsynaptic excitation alone or excitation combined with a decrease in tonic inhibition would cause depolarization. Such a change in synaptic input to a cell could be the result of alteration in the firing of presynaptic neurons, changes in the amount of transmitter released by presynaptic terminals, or an alteration in the number of transmitter-receptor complexes formed in the postsynaptic membrane. An alternative explanation for prolonged depolarizations is a change in the membrane properties of the cells in the epileptic focus. A change in the relative permeability of the membrane to different ions could depolarize the cell so that it has a tendency for either more rapid or sustained firing. Changes in the ionic environment of neurons could shift ionic equilibrium potentials in a depolarizing direction, producing depolarization. Another factor that may contribute to the potential across the neuron membrane is the electrogenic pumping of ions. The energy-requiring ionic pump that helps maintain differences in ionic concentration between the inside and outside of cells is generally assumed to be neutral. However, if more ionic charges are pumped in one direction than in another, an electromotive force is produced that contributes to the membrane potential. In recent years electrogenic ionic pumping has been demonstrated in neurons.

This is not the place to present each bit of evidence for and against each of the possible mechanisms, since the arguments are largely based on indirect measurements. However, the bulk of the evidence from single-cell studies suggests that postsynaptic excitation is enhanced during the paroxysmal depolarization shift. No changes in either the action potential mechanism or the membrane parameters controlling repetitive firing have been recorded from mammalian cortical cells in the focus with intracellular voltage-recording techniques. However, subtle changes in membrane properties are not easily detected with these techniques. Gasser once advised against making conclusions about the underlying neuronal mechanisms based only on potential recordings. More detailed voltage-clamp studies of the effects of epileptogenic agents on simpler systems such as invertebrate neurons indicate the presence of altered conductances of the voltage-dependent and time-dependent ionic channels in the presence of epileptogenic agents. Finally, ionic-specific electrodes indicate a significant increase in the extracellular potassium concentration during seizure activity. Because the change in concentration follows the initial epileptiform activity, it is assumed that the increased extracellular potassium is secondary to the synchronized excessive neuronal firing. Nevertheless, the change in the potassium equilibrium potential could be a contributing factor to the propagation of seizure activity.

One hypothesized role of the neuroglia is to regulate the ionic environment of neurons. If the glia in the regions of cortical gliosis do not adequately perform this function, altered neuronal behavior could ensue. Recent detailed studies in simple vertebrates have shown that the neuroglia are almost exclusively permeable to potassium ions. The resting potential of glial cells is near the potassium equilibrium potential, about 20 mV more negative than the transmembrane potential of neurons. Moreover, glial cells (astrocytes) are connected by low-resistance bridges (gap junctions), so that current can flow from one cell to another. In the region of increased extracellular potassium concentration, the potassium ions will flow into the glial syncytium. The potential gradient is established between the depolarized glia, where extracellular potassium is high, and adjacent glial cells. The resulting current flow through low-resistance bridges will tend to remove potassium from clefts where the concentration is high. This method of buffering the extracellular potassium concentration is one possible role of the glia and could be impaired in areas of glial scar formation. These are often sites of epileptic activity.

The cellular mechanisms of generalized seizure disorders are less well understood than those of partial seizures. In generalized epilepsy it appears as if the entire cortex suddenly does a flip-flop into an abnormal mode of behavior. There is insufficient time for abnormal activity to begin in one region of the cortex and spread by an intracortical mechanism to other portions of the cortex. It has therefore been postulated that the abnormal region is deep in the core of the cerebrum, near those areas that project symmetrically to wide regions of the cortex. Increased activity of neurons in deep structures could synchronously excite and induce epileptic activity bilaterally in the cortex. Experimental studies indicate that neurocircuits can transmit epileptic activity from one region to another. Focal stimulation of the cortex evokes seizures in the homotypical region of the cortex in the contralateral hemisphere by the pathways in the corpus callosum. On the other hand, recent experiments have shown that the symmetrical cortical epileptic foci cause bilaterally synchronous spike and wave activity. Similar results have also been demonstrated in animals with large islands of cortex disconnected by undercutting from subcortical structures. These experiments suggest that deep structures need not necessarily be the source of bilaterally synchronous cortical discharges.

Partial seizure disorders are sometimes difficult to distinguish from generalized epilepsy. If the focus is located far from the cerebral cortical surface, and in an area of the brain in which stimulation causes no subjective nor objective neurological changes, the first signs noted by the patient and recorded by the EEG may be a generalized motor convulsion. In these cases special placement of the EEG electrode frequently will reveal the initial focal spiking.

ADDITIONAL READING

Jasper, H. H., Ward, A. A., and Pope, A., eds. *Basic mechanisms of the epilepsies.* Boston, Little, Brown & Co., 1969.

Purpura, D. P., Penry, J. K., Tower, D. B., Woodbury, D. M., and Walters, R. D. *Experimental models of epilepsy*—A manual for the laboratory worker. New York, Raven Press, 1972.

Schmidt, R. P., and Wilder, B. J. *Epilepsy.* Philadelphia, F. A. Davis Co., 1968.

CHAPTER 25

SPECIAL CORTICAL FUNCTIONS

PHILLIP D. SWANSON

SPEECH AND SPATIAL PERCEPTION	DISCONNECTION SYNDROMES	THE NEUROLOGICAL BASIS OF MEMORY
	THE RIGHT CEREBRAL HEMISPHERE	

SPEECH AND SPATIAL PERCEPTION

It is well known that the majority of people are more dexterous with one hand (usually the right) than with the other. A person with an infarction or other lesion in the brain is much more likely to have a disorder of language (aphasia) when the lesion is located in the left cerebral hemisphere than in the right. These two facts have given rise to the concept of the dominance of the left cerebral hemisphere over the other. There have also been observations that suggest that lesions in certain parts of the dominant hemisphere are more likely to cause aphasia than lesions in other parts are. Moreover, the type of speech disorder may differ according to where the lesion lies. Some patients who have lesions in a cerebral hemisphere may have problems of perception rather than, or in addition to, speech disorders, such as inattention to stimuli on the side opposite the involved hemisphere, spatial disorientation, or failure to recognize common objects in the environment (agnosia). Although some of

the latter functions can be investigated in animals, it is obvious that study of speech mechanisms must depend upon observation of humans. It is important to remember that, as is also true of other symptoms or signs due to damage to the central nervous system, aphasias can be mild or severe, depending on the location of the pathologic lesion, on the acuteness of the damage, and often on the length of time that has passed since the damage occurred. Thus, infarction of a part of the left cerebral hemisphere may initially cause profound difficulty with use or understanding of words. After days or weeks improvement may be striking, so that the patient has very little deficit. It may be difficult to predict accurately the ultimate extent of recovery, since some unfortunate persons may improve very little. Probably it is correct to state that the earlier the onset of improvement, the better the ultimate prognosis. Anatomical–clinical correlations are obviously not always very precise, since the same lesion may be associated with aphasia of severe or mild degree, depending on the time of observation. Improvement in

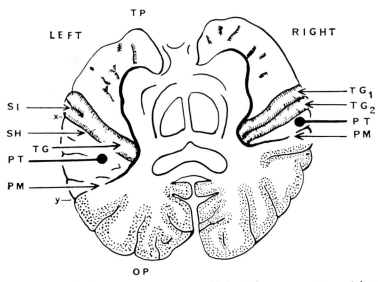

Figure 25–1. Asymmetry of the human superior temporal lobes. The upper surfaces of the temporal lobes are exposed by a horizontal section through the Sylvian fissures and removal of the parietal and frontal lobes. On the left the posterior margin (*PM*) of the planum temporale (*PT*) slopes posteriorly more sharply than on the right, the end of the Sylvian fissure (*y*) is posterior to the corresponding point on the right. The sulcus of Heschl (*SH*) slopes forward more sharply on the left so that the enclosed planum temporale (*PT*) is more extensive. On the left there is a single transverse gyrus of Heschl (*TG*); on the right, there are two (*TG$_1$* and *TG$_2$*). *TP*, temporal pole; *OP*, occipital pole. (From Geschwind and Levitsky, *Science*, 1968, *161*, 186–187. Copyright 1968 by the American Association for the Advancement of Science.)

speech may also be attributed erroneously to whatever therapeutic measures are being employed.

Speech disorders have been examined in most detail in patients with brain damage due either to infarction or to trauma. Even in left-handed individuals, the left hemisphere is usually the more important hemisphere for speech. Anatomically, in 65 per cent of brains a portion of the superior surface of the temporal lobe appears to be larger in the left hemisphere than in the right hemisphere (Fig. 25–1), and this area may be one of those that have particular importance for speech. This anatomical area is located behind the transverse gyrus (Heschl's gyrus), which receives auditory information from both ears. Asymmetry of size of these cortical regions is evident even in newborn infants, suggesting that anatomical specialization is a built-in feature of the cerebral hemispheres. Another important anatomical area for speech is located in the region of the operculum of the frontal lobe (Broca's area). Other parts of the left cerebral cortex in the temporal

and parietal lobes are also considered important for speech (Fig. 25–2). Further, damage to connections between the cortical areas involved with speech or to portions of the left thalamus may be associated with speech disturbances.

Confirmation that areas in the left cerebral hemisphere are important for speech has come from studies of Penfield and associates, who have applied electrical stimuli to areas on the exposed cerebral cortex at the time of a neurosurgical procedure (see Penfield and Roberts, 1959). Under local anesthesia, electrical stimuli are applied through surface electrodes in the form of saw-toothed or square waves with a frequency of 30 to 60 per second and variable voltage. Testing procedures include having the patient respond to a card picture by vocalizing or writing the name of the picture or asking the patient to count or read. Electrical stimuli applied to portions of the left hemisphere produce several alterations in speech: arrest of speech, hesitation and slurring of speech, distortion and repetition, confusion of numbers while counting,

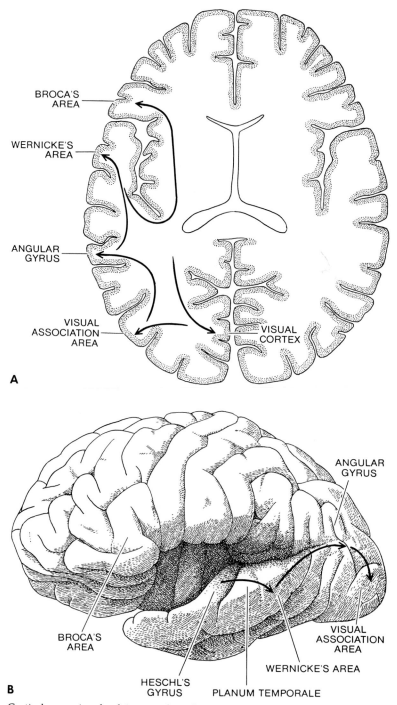

Figure 25–2. Cortical areas involved in speech and speech perception. *A,* Horizontal section through the brain. Naming a seen object involves transfer of the visual pattern from visual areas to the angular gyrus, and thence to Wernicke's area, where the auditory pattern is formed. Finally in Broca's area an articulatory pattern is generated that is passed on to the facial area of motor cortex, and the word is spoken.

B, Lateral view of left hemisphere, with Sylvian fissure pulled apart to expose Heschl's gyrus. Understanding the spoken name of an object involves sequential transfer of patterns from Heschl's gyrus to Wernicke's area to the angular gyrus to visual association cortex, where the appropriate visual pattern is generated. (From Language and the Brain, by Norman Geschwind. Copyright © 1972 by Scientific American, Inc. All rights reserved.)

inability to name, misnaming with or without perseveration, and vocalization. Speech arrest and vocalization may occur after stimulation of the primary and supplementary motor areas in either hemisphere, whereas the other speech abnormalities have been mainly produced by stimulation of the left hemisphere within the traditional Broca-Wernicke speech areas. Vocalization when the patient is silent has consisted of a sustained or interrupted cry. Arrest of speech and inability to name objects have more recently been reported during stereotactic surgery when electrical stimuli have been applied to thalamic nuclei on the dominant side.

The types of speech disorders that occur with lesions of the left hemisphere appear to depend on the speech areas involved. The usual classification divides aphasias into two broad types: expressive and receptive. Geschwind (1971) suggests that aphasias be classified according to the degree of loss of fluency: fluent and nonfluent. In *nonfluent* (expressive, motor, verbal) aphasias, the main difficulty appears to be related to expression in oral and written communication. Lesions that cause aphasias of this type are most often located in the region of the operculum of the inferior frontal lobe (Broca's area). In patients with persisting aphasia, the area of destruction usually includes part of the insula and adjacent white matter. Patients with nonfluent aphasias produce little speech and may be mute. Words are uttered slowly, with effort, and sentences may be telegraphic in style. *Fluent* (receptive, sensory) aphasias are usually caused by lesions further posterior in other association areas in either the parietal or temporal-parietal regions. These patients may produce either long phrases or sentences, but the content of the speech is affected and there may be difficulty in comprehending spoken or written language. Either an incorrect word or a word with incorrect syllables may be used. Geschwind further divides fluent aphasias into four subgroups; these are characterized and the locations of lesions described in Table 25–1. All of these aphasias are associated with difficulty in naming objects. In *anomic*, or *nominal*, aphasia, this is the predominant deficit. With lesions in both Broca's and Wernicke's areas (posterior superior temporal), a nonfluent aphasia may be combined with loss of comprehension and repetition and may be termed "global aphasia." Aphasias must also be considered more than disturbances of articulated speech, since expression in writing and reading comprehension are also affected, though sometimes to a different degree.

Clinical Cases

Case No. 1. (Case No. 6 from Head, 1926.) A 19-year-old soldier was struck by a piece of shrapnel in the left temple. He remained conscious and remembered everything that happened. When admitted to the hospital 4 days later he was speechless and silent. Shortly thereafter he began to make articulate noises, which seemed to bear no relation to the words he was trying to pronounce, such as "ho-nus" when asked his name and "ep" or "ons" when nodding his head in the affirmative. A negative response was accompanied by the sound "ong." He could understand simple commands but was slow to follow two or three consecutive orders. As he improved, he became able to say the alphabet and days of the week but pronounced words and letters poorly. He was soon able to write his own name and address but could not write that of his mother. He could not count but could write numbers to 21. When asked to write a simple phrase to dictation, he frequently failed to finish the sentence. Seven

TABLE 25–1. Geschwind's Subtypes of Fluent Aphasia

Type of Aphasia	Comprehension	Repetition	Location of Lesion
Wernicke's	Impaired.	Impaired.	Posterior superior temporal.
Conduction	Normal.	Impaired.	Suprasylvian-parietal.
Anomic	Normal.	Normal.	Angular gyrus or lower temporal lobe.
Isolation	Impaired.	Normal.	Surrounds intact speech areas.

months after the injury he still had great difficulty with verbalization. He was able to name objects well, but in spontaneous speech he had great difficulty in evoking words. Pronunciation was poor. Writing was done with difficulty, with defective word formation. Seven years later he still hesitated in finding words and showed defective enunciation and fluency in writing.

Though there was no pathologic confirmation of the site of damage, this patient's aphasia would be termed a nonfluent, expressive, or Broca's aphasia.

Case No. 2. A 55-year-old woman developed difficulties with speech over a period of several weeks. Her complaint was "I didn't have any memory in my arms or even to talk. I'd lost the ability to talk. I have lost all the use of the people I knew, except my own family and people I know real well, that's fine, I know them, but many, many people I used to know, I don't have their names. . . . There is a little bit of the regular things that I have lost the use of, some articles that I can't think of the name of."

On examination, she was able to talk rapidly, with long sentences. Most words were pronounced well, though she would occasionally substitute a word or a phrase that was not completely appropriate. She was able to read from a newspaper with some hesitation and mispronounced long words, such as "cancellation" She had moderate difficulty in understanding what she read. She was able to write her name and short sentences without spelling errors and she could calculate with little difficulty. Her most profound difficulty was an almost complete inability to name simple objects, such as a piece of chalk, a key, a pencil. She would say, "Oh, I should know; now what's the matter? I thought I knew." At times she would use an incorrect adjective. She was better able to find the correct name for a coin, but even here she sometimes was uncertain that the word she chose was correct. Shown a pair of glasses, she said, "It's what you look out of, I know what it's used for, and everything, but I cannot remember that name. It's used to see through."

This patient was found to have a gliomatous tumor in the left temporal lobe. Her aphasia was fluent, or receptive, and to a large degree could be characterized as a nominal, or anomic, aphasia.

Can aphasia result from lesions in the thalamus? Since thalamocortical projections are widespread and include "speech" areas of the brain, it is reasonable to ask this question. The answer is uncertain, though a few cases exist in which either infarction or tumor in the left thalamus has been associated with aphasic symptoms. Further, during certain neurosurgical operations for the treatment of involuntary movement disorders, it has been possible to pass electric current into the thalamus while the patients, who are awake, are reading from a series of words or are asked to name objects. Interruption of speech and inability to name objects are found when stimulation is in the region of the nuclei of the left thalamus.

DISCONNECTION SYNDROMES

Some important studies were carried out on patients who had undergone section of the corpus callosum as a treatment for epilepsy. (This procedure is very rarely performed even by neurosurgeons with special interests in the surgical treatment of epilepsy.) These patients had had their two cerebral hemispheres essentially disconnected, since the corpus callosum is the major interhemispheric commissure. On casual observation, the patients appeared quite normal, being able to swim, catch objects with both hands, or light a cigarette. In special test situations, however, it could be demonstrated that the two hemispheres were functioning quite independently (Fig. 25–3). It was found that if a patient had something placed in the right hand, or if an image was projected only into the right visual field (therefore, going via the left half of the retina into the left cerebral hemisphere), he was able to verbalize the name of the object he had felt in his hand or seen in his right visual field. In contrast, if an image was flashed in the left half of the visual field (information ultimately reaching the right hemisphere), the patient denied seeing the image. However, when the patient was directed to find with his left hand the object that he had seen, he was able to do this. His inability to report ver-

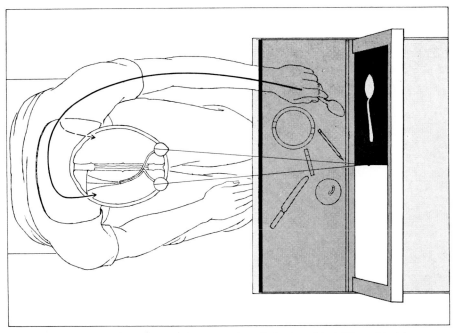

Figure 25–3. Diagram of visual-tactile association test in split-brain subject. The subject focuses on the center of the screen. A picture of a spoon is flashed on the left side of the screen, activating the right visual cortex, with the left hand the subject palpates objects below the table top and retrieves the spoon. Tactile information from the left hand projects mainly to the right hemisphere, the weak ipsilateral projection (*dotted line*) being inadequate for the subject to name the object selected (using only the left hemisphere). (From The Split Brain in Man, by Michael S. Gazzaniga. Copyright © 1967 by Scientific American, Inc. All rights reserved.)

bally about the visual input to the right hemisphere was due to the fact that he was unable to transfer the information in his right hemisphere over to the speech centers located in the left hemisphere. Similar findings occur when such a patient attempts to identify objects placed in the hand. If something is put into the left hand, he can match it on a nonverbal test but is unable to verbalize what he has felt. This indicates that the left hemisphere is indeed dominant for speech.

Certain clinical syndromes are sometimes encountered in which the symptoms are due in part to disconnection of one area of the brain from another. One such syndrome is characterized by *alexia* (word blindness) without *agraphia*, in which the patient has the ability to write but is unable to read. The patient also usually has a right homonymous hemianopsia but is able to name and recognize objects. This syndrome can occur with combined infarctions of the left primary visual cortex and the splenium of the corpus callosum, some-

times as a consequence of occlusion of the left posterior cerebral artery. Visual information comes to the right cerebral hemisphere but cannot be transferred to the left hemisphere and gain access to those parieto-occipital areas necessary for recognition of words. How can such an individual visually recognize objects other than words? The reason for this discrepancy is not certain but is suggested to be due to the nonverbal associations evoked by visual objects (touch, taste, smell), allowing transfer of information across callosal fibers located more anteriorly.

Another rare but instructive disconnection syndrome has been described in patients with destruction of the anterior four fifths of the corpus callosum due to ischemia in territories of branches of the anterior cerebral arteries. Visual information can pass between the two occipital lobes, so the patient can read in either visual field. An object held in the left hand cannot be named, however, since the somesthetic information from the right hemisphere cannot reach the left hemisphere speech centers. The patient cannot write correctly with the left hand or carry out commands with the left hand because of inaccessibility of verbal information to the right hemisphere.

THE RIGHT CEREBRAL HEMISPHERE

Some very interesting findings brought out in the studies on callosum-sectioned patients suggest that the right hemisphere can perform better than the left hemisphere in some test situations (Fig. 25–4).

The right hemisphere appears perfectly able to identify objects handled with the left hand if the patient is also shown a picture of the object. The right hemisphere also has some limited ability to understand language because when the word *pencil* is flashed in the left visual field (right hemisphere), the patient is able to pick out a pencil from among several other objects with his left hand, although he cannot verbalize what he is selecting. The right hemisphere is actually rather better than the left hemisphere when it comes to "visual-constructional" tasks. The left hand is better able to copy a drawing or to assemble blocks than is the right hand in callosum-

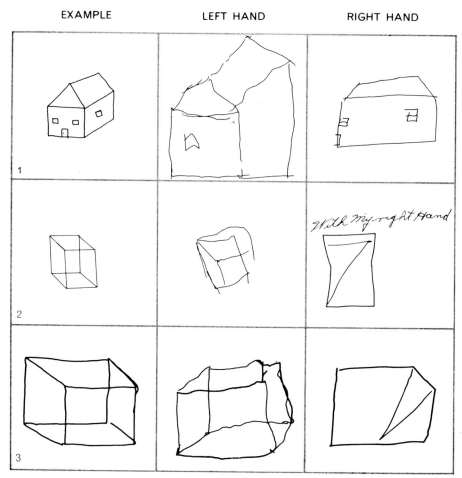

EXAMPLE   LEFT HAND   RIGHT HAND

Figure 25–4. Performance of visual constructional tasks by split-brain subject. He was asked to copy the drawings in the left column with the left hand (*middle column*) and the right hand (*right column*). Although the patient was right-handed, he copied the examples better with his left hand (right hemisphere). (From The Split Brain in Man, by Michael S. Gazzaniga. Copyright © 1967 by Scientific American, Inc. All rights reserved.)

sectioned patients. This observation helps explain the peculiar difficulty with spatial tasks that a patient has when the parietal area of the right hemisphere is damaged by an infarction or other lesion. For example, he may deny the existence of his left side, and he may ignore space on the left side of the body. Although such patients are able to speak quite well, they have great difficulty in drawing simple figures, such as a cube. These patients are often quite indifferent to their disability. Such "right parietal-lobe" patients may be more difficult to rehabilitate than the aphasic patient with a lesion in the left cerebral hemisphere.

Clinical Case

A 60-year-old former Air Force pilot with long-standing hypertension, while searching for his keys with his left hand, was noted by his wife to have difficulty in manipulating the keys. She also noted that he seemed rather lethargic, though he had no specific complaints. On examination by a neurologist, he appeared alert but was rather uninterested in performing well. He denied being ill and said he was in the hospital because his wife thought he had had a stroke. The only motor abnormalities were a mild weakness of the left face and some loss of precision on doing fine movements with the left hand. He performed accurately on testing of pinprick, light touch, position, and vibration sense. He could identify objects placed in his hands. He had similar difficulty on both sides with figure-writing on the skin. However, when touched on both sides simultaneously, he always denied feeling the stimulus on the left side, even when the stimulus occurred in the left field of vision.

He was able to read and write, and his speech was normal. He could not draw the simplest object accurately, failed to close a square, and put the numbers of a clock face outside the boundaries of the face. The inaccuracy was more pronounced on the left side of the drawn object. He drew a very inaccurate map of the state of Washington and paid little attention to boundaries that he drew. Asked to fill in gaps in a simple, incomplete drawing of a face, he ignored the absence of the right eye (to the patient's left). When inaccuracies were pointed out to him, he became somewhat hostile and asked the examiner to try to do better if he thought he could.

THE NEUROLOGICAL BASIS OF MEMORY

The ability to remember information that has been learned or experienced minutes, days, or years before is perhaps the most important function of the brain. We remain at a very primitive level of understanding both the neurophysiological and neurochemical bases of memory, though there are indications that certain anatomical regions are important for memory consolidation and recall. One problem that faces the student of learning and memory is the difficulty in reconciling information obtained from animal studies with that obtained from examination of humans. For example, in humans, damage to the medial portions of the temporal lobes, including the hippocampal regions, can be associated with profound memory deficits, whereas ablation of such regions in experimental animals may not alter performance on learning tests. Part of the problem may be due to difficulties in precisely subclassifying the varying types of memory. One classification differentiates memory into groups depending upon the interval between learning the information and recalling it, as in Table 25–2.

TABLE 25–2. Classification of Memory

	Duration of Recall	How Tested
Immediate recall	Seconds.	Repeat numbers, recall names of objects.
Short-term memory	Minutes to hours.	Recall names of objects or events of the recent past even after a distraction.
Long-term memory	Months to years.	Recall events remote in time.

Clearly, there are very broad time zones involved, and deciding at what point short-term memory blends into long-term memory is impossible. Even such a broad distinction is useful, however, since in certain situations one type of memory may be disturbed without effects on another. Certain clinical conditions encountered in man can be associated with rather striking deficits in the ability to learn and to recall recent events. This is called the *amnestic,* or *amnesic,* syndrome, or Korsakoff's psychosis, and is encountered in patients who have had *bilateral* damage to particular areas of the cerebral hemispheres.

In humans, the medial portions of the temporal lobes, including the hippocampal complexes, are generally accepted as being critical for memory formation. Agreement is less about the importance of connected areas, such as the fornix and mammillary bodies, though the brain of a patient with an amnestic syndrome due to thiamine deficiency will usually be found to have damage to the mammillary bodies. These areas appear to be of importance for the formation of a lasting record of events in other parts of the brain and for retrieval of memories from storage.

There have been several reports of marked deficits of memory in patients who have had surgical removal of both temporal lobes as a treatment for epilepsy and in patients with occlusions of both posterior cerebral arteries, resulting in infarction of the medial portions of the temporal lobes, including the hippocampus (Fig. 25–4).

A 29-year-old patient of Scoville and Milner (1957) had been incapacitated by intractable seizures since the age of 16 and was subjected to a neurosurgical procedure. At operation, the mesial surfaces of both temporal lobes were resected to about 8 cm posteriorly from the temporal tips.

After operation this young man could no longer recognize the hospital staff nor find his way to the bathroom, and he seemed to recall nothing of the day-to-day events of his hospital life. There was also a partial retrograde amnesia, inasmuch as he did not remember the death of a favorite uncle 3 years previously, nor anything of the period in the hospital, yet could recall some trivial events that had occurred just before his admission to the hospital. His early memories were apparently vivid and intact.

Even after 3 years this patient was unable either to learn a new address or to remember where objects in continued use were located. His memory deficit was the more remarkable since his intelligence quotient was 112 (prior to operation it had been recorded as 104). He appeared to a casual observer as relatively normal, since his understanding and reasoning were undiminished. He could retain a three-figure number or a pair of unrelated words for several minutes if undistracted, but if his attention was drawn to a new topic they were immediately forgotten. Psychological testing failed to reveal any deficits in either perception, abstract thinking, motivation, or personality.

Patients who have such lesions have difficulty in the process of storing memories. They can immediately remember a task (immediate recall) but are unable to consolidate it sufficiently to remember it a few minutes later. These patients are virtually unable to establish lasting new memories, although they can remember things that they have learned long before and may be able to remember small bits of information perfectly for seconds or a few minutes if undistracted. This type of memory consolidation, which requires the presence of the temporal lobes, is termed *recent* memory and is to be contrasted with long-term memory, which may not be dependent on the hippocampal areas. In animals, for example, lesions of the hippocampus that have been made a few days after the learning of a maze cause severe impairment in performance. Lesions made 6 or more days after learning produce no impairment in maze running; thus, it would appear that the "memory trace" has become independent of the hippocampus.

Implication of the hippocampal formation rather than either the parahippocampal cortex, amygdaloid nucleus, or uncus is strengthened by isolated cases of memory loss associated with discrete infarctions of both hippocampi, with sparing of these other areas. These regions lie in the supply territories of the posterior cerebral arteries and can be damaged with occlusion of these arteries by either thrombi or emboli.

When an amnesic syndrome occurs after a unilateral temporal lobectomy, it is usu-

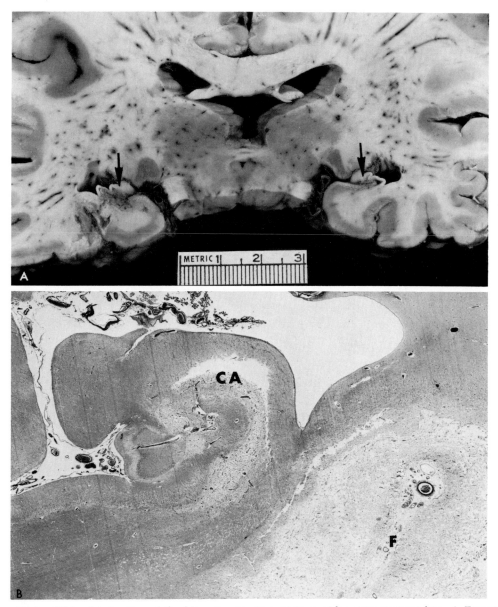

Figure 25-5. Bilateral infarction of the hippocampus in a patient with severe memory loss. *A.* Transverse section of the brain at the level of the lateral geniculate bodies. Arrows point to necrotic hippocampus. *B,* Microscopic section showing chronic infarct of Ammon's horn *(CA)* and of parahippocampal and fusiform gyri *(F).* (From DeJong *et al., Arch. Neurol.,* 1969, *20,* 339–348.)

ally assumed that prior damage has been present in the other hippocampal region, so that bilateral hippocampal dysfunction has resulted. In fact, the majority of patients with unilateral temporal lobectomies do not develop severe memory loss. Occasionally, however, a loss of recent memory occurs after unilateral temporal

lobectomy. One such patient became amnesic at age 46 after removal of the left hippocampus 5 years after removal of the anterior 4 cm of the same temporal lobe. At autopsy, the remaining right hippocampus was shrunken, pale, and firm, and there was severe loss of neurons in the pyramidal cell layer. These deficiencies probably occur at the time of birth and are frequently found in the brains of patients who have psychomotor seizures.

Only rarely has a profound memory disturbance occurred after damage to one cerebral hemisphere with pathologically confirmed absence of damage to the other side. One such patient had an extensive infarction in the territory of the left posterior cerebral artery (Caplan and Hedley-Whyte, 1974). She could write but was unable to read (alexia), had difficulty with calculations and with visual object and picture identification, and showed a severe defect in recent memory function. During the acute phase of her illness, she could recall 1 or 2 facts in a 10-part story after 3 min, but almost nothing of the story after 10 min. She could not recall being in a special room on 12 different occasions. Her memory gradually improved, so that after 7 months she could remember names and could report 7 of 10 facts of a story given 10 min before. She never regained memory for the onset of her illness or for events during her first hospital months.

The infarction included gray and white matter of the medial temporal lobe, extending into the occipital lobe and including the splenium of the corpus callosum, the posterior hippocampus, and geniculate bodies. An infarct was also present in the posteroventral lateral nucleus of the left thalamus. The left fornix and mammillary body were atrophic. It is possible that memory disturbance is more likely to occur with a unilateral lesion if the thalamus is involved in addition to the dominant temporal lobe.

When one goes beyond these anatomical considerations, discussions of memory mechanisms become even more difficult to relate to known physiological or biochemical phenomena. Memory consolidation may be impaired by electroshock. However, after deep coma, brought about by overdoses of sedative drugs, patients may remember events up to the time of drug ingestion. Persistence of memories may be found even after almost complete cessation of the electrical activity of the brain. This makes it unlikely that memory storage can be accounted for by reverberating electrical circuits. The establishment of memory traces must involve structural change that persists beyond the event that is remembered. Evidence is accumulating that a certain amount of plasticity exists at the level of fine nerve terminals, which can be demonstrated in electron micrographs to innervate areas that have been deprived of incoming connections.

Much of the biochemical work on memory has been difficult to reproduce, and there are widely divergent ideas about the chemical changes that occur with the making of memory. The most speculative workers envisage memory molecules that range from peptides to ribonucleic acid (RNA) and that code for specific memories. Claims of transfer of memories between animals and sometimes across species lines seem incredible. Less imaginative, but perhaps more likely to be correct, are the suggestions that biochemical changes at the synaptic level might occur in association with establishment of new and more lasting connections among nerve circuits.

ADDITIONAL READING

Caplan, L. R., and Hedley-Whyte, R. Cuing and memory dysfunction in alexia without agraphia — A case report. *Brain*, 1974, *97*, 251–262.

DeJong, R. N., Itabashi, H. H., and Olson, J. R. Memory loss due to hippocampal lesions. *Arch. Neurol.*, 1969, *20*, 339–348.

Gazzaniga, M. S. The split brain in man. *Sci. Amer.*, Aug. 1967, *217*, 24–29.

Geschwind, N. Language and the brain. *Sci. Amer.*, Apr. 1972, *226*, 76–83.

Geschwind, N. Aphasia. *New Engl. J. Med.*, 1971, *284*, 654–656.

Head, H. *Aphasia and kindred disorders of speech*, Vol. II. Cambridge, Cambridge University Press, 1926.

Penfield, W., and Roberts, L. *Speech and brain mechanisms*. Princeton, N.J., Princeton University Press, 1959.

Scoville, W. B., and Milner, B. Loss of recent memory after bilateral hippocampal lesions. *J. Neurol. Neurosurg. Psychiat.*, 1957, *20*, 11–21.

Victor, M. The amnesic syndrome and its anatomical basis. *Canad. med. Ass. J.*, 1969, *100*, 1115–1125.

Whitty, C. W. M., and Zangwill, O. L., eds. *Amnesia*. New York, Appleton-Century-Crofts, 1966.

CHAPTER 26

THE HYPOTHALAMUS

JOHN W. SUNDSTEN

ANATOMICAL SUBDIVISIONS	HYPOTHALAMIC REGULATORY FUNCTIONS	Behaviors Pituitary Gland
	Temperature Regulation Food and Water Intake	CLINICAL CASE

The hypothalamus is not a conspicuous part of the brain, yet more functions have been attributed to it than to any other region of the central nervous system (CNS) with comparable dimensions. It is the ventral part of the diencephalon, and its separation from the thalamus is clearly evident on a medial view of the forebrain (Fig. 26–1). The considerable expanse of the internal capsule that developed along with the cerebral hemispheres provides a lateral boundary throughout much of its rostrocaudal extent (see Figure 26–2). Medially, it faces the third ventricle. The hypothalamus is old phylogenetically, and its nuclear structure and connections are fairly consistent from species to species. In the fish the hypothalamus occupies practically the whole forebrain, but in higher groups of animals the hypothalamus is overshadowed in size by the development of the cerebral hemispheres.

The hypothalamus is essential for a variety of behaviors associated with emotion, and it is the region of the CNS that regulates the activity of the pituitary gland and, thereby, the metabolic functions of the en-docrine system. It accomplishes the latter both through *neural connections* with the posterior pituitary gland and through *humoral connections* with the anterior pituitary gland via the portal vessels. In addition, it modulates the various reflex functions of the autonomic nervous system that operate at the levels of the brainstem and spinal cord. It does this through descending pathways that impinge eventually on preganglionic neurons of the parasympathetic and sympathetic outflows. Because of this autonomic role it is sometimes referred to as the *head ganglion* of the autonomic nervous system. In addition, it is likely that specialized neural elements that perform sensor functions (*e.g.*, osmoreceptors, thermodetectors, hormone detectors) reside in this integrative part of the forebrain.

The hypothalamus receives input from all the sensory systems and in turn can be dominated by cortical and other forebrain structures that are usually considered together as the *limbic system*. It is clear then that its neuronal complexity is great. For example, it is not usual to find discrete iso-

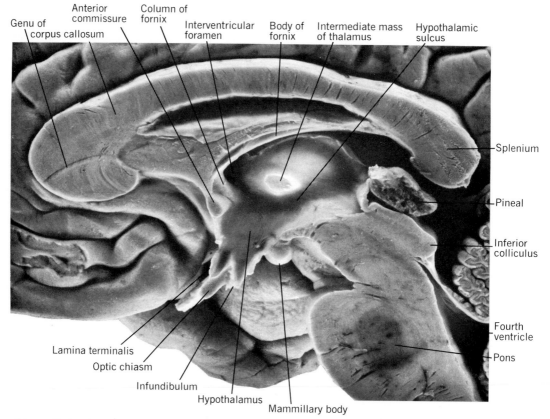

Figure 26–1. A sagittal view of the human brain, showing the hypothalamus and neighboring structures.

lated effects after either electrical stimulation or lesioning. Rather, patterns of responses are most commonly altered involving components of the endocrine, visceral motor, and somatic motor systems. The hypothalamic involvement in various regulatory functions will be summarized later as follows:

(1) Body temperature.
(2) Food and water intake.
(3) Selected behaviors.
  (a) Rage.
  (b) Sex.
  (c) Sleep.
(4) Pituitary gland.

ANATOMICAL SUBDIVISIONS

Before we go into the regulatory functions in any detail, it is worthwhile to summarize some of the major anatomical subdivisions of the hypothalamus. The hypothalamus is divided into medial and lateral parts; an approximate guide to these divisions is the position of the *fornix* (Fig. 26–2). The nuclei within the hypothalamus are located mainly in the medial division. The lateral part is primarily an area through which information is projected into and out of the hypothalamus by the *medial forebrain bundle* and is also the region in which fibers are projecting that interconnect different hypothalamic areas. For convenience, the hypothalamus is subdivided into three major areas by frontal planes of section as follows (refer to Figure 26–2):

(1) The supraoptic level above the optic chiasm.
(2) The tuberal level above the pituitary gland.
(3) The mammillary level above the mammillary body.

Most nuclear groups within the hypothala-

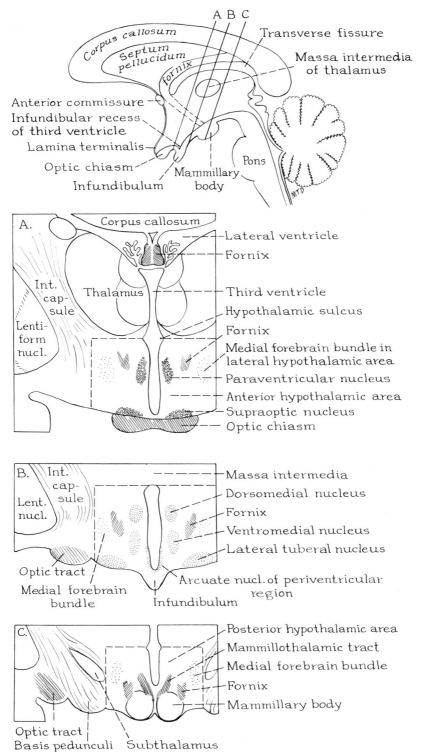

Figure 26–2. Representative frontal sections through the hypothalamus: *A,* supraoptic level; *B,* tuberal level; *C,* mammillary level. (From Everett, *Functional neuroanatomy,* Philadelphia, Lea & Febiger, 1971.)

mus are not clearly defined; as a result, they are often referred to as *areas,* or *regions,* rather than as nuclei. Thus, at the supraoptic level, the *anterior hypothalamic area* is found, as well as the two neurosecretory cell groups, the *supraoptic* and *paraventricular* nuclei. At the tuberal level, the major nuclei are the *ventromedial* and *dorsomedial* nuclei. At the mammillary level the major nuclei are the *mammillary bodies* themselves (composed of several subdivisions) and the *posterior hypothalamic area,* located dorsally. Although the lateral hypothalamus is composed mainly of fibers, neuron cell bodies are present, and the whole rostrocaudal extent of the lateral hypothalamus is referred to as the *lateral hypothalamic area.* The structural heterogeneity of hypothalamic connections is quite complex, as is evident from even the following simplified scheme:

(1) Any one part of the hypothalamus is connected to virtually any other part.

(2) The lateral hypothalamus receives major inputs from the amygdala (laterally), from the midbrain tegmentum (caudally), and from the limbic system (rostrally), especially via the medial forebrain bundle. The fornix (from the hippocampus) and the mammillary peduncle (from the midbrain) provide other major inputs to the medial hypothalamus.

(3) Interconnections are present between the medial and lateral parts of the hypothalamus.

(4) Hypothalamic efferents leave via both the lateral hypothalamus and the medial hypothalamus. The medial hypothalamus also has connections with the pituitary gland (vascular and neural) and with the anterior thalamic nucleus (via the mammillothalamic tract). In addition, a fine periventricular fiber system, in close proximity to the third ventricle, projects into the medial thalamus (dorsally) and midbrain (caudally).

These pathways are summarized in the block diagram shown in Figure 26–3.

It should be apparent that, because of the complex interconnections and poorly defined nuclear groups of the hypothalamus, it would be difficult to correlate any one individual hypothalamic function with any single underlying anatomical area. In part because of this difficulty, the concept of *centers* has evolved and is widely used. A *center* is usually not a precise, clearly defined nuclear group but rather is a general region that, on the basis of experiments with stimulation, lesioning, and recording techniques, seems to be involved in one (or more) fairly clear functions. There are many such *centers* in the hypothalamus, and they exist for the most part in pairs. Each member of the pair has the opposite regulatory function to its mate, and one would expect that each has reciprocal inhibitory interconnections. This simplified model is shown schematically in Figure 26–4.

A major difficulty in the interpretation of results of experimental manipulations of this part of the brain is due to its small size and interconnections. A measured effect may be either part of a regulatory mechanism under study or part of another that is not being looked at but that, in the hierarchy of behaviors, may be even more dominant. For example, lateral hypothalamic stimulation will increase food intake

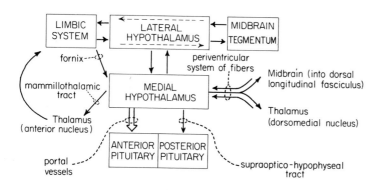

Figure 26–3. Summary diagram of hypothalamic connections. (See also Figures 27–4 to 27–6.)

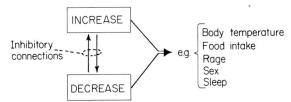

Figure 26-4. Schematic representation of how hypothalamic "centers" perform regulatory functions.

markedly, even in the satiated animal, and will also induce aggressive behavior if the option is available. Further, the same region has been referred to as a *pleasure center.* Animals can be trained to self-stimulate that area with electrical shocks and will do so in preference to sex or food. In humans undergoing neurosurgery, electrodes have on occasion been placed in the lateral hypothalamus, and the subjective reports have indicated that a very pleasurable feeling arises on electrical stimulation. Subjects will readily voluntarily press the switch that delivers the current and express a satisfaction that is difficult for them to describe. It is apparently something other than sexual gratification, perhaps best described as positively reinforcing, *i.e.,* very good indeed! Either changing the parameters of stimulation or moving the electrode a millimeter anterior can result in a negatively reinforcing effect. Thus, the model of reciprocally innervated opposing "centers" is in all likelihood very complex. However, it is certain that the hypothalamus is of critical importance in several regulatory functions and behaviors, even though the exact underlying neural mechanism is not clearly understood.

HYPOTHALAMIC REGULATORY FUNCTIONS

Temperature Regulation

It has long been known that the *anterior hypothalamic area* plays a decisive role in the regulation of body temperature. Destruction of this area results in the inability to maintain body temperature at normal levels by sufficient vasodilation or sweating, with the result that body temperature increases to a high, critical, and sometimes

fatal level. Regulation against cold stress remains intact, though core temperature may fluctuate about wider than normal limits. Conversely, the *posterior hypothalamic area* is thought to subserve heat conservation and production mechanisms. Carefully placed small lesions here result in insufficient vasoconstriction and shivering in response to cold exposure, with the result that body temperature falls. Larger lesions abolish both heat loss responses (because of interruption of descending pathways that originate more rostrally) and heat production responses, so that a tendency toward *poikilothermia* exists. The two regions, anterior hypothalamus and posterior hypothalamus, are interconnected, so that in the normal individual core temperature is maintained at an optimum value in the face of either a warm stress or a cold stress. It now seems certain that the anterior hypothalamus also contains thermosensitive elements that respond directly to the temperature of the blood bathing their environment. Thus, appropriate heat-loss mechanisms have been brought into play by a warming of this region and cold-defense mechanisms by a cooling of it; there are no thermosensitive elements in the posterior hypothalamus. The presence of such neural thermal "detectors" sensitive to temperature changes has also been demonstrated by single-unit recording techniques.

The effects of local variation of hypothalamic temperature provide a good example of the *patterns of responses* that occur with hypothalamic manipulation; *e.g.,* cooling the anterior hypothalamus results in shivering (a somatic motor response), vasoconstriction (a visceral motor response), and activation of the thyroid and adrenal glands (endocrine responses). Warming of the region results in the well-known heat-loss response, vasodilation, and the somatic behavioral response of seeking a cooler environment.

The above findings seem paradoxical since earlier lesion studies separated heat-loss and heat-conservation regions into the anterior and posterior hypothalamus, respectively. However, one may explain this seeming paradox by assuming that the "warm detectors" are the critical ones—the anterior hypothalamus is far more sensitive to increases in blood temperature than to decreases. The "cold detectors" in the anterior hypothalamus perhaps come into play only in severe hypothermic states; the normal responses to cold stress are initiated only by peripheral cold receptors. The more posterior lesions that block cold-defense responses can be assumed to interfere with the integrative mechanism receiving inputs from peripheral and central cold receptors; the posterior region normally has a dominant control over the sympathetic nervous system, loss of which would certainly impair defense against cold.

Clinical observations support these theories. Postoperative hyperthermia is not uncommon after surgical operations for hypophyseal tumors in which some damage (such as that from edema) has been done to the anterior hypothalamus. Furthermore, as mentioned earlier, evidence from patients with tumors in the anterior hypothalamic region has shown that it is an essential area for effective temperature regulation. Patients who have decerebrating lesions that isolate the hypothalamus from the midbrain commonly become poikilothermic and tend to take on the temperature of the environment, since the hypothalamic outflows regulating both heat loss and heat production have been interrupted.

Food and Water Intake

It has been postulated that the ventromedial nucleus is a *satiety center* and the lateral hypothalamic region at that level is a *feeding center*. Destruction of the ventromedial region bilaterally results in increased food intake (*hyperphagia*) and obesity in both animals and man, whereas destruction of the lateral hypothalamic region results in cessation of eating (*aphagia*). Conversely, electrical stimulation of the ventromedial area results in decreased food intake, even in the hungry animal, and stimulation of the lateral region causes increased food intake, even in the satiated animal.

Although not directly related to the regulation of food intake, it should be mentioned that because of the hypothalamus's major influence in controlling the digestive tract via the autonomic outflow, hypothalamic damage may result in gastric ulceration or hemorrhage or both. The exact area within the hypothalamus that is responsible has not been localized, most likely because autonomic effects can be elicited through stimulation of overlapping areas; the anterior hypothalamus is, however, predominantly a parasympathetic area. It is probable that the ordinary gastric ulcer occurs because of an imbalance between the parasympathetic and sympathetic outflows from the hypothalamus.

Hypothalamic *drinking centers* have been postulated but have not been worked out in as much detail as have those regions involved in the regulation of food intake. Certainly, water balance is a major function of the hypothalamus, both with respect to the regulation of antidiuretic hormone (ADH, or vasopressin) output by the supraoptic neurons (see later) and to the regulation of water intake by proposed hypothalamic integrative centers. The latter are in the same general regions as those proposed for food intake, *i.e.*, the *ventromedial* and *lateral hypothalamus*. Polydipsia, then, may be secondary to water loss resulting from impaired ADH release or may be a direct result of damage to a *thirst satiety* center somewhere in the (medial?) hypothalamus. Impaired regulation of water balance is also closely allied to altered plasma levels of sodium chloride; determining whether the primary involvement is electrolyte metabolism or water exchange is often a major clinical problem. However, when negative water balance (water loss) and hypernatremia develop in the conscious patient who is not thirsty, it is likely that the hypothalamic thirst-regulating mechanism is impaired.

Behaviors

Behaviors with strong emotional overtones are almost always expressed by components of both the somatic and visceral motor systems. Classic studies on the hypothalamus pointed to its role in two dominant behaviors necessary for the survival of the individual, rage or aggressive reactions and escape responses. In both of these there is considerable sympathetic discharge. (Sympathetic effects can readily be elicited by electrical stimulation of the more posterior and tuberal regions of the hypothalamus.) Stimulation posteriorly in the hypothalamus yields escape reactions, whereas stimulation laterally at the level of the ventromedial nucleus causes well-directed attack behavior, with snarling, scratching, and biting. In keeping with the "dual-center" concept, lesions in the ventromedial nucleus cause rage behavior, which can be thought of as normally keeping the lateral region in check. Note, however, that stronger stimulation of more anterior regions, including the preoptic and septal areas in the limbic system, also induce a rage reaction, which is called *sham rage*. The sham rage is different from the lateral hypothalamically induced rage in that the somatic motor components of the rage are poorly directed even if the animal is attacked. This has been explained on the basis that the stimulation is simultaneously activating the adynamic (parasympathetic) region, thus rendering the animal incapable of a well-directed and coordinated attack. Also, the lateral hypothalamic stimulation may be activating circuits in the medial forebrain bundle that are part of a motivational system. Thus in lateral hypothalamic rage the animal may really be "angry," whereas in sham rage the animal may be giving just a motor "display." Removing the forebrain rostral to the hypothalamus also results in sham rage, presumably because limbic system circuitry has been removed, allowing the hypothalamic motor rage mechanism to be released or disinhibited. The "jack-in-the-box" analogy fits well. The spring (hypothalamus) pushes the puppet (rage) out when the lid (limbic system) is removed.

Another hypothalamic mechanism that evolved along with the limbic system as a factor in the survival of the species is one that regulates sexual behavior. It has been proposed that a *sex center* resides in the anterior hypothalamus; lesions here in experimental animals have resulted in complete elimination of mating behavior (without affecting the hormonal balance in the animal). This is further substantiated by experiments in which testosterone has been implanted into the area in males and has resulted in increased mating behavior; the implantation of estrogen into the anterior hypothalamus in females has also elicited mating behavior. It has been suggested that the neurons in this region that are involved in the elicitation of sexual activity are chemosensitive to certain steroids.

Since the anterior hypothalamic region is interconnected with the limbic system (as most parts of the hypothalamus are), it is difficult to attribute such behaviors to only the hypothalamus, particularly when certain parts of the limbic system are well known to be involved in the expression of sexual activity. For example, animals with pyriform cortex lesions show rather bizarre hypersexuality, such as tandem mounting and inappropriate sexual responses to inanimate objects or members of different animal species (see Chapter 27). Also, some patients with temporal lobe epilepsy will show hypersexual activity in association with the aura preceding their seizure.

Behavioral phenomena are obviously composed of very complex patterns of responses involving a variety of neural and endocrine effectors. Whereas the mechanisms underlying these have not been resolved, the hypothalamus and the limbic system impinging on it are of critical importance.

It has been mentioned that sleep (Chap. 23) cannot be considered entirely as a passive process but that certain brain structures are involved actively. One of these may be the hypothalamus; note that the hypothalamus is considered by some to be the rostralmost part of the reticular formation. It was suggested early in this century on the basis of pathological studies of encephalitis that damage to the posterior hypothalamus (along with the rostral midbrain) resulted in sleep, whereas lesions in the anterior hypothalamus resulted in agitation and insomnia. Subsequent stimulation and lesion studies have implicated the anterior hypothalamus as a *sleep center* and the posterior hypothalamus as a *waking center*, but these definitions are probably too precise. If it is considered that various emotional behaviors as well as the metabolic and autonomic regulatory mechanisms in the hypothalamus would be readily altered with even small lesions or weak electrical stimulation, it is not surprising that changes in the animals' pattern of sleep and wakefulness could be interrupted also. The normal stages of the continuum between deep sleep and consciousness require the intactness of a number of CNS structures, including the brainstem caudal to the midbrain, the midbrain reticular formation, the hypothalamus, the thalamus, and the cortex.

Pituitary Gland

The pituitary gland is actually two glands with different embryological origins and modes of control. The anterior pituitary arises from the ectoderm in the primitive oral cavity and migrates upward to lie in contact with the developing posterior pituitary gland. The posterior pituitary originates from the neural ectoderm

at the base of the hypothalamus and remains attached to it by means of the infundibulum (pituitary stalk). The hypothalamus controls the output from these two glands in two different ways (Fig. 26–5). The anterior pituitary is under neural control by the hypothalamus but with the interposition of a portal system of vessels, the *pituitary portal vessels*, that drains the median eminence of *releasing factors* and supplies them to the anterior pituitary. The cells forming the releasing factors are believed to be located in the basal part of the hypothalamus, possibly in the arcuate and ventromedial nuclei. A separate releasing factor is formed for each of the pituitary tropic hormones, and under the appropriate neural or hormonal stimulus or both it is itself released into the portal vessels arising in the median eminence, thus reaching the anterior pituitary gland.

The posterior pituitary is under direct

A.

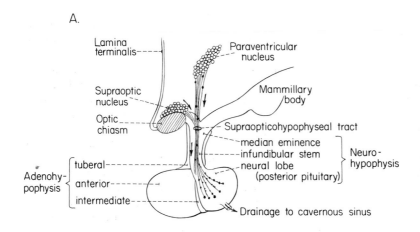

B.

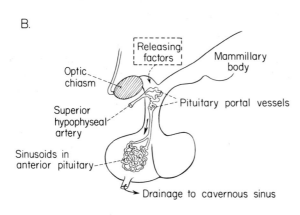

Figure 26–5. The two types of hypothalamic connections to the pituitary gland. Neural connections to the posterior lobe are shown in *A,* along with a terminology for the pituitary gland that is frequently used. The median eminence can be considered part of the neurohypophysis, or simply as the median eminence of the tuber cinereum; this latter is the floor of the hypothalamus. The pituitary portal vessels are shown in *B,* connecting the median eminence to the sinusoids of the anterior pituitary gland. The hypothalamic releasing factors enter the capillary bed of the median eminence. (*A,* After Everett, *Functional neuroanatomy*, Philadelphia, Lea & Febiger, 1971.)

neural control via the *supraopticohypophyseal* tract, which originates in the supraoptic (SO) and the paraventricular (PV) nuclei of the hypothalamus.

The supraoptic and paraventricular nuclei are composed of neurons that are *neurosecretory cells.* They behave as ordinary neurons elsewhere in the CNS, *i.e.,* they generate and conduct action potentials and, in addition, form, store, and release from their endings in the posterior pituitary the hormones vasopressin (antidiuretic hormone, ADH) and oxytocin. The supraoptic nuclei are primarily concerned with forming and secreting ADH, and the paraventricular nuclei with oxytocin. These hormones are formed in the cell bodies located in the two nuclei and pass down the axons of the supraopticohypophyseal tract to be stored in axonal swellings in the posterior pituitary. Release of hormone from these endings in the posterior pituitary is effected by the adequate stimulus of increased osmolarity of the blood for ADH, and suckling for oxytocin. For example, destruction of the supraopticohypophyseal tract by a tumor in the basal hypothalamus results in the loss of a large volume of water via the urine (diabetes insipidus), because without ADH water is not reabsorbed in the kidney. Secondary to the water loss, an increase in water intake (polydipsia) occurs as the body attempts to compensate for the dehydration. Several liters of water per day can be lost in patients with complete stalk section, a condition that must be corrected by either increased fluid intake or suitable ADH replacement therapy.

The major effect of oxytocin is to cause milk ejection from lactating mammary glands and is normally released by a suckling stimulus. Pituitary stalk section, which would cause diabetes insipidus, would also prevent oxytocin release but would only be of clinical importance in lactating mothers. A role for this hormone in males and nonlactating females has not been established.

Both supraoptic and paraventricular nuclear groups are subjected to control by other neural influences. For example, emotional stress can inhibit the reflex release of oxytocin and, conversely, lactating women will often eject milk in preparation for breast feeding before the infant has actually suckled. Presumably, such inputs would involve parts of the limbic system. Release of vasopressin is also enhanced by exercise and decreased extracellular fluid volume, the latter by way of ascending pathways from stretch receptors in the cardiovascular system.

CLINICAL CASE

It should now be apparent that a hypothalamic tumor would cause the interruption of several homeostatic and behavioral functions that are associated with the hypothalamus and its inputs and outputs. A selected case study (paraphrased from Reeves, A. G., and Plum, F., *Arch. Neurol.,* 1969, *20,* 616–624) is worthwhile describing in some detail, as it summarizes many of the topics covered in this chapter.

A 20-year-old, obese woman was first admitted to the hospital complaining of the following, which had been present for about a year: polyuria, polydipsia, hyperphagia, nonmenses, and frequent headaches.

The neurological examination, including the assessment of mental function, revealed no abnormalities. The results of laboratory tests confirmed that the patient had diabetes insipidus and hypogonadal and hypothyroid function. A pneumoencephalogram revealed a poorly outlined anterior part of the third ventricle. Because of a suspected hypothalamic tumor, a craniotomy and exploration was performed but no tumor was found. The patient was discharged from the hospital; her diabetes insipidus was controlled with vasopressin.

About 2 years later she was readmitted on the basis of pronounced behavioral alterations. She presented with bouts of laughing and crying, and, on occasion, rage behavior. According to her family, she held conversations with imaginary people and on several occasions had disrobed in public. Her vital signs were normal but she had gained about 30 lb. The neurological examination showed no focal neurological signs, but the visual fields could not be examined because of her uncooperativeness and aggressive out-

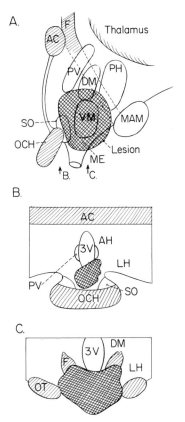

Figure 26–6. Reconstruction of hypothalamic damage caused by a tumor. *A*, Lesion (crosshatching) and hypothalamic nuclei projected onto a sagittal drawing of the hypothalamus. *B* and *C*, Frontal sections through the hypothalamus at the levels indicated in *C*, showing the lateral extent of the lesion. *AC*, Anterior commissure; *AH*, anterior hypothalamus; *DM*, dorsomedial nucleus; *F*, fornix; *LH*, lateral hypothalamic area; *MAM*, mammillary body; *ME*, median eminence; *OCH*, optic chiasm; *OT*, optic tract; *PH*, posterior hypothalamic area, *PV*, paraventricular nucleus; *SO*, supraoptic nucleus; *VM*, ventromedial nucleus, *3V*, third ventricle. (Redrawn from Reeves and Plum, *Arch. Neurol.*, 1969, 20, 616–624.)

bursts, at times reaching such violent proportions that she required sedation. Well-directed biting and hitting and throwing of objects were evident, which could be allayed by continual feeding; she was clearly hyperphagic. Her body temperature was irregular, frequently spiking to 104°F. Her mental alertness was at times seriously defective, including episodic confusion, memory loss, and disorientation. The laboratory examination revealed hypopituitary function, and her electroencephalogram showed 2 to 4 cycles/sec slow wave activity. The pneumoencephalogram now showed incomplete filling of portions of the ventral part as well as anterior part of the third ventricle. On craniotomy a tumor was found at the base of the third ventricle but was not removed because of its size and critical location. Postoperatively the patient's condition deteriorated, and she died 2 months later of a pulmonary embolus.

At autopsy a tumor was found protruding from the tuber cinereum (base of the hypothalamus), extending from the optic chiasm to the mammillary bodies (Fig. 26–6). It extended dorsally on both sides to the level of the dorsomedial hypothalamic nucleus and anteriorly to the supraoptic region, damaging to some extent the fornix bundles but sparing the lateral hypothalamic region.

Such tumors, restricted to these portions of the hypothalamus, are not common. The signs and symptoms this patient showed can be explained for the most part by the damage caused by the tumor's bilateral, basal, and medial position. Thus, the entire endocrine picture seen would be expected from destruction of the median eminence region with (1) its critical portal vessel connections to the anterior pituitary (presumably the cells producing releasing factors would also have been destroyed) and (2) its axons of the supraopticohypophyseal tract passing through, en route to the posterior pituitary. The easily provoked and well-directed aggressive reactions, as well as the hyperphagia, would follow from the damage to the ventromedial nuclei. Although the anterior hypothalamus-preoptic region was for the most part spared, an expanding mass encroaching on that heat-loss area would affect its outflow, thus accounting for the increases in body temperature.

It is more difficult to ascribe to a circumscribed area of the hypothalamus the severe deterioration of her mental functions—seen in her disrobing in public, disorientation, confusion, and impairment of memory. Both the fornices and more medial parts of the hypothalamus were damaged, including presumably interconnections with the medial part of the thalamus along the ventricle. The 2- to 4-cycles/sec waves in the electroencephalogram would indicate that functionally the cortex was also involved, although no lesion was evident there. A part of the disruptive process might be episodic as the tumor expanded, perhaps causing an abnormal discharge of neurons projecting to areas not directly damaged by the lesion. The disrobing in public and auditory hallucinations suggest this. The integrated role that these structures may normally play in mental activity is not clearly understood, although it is reasonable to predict that such a destructive lesion would alter normal mentation by disrupting the complex limbic system circuitry of which the hypothalamus is an essential part.

ADDITIONAL READING

Haymaker, W., Anderson, E., and Nauta, W. J. *The hypothalamus.* Springfield, Ill., Charles C Thomas, 1969.

Swaab, D. F., and Schadé, J. P., eds. Integrative hypothalamic activity. Vol. 41 in *Progress in brain research,* New York, American Elsevier Publishing Co., 1974.

CHAPTER 27

THE LIMBIC SYSTEM

JOHN W. SUNDSTEN

The limbic system houses the structures that are responsible for the affective aspect of emotions and also those involved in the behavioral expression of emotions. The name is credited to Broca (1879), who spoke of "le grand lobe limbique," since it is composed of a ring (thus the name *limbic*) of structures, both cortical and deeper-lying nuclear groups, that are found on the medial aspect of the cerebral hemisphere. The limbic system is sometimes equated with the term *rhinencephalon* (nose brain), but the latter is best used when relating to the development of the part of the brain that evolved along with the olfactory bulb, the sense of olfaction, and the structures subserving olfactory reflexes. Only a small part of the medial complex of limbic cortical and subcortical structures is involved in olfaction. The term *limbic system* was popularized so that the olfactory implications of the term *rhinencephalon* would be avoided and the limbic system's concern with emotional life would be emphasized.

The limbic structures and their interconnections, along with physiological responses attributed to them, are many and

complex. Only major anatomical groupings and functional aspects of the limbic system will be considered. Not to be lost sight of are the very dramatic changes in mentation, feeling tone, and behavior that can result when this part of the forebrain is altered by disease or experimental manipulation.

ANATOMICAL FEATURES

In keeping with the concept of a ring of structures on the medial aspect of the hemisphere, the following *cortical areas* can be described (Fig. 27–1). The most obvious are the *cingulate* and *parahippocampal gyri*, the *hippocampus* itself (rolled up in the temporal lobe), the *subcallosal gyrus*, part of the caudal *orbital cortex* of the frontal lobe, and the *temporal lobe cortex that adjoins* the orbital frontal cortex.

The *pyriform lobe* is a term used to describe the entire temporal lobe portions of the limbic system. Other terms often used are based on the cytoarchitecture of the cortical areas of portions of the limbic system, such as *entorhinal cortex* (covering

354

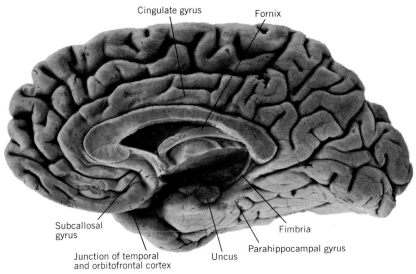

Figure 27–1. The medial aspect of the cerebrum. The brainstem has been removed by an oblique cut through the thalamus so that the fimbria and the parahippocampal gyrus are revealed.

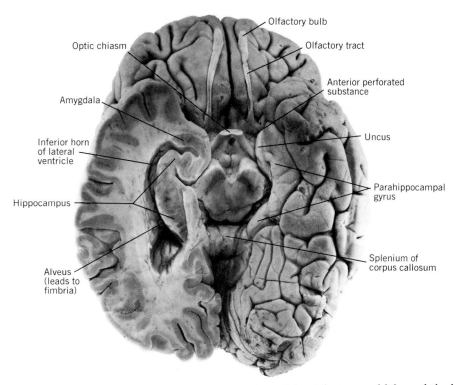

Figure 27–2. The inferior surface of the cerebrum. A portion of the right temporal lobe and the brainstem caudal to the midbrain have been removed. Note the relationship of the amygdala and hippocampus to the inferior horn of the lateral ventricle.

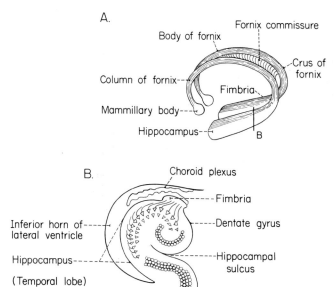

Figure 27–3. The fornix system of fibers and its hippocampus. *A,* Projection of the fornix from the hippocampus to the mammillary body. *B,* Coronal section through the hippocampus, showing its continuity with the dentate and parahippocampal gyri.

most of the parahippocampal gyrus), *pyriform cortex* (covering the *uncus,* which itself is the "hooked" portion of the parahippocampal gyrus), and *prepyriform cortex* (mainly related to the orbitofrontal gyri along the olfactory tract and the rostral tip of the parahippocampal gyrus).

The *hippocampus* is a phylogenetically old region of cortex (archicortex). In contrast to the six-layered cortex (neocortex) of most of the cerebral hemisphere, it is composed of only three layers. It is situated in the temporal lobe, continuous with the cortex of the parahippocampal gyrus (Fig. 27–2). Since it is rolled up on itself, bulging into the medial floor of the inferior horn of the lateral ventricle, it is not readily seen from the surface. In cross sections (Fig. 27–3) its appearance has been likened to a seahorse, ram's horn, or snail. It begins rostrally at the region of the uncus just behind the amygdala and extends caudally, arching upward to the level of the splenium of the corpus callosum, where it ends. At that point its efferent axons, which have been gathering together on its surface as the *fimbria,* pull free and form the *fornix* bundles (Figs. 27–2 and 27–3).

The major subcortical nuclear groups that are related to the limbic cortical areas are the *amygdala* and *septum.* The amygdala (amygdaloid body) is a large nuclear mass situated in the rostral part of the temporal lobe just in front of the hippocampus (Fig. 27–2). It underlies the uncus of the parahippocampal gyrus, immediately rostral to the inferior horn of the lateral ventricle. Several smaller nuclear subgroupings have been identified within it, but these need not be considered here. The septum is in the midline just in front of the preoptic region beneath the corpus callosum and blends imperceptibly into the septum pellucidum. In man, the septal nuclei extend laterally out into the subcallosal gyrus (Fig. 27–1).

All the complex connections within the limbic system will not be considered in detail. One example of a circuit is shown in Figure 27–4. The major efferent from the hippocampus is the *fornix,* which projects most of its fibers down through the hypothalamus to the mammillary body; the *mammillothalamic tract* projects from the mammillary body to the anterior nucleus of the thalamus, which in turn projects to the cingulate gyrus by way of the *anterior*

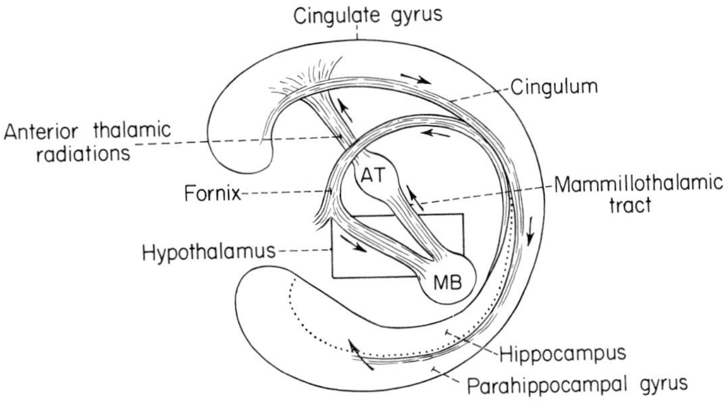

Figure 27–4. Possible feedback circuit linking the hypothalamus with the limbic system. The connection between the parahippocampal gyrus and the hippocampus is the temporal perforant path.

limb of the internal capsule. The cingulate gyrus projects by way of a cortical association bundle, the *cingulum*, to the parahippocampal gyrus; the latter has connections with the hippocampus. Whereas these pathways are shown as one-way, in some instances the connections are in both directions. For example, the fornix system receives fibers from the preoptic area just in front of the hypothalamus and carries them *to* the hippocampus. Note that the hypothalamus is a nodal point for many inputs from the limbic system; for limbic structures either to effect or to modify behavior, intact connections to the hypothalamus are necessary.

Another circuit is shown in Figure 27–5 that ties in the *amygdala* with the overlying pyriform cortex (of the parahippocampal gyrus) and the hypothalamus. The adjacent temporal lobe neocortex is also connected with the amygdala. In man the major efferent outflow of the amygdala is a diffuse pathway directed medially into the hypothalamus. The *stria terminalis* interconnects the amygdaloid nuclear masses on each side and also carries fibers connecting the amygdala with the hypothalamus, septal, and preoptic regions. The *anterior commissure* interconnects the rostral

parts of the temporal lobe cortex in general, just as the corpus callosum does for the greater expanse of the cerebral hemispheres. These complex circuits are summarized in Figure 27–6; also indicated is the bidirectional aspect of most of the fiber systems associated with the limbic system.

FUNCTIONAL ASPECTS

Olfaction

The sense of smell is of considerable importance among many animals in the phylogenetic scale, as it warns them of approaching enemies as well as guides them to an adequate food supply and an appropriate mate. Olfaction is of far less importance in man except as related to his own cultivated individual desires for food, drink, and sex. The hair-cell receptor neurons for the sense of smell lying in the olfactory epithelium convey input to the *olfactory bulb* and thence via the *olfactory* tract (Fig. 27–2) to the *prepyriform cortex.* The prepyriform cortex lies adjacent to the tract in the region of the *anterior perforated substance (olfactory trigone or tubercle)*

Figure 27–5. Connections in the limbic system that link the olfactory bulb, amygdala, septum, and hypothalamus.

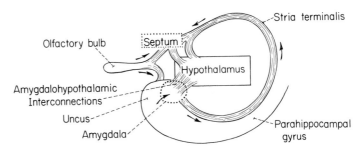

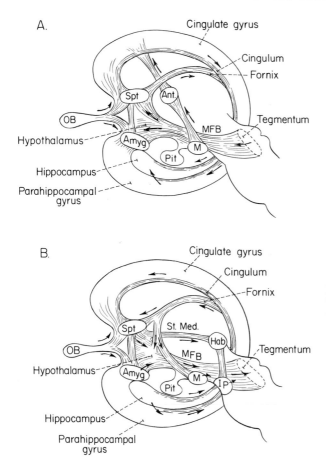

Figure 27–6. Limbic system circuitry, emphasizing the two-way interconnections of most of the limbic structures. The ascending paths from the midbrain tegmentum pass through the hypothalamus via the medial forebrain bundle *(A)*, and similarly, the descending paths from the rostral limbic areas *(B)*. *Amyg,* amygdala; *Ant.,* anterior nucleus of thalamus; *Hab,* habenula; *Ip,* interpeduncular nucleus; *M,* mammillary body; *MFB,* medial forebrain bundle; *OB,* olfactory bulb; *Pit,* pituitary gland; *Spt,* septum; *St. Med.,* stria medullaris. (After MacLean, *J. nerv. ment. Dis.,* 1958, *127,* 1–11.)

and is to some extent on the uncus of the temporal lobe. The prepyriform cortex is essential for the sense of smell; that is, it is the *primary olfactory receiving area.* Note that this is the only sensory modality that does not have a thalamic relay station.

Alterations in olfaction may be divided into two categories: (1) decreased ability to smell, most commonly due to local disease of the nasal mucosa (*e.g.,* colds), occasionally to trauma destroying the olfactory nerve fibers passing through the cribriform plate, and rarely to tumors involving the olfactory tracts; and (2) aberrations of smell as a hallucination that may occur, for example, in schizophrenia, or as the *aura* (initial perceptual manifestation) of an epileptic seizure. Clinically, an olfactory aura is usually part of an *uncinate fit,* in which auditory and visual hallucinations may also occur. This olfactory experience is seen in some cases with epileptic discharges originating in or near the *uncus.* These hallucinations are generally dis-

agreeable in nature and may be accompanied by smacking of the lips or other motor signs.

The Temporal Lobe

Bilateral removal of the temporal lobe in monkeys results in a number of signs and symptoms that are collectively called the *Kluver-Bucy syndrome.* This consists of several bizarre behavioral disturbances characterized by a loss of the ability to recognize common objects on the basis of visual criteria alone (visual agnosia) and, related to this, a compulsory exploratory behavior whereby all objects, familiar or not, are examined by mouth and by smelling. Profound changes of emotional behavior in the direction of passivity and unresponsiveness also occur. Objects that would normally evoke fear (*e.g.,* in monkeys a snake or a stranger) no longer do so. On the other hand, sexual activity is intensified and indiscriminate.

Many attempts have been made to fractionate this syndrome into its component parts by lesioning of different parts of the limbic system. To a certain extent, this has been accomplished. For example, bilateral removal of the amygdaloid nuclei reduces aggressive behavior (normally savage animals, such as the lynx, become very docile). Such operations also frequently increase sexuality, and it is thought that this latter is due to the removal of the cortex overlying the amygdala (pyriform cortex), not the amygdala itself.

A variety of somatic motor and autonomic responses have been elicited by stimulation of different parts of the amygdaloid nuclear complex. Several of these include:

(1) Cessation of spontaneous or cortically evoked movements.
(2) Alteration of spinal reflex activity.
(3) Turning movements of head and eye to the side opposite stimulation.
(4) Swallowing, licking, or chewing movements.
(5) Changes in cardiovascular, respiratory, or gastrointestinal functions.
(6) Micturition and defecation.
(7) Pupillary dilation and piloerection.

It has generally been concluded that these are components of fear or anger responses or both. Attempts have been made to fractionate the amygdala to determine which of its portions are responsible, but few clear-cut results have been obtained. However, taken as a whole, the stimulation experiments would complement the lesion experiments mentioned already in relation to the Kluver-Bucy syndrome. Thus, a view emerges that the amygdala integrates (along with other limbic and hypothalamic structures) various inputs, bringing about appropriate responses on a tameness-aggressiveness spectrum. Observations in man are relatively few, though stimulation of the amygdala has been done and commonly has given rise to a sensation of fear, disturbances of mood, sense of unreality, déjà vu, distortions of bodily perceptions, and other equally intense alterations of awareness. These alterations in man are difficult to localize to any one structure with absolute certainty, even though the site of the stimulating electrode is known. Such patients suffer from epilepsy or some other disease to begin with, and the stimulus could be triggering a seizure that spreads throughout the temporal lobe or eventually beyond. Nonetheless, it should not be forgotten that the patient's *experience* is *real*, whether evoked by his own disease or by a stimulating current.

Behaviors are exceedingly complex and difficult to quantify or to relate to specific nuclear groups in an exacting fashion. It was mentioned in Chapter 26 that lesions of the *ventromedial nucleus* of the hypothalamus induce rage behavior. Lesions in the *septal* region will also do this in animals that are normally placid. Further, animals that have undergone such an operation are made tame by removal of the amygdala. Limbic system structures, including the hypothalamus, are clearly involved in a variety of behaviors, but the manner in which such structures bring about coordinated responses is not known. There are two important factors that need to be taken into account and that complicate the interpretation of lesioning and stimulating experiments. (1) The first factor relates to the overall social and environmental set of the experimental subject. For example, baboons that have undergone amygdalectomy may show submissive behavior when they are in their own social group but show aggressive behavior when isolated. (2) The second factor relates to whether the behavior seen is part of an *affective experience* that is directing the behavior, or whether the behavior observed after experimental manipulation is composed of the *effector* side only, that is, the autonomic and somatic motor components of it. On the efferent side, the limbic system can be thought of as modulating or regulating hypothalamic behavioral mechanisms. The hypothalamus alone is probably not able to *initiate directed* emotional behaviors. Rather, it requires limbic system input for the appropriate operation and temporal coordination of its effects on lower brainstem autonomic and somatic outflows. Also, recall that the hypothalamus projects information upstream *to* the limbic system, thalamus, and cortex; when these are intact the message is rewarding to animals or pleasurable to humans that are receiving electrical current in the lateral part of the hypothalamus. Damage, then, to any one part of the limbic system-hypothalamic complex is very difficult to assess in terms of the exact structures involved.

The Hippocampus

Since antiquity, when it was named after the seahorse, the hippocampus has captured the imagination of poets and scientists alike. It was once thought of as the "seat of the soul" and more recently has been implicated in learning and memory processes. Bilateral hippocampal lesions cause a gross impairment in certain learning paradigms, particularly those involving the performance of sequential acts, such as pressing several levers in the proper order to gain a food reward. Although animals with hippocampal lesions may not show a defect in simple acquisition of task skills, *e.g.*, discriminating between two different symbols, they have difficulty in reversal learning, in which the former wrong choice is now made the correct one. These experiments and others have led to the view that animals with hippocampal lesions cannot categorize new sensory data correctly. Their "recent memory" is thought to be impaired because they do not have the full capacity for properly *acquiring* and *retaining* information encoded in new sensory stimuli.

Another complex function ascribed to the hippocampus is that of *goal-directed behavior*. When novel stimuli are presented to an animal, an electrical rhythm called the *hippocampal theta* (4 to 7 Hz) becomes dominant in their hippocampal electroencephalogram (EEG) records. This rhythm has been correlated with the approach behavior an animal shows before making his instrumental response (*e.g.*, lever pressing or lifting of a cup in order to gain a food reward). Disruption of pathways involving interconnections of the hippocampus and midbrain reticular formation, such as the medial forebrain bundle, will alter the hippocampal theta rhythm and block the response.

A simplified view is that the hippo-campus, interacting with the reticular formation and other parts of the limbic system, functions in the process of attention and the orderly acquisition and retention of new information.

CLINICAL EXAMPLES OF TEMPORAL LOBE DYSFUNCTION

Epileptic seizures that originate in the temporal lobes are relatively common. As mentioned earlier, the seizure may begin with an "aura" of acoustic or olfactory experience. Psychic experiences are sometimes described by patients with temporal lobe epilepsy, and they may carry out fairly complicated behavior, such as undressing or driving a car, but following the seizure they may have amnesia concerning what has just occurred. These are called *psychomotor attacks* (see Chapter 24). Two examples of clinical cases involving injury to the temporal lobe are contrasted below.

A 33-year-old engineer had developed seizures at age 22. . . . Attacks began with loss of consciousness and stare, followed by salivation, licking, swallowing, head turning to the left, impulse to run, searching movements, and rapid speech, followed by a return to consciousness with a feeling of intense hurt and depression. Treatment with anticonvulsants successfully controlled the early motor portions of the seizure, but the patient began to have frequent episodes of violent aggressive behavior. . . . He would proceed to brood aloud, dwell upon, and increasingly elaborate on [a] single theme with mounting anger, verbal abuse, and irrational accusations over a period of 3 or 4 hours, reaching a crescendo of rage, which was always climaxed by an outburst of physical aggression. . . . As the anger spent itself in physical violence, he rather suddenly seemed to come to himself, wept violently, feeling hurt and broken. Nearly total amnesia was claimed for the portion of the attack between the early complaint and the arousal with weeping and remorse. Immediately following the attacks, he always felt exceptionally well. . . . (From Stevens *et al.*, *Arch. Neurol.*, *21*, 157–169, 1969.)

The second example illustrates another aspect of temporal lobe dysfunction.

He remembered among other things that he always had one minute . . . when suddenly in the midst of sadness, spiritual darkness and oppression, there seemed . . . a flash of light in his brain, and with extraordinary impetus all his vital forces suddenly began working at their highest tension. The sense of life, the consciousness of self, were multiplied ten times at these moments which passed like a flash of lightning. His mind and heart were flooded with extraordinary light; all his uneasiness, all his doubts, all his anxieties were relieved at once; they were all merged in a lofty calm, full of serene, harmonious joy and hope. . . . That it really was the "highest synthesis of life" he could not doubt. . . . It was not as though he saw abnormal and unreal visions of some sort at that moment, as from hashish, opium, or wine, destroying the reason and distorting the soul. He was quite capable of judging of that when the attack was over. These moments were only an extraordinary quickening of self consciousness . . . and at the same time of the direct sensation of existence in the most intense degree. At that second, that is, at the very last conscious moment before the fit, he had time to say to himself clearly and consciously, "Yes, for this moment one might give one's whole life." (From Dostoyevsky, *The idiot.*)

ADDITIONAL READING

Adey, W. R., and Tokizane, T., eds. Structure and function of the limbic system. Vol. 27, in *Progress in Brain Research*. New York, American Elsevier Publishing Co., 1967.

Livingston, K. E., and Escobar, A. Anatomical basis of the limbic system concept. *Arch. Neurol.*, 1971, *24*, 17–21.

MacLean, P. D. The triune brain, emotion, and scientific bias. Chap. 33 in *The neurosciences; a second study program*, F. O. Schmitt, ed., New York, Rockefeller University Press, 1970.

Powell, E. W., and Hines, G. The limbic system: An interface. *Behav. Biol.*, 1974, *12*, 149–164.

CHAPTER 28

THE METABOLISM OF THE BRAIN AND RELATED DISORDERS

PHILLIP D. SWANSON

It is customary to view the functioning of the nervous system in anatomical and physiological terms. Similarly, the neuropathological processes and their clinical signs and symptoms are thought of in relation to the anatomical regions affected and to the resulting neurophysiological abnormalities. There are also, however, a variety of conditions that diffusely affect neural metabolism (metabolic encephalopathies). Moreover, certain congenital errors of either amino acid or lipid metabolism are associated with damage to neural elements. In addition, at least one condition, Parkinson's disease, was traditionally considered to be a disease of particular structures

(basal ganglia) but may now also be viewed as a disorder of neurons utilizing a specific class of neurotransmitters, the catecholamines. Other disorders of particular neuronal systems may come to be considered in such a way in the future.

The term *neurochemistry* is now used to encompass investigations that relate to the nervous system and in which biochemical techniques are used. The areas mentioned in the preceding paragraph are among those studied by neurochemists. Others include the neurochemical basis of memory, the biochemistry of excitability and ion transport, and the biochemical mechanism of axonal transport.

362

NEUROCHEMICAL METHODS

Many techniques used by neurochemists do not differ from those used by biochemists working with other tissues. However, some problems involving neural tissues require for their study the development of special procedures.

Electrical Stimulation of Brain Slices. Neural tissues can easily be sliced into thin sections, and these can be further studied during incubation in an oxygenated medium with a composition resembling that of cerebrospinal fluid. These isolated tissues consume oxygen and glucose for several hours and are able to maintain contents of high-energy phosphates and of potassium (K^+) ions that are much higher than the contents in the surrounding fluid. Metabolic rates are lower than those measured *in vivo*, however. McIlwain and coworkers found that one can markedly increase rates of respiration and glycolysis by passing electrical pulses of alternating polarity through such slices at frequencies of 10 to 1000 cycles per sec. One can apply electrical pulses by placing the slice between two grids, around each of which is wound an electrode connected to one pole of the stimulator. Other electrode designs can also be used. Slices that are stimulated are suitable for studies of the effects of drugs that probably act directly on outer cell membranes to reduce neuronal excitability, such as tetrodotoxin, anticonvulsants, and anesthetics. Release or uptake of ions or of neurotransmitters can also be studied in such preparations.

Isolation of Subcellular Particles by Differential and Density-Gradient Centrifugation. The central nervous system contains cells of several types. Further, neurons differ from other cells in having specialized processes, the dendrites and axons. The region of the synapse is specialized and contains identifiable vesicles that are thought to be repositories of neurotransmitter molecules. DeRobertis and Whittaker, using a combination of centrifugation at different speeds and centrifugation through a gradient of different densities, found it possible to separate homogenized brain tissue into subcellular fractions that could be distinguished under the electron microscope and that contained high concentrations of certain biochemical markers. For example, a subfraction that is sedimented through 1.2 M sucrose contains mitochondria and has the highest activity of the mitochondrial enzyme succinate dehydrogenase. Fractions enriched in nerve endings (synaptosomes) can be obtained by such techniques. These organelles have been sheared from the axons during the homogenization process. They apparently reseal, since they contain mitochondria, synaptic vesicles, and soluble enzymes after completion of the centrifugation procedures. Synaptosomes can be incubated in physiological media in the same fashion as brain slices. They are metabolically active and can respond to electrical stimuli by releasing neurotransmitter substances into the incubation medium. They can be used to study neurotransmitter release or uptake, ion transport, and other aspects of neural metabolism. Synaptosomes can be further fractionated by suspension in hypotonic media to release their contents. Fractions enriched in synaptic vesicles can be obtained and analyzed; so can fractions containing fragments derived from the outer synaptosomal membranes. As techniques become refined for detecting differences in protein compositions of different types of membranes, initial separation into purified subcellular fractions will be an essential first step.

Neuron-Glia Separations. Another goal of some neurochemists has been to characterize biochemically similarities and differences between glial cells and neurons. No technique is yet completely satisfactory for this purpose. One can use microdissection techniques on fresh or lyophilized tissues to isolate single cells and then analyze them by sensitive microtechniques. These techniques have the disadvantage of yielding only a few cells. More recent emphasis has been on macrotechniques aimed at obtaining larger quantities of cells. These techniques consist of disruption of tissues by sieving and/or by digestion of chopped tissue with trypsin, followed by collection of cells by density-gradient centrifugation. The validity of the separations is often difficult to establish, since the cells are identified by morphological distinctions and there may be disagreement about

TABLE 28–1.   Neurochemical Methods

Techniques	Developers
Electrical stimulation of brain slices	McIlwain
Isolation of nerve endings (synaptosomes) and synaptic vesicles by subcellular fractionation	DeRobertis, Whittaker
Neuron-glia separations	Hyden, Norton, Rose

the identity of particular cells. Further, cell processes are very likely sheared from cell bodies in some of these disruptions, and these fragments may contribute to biochemical findings attributed to cells of a particular type. Cells isolated by these techniques are not viable, so that reliable metabolic studies cannot be performed. Development of better separation techniques is being actively pursued at the present time.

Some of the special techniques used in neurochemistry and the key figures in their development are enumerated in Table 28–1.

THE BIOCHEMICAL BASIS OF EXCITABILITY

The property of action potential propagation is unique to nerve and muscle cells and must depend upon special properties of the nerve and muscle membrane. Thus far, analysis of membrane composition has not revealed differences between excitable and nonexcitable membranes that are sufficient to account for this property. Most lipids present in neuronal membranes are shared by other cell membranes and by mitochondria and other membrane organelles. A unique protein or polypeptide might be postulated to be present in excitable membranes, but an "excitability protein" has not yet been isolated. Of possible relevance, however, are studies of Rudin and Mueller, who have been able to produce transient potential changes resembling spikes in artificial membranes prepared from lipids to which has been added an *excitability-inducing* material, obtained from certain microorganisms.

Excitability can be abolished in certain ways, including making tissues anoxic and adding certain chemical substances, such as the puffer-fish poison, tetrodotoxin (once accidentally ingested, nonfatally, by Captain Cook). This substance binds to membranes and prevents the transient increase in permeability to sodium ions that initiates the action potential. The search for membrane fractions that specifically bind tetrodotoxin or an analogous substance may lead to isolation of excitability-conferring substances.

ENERGY METABOLISM

The brain has a very high requirement for metabolic energy when compared with other organs of the body. Although the brain's weight is only 2 per cent that of the whole body, yet the adult human brain commands 20 per cent of the cardiac output, 20 per cent of the oxygen consumption, and 70 per cent of the glucose consumption in man. In this section is discussed not only the ways in which energy is supplied to the brain but also the uses to which it is put and the effects of altered physiological states on its production and use.

Energy Production and Storage

In the brain, as in other tissues, energy is used to produce adenosine triphosphate (ATP), which is the high-energy compound used for the majority of energy-requiring processes. ATP is synthesized in the same way as in other tissues: by glycolysis and by oxidative phosphorylation. It is well accepted that glucose, supplied through the blood stream, is the primary substrate used for ATP production. The evidence for this is as follows:

(1) The amount of carbon dioxide (CO_2) that appears in venous blood from the brain in a given period of time (about 3.3 ml/100 g/min) can be entirely accounted for by the carbon of the glucose used by the brain, as determined from arteriovenous differences. In one study, the arteriovenous difference in glucose was 10.2 mg/100 ml of blood. Formed CO_2 was equivalent to 8.9 mg of glu-

cose/100 ml, lactic acid to 1.2 mg, and pyruvic acid to 0.2 mg, for a total of 10.3 mg/100 ml of blood. Thus, metabolism of all the carbons of glucose could be closely correlated with the appearance of CO_2, lactate, and pyruvate, the end products of oxidative and glycolytic metabolism.

(2) The respiratory quotient (RQ = ratio of volume of CO_2 formed to oxygen used over a given length of time at standard pressure and temperature) of one suggests the carbohydrate nature of the substrates. If lipid or protein composed a major portion of utilized substrate, there would be more oxygen used than CO_2 formed:

(a) For carbohydrate (glucose, etc.):

$$C_6H_{12}O_6 + 6O_2 \rightarrow 6CO_2 + 6H_2O,$$
$$RQ = 1$$

(b) For a lipid such as triolein (a triglyceride):

$$C_{57}H_{104}O_6 + 80\,O_2 \rightarrow$$
$$57\,CO_2 + 52\,H_2O,$$
$$RQ = 57/80 = 0.713$$

(3) Administration of glucose to hypoglycemic animals that have undergone hepatectomy rapidly restores the electroencephalogram to normal, even though other carbohydrates are without effect. Patients made hypoglycemic with insulin will also respond dramatically to administration of glucose.

(4) Infusion of ^{14}C-glucose intravenously into anesthetized animals is followed within an hour by production from the brain of $^{14}CO_2$ with specific activity equal to that of labeled glucose.

The brain relies primarily on oxidative metabolism for energy production. Glycogen is present in the brain, and the rate of glycolysis increases markedly when the brain is made hypoxic. However, glycolysis is not sufficient to maintain cerebral contents of high-energy phosphates. For example, anoxia produced by placement of a 10-day-old rat in a nitrogen chamber is accompanied by complete depletion of cerebral ATP and creatine phosphate after 10 min. Another important substance that is present in the brain in considerable quantities is creatine phosphate. ATP levels can be maintained for a short period of time by utilization of creatine phosphate through the enzyme creatine kinase, or ATP:creatine phosphotransferase:

$$\text{ADP} + \text{creatine phosphate} \rightleftarrows$$
$$\text{ATP} + \text{creatine}$$

Ischemia

When an artery to the brain is occluded by a thrombus, as in a patient with atherosclerotic arterial disease, or by other means, the brain areas supplied by that artery will not be able to obtain either oxygen or glucose. If the ischemia is prolonged beyond a period of a very few minutes, the cells will be irreversibly damaged (infarction). Data obtained from decapitated mice suggest that the effects of ischemia take place very rapidly. In adult animals at 1 min, creatine phosphate levels had fallen to zero and ATP had diminished to about 25 per cent of control values. It was of interest in this study that depletion of high-energy phosphates in 10-day-old immature animals took about twice as long as in adults; thus, it is possible that the immature brain has greater resistance to anoxia than does the mature brain.

Energy Utilization by the Central Nervous System

The reasons for the brain's high rate of energy consumption are not yet completely understood. Cell division, though occurring in glial cells as a response to adverse conditions, would not appear to be a major energy-utilizing process, except in the developing brain. Perhaps the best understood cerebral energy-requiring process is the coupled active transport of sodium and potassium across cell membranes. As most other cells do, nerve cells and their processes contain high levels of intracellular potassium and low levels of intracellular sodium ions. During a nerve impulse, a small amount of sodium moves into the cell, and a small amount of potassium goes out. These cation movements (downhill) do not require metabolic energy and are not abolished by metabolic inhibitors. However, energy in the form of ATP is required for extrusion of sodium ions and accumulation of potassium ions by the cells. This "active cation transport" very likely requires the presence of a membrane-bound enzyme, the sodium-requiring and potassium-requiring adenosine-triphosphatase (Na^+-, K^+-ATPase), which hydrolyzes ATP in the presence of Mg^{++}, Na^+, and K^+. From the rates of the energy-yielding processes and with the assumption of the validity of a P/O ratio (ratio of the number of ATP molecules formed for each oxygen atom utilized by mitochondria) of 3, the amount of energy available for energy-utilizing processes can be calculated. If we assume that each "energy-rich" phosphate bond provides 76,000 cal per mole, 25 to 36 per cent of the available energy is utilized for the rates of active cation movements observed in slices of cerebral cortex from the guinea pig.

Rates of energy consumption by other processes requiring metabolic energy are not available. Syntheses of substances required for neural transmission are probably energy-requiring processes. Acetylcholine is formed from choline and acetyl–coenzyme A. Other possible candidates as neurotransmitters include catecholamines, such as norepinephrine, glutamate, glycine, and gamma-aminobutyric acid (the last two are probable inhibitory transmitters). Transport of these substances back into nerve endings after their release into the extracellular space may be another way of maintaining concentrations of these substances and may be energy-requiring.

Synthesis of protein occurs rapidly in the brain. Proteins may need to be synthesized for the as yet uncharacterized process of memory consolidation, which might be envisaged as requiring the formation of tighter synapses between neurons.

Effects of Altered Physiological States on Energy Metabolism

The normal adult rate of respiration of 3.2 to 3.8 ml O_2/100 g of tissue/hour is,

TABLE 28–2. Cerebral Respiratory Rate

Condition	Respiratory Rate (ml O_2/100 g tissue/min)
Normal resting subjects	3.2–3.8
Natural sleep	3.4
Thiopentone anesthesia	1.9
Uremia	2.3
Diabetic coma	1.7
Insulin coma (arterial glucose level 9 mg/100 ml)	1.9
Insulin hypoglycemia (arterial glucose level 19 mg/100 ml)	2.6

interestingly, the same during sleep but is diminished in a variety of pathophysiological states (Table 28–2).

It should be remembered that depression of the metabolic rate might result either from a depression of energy production or from a decrease in energy utilization that lessens the requirement for metabolic energy. Thus, marked diminution in blood glucose levels by administration of insulin or other hypoglycemic agents is followed by coma and by reduction in cerebral metabolism, presumably because of the lack of substrate necessary for glycolysis and oxidative metabolism.

An example of a depression of metabolic rate due to an inhibition of energy utilization is anesthesia. In animals anesthetized with barbiturates, the brain content of high-energy phosphates is high. Creatine phosphate is a third above its normal level, and adenosine triphosphate is slightly increased, presumably because of decreased utilization. *In vitro* studies suggest that depressant agents, such as barbiturates, diminish the excitability of the brain, presumably by an effect on the cell membrane that prevents cells from depolarizing and that thus blocks the passage of nerve impulses.

Brain dysfunction may be an indirect effect of a number of so-called "metabolic disorders." The associated symptoms and signs are not specific and include alteration in the level of consciousness and sometimes either seizures or twitching movements, called myoclonus.

Reasons for the depression of metabolism in metabolic coma, such as uremia, hepatic coma, or acidosis, are not clearly understood. Acidosis does not alter the excitability of isolated brain slices but lowers levels of creatine phosphate and ATP; thus, it may interfere with energy production.

Increased Cerebral Metabolism with Seizures

Generalized convulsions brought about by electroshock or other means are accompanied by profound changes in the levels of several brain constituents. Within 3 sec of application of electric shock to a mouse, a reduction in brain levels of creatine phosphate can be demonstrated. In one series of experiments, ATP levels fell by one-half and creatine phosphate by two-thirds when these substances were measured 20 sec after a 1-sec period of electrical stimulation. It appears that when the metabolic rate is increased during a generalized convulsion, the normal energy-producing mechanisms may not be able to replenish high-energy phosphates at a rate rapid enough to prevent a drop in their levels. In mice, it can be calculated that seizures increase the utilization of high-energy phosphates from 30 to 105 mmol of high-energy phosphate per kg of brain per min.

VITAMINS AND THE NERVOUS SYSTEM

Several vitamins are vital for the normal function of the nervous system. When deficiency states develop, neurological syndromes occur that are quite characteristic for the particular vitamin. In their active forms, vitamins usually function as coenzyme units for certain enzyme systems. Thus, the consequences of vitamin deficiency probably result from reduction in activities in one or more enzyme systems that require the particular vitamin. It may be difficult to understand the pathogenesis of a disorder when the vitamin serves as a coenzyme for several enzyme systems.

In addition to the disorders that occur as a consequence of reduction in the amounts of vitamins available to the tissues, a number of "vitamin-dependent" diseases have been discovered in recent years; and a new approach has been opened to the treatment of genetically determined inborn errors of metabolism. In these disorders an alteration in a reaction requiring utilization of a vitamin results in clinical symptoms that can be overcome by administration of much greater amounts of the vitamin than are normally required.

Vitamin Deficiencies

Thiamine (Vitamin B_1). The term "biochemical lesion" was coined by Sir Rudolph Peters for the consequences of thiamine deficiency. Pigeons that were fed on polished rice were found in a few weeks to develop neurological abnormalities characterized by head retraction and arching of the back (opisthotonus). It was discovered that administration of thiamine could reverse the symptoms within 15 to 30 min. The human patient with acute thiamine deficiency exhibits limitation of extraocular movement because of hemorrhage and necrosis of cellular elements in the regions of the brainstem where the cell bodies that give rise to the cranial nerve nuclei are located. Damage in the mammillary bodies and possibly the thalamus may be responsible for the deficits in memory consolidation and recall that are seen in the Wernicke-Korsakoff syndrome (see Chapter 27).

In mammalian tissues, normally about 90 per cent of the total thiamine is thiamine pyrophosphate. Thiamine pyrophosphate is formed from free thiamine and ATP. When animals are made thiamine-deficient, a decrease in thiamine pyrophosphate levels of 50 to 75 per cent can be demonstrated in some brain areas. It is not, however, certain which of the three enzymes that require thiamine pyrophosphate as a cofactor is the most important for neurological functioning. The three enzymes are: pyruvate dehydrogenase, alpha-ketoglutarate dehydrogenase, and transketolase. Each of these enzyme systems is present in peripheral and central nervous tissues. Pyruvate dehydrogenase has been traditionally considered to be the most important of the three enzymes, since it is required for the formation of acetyl–coenzyme A, the compound that is pivotal in linking the glycolytic pathway to the tricarboxylic cycle. In the early studies of Sir

Rudolph Peters, the brains from thiamine-deficient birds contained more lactic acid than normal, suggesting diversion of pyruvate. Alpha-ketoglutarate dehydrogenase is a Krebs-cycle enzyme system that is important for catalyzing the formation of succinyl-coenzyme A from alpha-ketoglutarate. The product is then utilized in the formation of succinate and another high-energy phosphate, guanosine triphosphate (GTP). In some experimental animals that have been made thiamine-deficient by administration of a thiamine antagonist, pyrithiamine, alpha-ketoglutarate levels rose in the brain prior to the development of clinical symptoms. The third enzyme requiring thiamine triphosphate is transketolase, which is important for the function of the hexose-monophosphate shunt. In contrast to the others, this enzyme may be a predominantly glial enzyme, since activity is higher in white matter than in gray matter.

Why particular brain regions are particularly susceptible to thiamine deficiency is not completely understood. It seems likely that quite low levels of thiamine pyrophosphate have to be reached before the critical enzyme systems become nonfunctional.

Vitamin B_{12}. Subacute combined degeneration of the spinal cord and peripheral nerves is one of the classic neurological disorders and has long been known to result from systemic vitamin B_{12} deficiency, usually associated with pernicious anemia. A good deal has been learned about the role of this vitamin in metabolic processes. In contrast, almost nothing is known about the reasons for the neurological degenerative changes that occur with vitamin B_{12} deficiency.

There are two forms of B_{12} compounds that are biologically active. These are sometimes called the *coenzyme form* and the *vitamin form*. Both contain a cobalt atom, but in the coenzyme form the cobalt atom is covalently bound to a 5'-deoxyadenosine moiety. The coenzyme form usually acts to replace a carbon atom of a molecule with a hydrogen atom from an adjacent carbon, whereas the vitamin form catalyzes several reactions in which a methyl group is transferred from one compound to another. In mammalian tissues there are only two enzymes that require B_{12} cofactors. One of these is methylmalonyl–coenzyme A mutase, which catalyzes a reversible reaction between methylmalonyl–coenzyme A and succinyl–coenzyme A. Patients with vitamin B_{12} deficiency do excrete increased amounts of methylmalonic acid and its precursor in the urine. However, it is not established that interference with this reaction is critical to the function of the nervous system. The enzyme methionine synthetase catalyzes the methylation of homocysteine to methionine. The methyl group is transferred from methyltetrahydrofolate.

Pyridoxine. The active form of pyridoxine is pyridoxal phosphate, which requires ATP for its formation. Pyridoxal phosphate is a coenzyme for a variety of enzymatic reactions; hence it is difficult to determine just which enzyme is critical. Seizure activity appears to be the principal consequence of pyridoxine deficiency. Infants on pyridoxine-deficient diets can develop seizures, as can experimental animals. Pyridoxal phosphate–requiring enzymes include phosphorylase, enzymes involved in amino acid decarboxylation, and transaminases. A candidate for attention in pyridoxine deficiency states is glutamate decarboxylase. This enzyme is responsible for the formation of gamma-aminobutyric acid, which is a probable inhibitory transmitter in parts of the nervous system. This enzyme is inhibited in other ways by pharmacological compounds such as allylglycine, which when injected into experimental animals also can cause seizures. Decreased amounts of gamma-aminobutyric acid (GABA) have been found in the brains of vitamin B_6–deficient animals, and the finding has given some indirect support to the suggestion that a reduction in this inhibitory transmitter as a consequence of pyridoxine deficiency might be responsible for seizure activity.

Nicotinic Acid. The coenzymes nicotinamide adenine dinucleotide and nicotinamide adenine dinucleotide phosphate are vital for the function of the dehydrogenase enzymes that transport electrons from organic substrates to electron-acceptors in the major oxidation-reduction reactions that take place in all cells. Nicotinic acid is required for enzymatic synthesis of the coenzymes. Deficiency of this

TABLE 28–3. Neurological Syndromes Associated with Vitamin Deficiencies

Vitamin	Clinical Syndrome in Man
Thiamine	Wernicke-Korsakoff syndrome. Polyneuritis.
Cobalamin (B_{12})	Subacute combined degeneration of the spinal cord.
Pyridoxine	Seizures.
Nicotinic acid	Pellagra (polyneuritis, dementia).

vitamin causes *pellagra,* which is characterized by dermatitis and disturbances in mentation. Classic pellagra occurred in a large number of individuals in mental institutions in which corn made up a large part of the diet. Corn is deficient in the amino acid tryptophan. It is now known that tryptophan can serve as substrate for the endogenous synthesis of nicotinic acid and that tryptophan deficiency can accelerate the development of nicotinic acid deficiency. Hartnup disease is a recessively inherited disorder associated with a defect in intestinal transport of tryptophan and some other amino acids. Some of the symptoms of this disease resemble those of pellagra.

Vitamin-Responsive Inherited Disorders

A new field of investigation has developed since the discovery that seizures occurring in a newborn infant could be controlled by administration of pyridoxine. An infant was jittery at birth and began to have generalized seizures on day 5. The seizures stopped after parenteral administration of a multivitamin preparation. It was eventually determined that pyridoxine was the effective vitamin in preventing seizures in this infant. The syndrome of pyridoxine-dependent seizures is probably inherited as an autosomal recessive disorder. It is postulated that the enzyme glutamate decarboxylase may be structurally abnormal and only able to convert glutamate to gamma-aminobutyric acid in the presence of excessive amounts of pyridoxal phosphate. This idea is supported by the finding in another child with this dis-

order that glutamate decarboxylase activity was reduced in kidney tissue obtained by biopsy but could be restored by inclusion of high concentrations of pyridoxal phosphate in the incubation medium for the enzyme assay.

Other inherited disorders are now being recognized in which a metabolic abnormality can be corrected by administration of large amounts of a single vitamin. Pyridoxine, thiamine, vitamin B_{12}, folic acid, biotin, nicotinamide, and vitamin D have each been implicated in one or more vitamin-dependent disorders. Some of these conditions are associated with neurological symptoms (Table 28–4), others affect other organ systems, and some produce no clinical symptoms at all. When neurological symptoms are present they may or may not resemble the symptoms that occur with deficiency of the vitamin in an otherwise normal individual. The symptoms, for example, in the inherited disorders that respond to vitamin B_{12} administration, do not resemble those of subacute combined degeneration due to B_{12} deficiency. This difference may in part be due to the different ages of onset of the two types of disorders.

Most of the vitamin-dependent disorders can be viewed as examples of genetic heterogeneity, since defects in the same enzymes occur that do not respond to vitamin administration. When it is possible to isolate and characterize the abnormal enzyme, as has been done with families of patients with the clinical condition termed *homocystinuria,* it may be possible to demonstrate several different genetically determined abnormalities of the enzyme protein, each one with similar clinical symptoms. Unfortunately, only a minority of these defects have been found to be vitamin-responsive (Table 28–4).

CEREBRAL NEUROTRANSMITTERS

In Chapter 25 the criteria deemed important for assigning a neurotransmitter role to a particular substance are discussed. It is fair to say that proof that most possible neurotransmitters do indeed function in this capacity has not been achieved. Never-

TABLE 28–4.   Some Vitamin-Responsive Disorders that Affect the Nervous System

Vitamin	Disease	Enzyme Defect	Neurological Manifestations
Pyridoxine (vitamin B_6)	Pyridoxine-dependent seizures.	Glutamate decarboxylase.	Infantile seizures.
	Homocystinuria.	Cystathionine synthase.	Mental retardation, vascular occlusions, psychoses.
Thiamine (vitamin B_1)	Branched-chain keto-aciduria.	Branched-chain ketoacid decarboxylase.	Lethargy, coma.
	Lactic acidosis.	Pyruvate decarboxylase.	Mental retardation.
	Pyruvic acidemia.	Pyruvate dehydrogenase.	Cerebellar ataxia.
Cobalamin (vitamin B_{12})	Methylmalonic aciduria.	$5'$-deoxyadenosyl-B_{12} synthesis.	Lethargy, coma.
	Methylmalonic aciduria and homocystinuria.	$5'$-deoxyadenosyl-B_{12} and methyl-B_{12} synthesis.	Developmental arrest, ataxia.
Nicotinamide	Hartnup disease.	Intestinal absorption of tryptophan.	Cerebellar ataxia, psychosis.
Folic acid	Formiminotransferase deficiency.	Formiminotransferase.	Mental retardation.
	Homocystinuria and hypomethioninemia.	N^5, N^{10}-methylenetetrahydrofolate reductase.	Mental retardation, psychosis.

theless, a strong case can be made for a neurotransmitter role in the central nervous system for the following substances: acetylcholine (ACh), gamma-aminobutyric acid (GABA), glycine, aspartate, glutamate, norepinephrine, dopamine, and 5-hydroxytryptamine (serotonin). Other substances that have also been found to have effects on neuronal excitability and that are present in the central nervous system are adenosine, histamine, and taurine.

Many investigations to better define pathways utilizing a particular neurotransmitter are now being carried out. A widely accepted tenet that is not necessarily always true is that a neuron will utilize only a single neurotransmitter at all of its terminals. Another important principle, and one to which exceptions have not yet been found, is that an enzyme directly involved in catalyzing the synthesis of a particular transmitter is only found in the neuron that uses this transmitter. In contrast, degradative enzymes are much more widely distributed. In the instance of acetylcholine, for example, the enzyme choline acetylase (choline acetyltransferase), which synthesizes the transmitter from acetyl CoA and choline, will only be found in cholinergic neurons, whereas the degradative acetylcholinesterase may be present in membranes from neurons using other transmitters as well. The evidence for this principle is being obtained by analysis of physiologically characterized single cells from organisms such as gastropods and arthropods. The evidence is best for the transmitters acetylcholine and gamma-aminobutyric acid.

The skeletal muscles of the lobster are innervated by both excitatory and inhibitory axons. Kravitz and coworkers have shown that inhibitory axons accumulate gamma-aminobutyric acid. By analyzing individual axons they have shown that only inhibitory axons contain the enzyme glutamate decarboxylase. In contrast, the degradative enzyme GABA:transaminase is found also in excitatory axons and in the sensory axons of the lobster. The sensory neurons contain acetylcholine and contain 500 times the amount of choline acetylase than the excitatory and inhibitory motoneurons do, and acetylcholinesterase is also distributed among all three systems. The probable third transmitter in the excitatory motoneurons of the lobster is glutamate, but in this instance there is not a single pathway for synthesis or degradation.

A new field termed *biochemical neuroanatomy* may now be identified in which biochemical and anatomical techniques are used together in the definition of pathways utilizing particular neurotransmitters. The techniques used in complex nervous systems include histochemical identification of biogenic amines, localization of neurotransmitter-synthesizing enzymes by immunochemical techniques, examination of the anatomical distributions of possible neurotransmitters, and study of the changes in such distributions after destructive lesions are placed. The enzyme dopamine β-hydroxylase is important for forming norepinephrine from dopamine. Destruction of the *locus coeruleus* is followed by a 90 per cent drop in this enzyme in cerebral cortex and hypothalamus; thus, it appears that most cerebral noradrenergic fibers originate in the *locus coeruleus.*

In more complex nervous systems, a variety of anatomical and biochemical techniques have been used in the identification of pathways using particular neurotransmitters. It has been suggested that certain degenerative diseases may involve particular pathways that are defined not only by sites of origin and destination but also by the type of neurotransmitter used by neurons in those pathways. The clearest example is the nigrostriatal pathway, which has cell bodies in the substantia nigra and nerve endings in the corpus striatum. Surgical sectioning of these fibers results in a decrease in content of dopamine in the corpus striatum. This pathway is thus probably *dopaminergic.* In *Parkinson's* disease, analysis of postmortem tissues has shown sharply reduced dopamine contents of the striatum and the substantia nigra. This observation has led to the use of L-dopa (dihydroxyphenylalanine), which crosses the blood-brain barrier and is converted to dopamine by a reaction catalyzed by the enzyme L-aromatic amino acid decarboxylase:

L-*Dopa*

Dopamine

TABLE 28–5. Probable Neurotransmitters and Their Synthesizing Enzymes

Neurotransmitter	Synthesizing Enzymes
Acetylcholine (ACh)	Choline acetylase.
Gamma-aminobutyric acid (GABA)	Glutamate decarboxylase.
Norepinephrine	Tyrosine hydroxylase. Dopa decarboxylase. Dopamine β-hydroxylase.
Dopamine	Tyrosine hydroxylase. Dopa decarboxylase (L-aromatic acid decarboxylase).
Serotonin (5-hydroxytryptamine)	Tryptophan hydroxylase. Aromatic amino acid decarboxylase.

Another recent addition to the treatment of Parkinson's disease is carbidopa, an inhibitor of aromatic amino acid decarboxylation. This agent does not enter the central nervous system. By blocking peripheral decarboxylation of L-dopa, the carbidopa increases the effectiveness of low doses of L-dopa.

Huntington's chorea is a genetic disorder transmitted as an autosomal dominant trait that is associated with loss of neurons in the corpus striatum and also to a lesser degree in the cerebral cortex. Biochemical analyses have shown striatal reductions in levels of the enzymes glutamate decarboxylase and choline acetylase. Other abnormalities are found as well, but mentioned enzyme losses may be regarded as indicating loss of neurons that utilize gamma-aminobutyric acid and acetylcholine as transmitters in the striatal region. This information may give clues to therapeutic approaches to this disease.

LIPID METABOLISM AND ASSOCIATED DISORDERS

Many reviews of normal and abnormal nervous system lipid metabolism have been written. The subject is especially important because of the high lipid content of the myelin sheath (80 per cent of the dry weight) and because of the occurrence of diseases that affect the nervous system that are associated with lipid accumulation.

Lipids in the Central Nervous System

Brain lipids can be separated into three groups: cholesterol, glycerophospholipids, and sphingolipids. Cholesterol is found in the nonesterified form in significant amounts in all brain membranes. All phospholipids except sphingomyelin consist of glycerol linked to two fatty acids by acyl ester linkages, with the third hydroxyl group of glycerol linked to the phosphate moiety of the group by which the compound is named. Other important phospholipids are lecithin (phosphatidylcholine) and phosphatidylethanolamine. The sphingolipids utilize the long-chain amino alcohol sphingosine rather than glycerol as the building block.

Each sphingolipid has a long-chain fatty acid linked to the sphingosine nitrogen. To this fatty acid-sphingosine complex (ceramide) is attached an additional component at carbon-1. This component is characteristic of the individual sphingolipid, and can be galactose, glucose, more complex sugars, or phosphorylcholine.

Disorders of Lipid Metabolism

There is a group of genetic diseases in which an enzyme that normally catalyzes the breakdown, or catabolism, of a type of lipid is defective.

The consequence of this catabolic defect is usually accumulation of large amounts of the particular lipid. Since these catabolic enzymes are normally contained in intracellular organelles called *lysosomes*, the disorders are sometimes called *lysosomal diseases*. Other synonyms are *lipid storage diseases* and *lipidoses*. Further, most of the conditions are associated with abnormal metabolism of a sphingosine-containing lipid, and hence the term *sphingolipidosis* is also used for the group of conditions.

Several general points can be made about these disorders. First, none of them is inherited as an autosomal dominant trait. Most are autosomal recessive, though Fabry's disease is sex-linked recessive. Since one gene is capable of directing the formation of normal enzyme, heterozygotes for these conditions will make half the usual amount of enzyme, and this amount will suffice for catabolism of its particular lipid. A second point about these disorders is that in those instances in which it has been possible to purify the lipid-degrading enzyme and to prepare antibody to it, it has been found that in the disease state, a protein is present that will complex with the antibody. Thus in tissues of the patient with the disorder, the enzyme protein is being made but is structurally abnormal and incapable of carrying out its enzymatic function. A third feature of many of these conditions is the possibility of substituting a synthetic substrate for the natural substrate in the enzyme assay, so that diagnosis of the disorder is facilitated. Diagnosis has also been facilitated by the discovery that the defect in the enzyme is often detectable in easily accessible tissues, such as skin fibroblasts and blood leukocytes. It is now possible to diagnose many of these conditions *in utero* by procurement of specimens of amniotic fluid and assaying of cells cultured from this fluid for enzyme activity.

Heterozygotes whose tissues contain about half the normal amount of enzyme activity can also be detected. Exploration of the feasibility of infusing exogenous enzymes into patients with some of these disorders is underway, and in Gaucher's disease and Fabry's disease some reduction

TABLE 28–6. Lipid Storage Diseases

Condition	Stored Lipid	Enzyme Deficiency
Gaucher's disease	Glucocerebroside.	Glucocerebrosidase.
Tay-Sachs disease	G_{M2} ganglioside.	G_{M2} hexosaminidases.
G_{M1} gangliosidosis	G_{M1} ganglioside.	G_{M1} β-galactosidases.
Metachromatic leukodystrophy	Sulfatide.	Sulfatidase.
Krabbe's disease	Galactosyl ceramide.	Galactocerebrosidase.
Niemann-Pick disease	Sphingomyelin.	Sphingomyelinase.
Fabry's disease	Ceramide trihexoside.	α-Galactosidase (ceramidetrihexosidase).

in levels of circulating lipid has been achieved.

AXONAL TRANSPORT

The cell body is the site for most of the protein synthesis that takes place within neurons. Materials must move long distances if they are to be utilized at the nerve ending. Axonal transport can be examined by exposure of a cell body to a radioactively labeled substance that is incorporated into the material being transported. For example, proteins can be tagged with a labeled amino acid precursor, such as [^{3}H]leucine. At intervals of time, the nerve can be sectioned into small segments, and the distribution of radioactivity can be determined. Rates of movement of the front of the radioactive label can then be easily calculated. There are at least two proximodistal transport systems that are separable by their fast and slow rates. Substances that move with the slow transport system travel approximately 1 to 3 mm per day. Rapid transport proceeds at a rate of 40 to 1000 mm per day. The latter system has been examined intensively in recent years and can be demonstrated in peripheral motor or sensory fibers, in sympathetic nerves, in optic nerves and in some other central nervous system neurons. Systems for transporting substances in a distal–proximal direction have also been demonstrated.

The slow movement of substances down the axon was first demonstrated by Weiss and Hiscoe in 1948. They constricted the peripheral nerves by slipping over the cut nerve ends short segments of arteries with luminal diameters smaller than those of the nerves. The axons proximal to the obstruction became enlarged, and after release the accumulated axoplasm could be observed to move at rates of 1 to 3 mm per day. Later, they used radioautographic techniques to show movement of ^{32}P- and ^{3}H-labeled precursors at about 3 mm per day.

No disease has yet been shown to result from interference with these transport systems. It might be predicted, however, that some peripheral neuropathies could be caused in this way. Rapid transport can be blocked by interference with the metabolism of the axon, by treatment with inhibitors of cation transport, and by application of very high concentrations of local anesthetics.

ADDITIONAL READING

Cohen, M. M., ed. *Biochemistry of neural disease.* Hagerstown, Md., Harper & Row, 1975.

McIlwain, H., and Bachelard, H. S. *Biochemistry and the central nervous system.* Edinburgh, Churchill-Livingstone, 1971.

Siegel, G. J., Albers, R. W., Katzman, R., and Agranoff, B. W., eds. *Basic neurochemistry.* Boston, Little, Brown & Co., 1976.

CHAPTER 29

THE VASCULATURE OF THE BRAIN AND SPINAL CORD

JOHN W. SUNDSTEN
and PHILLIP D. SWANSON

Diseases of the vascular system are responsible for the largest proportion of neurological illnesses. Some of these conditions are treatable by medical or surgical means, especially if recognized before irreversible damage to the nervous system has occurred. Most vascular disorders are either *occlusive* or *hemorrhagic*. In occlusive cerebrovascular disease, the neurological symptoms result from *ischemia*, due to reduction in blood flow. In hemorrhagic conditions, tissue destruction results from the pressure and volume of ejected blood. Secondary effects of increased intracranial pressure are more common in hemorrhages, but they can also occur with large ischemic infarctions that are accompanied by brain swelling.

THE BLOOD SUPPLY TO THE BRAIN

Two paired systems of vessels, the internal carotid and the vertebral arteries, carry blood to the cerebral hemispheres and brainstem (Figs. 29–1 and 29–2). The internal carotids arise from the common carotid arteries and the vertebrals from the subclavian arteries. These vascular streams join together at the base of the brain through a network of vessels called the *circle of Willis.* The circle of Willis is formed of the first segments of the two anterior cerebral arteries joined by the anterior communicating artery, the first segments of the two posterior cerebral arteries as they arise from the basilar artery, and the two posterior communicating arteries, connecting the posterior cerebrals with the internal carotid arteries. The circle of Willis provides a shunting mechanism between the two systems that enables a continual blood supply to the brain when one system or the other is compromised. If pressure falls in one of the systems, blood will flow into it from the other. This mechanism operates even under normal conditions. It should be remembered, however, that perfect symmetry of the circle of Willis

374

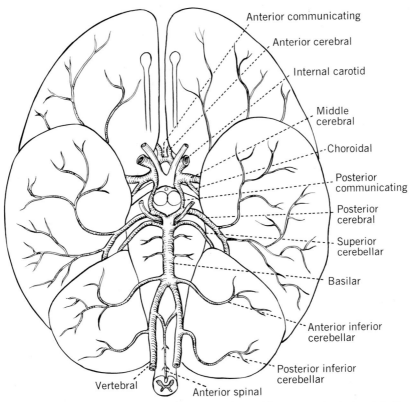

Figure 29–1. Major branches of the vertebral and internal carotid systems of arteries at the base of the brain.

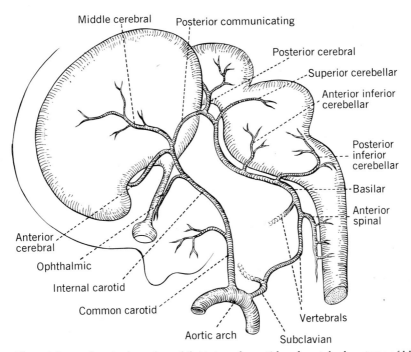

Figure 29–2. The origins and major branches of the internal carotid and vertebral systems of blood supply to the fetal brain.

is an exceptional occurrence, and that one or more of the connecting vessels may be hypoplastic. One of the posterior communicating arteries is particularly likely to be hypoplastic. Variations in the circle of Willis and hypoplasia in other vessels, such as the vertebral artery, make the results of occlusion of an artery supplying the forebrain or brainstem somewhat unpredictable.

Potential anastomotic channels also exist extracranially, especially through the facial branches of the external carotid artery with orbital branches of the ophthalmic artery. The ophthalmic artery arises from the internal carotid artery. Potential channels of less importance can develop through the occipital branch of the external carotid with the vertebral artery. Leptomeningeal anastomoses between major cerebral end arteries form additional shunting routes that are considered secondary to those of the circle of Willis. The major individual branches of the internal carotid and verte-

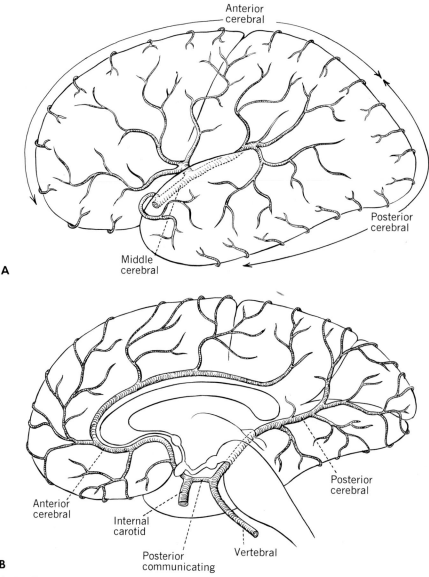

Figure 29–3. Distribution of the anterior, middle, and posterior cerebral arteries on the surface of the cerebral hemispheres. *A*, Lateral view. *B*, Medial view.

bral arterial systems are illustrated in Figures 29–1 and 29–2 and discussed below.

The Internal Carotid System

The *internal carotid artery* enters the skull through the carotid canal and foramen lacerum to gain access to the middle cranial fossa. It then passes through the cavernous sinus (supplying the pituitary gland) and makes an S-turn back on itself (the carotid siphon) in relation to the anterior clinoid process of the sphenoid bone and to the optic chiasm. Here it enters the subarachnoid space and gives off the *ophthalmic artery*. The internal carotid artery gives off the *posterior communicating* and *anterior choroidal arteries* under the anterior perforated substance and then divides into its terminal and largest branches, the *anterior* and *middle* cerebral arteries (Figs. 29–2 and 29–3). The posterior communicating artery joins the *posterior* cerebral artery linking the carotid and vertebral systems. The

anterior choroidal artery feeds the choroid plexus along with *posterior choroidal* branches of the posterior cerebral artery. The anterior choroidal artery travels posteriorly along the optic tract and enters the choroid fissure, from which it has access to structures deep in the temporal lobe, such as the amygdala and hippocampus. Its branches reach parts of the globus pallidus, thalamus, internal capsule, and cerebral peduncle (see Figs. 29–4 and 29–5).

The anterior cerebral arteries are joined together by the *anterior communicating artery* and proceed around the medial aspect of the hemispheres in relation to the corpus callosum (Fig. 29–3). They meet the posterior cerebral circulation in the occipital lobe. The anterior cerebral artery supplies the medial aspect of the frontal and parietal lobes and the corpus callosum. Early in the course, it gives off *striate* branches that penetrate the anterior perforated substance to reach anterior parts of the basal ganglia and internal capsule.

The *middle cerebral artery* passes through

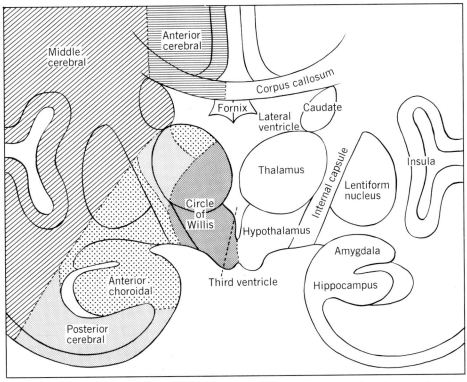

Figure 29–4. A frontal section through the forebrain, showing the general distribution of major cerebral arterial branches to deep structures. (After Haymaker, *Bing's local diagnosis in neurological diseases*, St. Louis, The C. V. Mosby Co., 1969).

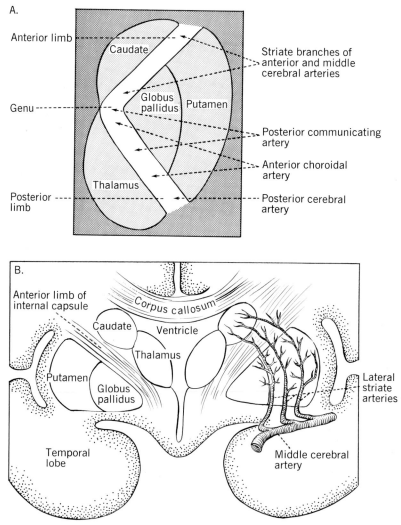

Figure 29–5. Arterial supply to the internal capsule and striatum. *A,* A horizontal section showing the internal capsule (anterior limb, genu, and posterior limb), surrounding structures, and blood supply. *B,* A frontal section through the anterior limb of the internal capsule, showing the lateral striate branches of the middle cerebral artery.

the lateral fissure, and, after giving off perforating *striate* branches to the internal capsule and corpus striatum, supplies most of the lateral surface of the hemisphere (Figs. 29–2, 29–3, 29–4, and 29–5). Because of its large area, the brain tissue supplied by the middle cerebral artery is more prone to infarction than brain tissue in other circulatory territories. Subsequent to occlusion of the middle cerebral artery there may follow hemiparesis and hemianesthesia (the lower extremity is less involved because most of the leg area is located medially and is supplied by the anterior cerebral artery). Hemianopia or

quadrantanopia may result from damage to the optic radiations, and aphasia can occur with lesions in the left hemisphere. Occasionally, individual branches of the middle cerebral artery are affected, but most occlusions are proximal. The extent of infarction will vary, depending on the amount of collateral flow from other vessels. Blood can sometimes be demonstrated to flow retrograde from other major arterial supply areas. The general regions of blood supply that the above vessels provide to deep structures are shown in a selected frontal section through the forebrain (Fig. 29–5).

The Vertebrobasilar System

The vertebral arteries (Figs. 29–1 and 29–2) enter the cranial vault through the foramen magnum. They ascend along the anterior surface of the medulla, giving off *meningeal branches* to the posterior cranial fossa and the *anterior spinal* and *posterior inferior cerebellar arteries*. They end by joining together at the pons to form the anteriorly placed *basilar artery*. The basilar artery ends in the interpeduncular fossa between the two cerebral peduncles, where it divides into the two *posterior cerebral arteries*. The basilar artery gives off several branches as it ascends: the *anterior inferior cerebellar, auditory, pontine*, and *superior cerebellar arteries*. Note that the oculomotor nerve begins its intracranial course by exiting from the brainstem between the superior cerebellar and posterior cerebral arteries (Fig. 29–1). As the posterior cerebral artery ascends around the cerebral peduncle, it gives off branches to that structure and to the midbrain; and as it reaches the hemisphere, it supplies the occipital lobe and the inferior and medial aspects of the temporal lobe. Deeper branches supply the thalamus and hippocampus. Its posterior choroidal branch reaches the choroidal fissure and supplies, along with the anterior choroidal artery, the choroid plexus.

The regional distributions of the above vessels are indicated by their names. The cross-sectional area of vascular supply to the brainstem is either *paramedian* or *circumferential* in position. The paramedian branches supply the medial regions of the stem; the circumferential vessels supply more lateral parts (short circumferential vessels) and suprasegmental structures (long circumferential vessels), i.e., the cerebral hemispheres, the cerebellum, and the colliculi. These distributions have their clinical counterparts in the different syndromes that a patient may present with. Two cases in point are the medial and lateral medullary plate syndromes due to infarction in the paramedian and circumferential portions of the medulla (Fig. 29–6). Paramedian branches of the vertebral artery supply the region of the pyramid, medial lemniscus, and exiting hypo-

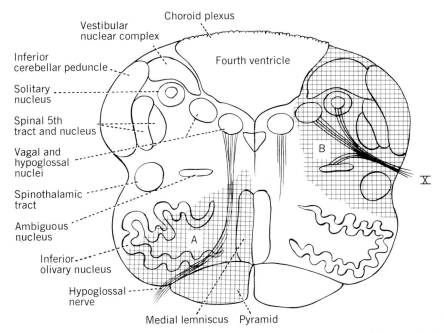

Figure 29–6. Examples of infarcts in the medulla. *A,* Paramedian infarct (branches of the vertebral or anterior spinal arteries). *B,* Circumferential infarct (branches of the vertebral or posterior inferior cerebellar arteries). See text for description of signs and symptoms. (After Haymaker, *Bing's local diagnosis in neurological diseases,* St. Louis, The C. V. Mosby Co., 1969.)

glossal nerve. Occlusion of these branches results in the *medial medullary plate syndrome,* characterized by contralateral hemiplegia (pyramid and other descending fibers), contralateral decrease in the proprioceptive and tactile discriminatory sensibilities (medial lemniscus), and ipsilateral paralysis and atrophy of the tongue (hypoglossal nerve).

The lateral part of the medulla is supplied by the posterior inferior cerebellar artery as it courses in a circumferential manner to the cerebellum (Figs. 29–1, 29–2, and 29–6). Occlusion of this vessel or of the vertebral artery may produce infarction in the lateral medulla. The resulting clinical syndrome is termed the *lateral medullary plate syndrome* (of Wallenberg). The patient presents with contralateral loss of pain and temperature below the head (spinothalamic tract), ipsilateral loss of pain and temperature on the face (spinal tract and nucleus of the trigeminal nerve), hoarseness and difficulty in phonation (nucleus ambiguus), ataxia (spinocerebellar tract and cerebellum), dizziness (vestibular nuclei), ipsilateral warm, dry face, ptosis and small pupil (reticulospinal fibers descending to sympathetic outflow), and ipsilateral loss of the gag reflex (solitary nucleus and tract). Such lesions in the paramedian or circumferential regions of vascular supply can occur anywhere throughout the brainstem and forebrain; the signs and symptoms that the patient develops will result from damage to the long motor and sensory paths passing through the region and from damage to specific structures located only at the particular level involved, such as the cranial nerves (see Figures 29–7 and 29–8).

The Venous System

The venous return from the brain is divided into an external and internal group of vessels that drain, respectively, the surface and deep regions of the hemisphere. Both sets end in a system of venous sinuses in the dura that ultimately empty into the *internal jugular vein* (Fig. 29–9). The *external cerebral veins* may enter the dural sinuses directly by bridging the subarachnoid space and piercing the dura or indirectly by forming larger vessels that first travel some distance in the subarachnoid space. These longer channels are divided into superior, middle, and inferior groups that for the most part follow sulci and fissures.

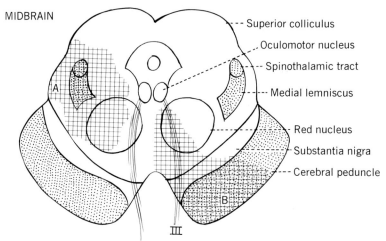

Figure 29–7. Examples of infarcts in the midbrain. *A,* Tegmental infarct (circumferential branches of posterior cerebral artery), producing contralateral cerebellar signs and hypesthesia. The cerebellar signs may instead be accompanied by ipsilateral oculomotor paralysis if the lesion is more medially placed. *B,* Peduncular infarct (paramedian branches of posterior cerebral artery), producing ipsilateral oculomotor paralysis and contralateral hemiparesis. A somewhat larger lesion could involve also the red nucleus, resulting in contralateral cerebellar signs. Note that sometimes the cerebral peduncle may be spared. (After Haymaker, *Bing's local diagnosis in neurological diseases,* St. Louis, The C. V. Mosby Co., 1969.)

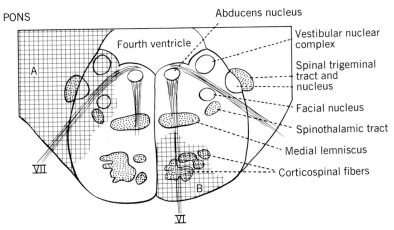

Figure 29–8. Examples of infarcts in the pons. *A,* Tegmental infarct (circumferential branches of the anterior inferior cerebellar artery), producing contralateral hypalgesia and thermohypesthesia below the head (spinothalamic tract), ipsilateral pain and temperature loss on the face (spinal trigeminal tract), ipsilateral facial paralysis (facial nerve), ipsilateral cerebellar signs such as ataxia (cerebellar peduncles), nausea and vertigo (vestibular complex), and ipsilateral deafness (if the lesion extends caudally to include the cochlear nuclei). *B,* Basal pontine infarct (paramedian branches of the basilar artery), producing contralateral hemiparesis and abducent nerve palsy. (After Haymaker, *Bing's local diagnosis in neurological diseases,* St. Louis, The C. V. Mosby Co., 1969.)

The *internal cerebral veins* begin at the interventricular foramen by forming a pair of vessels that extend posteriorly in the transverse cerebral fissure. They unite below the splenium of the corpus callosum to form the *great cerebral vein,* which empties into the straight sinus (Fig. 29–9).

Communications of veins located outside

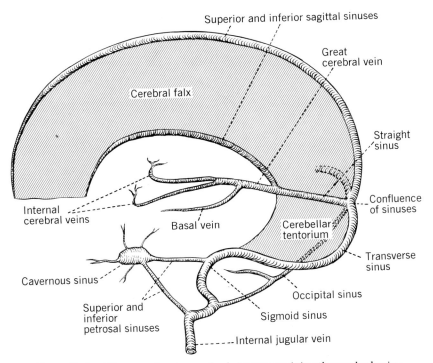

Figure 29–9. Diagram of major cerebral sinuses receiving the cerebral veins.

TABLE 29–1. Potential Sites of Communication between Extracranial and Intracranial Venous Channels

Extracranial	Communication	Intracranial
Facial vein	Ophthalmic veins	Cavernous sinus
Occipital vein	Mastoid vein	Sigmoid sinus
Scalp veins	Parietal vein	Superior sagittal sinus
Internal jugular vein	Hypoglossal venous plexus	Sigmoid sinus
Pterygoid plexus	Plexus in foramen ovale	Cavernous sinus
Internal jugular vein	Internal carotid venous plexus	Cavernous sinus
External jugular vein	Petrosquamous sinus	Transverse sinus

and inside the skull provide routes through which inflammatory processes may spread from extracranial structures and cause thrombosis of sinuses. The orbit and variable *emissary veins* that pass through small foramina in skull bones are the most common sites for potential communication. Major examples of such venous anastomoses are listed in Table 29–1.

CONTROL OF CEREBRAL BLOOD FLOW

Cerebral blood flow in man and animals can be estimated accurately. The rate in an adult human male is 54 to 62 ml per 100 g of brain per min during both wakefulness and sleep. The rate is almost double in a 6-year-old child. Under normal circumstances cerebral blood flow remains remarkably constant in spite of alterations in heart rate or blood pressure. The blood flow can rise or fall, however, in response to increase or decrease in the metabolic demands of the brain. For example, during seizures, when the rate of oxygen consumption may increase severalfold, cerebral blood flow will increase proportionately. Conversely, during anesthesia, when metabolic demands diminish, cerebral blood flow falls.

The volume of blood that enters the brain during a given period of time will be governed by the effective perfusion pressure and by the cerebral vascular resistance. The effective perfusion pressure is the difference between arterial and venous pressures and depends particularly on the level of the systemic arterial blood pressure. Above mean arterial pressure of about 80 mm Hg, the rate of blood flow to the brain is controlled by intrinsic mechanisms.

The cerebral vascular resistance is able to adjust to changing metabolic needs of the brain and to changes in arterial blood pressure by means of at least three mechanisms: (1) arteriolar constriction or dilatation secondary to changes in arterial pressure; (2) adjustment of resistance to alterations in tissue metabolism; and (3) neurogenic control. Cerebral arterioles respond to a rise in systemic arterial pressure by constriction. When systemic pressure falls, the cerebral arterioles dilate. This *autoregulation* of blood flow in response to blood pressure changes allows the treatment of essential hypertension without reduction in cerebral blood flow.

Adjustment of cerebral blood flow to cerebral metabolism is well documented. Increases in carbon dioxide or hydrogen ion concentration will dilate cerebral arterioles and thereby increase flow; this may be the principal factor in metabolic regulation. More recently developed techniques have enabled increases in blood flow to discrete brain regions to be demonstrated to occur when there is increased functional activity in these regions. In animals visual stimulation is associated with increased blood flow to the visual cortex and lateral geniculate bodies. It has even been demonstrated in humans that mental effort can raise blood flow to cortical gray matter by 8 per cent.

A third influence on cerebral blood flow is termed *neurogenic control.* Cerebral arteries and arterioles are innervated by autonomic nerve fibers that utilize noradrenaline as a neurotransmitter. Fibers to the extraparenchymal vessels arise from the superior cervical ganglion. Some of the small intraparenchymal vessels may be supplied by noradrenergic nerves whose cell bodies are located in the locus ceruleus of the midbrain.

The relative importance of the three mechanisms for control of blood flow is not certain. The neurogenic system is being studied most intensively at the present time, in part because of the possibility of improving cerebral blood flow in pathologic states by the use of drugs that influence the action of catecholamines.

DISORDERS OF THE CEREBRAL CIRCULATION

Ischemic or hemorrhagic disorders can occur in either the carotid or vertebrobasilar circulations. The precise symptoms will be determined by the anatomical area of ischemia or hemorrhage and by secondary effects of increased intracranial pressure. The symptoms of vascular diseases usually come on rapidly, in periods ranging from seconds to a few hours.

Ischemia

Atherosclerotic narrowing of arteries can occur either extracranially or intracranially. Because of the anastomotic connections, complete occlusions of one or more major extracranial vessels can sometimes take place without producing any clinical symptoms whatsoever. In some patients, *transient ischemic attacks* occur, due either to temporary reduction in blood flow or to breaking off of small fibrin or atheromatous emboli, which then travel to distal arterioles and produce ischemic symptoms that often last only a few seconds or minutes.

When ischemia persists beyond a few minutes, necrosis of tissue elements will occur. Pathologic specimens will show "softening," or *encephalomalacia*, in the area of infarction. The clinical symptoms will obviously be determined by the territory supplied by the occluded vessel. If a small infarct occurs from occlusion of a small arteriole in the prefrontal cortex, there may be virtually no clinical symptom or sign. In contrast, a strategically placed small infarction in a major pathway might produce profound neurological dysfunction.

Clinical case. A 71-year-old retired Army colonel noticed he was unable to stand after a morning bath. He was dizzy and would fall off to the left. He was helped to bed and began to notice a numb feeling on the left side of his lips, cheek, and throat. Within ½ hour he was unable to walk even with help. He had a moderate headache (located behind the left ear). His voice seemed hoarser than usual, and he noted that his throat was "paralyzed." He could swallow small quantities down the right side of his throat. His tongue worked well, and he was fully alert.

After 2 days his ability to swallow improved, and he was able to walk with assistance. At that time, on neurological examination, his speech, though clearly enunciated, was hoarse. The left pupil was smaller than the right, and there was mild left ptosis. The left side of the face was dryer than the right. Corneal reflex could not be elicited on the left, and sensation to pinprick and temperature was impaired over the left face in the distribution of all three divisions of the left fifth cranial nerve. Sensation to pinprick was also impaired on the left side of the tongue. The left side of the soft palate moved less well than the right, and the gag reflex could not be elicited from the left side of the oropharynx. There was no weakness of either tongue or face or of either the sternocleidomastoid or trapezius muscles. Over the body, sensation to pinprick and temperature was impaired on the right side, but light touch, vibratory, and position sensations were intact. There was no weakness, though a moderate degree of clumsiness was present in the left hand, and the patient was markedly ataxic when he attempted to walk.

This patient's symptoms and signs are those described earlier as characterizing the *lateral medullary plate syndrome* (Fig. 29–6).

Venous Occlusion

Thrombosis of cerebral veins or of venous sinuses is a rarer occurrence than arterial obstruction. Cerebral venous occlusions can occur in acutely ill, dehydrated individuals; hemorrhagic infarction may result, often with accompanying seizures. In some instances obstruction of the venous sinuses produces increased intracranial pressure because of reduced absorption of cerebrospinal fluid.

Hemorrhage

Spontaneous hemorrhage from cerebral arteries can produce devastating, often fatal, consequences. Rupture of large surface arteries directly into the subarachnoid space may occur, producing symptoms of headache, stiff neck, and alterations in the level of consciousness. The most common associated abnormality in a cerebral artery is a saccular, or *berry*, aneurysm. These dilatations occur most commonly at arterial bifurcations and junctions, especially at the junction of the internal carotid and posterior communicating arteries, on the anterior communicating arteries, and on the middle cerebral artery. It is uncertain whether there is a congenital defect in the vessel wall that predisposes to formation of an aneurysm. Pathologic specimens often show degenerative changes in the internal elastic lamina. Expansion of the aneurysm may produce signs due to pressure on neighboring structures. Internal carotid–posterior communicating aneurysms (Fig. 29–10) typically compress the third cranial nerve, resulting in a dilated pupil, ptosis, and weakness of appropriate extraocular muscles. These may occur suddenly just before or at the time of rupture.

Intracerebral hemorrhage usually occurs in patients with hypertension. Hyaline degeneration of small perforating arteries and arterioles may result in the development of small microaneurysms. These microaneurysms may thrombose, resulting in small "lacunar" infarctions. Or they may rupture into the brain substance. The most

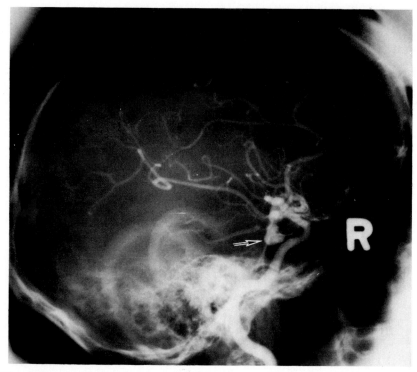

Figure 29–10. Angiogram showing an aneurysm that arises at the internal carotid–posterior communicating arterial junction. The fundus of the aneurysm is indicated by the arrow.

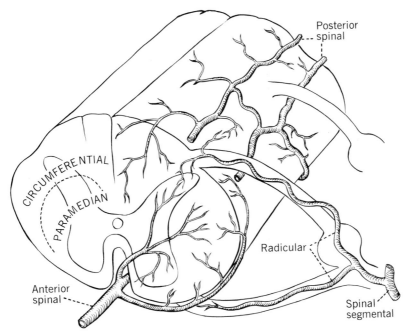

Figure 29–11. Arterial supply to the spinal cord.

common site for rupture is the striatum (see Figure 29–5). Intracerebral hemorrhages also occur in the cerebellum, pons, subcortical white matter, and thalamus. They frequently enlarge over a period extending from minutes to a few hours and may rupture into the ventricle or subarachnoid space. The morbidity of intracerebral hemorrhage is high because of the destruction of tissue that occurs. Mortality is especially high in pontine hemorrhages and in hemorrhages that rupture into the ventricles.

Subarachnoid and intracerebral hemorrhages can also occur from *arteriovenous* malformations. Usually the prognosis is better after this type of hemorrhage than after aneurysmal rupture or hypertensive intracerebral hemorrhage.

VASCULAR SUPPLY OF THE SPINAL CORD

Blood reaches the spinal cord by three routes: the *anterior* and *posterior spinal arteries* and the *radicular arteries* (Fig. 29–11). The anterior spinal artery is connected with the vertebral arteries on the anterior surface of the medulla but also receives blood from radicular arteries. The anterior spinal artery extends the length of the spinal cord in the anteromedian fissure and supplies paramedian branches to the anterior and posterior gray matter and the central portions of the anterior and lateral white matter. Thus, the anterior spinal artery nourishes most of the cross-sectional area of the cord. The posterior spinal arteries arise from the posterior inferior cerebellar artery or the vertebral artery. They form a pair of longitudinal channels on either side of the posterior roots but may terminate anywhere along the cord. They supply the posterior white columns and part of the posterior gray. The radicular arteries arise from spinal intersegmental arteries and reach the spinal cord by coursing along the posterior and anterior roots. They are variable in number and are smaller than the other vessels; they may terminate in the roots. However, there are usually three or so that form larger vessels that do link with the spinal arterial system. A plexus of vessels is formed in the pia mater by anastomotic branches of all three sources of blood supply. These channels supply the circumferential parts of the white matter.

Blood flows both rostrally and caudally

in spinal arteries, depending on the relation to the major feeding radicular vessels. There are therefore anastomotic "watershed areas" between the territories supplied by the radicular arteries. Ischemia to the spinal cord can occur either with occlusion of the anterior spinal artery or from impairment of supply through a major radicular vessel after aortic surgery or secondary to a dissecting aneurysm in the aorta.

The veins draining the intramedullary region of the spinal cord form a tortuous plexus on the cord's surface in the pia mater. The deep veins and the plexus empty into four longitudinal channels. Two are situated in the midline, the *posterior spinal vein* along the posteromedian sulcus and the *anterior spinal vein* along the anteromedian sulcus. Two are related to the laterally placed sulci along which the roots of the spinal nerves attach, the *posterolateral spinal vein* and the *anterolateral spinal vein*. The spinal veins communicate freely with the *internal vertebral plexus of veins* in the vertebral canal and exit through the intervertebral foramina as *intervertebral veins*. The intervertebral veins drain into the *external vertebral plexus* of veins around the vertebra, the *vertebral vein, intercostal, lumbar* and *sacral segmental veins*. The intervertebral veins have no valves and, with changes in pressure in the body cavities, tumor cells or other foreign material can easily reach the vertebral bodies by retrograde flow into the voluminous spinovertebral venous anastomoses. Vertebral body metastases can extend into the spinal epidural space and produce compression of the spinal cord.

ADDITIONAL READING

Kaplan, H. A., and Ford, D. H. *The brain vascular system.* New York, American Elsevier Publishing Co., 1966.

A Glossary of Neurological Terms and Word Roots and Their Origins

Harry D. Patton and John W. Sundsten

adeno.   Prefix meaning *like an acorn*. Pertains to a gland; thus, the *adenohypophysis* is the glandular part of the hypophysis, as distinguished from the neural posterior lobe, or *neurohypophysis*.

ageusia.   Loss of the sense of taste.

alar.   Winglike, e.g., the alar plate of the developing nervous system.

alexia.   Loss of the ability to read.

algesia.   Suffix meaning *pain*. Examples: *analgesia*, lack of sensitivity to pain; *hypalgesia*, diminished sensitivity to pain; *hyperalgesia*, increased sensitivity to pain. An *analgesic* drug is one that relieves pain.

amblyopia.   Dull eye; thus, dimness of vision; partial loss of sight.

amnestic.   Amnesic; lack or loss of memory.

ampulla.   A little bottle or rounded flask; hence, a bottle-shaped swelling in semicircular canals.

amygdaloid.   Almond-shaped, as the *amygdaloid nucleus*, or *amygdala*.

angio.   Prefix referring to blood vessels. Thus, an *angioma* is a tumor of blood vessels, and an *angiogram* is a radiogram taken while the vessels contain a radiopaque dye.

anoxia.   Oxygen deprivation. Also, hypoxia, a condition of reduced oxygen.

ansa.   Handle of an urn; hence, a loop or curve, as the *ansa lenticularis*, the loop of fibers around the lens-shaped (lenticular) nucleus.

aphakia.   Literally, lacking a lentil. Neurologically, lacking a lens (which is lentil-shaped).

aphasia.   Without speech. Used broadly to denote impairment of communication by language in any form — reading (alexia), writing (agraphia), or speaking.

apraxia.   Literally, lack of action. Inability to carry out motor acts on command in the absence of paralysis.

aqueduct.   A passage or channel for conduction of water or fluid. Example: the cerebral aqueduct (of Sylvius) between the third and fourth cerebral ventricles.

arachnoid.   Like a cobweb; thus, the delicate arachnoid meningeal membrane.

artifact.   Literally, made by art, *i.e.*, man-made. Therefore, an artificial structure or feature introduced into a record or preparation by the experimental procedure. Eschewed by natural and physical scientists, who study nature, artifacts are cherished by anthropologists and archeologists, who study man and his artistic products.

astro.   Prefix meaning *starlike, stellar*. An *astrocyte* is a star-shaped glial cell.

ataxia.   Literally, want of order or arrangement; specifically, awkwardness in motor behavior associated with loss of afferent information from the moving part or with loss of control mechanism of the cerebellum.

athero.   Prefix meaning *like groats* or *porridge*. An *atheroma* is a fatty growth in the arterial wall resembling oatmeal. *Atherosclerosis* is hardening of the arteries associated with atheromas (see *sclerosis*, under *scler, sclero*).

athetosis. Not fixed; thus, continually moving or changing position. Refers to sinuous involuntary movements of some patients with disease of the basal ganglia.

aura. Literally, a breath or a breeze. Neurologically, sensation or feeling states preceding an epileptic seizure (sometimes a feeling of cold air).

axon. Axis; hence, the straight, relatively unbranched process of a nerve cell.

ballism. [From the Greek *ballo*, to throw.] Neurologically, violent involuntary tossing or throwing movements.

biopsy. View of life. Removal of tissue from living subjects for diagnostic purposes. Contrasted with *necropsy* (*cf.* under *necro*).

bouton. [French for *button*.] Synaptic knobs are sometimes called *boutons terminaux* (terminal buttons).

brachium. Arm; thus, *brachium conjunctivum*, the arm of the cerebellum (superior cerebellar peduncle) joining with the midbrain.

brady. Prefix meaning *slow;* thus, *bradykinesia*, slowness of movement; *bradycardia*, slow pulse.

callosum. Literally, hard or tough. The *corpus callosum* is so called because of its density and toughness.

calvaria. Literally, the hairless scalp. The roof of the skull above the orbits, the auditory meatus, and the occipital protuberance. *Calvaria* is singular, not *calvarium*, although the latter is almost universally incorrectly used.

carotid. [From the Greek verb *karoo*, to plunge into sleep or stupor.] Compression of the carotid arteries causes unconsciousness.

cataplexy. Literally, a striking down. Neurologically, a transient attack of weakness precipitated by emotional excitement or hearty laughter. The patient falls as if struck down. Attacks usually occur in patients who also have narcolepsy.

cauda. Tail; thus, the *cauda equina* resembles a horse's tail, and the *caudate nucleus* forms a tail around the lenticular nucleus. *Caudal* and *caudad* mean *toward the tail. Cf. rostral* or *rostrad.*

cele (or **coele**). A tumor or hernia. Describes a swelling caused by herniation of a soft part. Thus, a *meningocele* is a herniated meningeal sac, and a *meningomyelocele* is one in which neural tissue herniates along with its meningeal covering.

cerebellum. The little brain.

ceruleus. Blue. The locus ceruleus of the brainstem contains a blue pigment.

chiasm. Like the Greek letter χ or *chi*. Descriptive of the crossing of optic nerve fibers.

chorea. Dance, describing the terpsichorean involuntary movements of patients with disease of the basal ganglia.

choroid (chorioid). Like the chorion, the vascular membrane surrounding the fetus. The resemblance is at best tenuous in the choroid coat of the eye and the choroid plexus of the cerebral ventricular system.

cinereum. Ash gray. The *tuber cinereum* (ash gray bump or nodule) is a gross anatomical term descriptive of the base of the hypothalamus as seen from the outside.

cingulum. Girdle or belt. The *cingulate gyrus* girdles or surrounds the corpus callosum.

cistern. A closed space serving as a reservoir of fluid, especially one of the enlarged subarachnoid spaces containing cerebrospinal fluid.

claustrum. A barrier. Fancifully, the claustrum stands as an outer wall or barrier to the medially situated lentiform nucleus.

clava. Club. Describes the clubbed or hockey-stick appearance of the rostral extent of the fasciculus and nucleus gracilis viewed in gross dissection of the bulbospinal junction.

clinoid. Like a bed. The clinoid processes surround the pituitary fossa, thus resembling the knobs on bedposts.

clonus. Turmoil. The oscillatory contraction and relaxation of muscle in spasticity suggests agitation or turmoil.

cochlea. Snail shell. Describes the architecture of the bony part of the inner ear.

coele. See *cele*.

colliculus. Little hill, or mound. The superior and inferior colliculi are two pairs of hills forming the roof of the midbrain.

commissure. Putting together or joining. Thus, a tract of fibers binding the two sides, *e.g.*, the anterior and posterior commissures in the forebrain.

contralateral. On the opposite side. A crossed pathway is contralateral to its site of origin.

corona. Crown. The *corona radiata* is a radiating crown. The coronal suture between the frontal and parietal bones follows less the plane of conventional royal haberdashery than that of a pair of earmuffs or headphones. A coronal section of brain is in the plane of the coronal suture, *i.e.*, a frontal section.

corpus. Body. The *corpus callosum* is the largest forebrain commissure.

cortex. Bark. The outermost layers of the cerebral or cerebellar hemispheres.

corticifugal. Fleeing from the cortex. The pyramidal tract is a corticifugal pathway.

corticipetal. Seeking, *i.e.*, running toward, the cortex. The thalamocortical projections are corticipetal fibers.

cribriform. Like a sieve, perforated. The *cribriform plate* is the perforated part of the ethmoid bone through which the primary olfactory nerve fascicles enter the cranial cavity.

crista. Crest. The *crista ampullaris* is a crest on the inner surface of the ampulla of the semicircular ducts; its surface contains hair cells.

culmen. Summit. The *culmen monticuli* (peak of the mountain) is the high point on the cerebellar sphere.

cuneate. Wedge-shaped. Describes the shape of the *cuneate fasciculus* seen in cross section.

cupula. Literally, a little tub. Used to describe a cuplike structure or dome (an inverted cup or tub). Applied to the apex of the cochlea (*cochlear cupula*) and to the domelike gelatinous mass capping the hair cells of the cristae ampullaris of the semicircular ducts.

cyto. Prefix meaning literally *hollow*, but generally pertaining to cells. Hence, *cytochrome*, cell color, and *cytoarchitecture*, cell architecture. Also used as a suffix (*cyte*), *e.g.*, astrocyte, lymphocyte.

declive. Sloping downward. A lobe of the cerebellum on its downward slope.

decussation. A division crosswise or in the form of an X; thus, a crossing from one side of the brain to the other, *e.g.*, decussation of the superior cerebellar peduncle.

déjà vu. [French.] Already seen. The illusion of having previously experienced something actually being encountered for the first time. This may occur at the onset of a psychomotor seizure arising in the temporal lobe.

dendrite. Like a tree. *Dendro* is used as a combining form. An *axodendritic synapse* is a synapse between an axon and a dendrite.

dentate. Like a tooth; thus, notched or serrate. Examples: dentate membrane, dentate nucleus.

dermatome. A slice of skin. Describes the laminar segmental arrangement of the distribution of dorsal roots to cutaneous areas.

diabetes insipidus. *Diabetes* means *siphon*, descriptive of the prompt excretion of ingested water as through a siphon; *insipidus* means *tasteless*, describing the dilute urine and distinguishing it from the sweet-tasting urine of diabetes mellitus. Urine tasting, once employed diagnostically, has fortunately been supplanted by more hygienic chemical tests.

diadochokinesis. Literally, a succession or sequence of movements; hence, the ability to carry out repeated alternating movements, such as rapid pronation and supination of the hand. Loss of or impairment of this function is called *adiadochokinesis* or *dysdiadochokinesis*, respectively.

diplopia. Literally, double eye. Double vision.

dromic. Pertaining to the layout of a race course. Used as a suffix to describe the direction of conduction in a nerve fiber: *orthodromic*, in the direction of normal conduction; *antidromic*, in a direction opposite to that of normal conduction.

dura mater. Hard mother. The thick, tough protective covering of the brain. The familial reference "mother" was used by the Arabs to indicate the importance of the meningeal coverings; thus, the "thick mother" (dura mater) and the "thin mother" (pia).

dys. Prefix meaning *difficult, defective*, or *bad*. Examples: *dystonia*, disturbance of tone; *dysesthesia*, disturbance of sensation; *dyspnea*, labored respiration; *dystrophy*, defective nutrition.

ectomy. Suffix meaning *removal of*. Examples: *cerebellectomy*, removal of the cerebellum; *laminectomy*, removal of the vertebral laminae (to expose the spinal cord).

emboliform. Shaped like a plug or a wedge. Example: the *emboliform nucleus* of the cerebellum. An *embolus* is a dislodged blood clot that plugs a vessel too small to permit its passage.

emmetropia.   Literally, vision in proper measure. Normal vision, *i.e.*, vision in which the relaxed eye accurately focuses parallel rays on the retina.

encephalon.   In the head; thus, brain. Examples: *rhinencephalon*, nose brain; *prosencephalon*, forebrain; *diencephalon*, between brain; *telencephalon*, end brain; *mesencephalon*, midbrain; *rhombencephalon*, rhombus brain; *myelencephalon*, marrow brain; *metencephalon*, after brain.

endo.   Prefix meaning *within*. *Endolymph* is the fluid within the membranous labyrinth. *Endoneurium* is the connective tissue supporting nerve fibers within a fasciculus.

ependyma.   Put over; thus, a covering or a lining. Describes the lining of the brain and spinal cavities.

epilepsy.   Take a hold on; hence, a seizure.

esthesia.   Suffix meaning *sensation*. Examples: *anesthesia*, lack of sensation; *dysesthesia*, disturbance of sensation; *paresthesia*, abnormal spontaneous sensation; *pallesthesia*, appreciation of vibration; *kinesthesia*, sensation of movement; *thermesthesia*, thermal sensation.

ethmoid.   Like a sieve. The bone is perforated for the passage of olfactory nerve bundles; *cf.* under *cribriform*.

falx.   Sickle. Describes the shape of the dural partitions. The *cerebellar falx*, or alternatively the *tentorium cerebelli*, is between the cerebellum and the cerebrum.

fasciculus.   Little bundle. Used to describe bundles of nerve fibers in the central nervous system, *e.g.*, the fasciculus gracilis and fasciculus cuneatus.

fastigial.   Pointed like a gabled roof. Example: the *fastigial nucleus* in the cerebellum.

festination.   Hastening. Describes the rapid shuffling gait in Parkinson's disease.

filum.   Thread (plural *fila*). Examples: *fila olfactoria*, olfactory nerve fibers; *filum terminale*, the terminal thread of the spinal cord.

fimbria.   Fringe. Example: the fimbria of the hippocampus.

fissure.   [From the Latin verb meaning *to cleave*.] Hence, a cleft, as the central fissure, lateral fissure, etc.

flocculus.   A little flock of wool. Describes the appearance of one of the cerebellar lobes.

folium.   A leaf. The *folia* of the cerebellum are the narrow leaflike gyri.

fornix.   Arch or vault. Describes the shape of the structure so named.

fovea.   Pit; hence the name of the central pit of the retina, *fovea centralis*.

fundus.   Bottom. Describes the part of the retina around the posterior pole, *i.e.*, the part readily examined with the ophthalmoscope.

funiculus.   Cord. A bundle or cord of nerve fibers in a nerve trunk.

fusiform.   Spindle-shaped. Describes the shape of some neurons and of the muscle spindle. *Fusal* is used as a suffix: *intrafusal muscle fibers* are the small muscle fibers within the muscle spindle; *extrafusal* fibers are the muscle fibers outside the spindle. Fusimotor nerve fibers are the small fibers that innervate intrafusal muscle fibers.

ganglion.   A swelling, or knot. A nodular accumulation of neuron cell bodies outside the central nervous system.

genu.   Knee. Examples: *geniculate* (knee-shaped) ganglion, *genu* of the internal capsule, *genu* of the corpus callosum.

glabrous.   Bald, or hairless. Applied to some areas of skin.

glia.   Glue; hence, the cells that "glue" the nervous system together.

globose.   Like a ball or sphere. Example: *globose nucleus* of the cerebellum.

gnosis.   Suffix meaning *knowledge*. Examples: *stereognosis*, recognition of shapes; *topognosis*, recognition of the location of stimuli. Loss of these capabilities is indicated by the prefix *a*: *astereognosis, atopognosis*.

gracile.   Slender. Examples: the *fasciculus gracilis*, the *nucleus gracilis*.

grand mal.   [French.] Big sickness. Epileptic seizure with generalized convulsions and loss of consciousness.

griseum.   Gray. The *indusium griseum* resembles a gray undergarment.

gyrus.   Circle; hence, a convolution.

habenula.   A little strap, or rein.

helicotrema.   Spiral hole. The communicating hole joining the scala vestibuli and the scala tympani at the apex of the cochlea.

hemianopsia (or **hemianopia**).   Half-blindness. Blindness in half the visual field.

hippocampus.   Sea horse. The neural structure is S-shaped, like a seahorse.

homo or **homeo.** Prefix meaning the same, or invariant. *Homolateral* means ipsilateral. A *homeotherm* is an animal with constant body temperature (a warm-blooded animal). *Homeostasis* (standing steady) refers to the sum total of regulatory mechanisms that keeps the environment of cells relatively constant in composition and physical state.

hydrocephalus. Literally, water brain. Abnormal accumulation of cerebrospinal fluid due to abnormalities in the production or absorption of cerebrospinal fluid.

hypophysis. Undergrowth. The pituitary gland.

hypoxia. See *anoxia.*

idiopathic. Literally, one's own disease. Denotes a disease of unknown origin.

incus. Anvil. The middle auditory ossicle. To the imaginative, it resembles an anvil.

infarct or **infarction.** [From the Latin verb meaning *to stuff.*] Death or necrosis of tissue that occurs when its arterial supply is insufficient to meet its metabolic needs, as when the artery is "stuffed" with a clot or other mass.

infundibulum. A funnel. Describes the shape of the pituitary stalk.

insula. Island. The island of Reil.

inter. Prefix meaning *between. Intercellular* means *between cells,* as *intercellular bridges.* An *interneuron* is a neuron interposed between primary afferent neurons and motoneurons.

intra. Prefix meaning *within. Intracellular* means *inside the cell.* Examples: *intracellular electrodes; intracellular inclusions,* as mitochondria, Golgi bodies, and so forth.

ipsilateral. On the same side. The dorsal columns are ipsilateral ascending paths; *i.e.,* they ascend in the cord without crossing.

ischemia. Literally, keep back blood. Pathological reduction of blood flow to an organ or tissue.

juxta. Next to or near. Example: *juxtarestiform body,* a bundle of fibers near the inferior cerebellar peduncle.

karyon. A nut or kernel; hence, nucleus.

kinesis or **kinesia.** Movement. *Kinesia* is often used as a suffix, as in *bradykinesia, dyskinesia,* and *akinesia* (slow, disturbed, and lacking movement, respectively).

leio. Smooth. Used with *myo* to mean *smooth muscle.* Thus, a *leiomyoma* is a tumor of smooth muscle.

lemma. Husk. Thus, *neurolemma* and *sarcolemma* are the surrounding membranes of nerve and muscle fibers, respectively.

lemniscus. Ribbon or fillet. Example: *medial lemniscus,* a ribbon of fibers.

lentiform. Like a lentil. The lens is named for its shape; hence, *lentiform* also means *like a biconvex lens.*

lepto. Thin. The *leptomeninges* are the thin pial and cobweblike arachnoid membranes.

leuko. White. *Leukodystrophy* is disturbance of the white matter of the brain.

limbus. Border or edge. The limbic cortex is so called because it is the bounding neck or hilus between the neocortex and the diencephalon, from which it grows.

limen. Threshold. Examples: *liminal stimulus, difference limen.* Also used to denote a transition area, *e.g., limen insulae.*

lingula. Tongue. The *cerebellar lingula* resembles a tongue.

lutea. Yellow. The *macula lutea* is the yellow spot in the center of the retina (see *macula*).

macula. Spot. The *macula lutea* is the yellow spot of the retina. A *macular* rash is a spotty rash.

malleus. Hammer. The malleus of the middle ear is hammer-shaped.

manubrium. Handle. Describes the handle of the malleus (hammer), which attaches to the tympanum.

meatus. A passage. Used especially for the openings of a canal, as the *external* and *internal auditory meatus.* (Note that the plural is *meatus.*)

medulla. Marrow. The *medulla oblongata* is the "rather long marrow." The *lateral medullary plate syndrome* occurs with damage to a portion of the medulla.

meninges. Membranes. The covering membranes of the brain.

meso or **mes.** Prefix meaning *middle* or *intermediate.* The *mesencephalon* is the midbrain. A *mesial location* is near the midline.

meta or **met.** Prefix meaning *after.* The *metencephalon* is the afterbrain.

milieu intérieur or **interne.** [French.] Literally, the interior middle place. The internal environment of the cells of multicellular organisms, *i.e.,* the interstitial fluid.

miosis. Literally, a lessening. Denotes constriction of the pupil.

mitochondrion. From *mitos*, thread, and *chondros*, granule or grits; hence, a thread-bearing granule.

modiolus. The nave or hub of a wheel. Describes the central supporting column of the cochlea.

myasthenia gravis. Literally, severe muscle weakness. A disorder of neuromuscular transmission characterized by muscle weakness aggravated by exercise.

mydriasis. Pupillary dilatation. A *mydriatic* is a drug that dilates the pupil, *e.g.*, atropine.

myelo. Prefix meaning *marrow*. Pertaining to the spinal cord, *e.g.*, *myelogram*, a diagnostic radiologic procedure used to outline the spinal cord. Also used to refer to bone marrow, *e.g.*, *myeloma*, a tumor of bone marrow origin.

myo. Prefix meaning *muscle*. Examples: *myocardium*, heart muscle; *myoclonus* (muscle turmoil), rhythmic twitching of muscle.

myopia. Literally, shut the eye. Nearsightedness.

myotatic. Literally, muscle stretching. The *myotatic reflex* is the stretch reflex.

narcolepsy. A seizure of numbness. A syndrome characterized by uncontrollable disposition to sleep, often at inappropriate times.

necro. Prefix meaning *corpse*. A *necropsy* (view of the dead) is a postmortem examination. *Necrosis* refers to death of cells in an otherwise living organism.

neuron. Literally, a nerve. Specifically, a nerve cell. Often used as a prefix or as a combinant, as in *neuronophagia*, phagocytosis of nerve cells; *neuronatrophy*, atrophy of nerve cells.

neuropil (or **neuropile**). Nerve felt. The mesh of fine fibers surrounding cell bodies in the central nervous system. An area of many synapses.

nigra. Black. The *substantia nigra* has a dark color because of melanin in the cells.

nystagmus. A nodding. Oscillation of the eyeballs.

occult. Hidden, or concealed. Occult blood in spinal fluid is detected only by microscopic examination or chemical testing.

oligo. Prefix meaning *few*. Thus, an *oligodendroglia* is a glial cell with few dendrites, and *oligophrenia* is little or feeblemindedness (see *phrenic*).

oma. Suffix meaning *tumor* or *swelling*. Thus, a *neuroma* is a nerve tumor; a *glioma* is a glial cell tumor; a *meningioma* is a meningeal tumor.

operculum. A lid or cover. Describes those portions of cortex along the lateral sulcus covering the insula.

opisthotonos. Back (*opistho*) plus stretching (*tonos*). Spasms in which the spine, neck, and extremities are bent backward, arching the body.

ortho. Prefix meaning *correct* or *straight*. *Orthotonos* is a spasm in which the body is held straight (*cf. opisthotonos*). *Orthopaedics* literally means "straight children." For *orthodromic*, see under *dromic*.

osis. Suffix meaning a *process, condition,* or *state*, usually pathological. *Neurofibromatosis*, the condition of multiple neuromas or neurofibromas (von Recklinghausen's disease); *tuberculosis*, afflicted with tubercles; *phagocytosis*, the process of ingestion of cells, and so forth.

pachy. Prefix meaning *thick*. *Pachymeninx*, the dura mater; *pachymeningopathy*, disease of the dura mater.

pallesthesia. Literally, sensation of quivering. Vibratory sensation.

pallidus. Pale. The *globus pallidus*, "pale ball," is so called because of its pallid appearance in unstained sections, which is due to its associated myelinated fibers.

pallium. Cloak, or mantle. Used to describe the cortex that cloaks the cerebrum. *Neopallium* (new mantle) and *archipallium* (old cloak) refer to the phylogenetic ages of parts of the pallium.

para. Prefix meaning *near* or *beside*. Thus, a *parasagittal section* is a longitudinal section near, but not in, the midline, as opposed to a *midsagittal section*. The *paraventricular nuclei* are near the ventricle.

paresis. A letting go, or slackening. Denotes motor weakness, partial or incomplete paralysis.

peduncle. A little foot. Name for a stalk, stem, or base, *e.g.*, the cerebral peduncles.

pellucidum. Clear, transparent. Hence, the *septum pellucidum* is the transparent wall or partition situated between a portion of the lateral ventricles.

peri. Prefix meaning *around*. Not to be confused with *para*, which means near or alongside. *Perikaryon* means around the kernel, *i.e.*, the body surrounding the nucleus.

Perimysium and *perineurium* are fibrous sheaths surrounding bundles of muscle and nerve fibers, respectively. *Perilymph* is the fluid surrounding the membranous labyrinth.

perimeter. Literally "measure around"; hence, circumference. *Perimetry* plots the circumference of the visual field.

petit mal. [French.] Little sickness. Seizures characterized by momentary lapses of consciousness without generalized convulsions. *Cf. grand mal.*

phago. Prefix or combining form meaning *to eat.* Hence, *neuronophagia* is ingestion of neurons by phagocytes, or cell-eating cells; *hyperphagia* is excessive eating; *dysphagia* is difficulty in swallowing.

pheo. Dusky. A *pheochromocytoma* is a tumor of dusky-colored cells, from sympathetic or adrenomedullary cells that contain melanin.

phrenic. The midriff or diaphragm; more abstractly, the heart, mind, or soul. Hence, the *phrenic nerve* innervates the diaphragm; *schizophrenia* means *split mind.*

pia. Tender, soft. The *pia mater* is the soft or tender mother. *Cf. dura mater.*

pilo. Prefix meaning *hair.* Hence, *piloerection* is elevation of the hairs, and *pilomotor fibers* are nerve fibers innervating the erector muscles of the hairs.

pineal. Relating to the pine. The pineal body is shaped like a pine cone.

pino. Prefix meaning *to drink.* Hence, *pinocytosis* is cellular drinking, *i.e.,* engulfment of liquids by membrane invaginations that separate to become intracellular vesicles.

pituitary. [From *pituita,* meaning *phlegm, slime,* or *mucus.*] The gland is so named because the ancients thought it was the source of nasal secretions.

plasm or **plasma.** Suffix or combining form meaning *a thing formed* or *molded. Cytoplasm, axoplasm,* and *sarcoplasm* are materials made by the cell, the axon, and the muscle cell, respectively. *Dysplasia* is defective tissue formation.

plegia. Suffix meaning *paralysis. Hemiplegia* is paralysis of one side of the body; *paraplegia* is paralysis of both lower extremities; *quadriplegia* is paralysis of all four extremities. *Ophthalmoplegia* is paralysis of eye movements.

plexus. A braid; hence, a network or rete of nerve fibers, blood vessels, or lymphatics.

poikilo. Prefix meaning *varied.* Hence, a *poikilothermic* animal is one with variable body temperature, *i.e.,* a cold-blooded animal.

polio. Prefix meaning *gray. Poliomyelitis* is inflammation of the gray marrow.

pons. Bridge. The pons bridges the midbrain and the medulla.

proprio. Prefix meaning *of one's own. Propriospinal fibers* are fibers arising from cells within the spinal cord. *Proprioceptors* are receptors detecting changes within the body itself, *e.g.,* the muscle spindles that monitor length of muscle fibers.

ptosis. A falling. Describes drooping of the eyelid. Also used as a combining form to describe drooping or sagging of an organ: *visceroptosis* is sagging of the viscera.

presbyopia. Literally, old vision. Farsightedness due to loss of elasticity of the lens, which occurs with aging.

pulvinar. A couch made of cushions. Describing fancifully the large nuclear mass of the posterior thalamus.

purulent. Festering, suppurative, forming pus.

putamen. That which falls off when a tree is pruned. The outer part of the lenticular nucleus.

pyo. Prefix meaning *pus. Pyogenic* organisms are pus-producing organisms.

pyramis. Pyramid. Describes the shape of a cerebellar lobe.

pyriform. Pear-shaped. Describes the shape of a portion of the ventral surface of the temporal lobe.

quadrigemina. Four twins. The *corpora quadrigemina* are really two pairs of twins (the two superior and the two inferior colliculi), making four bodies.

raphe. A seam; hence, the line of junction between adjacent structures. For example, *raphe nuclei* of the brainstem, which are located in the midline.

restiform. Ropelike. The *restiform body* is the ropelike inferior cerebellar peduncle.

reticulum. A little rete or network. The *reticular formation* is a complex network of nuclei and fibers.

rhabdo. Prefix meaning *a rod,* or *a strip.* Refers to striated muscle; a *rhabdomyosarcoma* is a malignant tumor of skeletal muscle.

rhino. Prefix meaning *nose.* The *rhinencephalon* is the "nose brain," because of its olfactory connections.

rhizo.   Prefix meaning *root. Rhizotomy* is section of a root of the spinal cord.

rhodopsin.   Literally, rose eye. The purplish or pinkish photosensitive pigment of the rods.

rhombo.   Prefix meaning *lozenge-shaped.* Describes the appearance of the hindbrain viewed from above.

rostral or **rostrad.**   Toward the beak. Used in opposition to *caudal* or *caudad*, toward the tail.

rrhea.   Suffix meaning *a flowing.* Thus, *diarrhea* is a flowing through; *rhinorrhea*, running nose; *sialorrhea*, drooling.

ruber.   Red. The *nucleus ruber*, or *red nucleus*, has a reddish tinge in fresh specimens. Also used as a combining form, *e.g.*, *rubefacient* (make red), an irritant that reddens the skin.

saccade.   A jerk on the reins to check a horse. Describes the jerky movements of the eyes in visual scanning.

sacculus.   A little sac. Describes the shape of the smaller of the two membranous structures of the vestibule.

sagittal.   Like an arrow; hence, in the line of an arrow, *i.e.*, anteroposterior or longitudinal.

saltatory.   Hopping, leaping. Descriptive of conduction of the nerve impulse, which hops from node to node.

sarco.   Prefix meaning *flesh.* Usually refers to muscle. Examples: *sarcomere*, a unit of skeletal muscle between two adjacent Z bands; *sarcolemma*, muscle fiber plasma membrane; *sarcoma*, a malignant tumor of mesodermal origin, as opposed to *carcinoma*, which derives from epithelium.

scala.   A stairway. Describes the cavities within the cochlea winding around the modiolus.

scler, sclero.   Combining form meaning *hard.* The *sclera* is the tough or hard coat of the eyeball. *Sclerosis* is a hardening, as in *multiple sclerosis*, in which patchy demyelination leads to hard scars, and as in *atherosclerosis*, in which the pathological process hardens or stiffens the arteries. Areas of cerebral cortex damaged by ischemia may become sclerotic because of astroglial proliferation.

scotoma.   Darkness. A blind or semiblind area in the visual field.

sella turcica.   Turkish saddle. The saddlelike pit in the sphenoid bone in which the hypophysis sits.

sialo.   Prefix meaning *saliva.* Thus, *sialorrhea* means drooling, and a *sialogogue* is a drug or agent that stimulates salivation.

soma.   Body. The cell body, or perikaryon, of a neuron. The *somatic nervous system* is that part devoted to innervation of the body surface, as opposed to the *visceral nervous system*, which serves the viscera.

spasticity.   A drawing in. The syndrome of hypertonus with exaggeration of stretch reflexes following certain central neural lesions.

sphingo.   Prefix meaning *to bind tight. Sphingosine* is a long-chain basic amino alcohol present in several sphingolipids.

splenium.   A bandage. The splenium of the corpus callosum resembles a bandage.

stapes.   Stirrup. The stirrup-shaped auditory ossicle that rocks in the oval window.

steno.   Prefix meaning *narrow;* hence, *stenosis* is a condition of narrowing of a duct canal or sphincter. Stenosis of the aqueduct produces hydrocephalus.

stereo.   Prefix or combining form meaning *solid;* hence, it refers to the form of tridimensional objects. *Stereognosis* refers to recognition of objects by the feeling of their shape and form (*cf. gnosis*).

stomy.   Suffix meaning *mouth* and hence *to create an opening into a hollow organ*, as in *ventriculocisternostomy*, an opening from the ventricles to the subarachnoid space, or in *gastrostomy*, an external opening into the stomach.

strabismus.   A twisted distortion. Imbalance of extraocular muscles interfering with binocular vision (cross-eyes, walleyes, squint).

stria.   A channel or furrow. Usually used to describe a stripe or strip. The *striate cortex* has a striped appearance because of fiber tracts.

sudo.   Prefix meaning *sweat. Sudomotor fibers* are sympathetic fibers innervating sweat glands.

sulcus.   A furrow or ditch; a gross anatomical term for a shallow fissure.

synapse.   A connection or junction; hence the functional contact of one neuron with another.

syncope.   A cutting short. Fainting due to a sudden fall of blood pressure below the level required to maintain oxygenation of brain tissue.

synergy.   A working together. *Synergistic muscles* act on the same joint in the same way, in contrast to *antagonistic muscles*, which pull the joint in opposing directions.

syringo.   Prefix meaning *like a tube* (syrinx). *Syringomyelia* is a disease in which cystic tubes form about the central canal of the spinal cord.

tabes.   A wasting away. *Tabes dorsalis* is so called because the destruction of dorsal root cells leads to atrophy of the dorsal columns.

tachy.   Prefix meaning *quick* or *rapid. Tachycardia* is a rapid pulse (over 100 beats per minute). *Tachypnea* is rapid breathing.

tectum.   Roof or covering. Describes the roof portion of the midbrain.

tegmentum.   A cover; hence, the covering of the cerebral peduncles and basal pons as seen in cross section.

tel, tele, telo.   Prefix meaning distance or end. The *telencephalon* is the endbrain. *Teleceptors* are receptors that provide information about the remote environment: eyes, ears, nose.

tentorium.   Tent. The *tentorium cerebelli* is a tent covering the cerebellum (also called the *falx cerebelli*).

tetanus.   Convulsive tension. A disease caused by the toxin of *Clostridium tetani,* which blocks release of inhibitory transmitter from presynaptic terminals. *Tetanus* also means the sustained muscular contraction caused by stimulation of the motor nerve trunk at frequencies so high that individual muscle twitches are fused.

tetany.   [From the same root as *tetanus* but with a different usage.] Refers to the hyperexcitability of nerve and muscle when the concentration of extracellular ionized calcium is decreased.

thalamus.   An inner chamber. The thalamus was believed by Galen to be a chamber from which vital spirits flowed into the optic nerves.

tic.   A French word of uncertain origin describing repeated involuntary twitches or spasms of related muscle groups. *Tic douloureux* (painful tic), or trigeminal neuralgia, is characterized by paroxysms of pain in the face, often triggered by minor stimuli and accompanied by facial grimacing.

titubation.   Staggering. Describing the ataxic gait of the tabetic patient, or of patients with cerebellar disease.

tomy.   Suffix meaning *to cut* or *incise.* Examples: *vagotomy,* vagal section; *craniotomy,* opening of the cranium; *tympanotomy,* incision of the tympanum.

tone or **tonus.**   In muscle, resistance to stretch, partly due to the stretch reflex. *Hypertonus* is abnormal resistance associated with exaggerated stretch reflexes. *Hypotonus,* or atonia, is deficient or absent resistance, with depressed stretch reflexes. In nerve trunks, a *tonic discharge* is a continuous repetitive asynchronous discharge similar to that producing tone in normal muscle.

trochlea.   Pulley. The *trochlear nerve* is so named because it innervates the superior oblique muscle, which pulls on the eyeball through a fibrous loop or pulley in the anteromedial part of the orbit.

trophy.   Suffix meaning *nutrition.* Thus, *atrophy* means without nutrition, and *dystrophy* means defective nutrition. The latter usually refers to a progressive degenerative process, as in *muscular dystrophy.*

tympanum.   A kettle drum. The name for the eardrum.

umbo.   The base of a shield, a knob. The depression in the tympanum where the manubrium of the malleus is attached.

uncus.   Hook; hence, the hook-shaped extremity of the parahippocampal gyrus.

utricle.   A skin bag. The larger of the two dilatations of the membranous labyrinth in the vestibule.

vagus.   Wandering. The *vagus nerve* is so named because of the wide extent of its field of innervation.

velum.   Veil or sail. The *medullary vela* are so called because of their thin, veillike appearance.

ventricle.   A small cavity.

vermis.   Worm. The middle portion of the cerebellum, which is wormlike in appearance.

vertigo.   Dizziness. An illusion of movement of the environment about the body, or vice versa.

vesicle.   A blister, bleb, or bladder. The *synaptic vesicles* are little intracellular "bladders" believed to be filled with synaptic transmitter substances.

vestibulum.   An antechamber. The *vestibule* is the bony chamber between the semicircular canals and the cochlea.

villus.   The shaggy hair of a beast. The *arachnoid villi* resemble hairs.

viscus.   A soft internal organ. The plural is *viscera.*

xanthochromic.   Yellow-colored. Describes cerebrospinal fluid drawn hours after a hemorrhage; the yellow color is due to products of the breakdown of hemoglobin.

Appendix II

Atlas of the Spinal Cord and Brainstem

John W. Sundsten

This schematic atlas of transverse sections is provided as an outline of major fiber systems and nuclei within the spinal cord and brainstem. The brainstem sections are drawn at levels selected to show the origin and formation of the cranial nerves. In some instances the size of an internal structure has been slightly exaggerated for illustrative purposes. The drawings have been adapted from transverse sections of the central nervous system that appear in Everett, *Functional neuroanatomy,* Philadelphia, Lea & Febiger, 1971, and in DeArmond, Fusco, and Dewey, *Structure of the human brain: A photographic atlas,* New York, Oxford University Press, 1974. Atlases such as these should be consulted for a more detailed anatomical treatment of the brainstem.

See illustrations on following pages.

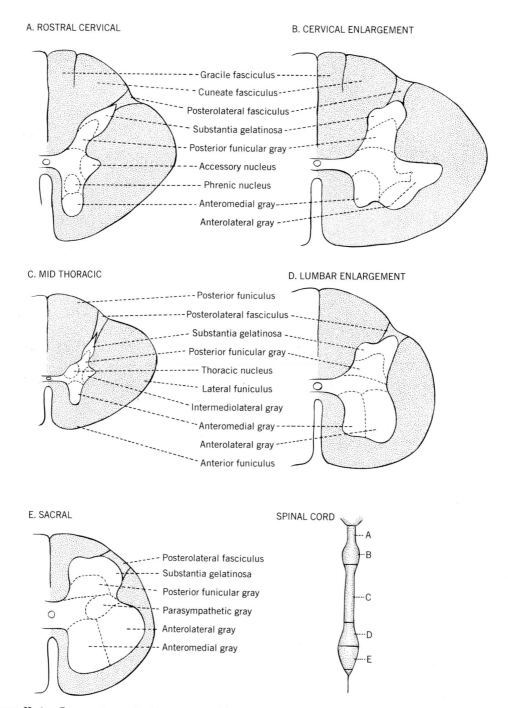

A. ROSTRAL CERVICAL

B. CERVICAL ENLARGEMENT

Gracile fasciculus
Cuneate fasciculus
Posterolateral fasciculus
Substantia gelatinosa
Posterior funicular gray
Accessory nucleus
Phrenic nucleus
Anteromedial gray
Anterolateral gray

C. MID THORACIC

D. LUMBAR ENLARGEMENT

Posterior funiculus
Posterolateral fasciculus
Substantia gelatinosa
Posterior funicular gray
Thoracic nucleus
Lateral funiculus
Intermediolateral gray
Anteromedial gray
Anterolateral gray
Anterior funiculus

E. SACRAL

SPINAL CORD

Posterolateral fasciculus
Substantia gelatinosa
Posterior funicular gray
Parasympathetic gray
Anterolateral gray
Anteromedial gray

A
B
C
D
E

Figure II–1. Gray matter and white matter of the spinal cord, as seen in representative cross sections. The inset at the lower right indicates the approximate level in the spinal cord for each of the sections.

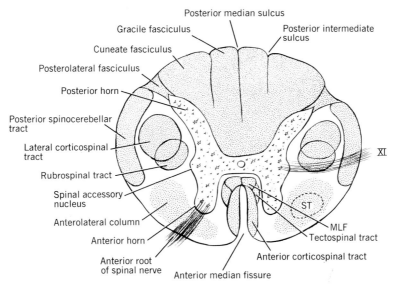

Posterior median sulcus

Gracile fasciculus

Posterior intermediate sulcus

Cuneate fasciculus

Posterolateral fasciculus

Posterior horn

Posterior spinocerebellar tract

Lateral corticospinal tract

Rubrospinal tract

Spinal accessory nucleus

Anterolateral column

Anterior horn

Anterior root of spinal nerve

Anterior median fissure

XI

ST

MLF

Tectospinal tract

Anterior corticospinal tract

Figure II–2. The rostral cervical cord. The posterior white columns are divided into a medially placed gracile fasciculus and a laterally placed cuneate fasciculus (carrying fibers from the lower and upper limbs, respectively). The lateral white columns contain rubrospinal, corticospinal, and spinocerebellar fibers. The spinocerebellar fibers form a posterior and an anterior spinocerebellar tract. The anterior spinocerebellar tract is not shown in these drawings; it is positioned lateral to the spinothalamic fibers at the lateral margin of the anterolateral quadrant. It enters the cerebellum through the superior cerebellar peduncle (see Chapter 21). The spinothalamic tract *(ST)* is in the anterolateral white column. The anterior white column contains the medial longitudinal fasciculus *(MLF),* the tectospinal tract, and the uncrossed anterior corticospinal tract. Fibers of the spinal accessory nerve *(XI)* are exiting laterally, and anterior root fibers of a spinal nerve, anteriorly.

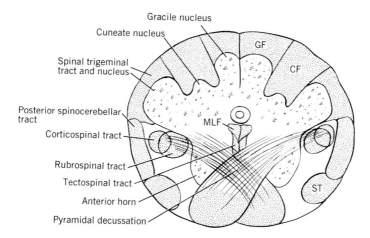

Gracile nucleus

Cuneate nucleus

Spinal trigeminal tract and nucleus

Posterior spinocerebellar tract

Corticospinal tract

Rubrospinal tract

Tectospinal tract

Anterior horn

Pyramidal decussation

GF

CF

MLF

ST

Figure II–3. The caudal medulla at the level of the pyramidal decussation. The decussating pyramidal fibers will take up a position in the lateral white columns as the corticospinal tract, intermixed somewhat with the rubrospinal fibers. The posterior column fibers, the cuneate and gracile fasciculi, are reaching the cuneate and gracile nuclei. The spinothalamic fibers are in the anterolateral part of the field. The spinal trigeminal tract and nucleus will overlap with the posterolateral fasciculus and the substantia gelatinosa of the posterior gray matter of the spinal cord caudal to this section. Some of the anterior gray matter of the cervical spinal cord appears just lateral to the pyramidal decussation. *CF,* cuneate fasciculus; *GF,* gracile fasciculus; *ST,* spinothalamic tract.

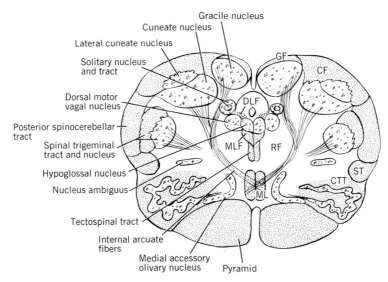

Figure II–4. The caudal medulla at the level of the sensory decussation. Most of the fibers of the gracile fasciculus *(GF)* have already synapsed in the gracile nucleus. Internal arcuate fibers from the cuneate and gracile nuclei are crossing to form the medial lemniscus *(ML)*. Second-order fibers from the spinal trigeminal nucleus are extending toward the midline. They will cross, some forming a component of the medial lemniscus and others mixing with the spinothalamic fibers (see Chapter 13). The spinothalamic tract *(ST)* is in the lateral tegmental field. The posterior spinocerebellar tract is lateral to the spinal trigeminal tract and will enter the inferior cerebellar peduncle rostral to this level. *CF,* cuneate fasciculus; *CTT,* central tegmental tract; *DLF,* dorsal longitudinal fasciculus; *MLF,* medial longitudinal fasciculus; *RF,* reticular formation.

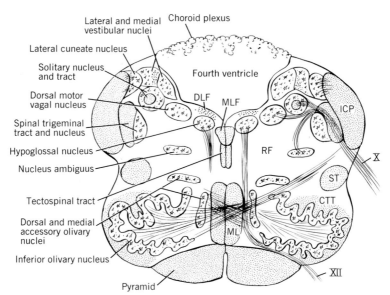

Figure II–5. The midmedulla at the level of the vagus *(X)* and hypoglossal *(XII)* nerves. The vagus nerve exits lateral to the inferior olivary nucleus, whereas the hypoglossal nerve exits between it and the pyramid. Motor components of the vagus are shown coming from the dorsal motor vagal nucleus and nucleus ambiguus; visceral afferents are forming the solitary tract. The medial lemniscus is oriented dorsoventrally along the midline above the pyramid; the spinothalamic tract *(ST)* is in the lateral part of the tegmental field. Olivocerebellar fibers are crossing and will enter the inferior cerebellar peduncle *(ICP)*. The lateral cuneate nucleus is also sending fibers into the inferior cerebellar peduncle. The descending corticospinal and corticobulbar fibers have grouped together to form the pyramids. *CTT,* central tegmental tract; *DLF,* dorsal longitudinal fasciculus; *ML,* medial lemniscus; *MLF,* medial longitudinal fasciculus; *RF,* reticular formation.

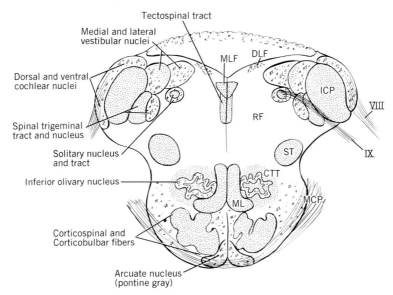

Tectospinal tract

Medial and lateral
vestibular nuclei

Dorsal and ventral
cochlear nuclei

Spinal trigeminal
tract and nucleus

Solitary nucleus
and tract

Inferior olivary nucleus

Corticospinal and
Corticobulbar fibers

Arcuate nucleus
(pontine gray)

MLF   DLF

ICP

VIII

RF

ST

IX

CTT

ML   MCP

Figure II–6. The rostral medulla at the level of the vestibulocochlear *(VIII)* and glossopharyngeal *(IX)* nerves. The cochlear nuclei cap the lateral surface of the inferior cerebellar peduncle *(ICP)*. The medial lemniscus *(ML)* is still situated medially along the midline. Its trigeminolemniscal components (not shown) would be in its most dorsal part; the laterally placed spinothalamic tract *(ST)* would also contain trigeminothalamic components (see Chapter 13). The rostral pole of the inferior olivary nucleus appears in the course of the descending central tegmental tract *(CTT)*, some of whose fibers terminate there; another component of the central tegmental tract will continue its descent to the spinal cord (rubrospinal tract). The corticospinal and corticobulbar fibers are closely grouped as the pontine gray matter thins out; just caudal to this section they will form the medullary pyramids. The caudalmost edge of the middle cerebellar peduncle *(MCP)* is present. *DLF,* dorsal longitudinal fasciculus; *MLF,* medial longitudinal fasciculus; *RF,* reticular formation.

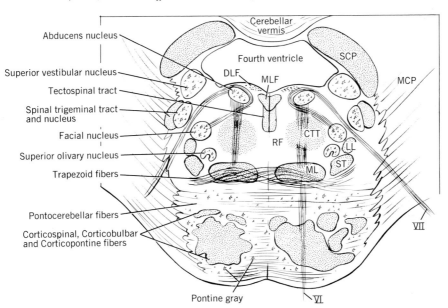

Abducens nucleus

Superior vestibular nucleus

Tectospinal tract

Spinal trigeminal tract
and nucleus

Facial nucleus

Superior olivary nucleus

Trapezoid fibers

Pontocerebellar fibers

Corticospinal, Corticobulbar
and Corticopontine fibers

Cerebellar
vermis

Fourth ventricle

SCP

MCP

DLF   MLF

RF   CTT   LL

ST

ML

VII

Pontine gray   VI

Figure II–7. The caudal pons at the level of the abducens *(VI)* and facial *(VII)* nerves. The abducens nerve exits ventrally through the basal pons near the midline; the facial nerve loops medially around the abducens nucleus and then courses laterally to exit at the caudal edge of the middle cerebellar peduncle *(MCP)*. The pontine gray matter is sending pontocerebellar fibers across the midline to form the middle cerebellar peduncle. The superior cerebellar peduncle *(SCP)* is projecting toward the midbrain. The medial lemniscus *(ML)* has rotated to a mediolateral position and is obscured by trapezoid fibers of the auditory system that cross the midline; the trapezoid fibers will turn rostrally to ascend in the lateral lemniscus. Primary afferents from the trigeminal nerve have formed the spinal trigeminal tract. *CTT,* central tegmental tract; *DLF,* dorsal longitudinal fasciculus; *LL,* lateral lemniscus; *MLF,* medial longitudinal fasciculus; *RF,* reticular formation; *ST,* spinothalamic tract.

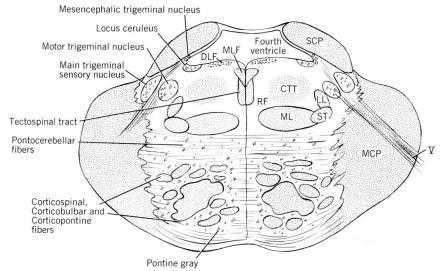

Figure II–8. The midpons at the level of the trigeminal *(V)* nerve. Fibers of the trigeminal nerve separate the main sensory trigeminal and motor trigeminal nuclei. The cell bodies of proprioceptive trigeminal afferents constitute the mesencephalic nucleus. The trigeminal nerve exits through the middle cerebellar peduncle *(MCP)*. The medial lemniscus *(ML)* has begun to move laterally toward the spinothalamic tract *(ST)*. The superior cerebellar peduncle *(SCP)* forms the lateral wall of the fourth ventricle as it descends from the cerebellum toward the midbrain tegmentum. Pontocerebellar fibers (receiving input from the corticopontine fibers) are streaming across the midline to form the middle cerebellar peduncle. The corticospinal, corticobulbar, and corticopontine fibers are scattered throughout the basilar pontine gray matter. *CTT*, central tegmental tract; *DLF*, dorsal longitudinal fasciculus; *LL*, lateral lemniscus; *MLF*, medial longitudinal fasciculus; *RF*, reticular formation.

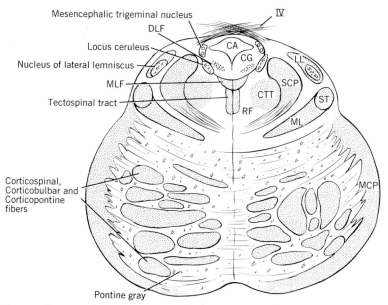

Figure II–9. The rostral pons at the isthmus. Fibers of the trochlear nerve *(IV)* are crossing as they exit dorsally. The medial lemniscus *(ML)* is moving laterally and beginning to rotate to a dorsoventral position. The superior cerebellar peduncle *(SCP)* is moving toward the midline. The rostralmost edge of the middle cerebellar peduncle *(MCP)* is present. The corticospinal, corticobulbar, and corticopontine fibers, which constituted the cerebral peduncle, are separating as they plunge into the basilar pontine gray matter. *CA*, cerebral aqueduct; *CG*, central gray matter; *CTT*, central tegmental tract; *DLF*, dorsal longitudinal fasciculus; *LL*, lateral lemniscus; *MLF*, medial longitudinal fasciculus; *RF*, reticular formation; *ST*, spinothalamic tract.

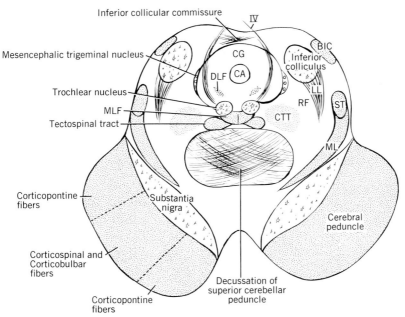

Figure II–10.   The midbrain at the level of the inferior colliculus and the trochlear nerve *(IV)*. Fibers of the trochlear nerve are exiting dorsally. The medial lemniscus *(ML)* is rotating into a dorsoventral position in the lateral tegmental field. The lateral lemniscus *(LL)* is entering the nucleus of the inferior colliculus. Fibers from the cerebellum are crossing through the tegmentum as the decussation of the superior cerebellar peduncle. *BIC,* brachium of inferior colliculus; *CA,* cerebral aqueduct; *CG,* central gray matter; *CTT,* central tegmental tract; *DLF,* dorsal longitudinal fasciculus; *MLF,* medial longitudinal fasciculus; *RF,* reticular formation; *ST,* spinothalamic tract.

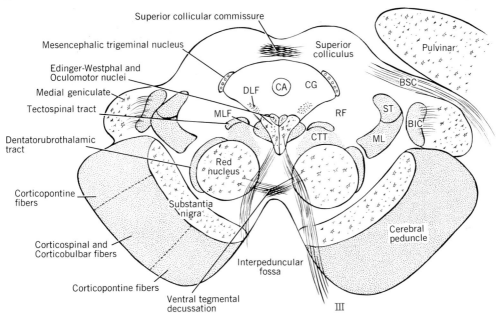

Figure II–11.   The midbrain at the level of the superior colliculus and oculomotor nerve *(III)*. Fibers of the oculomotor nerve are exiting into the interpeduncular fossa. The medial lemniscus *(ML)* is in the lateral part of the tegmental field. The brachium of the inferior colliculus *(BIC)* is entering the medial geniculate, and the brachium of the superior colliculus *(BSC)* is entering the superior colliculus. Fibers from the decussation of the superior cerebellar peduncle have formed at the lateral margin of the red nucleus as the dentatorubrothalamic tract; it sends fibers to the red nucleus and to the ventralis lateralis nucleus of the thalamus. Rubrospinal fibers from the red nucleus cross as the ventral tegmental decussation, and at a more caudal level will join the fibers in the central tegmental tract *(CTT)*, finally ending in the spinal cord. *CA,* cerebral aqueduct; *CG,* central gray matter; *MG,* medial geniculate; *MLF,* medial longitudinal fasciculus; *RF,* reticular formation; *ST,* spinothalamic tract.

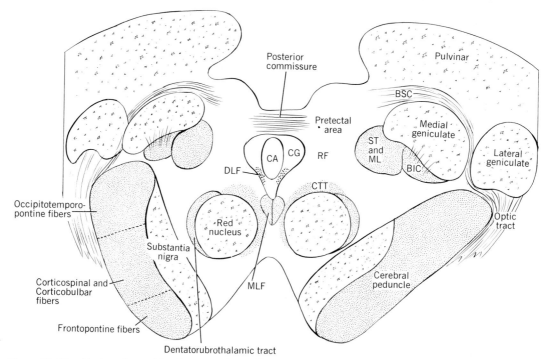

Figure II–12. Region of transition between the midbrain and the diencephalon. The spinothalamic and medial lemniscal fibers are intermingled here before entering the thalamus. The optic tract enters the lateral geniculate, sending some of its fibers beyond it as the brachium of the superior colliculus (*BSC*) to the pretectal region. The brachium of the inferior colliculus *(BIC)* is entering the medial geniculate. The posterior commissure is interconnecting the pretectal region on the two sides. The central tegmental tract *(CTT)* contains a variety of descending fiber systems from the red nucleus and the reticular formation *(RF)* throughout the tegmental field of the brainstem. In the cerebral peduncle, the corticospinal and corticobulbar fibers separate two groups of corticopontine fibers, the occipitotemporopontine and the frontopontine fibers. *CA,* cerebral aqueduct; *CG,* central gray matter; *DLF,* dorsal longitudinal fasciculus; *ML,* medial lemniscus; *MLF,* medial longitudinal fasciculus; *ST,* spinothalamic tract.

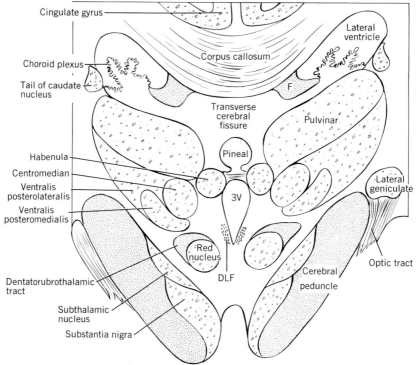

Figure II–13. The caudal diencephalon at the level of the somatosensory relay nuclei of the thalamus: the nucleus ventralis posteromedialis and nucleus ventralis posterolateralis. The optic tract is entering the lateral geniculate nucleus. Fibers of the dorsal longitudinal fasciculus *(DLF),* from the hypothalamus, are clustered in the gray matter near the third ventricle *(3V). F,* fornix.

INDEX

In this index illustrations are indicated by *italic* page numbers, tables by (t), and glossary entries by (g).

Brain scan, mechanism of, 20
Brainstem, anatomy of, 44–46, 397, *399–404*
  and consciousness, *321*
Brainstem, definition of, 7
  development of, 7
  in motor systems, *270*
  internal, morphology of, 43–44, *44–46*
  lesions of, 278–279
    vs. cord lesions, 186
  sensory paths through, *184*
Brainstem nuclei, and parasympathetic innervation, 140, 144(t)
  morphology of, 44, *44–46*
Brainstem pathways, 186–187
Branched-chain ketoaciduria, thiamine for, 370(t)
Branchial efferents, of cranial nerves, *44–46*
Broca's area, and speech, 333–335, *334*
Brodmann areas, in sensory pathways, 190(t), 193
  in suprasegmental pathways, 272
  in vision, 246–247
  map of, *314*
Brown-Séquard syndrome, neuropathy in, 180–186
Bulb(s), at nerve endings, 26, *26*
  neuronal. See *Axon terminals.*
Bundle, medial forebrain. See *Medial forebrain bundle.*
α-Bungarotoxin, and neuromuscular transmission, 88–89
Burn, nerve conduction in, 172
Buttons, terminal. See *Axon terminals.*
Butyrophenones, and Parkinsonism, 287

C fibers, histological composition of, 115
  polymodal response of, 172
  polysynaptic connections by, 116
Cable-property of membranes, definition of, 51
Calcium ions, in muscle contraction, 74–75
  at initiation, 75–77
  smooth, 91
  in neuromuscular transmission, 78
  drug effects on, 81–82
  in retina, 226, *226*
Callosum, definition of, 388(g)
Caloric test, 311–312
Calvaria, definition of, 388(g)
Canal(s), auditory, anatomy of, 252, *252*
  of Cloquet, *205*
  semicircular, *307*
  anatomy of, *252, 254, 254*
Capacitance, definition of, 66
Capsule, external, 282
Capsule, internal. See *Internal capsule.*
Carbidopa, for Parkinson's disease, 371
Carbon dioxide (CO_2), in cerebrospinal fluid, 14
Cardiac muscle, autonomic nervous system and, 138, 139, *139*
  innervation of, *44–46*, 144(t)
Cardiac output, utilized by brain, 364

Carotid, definition of, 388(g)
Carotid arteries, internal, anatomy of, 374, *375–376*, 377–378
Carotid sinus reflex, 150–151, *151*
Cataplexy, definition of, 388(g)
  in narcolepsy, 324
Cataract, congenital vs. acquired, 244
Catecholamines, and Parkinson's disease, 285–286, 362
  in synaptic transmission, 104
  synthesis of, metabolic pathway for, *286*
Cation(s), in cellular fluids, 53, 53(t)
Cation pump, 57–60. See also *Ion pump.*
Cauda, definition of, 388(g)
Cauda equina, definition of, 388(g)
  morphology of, 41, *41*
Caudad, definition of, 388(g)
Caudal, definition of, 388(g)
Caudal foramen (of Magendie). See *Median foramen (of Magendie).*
Caudate nucleus, and basal ganglia, 6, 281–282, *281*
  definition of, 388(g)
  development of, 6, *9*
  dopamine in, 286(t)
  Huntington's chorea and, 283
Cele, definition of, 388(g)
Cells, amacrine, 225, 228
  basket, cerebellar, *293–294, 294*
  Betz, morphology of, *314*
  bipolar, 212, 224, *225*
  Claudius', in auditory anatomy, *255, 256*
  Deiters', in auditory anatomy, *255, 256*
  ependymal, 4, *4, 30*
  excitability of, 49, 67
  fusiform, morphology of, *315*
  ganglion. See *Ganglion cells.*
  glial, *19, 30*. See also *Schwann cells.*
  Golgi, cerebellar, *293, 294, 294*
  granule. See *Granule cells.*
  hair. See *Hair cells.*
  Hensen's, in auditory anatomy, *255, 256*
  horizontal. See *Horizontal cells.*
  Martinotti's, morphology of, *315*
  mastoid, in auditory anatomy, *252, 254*
  neuroglial, 28–29
  neurosecretory, in hypothalamic regulation, 351
  nuclear, cerebellar, *292, 293*
  phalangeal, in auditory anatomy, 256
  Purkinje. See *Purkinje cells.*
  pyramidal. See *Pyramidal cells.*
  receptor, *225*
  retinal, *225*
  Schwann, 29, *29, 30*. See also *Glial cells.*
  stellate. See *Stellate cells.*
  tract, in posterior gray columns, 42
Center(s), hypothalamic, and body regulation, 346–347, *347*
  optical, definition of, 204
Central auditory pathways, 267–268, *267*
Central gray matter, anatomy of, *402–404*
Central nervous system (CNS), anatomy of, 1–11, *2–10, 398–404*
  components of, 1
  development of, 1–11